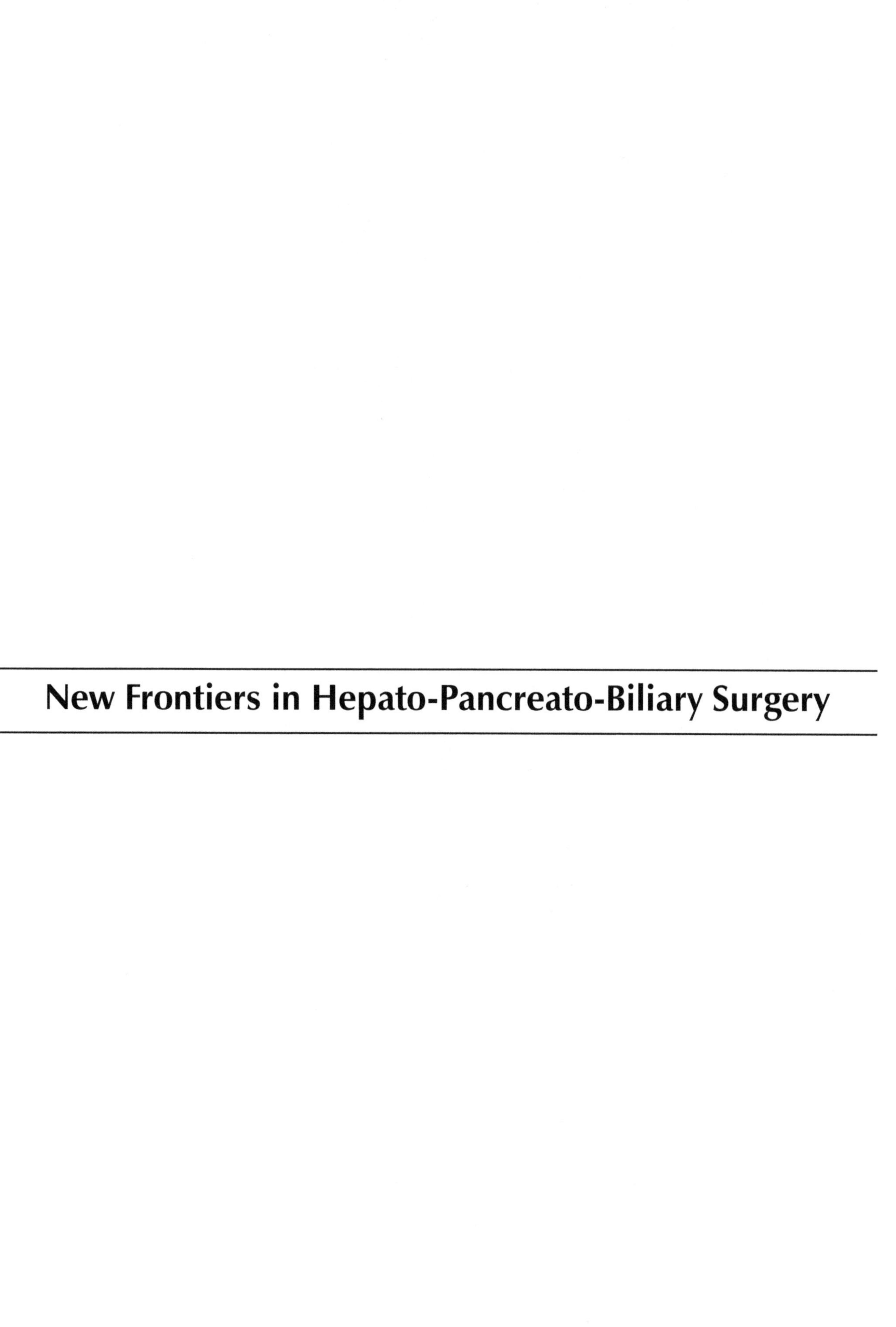

New Frontiers in Hepato-Pancreato-Biliary Surgery

New Frontiers in Hepato-Pancreato-Biliary Surgery

Editor: Isaac Stanton

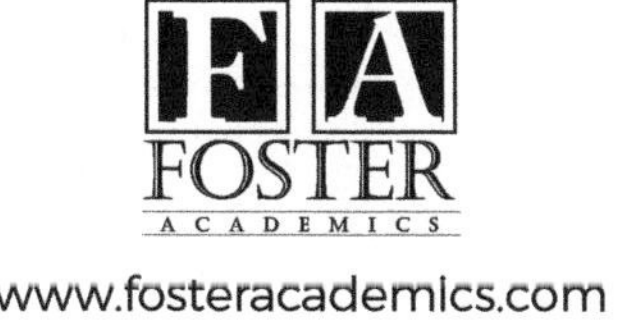

www.fosteracademics.com

www.fosteracademics.com

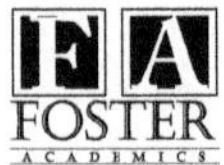

Cataloging-in-Publication Data

New frontiers in hepato-pancreato-biliary surgery / edited by Isaac Stanton.
p. cm.
Includes bibliographical references and index.
ISBN 978-1-63242-813-4
1. Liver--Surgery. 2. Biliary tract--Surgery. 3. Pancreas--Surgery. I. Stanton, Isaac.
RD546 .N48 2019
617.556 205 92--dc23

Foster Academics,
118-35 Queens Blvd., Suite 400,
Forest Hills, NY 11375, USA

ISBN 978-1-63242-813-4 (Hardback)

Contents

Preface

Over the recent decade, advancements and applications have progressed exponentially. This has led to the increased interest in this field and projects are being conducted to enhance knowledge. The main objective of this book is to present some of the critical challenges and provide insights into possible solutions. This book will answer the varied questions that arise in the field and also provide an increased scope for furthering studies.

The specialized domain of hepato-pancreato-biliary surgery encompasses the surgical solutions and interventions for the treatment of liver, pancreas and biliary tract related conditions. Such conditions include neoplastic liver disease, congenital and acquired non-neoplastic liver disease, neoplastic biliary disease, congenital and acquired non-neoplastic biliary disease, neoplastic pancreatic diseases, congenital and acquired non-neoplastic pancreatic disease and diseases of the duodenum, among others. The surgical procedures involved in transplantation, surgical oncology and trauma surgery in the regions of the pancreas and duodenum, the biliary tract and the liver are also part of hepato-pancreato-biliary surgery. This book is compiled in such a manner, that it will provide in-depth knowledge about hepato-pancreato-biliary surgery. The aim of this book is to present researches that have transformed this discipline and aided its advancement. The readers would gain knowledge that would broaden their perspective about this field of surgery.

I hope that this book, with its visionary approach, will be a valuable addition and will promote interest among readers. Each of the authors has provided their extraordinary competence in their specific fields by providing different perspectives as they come from diverse nations and regions. I thank them for their contributions.

Editor

1

The Underlying Mechanisms: How Hypothyroidism Affects the Formation of Common Bile Duct Stones

Johanna Laukkarinen, Juhani Sand, and Isto Nordback

Department of Gastroenterology and Alimentary Tract Surgery, Tampere University Hospital, Teiskontie 35, FIN-33521 Tampere, Finland

Correspondence should be addressed to Johanna Laukkarinen, johanna.laukkarinen@fimnet.fi

Academic Editor: J. R. Izbicki

For decades, one well-known risk factor for the development of gallbladder stones has been hypothyroidism. Recent studies have interestingly reported that the risk in particular for common bile duct (CBD) stones increases in clinical and subclinical hypothyroidism. There are multiple factors that may contribute to the formation and/or accumulation of CBD stones in hypothyroid patients, including decreased liver cholesterol metabolism, diminished bile secretion, and reduced sphincter of Oddi relaxation. This paper focuses on the mechanisms possibly underlying the association between hypothyroidism and CBD stones. The authors conclude that when treating patients with CBD stones or microlithiasis, clinicians should be aware of the possible hypothyroid background.

1. Introduction

Several factors affecting bile content and bile flow are involved in the complex pathogenesis of gallstones. In hypothyroidism, not only the risk for gallbladder stones [1, 2], but also the risk for common bile duct (CBD) stones in particular is increased [3–5]. Impaired liver cholesterol metabolism [6], diminished bile secretion [7], and reduced sphincter of Oddi (SO) relaxation [8, 9] may contribute to the formation and/or accumulation of CBD stones in hypothyroid patients. In this paper the possible mechanisms underlying the association between hypothyroidism and CBD stones are being discussed.

2. Review Criteria

PubMed was searched in April 2011 with the terms "hypothyroidism," "subclinical hypothyroidism," "thyroxine," "thyroid function," "gallstones," "bile duct stones," "sphincter of Oddi," "biliary motility," "cholesterol metabolism," and "hepatic secretion" for full-length English language original publications and review articles published between 1950 and 2010 (initial inclusion criteria). Abstracts and articles not relevant to the topic were excluded. A total of 3472 publications were identified at the initial step, out of which 3396 were excluded and 76 were finally considered. The search was updated in August 2012.

3. Prevalence of Clinical and Subclinical Hypothyroidism in CBD Stone Patients

Several recent studies report an association between hypothyroidism, or subclinical hypothyroidism, and CBD stones (Table 1). In a retrospective study on patients over 60 years of age [3], it was noted for the first time that CBD stone patients have significantly more diagnosed hypothyroidism (11%), not only when compared to control patients from whom gallstones had been excluded (2%), but also when compared to gallbladder stone patients without CBD stones (6%). In this study, there was no difference between groups in the frequency of other diseases. This finding suggested that factors other than merely those affecting cholesterol metabolism, for example, specific effects on bile flow, might be behind the association between CBD stones and hypothyroidism.

A prospective study [4] showed that even subclinical hypothyroidism is more common among CBD stone patients. This study investigated the prevalence of previously

Table 1: Data of the studies published over the last ten years, reporting an association between hypothyroidism, or subclinical hypothyroidism, and CBD stones.

Author	Year	Journal	Study type	Patient population	Patient number	Gender	Age (years)	Main finding	Risk factors other than hypothyroidism contributing to development of CBD stones
Inkinen et al. [8]	2001	Hepato-gastroenterol	Retrospective	CBD stone patients, age and sex matched GB stone patients and controls	168	65% F	>60	Hypothyroidism: CBD 11%, GB 6%, controls 2%	Groups did not differ in any other diagnosed diseases
Laukkarinen et al. [4]	2007	J. Clin. Endocrinol. Metab.	Prospective, multicenter	Clinically euthyreotic CBD stone patients and nongallstone controls	445	61% F	median 67 (range 18–98)	Subclinical hypothyroidism (TSH > 6.0 mU/L): CBD 5.3%, control 1.4%.	Groups did not differ in any other diagnosed diseases
					161	F	>60	Subclinical hypothyroidism: CBD 11.4%, control 1.8%	Groups did not differ in any other diagnosed diseases
Laukkarinen et al. [5]	2010	Scand. J. Gastroenterol.	Medical registry-based cohort	Hypothyroid patients and age, sex, and area of residence adjusted glaucoma (control) patients	28.668	68% F	median 62 (range 18–88)	CBD stone treatments: hypothyroid cohort 0.23%, control cohort 0.16%. After diagnosing hypothyroidism 56% more CBD stone treatments than after diagnosing glaucoma.	Patients with other diseases were excluded from the cohort to create a "purely" hypothyroid (or glaucoma) cohort of patients. Also no difference in any other medications between the groups.

undiagnosed subclinical hypothyroidism in clinically euthyreotic CBD stone patients compared to nongallstone controls. It was found that 5.3% of the CBD stone patients had subclinical hypothyroidism, defined as serum thyrotropin above the normal upper limit (6.0 mU/L), compared to only 1.4% in the control group. In women over 60 years, the prevalence of subclinical hypothyroidism was as high as 11.4% in the CBD stone group compared to 1.8% among the control patients.

Finally in 2010, a large, medical registry-based study from Finland [5] confirmed that hypothyroid patients did indeed seem to have a higher likelihood for CBD stone treatment. In this study, the prevalence of CBD stone treatments was investigated in patients with diagnosed hypothyroidism and compared to age, sex, and area of residence adjusted glaucoma (control) patients. Patients with other diseases were excluded to create a "purely" hypothyroid (or glaucoma) cohort of patients. Out of 14,334 patients in each group who met the inclusion criteria, 0.23% in the hypothyroid cohort and 0.16% in the control cohort had been treated for CBD stones. The groups did not differ in the number of CBD stone treatments before the diagnosis of hypothyroidism or glaucoma, but after these diagnoses there were 56% more CBD stone treated individuals in the hypothyroid cohort than in the control cohort. This may suggest that the higher risk for CBD stones in hypothyroid patients may increase after taking medication for hypothyroidism. As the process of bile stone formation takes time, stone formation may have started during the untreated period of hypothyroidism and have been completed regardless of thyroxine replacement therapy. This hypothesis is supported by the findings that both subclinical [4] and clinical [3] hypothyroidism are more common in CBD stone patients. However, the question remains whether thyroxine replacement therapy is sufficient to cause the physiological effects of thyroxine, as it seems that even though thyroxine replacement therapy has been initiated, the CBD stones do indeed form or continue to grow. Earlier studies with subclinical hypothyroid patients have demonstrated that a positive effect on changes in the cholesterol level, cardiovascular effects, or neuromuscular symptoms may be achieved with early replacement treatment with thyroxine [10, 11]. It has also been reported that gallstones have dissolved after initiation of thyroxine therapy [12]. It is possible that thyroxine replacement therapy is not sufficient, or not sufficient at all times of the day, in all patients to maintain normal sphincter of Oddi function, causing the formation of CBD stones.

These interesting findings raise a question about the mechanisms underlying the association, which is stronger between hypothyroidism and CBD stones than between hypothyroidism and gallbladder stones.

4. How Hypothyroidism May Affect the Formation of CBD Stones?

In general, the pathogenesis of gallstones is a complex process involving mechanisms affecting bile content and bile flow. There are several factors that may contribute to the formation of CBD stones in hypothyroid patients. Based on the investigations currently available, it cannot be concluded whether hypothyroid individuals develop isolated CBD stones or present with CBD stones in addition to gallbladder stones. However, based on what is known about the effects of hypothyroidism on the formation of gallbladder and CBD stones, it seems likely that in hypothyroidism both the risk for gallbladder-originated as well as for de novo CBD stones is increased. In hypothyroidism, the lack of thyroxine (1) decreases liver cholesterol metabolism [6] resulting in bile cholesterol supersaturation, which in turn impairs the motility [13], contractility [14], and filling [15] of the gallbladder, contributing to the retention of cholesterol crystals and to the nucleation and growth of gallstones [13]; (2) diminishes bile secretion from hepatocytes [7] resulting in impaired clearance of precipitates from the bile ducts; (3) reduces SO relaxation [8, 9] resulting in delayed bile flow [16, 17] and thus the formation and accumulation of CBD stones.

THs regulate multiple functions in virtually every type of vertebrate tissue [18, 19]. Most actions of THs can be explained by their interaction with nuclear receptors, which are expressed in a tissue- and development stage-specific fashion [20–24]. In human, the SO expresses both TR β_1 and β_2 [9]. Any acute-type response of a cell to THs is unlikely to involve a transcriptional mechanism but is rather a result of nongenomic mechanisms involving extranuclear sites of action [25–35]. In general, thyroid hormone actions are largely intracellular events that require transport across the plasma membrane. Recently, several active and specific thyroid hormone transporters have been identified, including monocarboxylate transporter 8 (MCT8), MCT10, and organic anion transporting polypeptide 1C1 (OATP1C1) [36, 37].

4.1. Hypothyroidism Decreases Liver Cholesterol Metabolism. A 90% of hypothyroid patients have elevated cholesterol levels, triglyceride levels, or both [38–42]. Treatment of hypothyroid patients with concomitant hyperlipidemia will have beneficial effects on serum cholesterol levels [40]. In hypothyroidism, decreased LDL receptor activity leads to impaired removal of cholesterol from the serum [38, 43, 44], and reduced regulation of HMG-CoA reductase expression leads to decreased cholesterol synthesis [45, 46]. Even though THs reduce the synthesis of bile salts in human hepatocytes [46], a decrease in biliary bile salt concentration in hypothyroidism has been reported [47]. Hypothyroidism lowers biliary cholesterol secretion in rat, while thyroxine replacement in hypothyroid animals markedly increases cholesterol secretion [48]. However, in cholesterol-fed hypothyroid rat, biliary cholesterol content is significantly increased and the rate of bile secretion decreased [7].

Serum hypercholesterolemia in hypothyroidism may cause bile to supersaturate in cholesterol. A direct consequence of cholesterol supersaturated bile is reduced motility [13], depressed contractility [14], and impaired filling [15] of the gallbladder, giving rise to prolonged residence of bile in the gallbladder. This may contribute to the retention of cholesterol crystals, thereby allowing sufficient time for nucleation and continuous growth into mature gallstones [1, 3]. In one prospective study [17], biliary transabdominal ultrasonography was performed in patients with gallbladder *in situ* in the euthyreotic phase, and then again 2–4 weeks after thyroidectomy in the hypothyroid stage. In these ultrasonography studies no gallstones, sludge, or dilatation of the bile ducts were seen in the hypothyroid stage compared to the euthyreotic stage. Thus, the 2–4 week period of hypothyroidism following thyroidectomy was not long enough to cause the formation of such cholesterol crystals which could be detected in transcutaneous ultrasonography; a longer period of time is needed. Gallbladder fasting volume and gallbladder ejection fraction measured by conventional ultrasonography have also been reported to remain unchanged between euthyreotic, hypothyroid, and hyperthyroid patients [49]. In one patient report, gallstones were shown to disappear after thyroxine treatment [12]. Extremely high doses of thyroxine have also been reported to induce gallbladder stones in hamsters [50], but this has not been reported with physiological doses of thyroxine.

4.2. Hypothyroidism May Reduce Hepatic Bile Secretion. In a prospective study in humans, the dynamic Tc^{99m} HIDA biligraphy performed in the acute hypothyroid stage after thyroidectomy showed that the hepatic maximal uptake and appearance of radioactivity in the large bile ducts at the hepatic hilum was similar to the euthyreotic stage in the same patients [17]. This suggested that hepatocytic bile secretion may not be significantly reduced in humans in the early phase of hypothyroidism. However, in rats, where bile secretion rate can be measured by cannulating bile ducts proximal to the SO (to block out the SO effect), decreased bile secretion in prolonged hypothyroidism has been reported, whereas hyperthyroidism seems to have no effect [7, 51]. Thus decreased bile hepatic secretion may have at least some impact on the delayed bile flow in prolonged hypothyroidism.

4.3. Hypothyroidism Reduces Bile Flow into the Duodenum. In a rat study where the effect of SO was not excluded by cannulation, hypothyroidism reduced and hyperthyroidism increased the bile flow into the duodenum [16]. Similarly, in a prospective human study [17], hepatic clearance was significantly decreased and the hilum-duodenum transit time had a tendency to increase in the hypothyroid stage after thyroidectomy, when compared to the euthyreotic stage in the same patients. As the hepatic maximal uptake and the appearance of radioactivity in the large bile ducts at the hepatic hilum were similar in the hypothyroid and euthyreotic stages of this study, the findings are hardly attributable to different hepatic secretion but strongly suggest that bile flow into the duodenum is reduced in the hypothyroid stage [17]. This could be due to changes in bile composition and gallbladder motility, and because of changes in the resistance to flow, that is, in the SO motility.

4.4. Hypothyroidism Leads to Impaired SO Relaxation. The existence of gastrointestinal hypoactivity in hypothyroidism has been well known for decades [52–58]. For example, the effect of thyroxine has been documented in anal canal pressure and in lower esophageal sphincter pressure [59, 60]. The effect of THs on smooth muscle contraction depends on the smooth muscle type and the species studied. THs have a direct, relaxing effect on vascular smooth muscle contractility [31, 61, 62]. This effect is mediated by intranuclear binding of TH to the TR [61, 63, 64], and partly by nongenomic mechanisms involving extranuclear sites of action [25]. The potassium (K^+) channel blocker glibenclamide attenuates triiodothyronine-induced vasodilatation in rat skeletal muscle arteries, and triiodothyronine-induced vasodilatation may thus be mediated by ATP-sensitive K^+-channels [65].

Since Sandblom et al. [66] first demonstrated the hormonal action of cholecystokinin (CCK) on the SO in 1935, several other hormones have been shown to affect SO activity [67–71]. In 2001 [8], it was shown for the first time that thyroxine has a direct effect on SO contractility in physiological concentrations in pig experiments. Triiodothyronine had a similar effect on thyroxine, whereas cortisone, estrogen and testosterone had no effect. Thus the effect of THs is not an unspecific effect of any hormone. Progesterone, which is thought to be involved in the smooth muscle relaxation seen in pregnancy [72], reduced not only the ACh- and Hist-induced but also KCl-induced SO contractions. Thus, its effect on SO relaxation differs from the more specific effect of thyroxine. Thyroxine reduced receptor-mediated acetylcholine and histamine-induced SO contraction, but had no effect on unspecific, KCl-induced SO contraction, which suggests a direct effect of thyroxine on the control mechanisms of SO motility. Since the effect of thyroxine on the precontracted SO is relaxing, the absence/insufficient concentration of thyroxine may result in increased tension of the SO in hypothyroidism [9]. A similar relaxant effect of thyroxine was also shown in human SO specimens, indicating that the finding may also be of clinical significance [9].

5. Mechanisms by Which Thyroxine Mediates SO Relaxation

Several examinations were performed to determine how the relaxant effect of thyroxine on SO is mediated [9]. The experiments with α- and β-adrenoceptor antagonists, NO-synthesis inhibitor, and the elimination of nerve function with tetrodotoxin showed that the thyroxine-induced relaxation of SO is not mediated via neural effects. Human SO was shown to express TR β_1 and β_2. The presence of TRs [9] in the SO is necessary but not sufficient evidence that thyroxine exerts its prorelaxant effect via a hormone-receptor complex action. However, the experiments with different incubation times of thyroxine showed that the underlying cellular mechanisms involved do not act immediately but require a certain time lag, supporting the theory that at least part of the action of thyroxine is TH-TR mediated [9]. The passage of TH through cell membrane, cytoplasm, and nuclear membrane and binding to a nuclear protein (TR) is a relatively fast event, whereas the resulting transcriptional and translational regulation is time-consuming, and probably explains why the relaxant effect is not immediate. Thus, the effect of thyroxine could be mediated by regulatory proteins partly synthesized as a result of thyroxine-induced gene expression.

Estrogen is one hormone known to affect the synthesis prostaglandins [73], which, in turn, can relax smooth muscle [74]. However, in prostaglandin synthesis inhibition experiments it was shown that prostaglandin synthesis is not required in the mediation of the prorelaxant effect of thyroxine.

K^+ channels can be modulated by neurotransmitters and other messengers in smooth muscle cells, and these effects are often functionally important in the whole tissue [75]. Similarly to what has been shown in rat skeletal muscle arteries, where triiodothyronine-induced vasodilatation is mediated by ATP-sensitive K^+ channels [65], it was shown in SO that the effect of thyroxine on SO smooth muscle is mediated via the opening of ATP-sensitive K^+ channels [9]. This results in hyperpolarisation, which closes all membrane Ca^{2+} channels and reduces Ca^{2+} influx, allowing only limited contraction of the smooth muscle [76].

The prorelaxant effect of thyroxine is probably partly mediated via transporter proteins [36, 37], and partly via binding to nuclear receptors, subsequently leading to the activation of K^+ channels [9]. The opening of K^+ channels is followed by hyperpolarisation, which closes cell membrane Ca^{2+} channels, reduces Ca^{2+} influx, and results in reduced contraction of the SO smooth-muscle cell in response to any specific stimulus.

6. Conclusions and Clinical Implications

In summary, several recent studies report an association between hypothyroidism, or subclinical hypothyroidism, and CBD stones. The higher prevalence of hypothyroidism in CBD stone patients compared to gallbladder stone patients suggests that not only changes in the cholesterol metabolism, or bile excretion rate, but particularly changes in the function of the SO that may underline the association between CBD stones and hypothyroidism. It remains to be investigated whether hypothyroid individuals who have had their gallbladder removed are at an increased risk to develop CBD stones when compared to euthyroid individuals in the same situation.

It seems likely that the lack of thyroxine in hypothyroidism gives rise to a reduction in bile flow in many ways. In addition to the increased cholesterol load in bile and the reduced bile secretion rate, the deficiency of the prorelaxant effect of thyroxine on the SO appears to be a crucial factor leading to the reduced bile flow in hypothyroidism.

The initial formation of bile cholesterol crystals may begin during the untreated period of hypothyroidism, and the stones may continue to develop or mature even after the thyroxine replacement therapy has begun. It is possible that thyroxine replacement therapy is not sufficient in all patients to maintain normal SO function, causing increased risk of CBD stone formation. Studies with subclinical hypothyroid patients have demonstrated that a positive effect on the changes in the serum cholesterol level, on cardiovascular effects, or on neuromuscular symptoms may be achieved with early replacement treatment with thyroxine [10, 11], and it can be assumed that patients at risk of forming CBD stones due to subclinical hypothyroidism may also benefit from such early treatment. Most importantly, when treating patients with CBD stones or microlithiasis, clinicians should be aware of the possible hypothyroid background and consider examining the thyroid function, at least in female patients over 60 years of age, in which group the prevalence of clinical and subclinical hypothyroidism is the highest.

Authors' Contribution

J. Laukkarinen has written this paper, and J. Sand and I. Nordback have Critically reviewed the paper for the important intellectual content.

Acknowledgment

This work was financially supported by the Medical Research Fund of Pirkanmaa Hospital District, Finland.

References

[1] L. H. Honore, "A significant association between symptomatic cholesterol cholelithiasis and treated hypothyroidism in women," *Journal of Medicine*, vol. 12, no. 2-3, pp. 199–203, 1981.

[2] S. M. Strasberg, "The pathogenesis of cholesterol gallstones—a review," *Journal of Gastrointestinal Surgery*, vol. 2, no. 2, pp. 109–125, 1998.

[3] J. Inkinen, J. Sand, and I. Nordback, "Association between common bile duct stones and treated hypothyroidism," *Hepato-Gastroenterology*, vol. 47, no. 34, pp. 919–921, 2000.

[4] J. Laukkarinen, G. Kiudelis, M. Lempinen et al., "Increased prevalence of subclinical hypothyroidism in common bile duct stone patients," *Journal of Clinical Endocrinology and Metabolism*, vol. 92, no. 11, pp. 4260–4264, 2007.

[5] J. Laukkarinen, J. Sand, V. Autio, and I. Nordback, "Bile duct stone procedures are more frequent in patients with hypothyroidism. A large, registry-based, cohort study in Finland," *Scandinavian Journal of Gastroenterology*, vol. 45, no. 1, pp. 70–74, 2010.

[6] J. P. Andreini, W. F. Prigge, C. Ma, and R. L. Gebhard, "Vesicles and mixed micelles in hypothyroid rat bile before and after thyroid hormone treatment: evidence for a vesicle transport system for biliary cholesterol secretion," *Journal of Lipid Research*, vol. 35, no. 8, pp. 1405–1412, 1994.

[7] F. J. Field, E. Albright, and S. N. Mathur, "Effect of dietary cholesterol on biliary cholesterol content and bile flow in the hypothyroid rat," *Gastroenterology*, vol. 91, no. 2, pp. 297–304, 1986.

[8] J. Inkinen, J. Sand, P. Arvola, I. Pörsti, and I. Nordback, "Direct effect of thyroxine on pig Sphincter of Oddi contractility," *Digestive Diseases and Sciences*, vol. 46, no. 1, pp. 182–186, 2001.

[9] J. Laukkarinen, J. Sand, S. Aittomaki et al., "Mechanism of the prorelaxing effect of thyroxine on the sphincter of Oddi," *Scandinavian Journal of Gastroenterology*, vol. 37, no. 6, pp. 667–673, 2002.

[10] R. Gärtner, "Subclinical hyperthyroidism—does it have to be treated?" *MMW-Fortschritte der Medizin*, vol. 146, no. 39, pp. 37–39, 2004.

[11] B. Biondi and I. Klein, "Hypothyroidism as a risk factor for cardiovascular disease," *Endocrine*, vol. 24, no. 1, pp. 1–13, 2004.

[12] J. S. Vassilakis and N. Nicolopoulos, "Dissolution of gallstones following thyroxine administration. A case report," *Hepato-Gastroenterology*, vol. 28, no. 1, pp. 60–61, 1981.

[13] J. M. Donovan, "Physical and metabolic factors in gallstone pathogenesis," *Gastroenterology Clinics of North America*, vol. 28, no. 1, pp. 75–97, 1999.

[14] L. Behar, K. Y. Lee, W. R. Thompson, and P. Biancani, "Gallbladder contraction in patients with pigment and cholesterol stones," *Gastroenterology*, vol. 97, no. 6, pp. 1479–1484, 1989.

[15] R. P. Jazrawi, P. Pazzi, M. L. Petroni et al., "Postprandial gallbladder motor function: refilling and turnover of bile in health and in cholelithiasis," *Gastroenterology*, vol. 109, no. 2, pp. 582–591, 1995.

[16] J. Laukkarinen, P. Kööbi, J. Kalliovalkama et al., "Bile flow to the duodenum is reduced in hypothyreosis and enhanced in hyperthyreosis," *Neurogastroenterology and Motility*, vol. 14, no. 2, pp. 183–188, 2002.

[17] J. Laukkarinen, J. Sand, R. Saaristo et al., "Is bile flow reduced in patients with hypothyroidism?" *Surgery*, vol. 133, no. 3, pp. 288–293, 2003.

[18] R. Polikar, A. G. Burger, U. Scherrer, and P. Nicod, "The thyroid and the heart," *Circulation*, vol. 87, no. 5, pp. 1435–1441, 1993.

[19] M. I. Surks and R. Sievert, "Drugs and thyroid function," *The New England Journal of Medicine*, vol. 333, no. 25, pp. 1688–1694, 1995.

[20] C. K. Glass and J. M. Holloway, "Regulation of gene expression by the thyroid hormone receptor," *Biochimica et Biophysica Acta*, vol. 1032, no. 2-3, pp. 157–176, 1990.

[21] M. A. Lazar and W. W. Chin, "Nuclear thyroid hormone receptors," *Journal of Clinical Investigation*, vol. 86, no. 6, pp. 1777–1782, 1990.

[22] V. K. K. Chatterjee and J. R. Tata, "Thyroid hormone receptors and their role in development," *Cancer Surveys*, vol. 14, pp. 147–168, 1992.

[23] M. A. Lazar, "Thyroid hormone receptors: multiple forms, multiple possibilities," *Endocrine Reviews*, vol. 14, no. 2, pp. 184–193, 1993.

[24] W. W. Chin, "Molecular mechanisms of thyroid hormone action," *Thyroid*, vol. 4, no. 3, pp. 389–393, 1994.

[25] D. R. Salter, C. M. Dyke, and A. S. Wechsler, "Triiodothyronine (T3) and cardiovascular therapeutics: a review," *Journal of Cardiac Surgery*, vol. 7, no. 4, pp. 363–374, 1992.

[26] J. Segal, "A rapid, extranuclear effect of 3,5,3'-triiodothyronine on sugar uptake by several tissues in the rat in vivo. Evidence for a physiological role for the thyroid hormone action at the level of the plasma membrane," *Endocrinology*, vol. 124, no. 6, pp. 2755–2764, 1989.

[27] C. A. Siegrist-Kaiser, C. Juge-Aubry, M. P. Tranter, D. M. Ekenbarger, and J. L. Leonard, "Thyroxine-dependent modulation of actin polymerization in cultured astrocytes. A novel, extranuclear action of thyroid hormone," *Journal of Biological Chemistry*, vol. 265, no. 9, pp. 5296–5302, 1990.

[28] P. R. Warnick, P. J. Davis, F. B. Davis, V. Cody, J. Galindo Jr., and S. D. Blas, "Rabbit skeletal muscle sarcoplasmic reticulum Ca^{2+}-ATPase activity: stimulation in vitro by thyroid hormone analogues and bipyridines," *Biochimica et Biophysica Acta*, vol. 1153, no. 2, pp. 184–190, 1993.

[29] W. D. Lawrence, M. Schoenl, and P. J. Davis, "Stimulation in vitro of rabbit erythrocyte cytosol phospholipid-dependent protein kinase activity. A novel action of thyroid hormone," *Journal of Biological Chemistry*, vol. 264, no. 9, pp. 4766–4768, 1989.

[30] K. Sterling, "Direct thyroid hormone activation of mitochondria: the role of adenine nucleotide translocase," *Endocrinology*, vol. 119, no. 1, pp. 292–295, 1986.

[31] T. Ishikawa, T. Chijiwa, M. Hagiwara, S. Mamiya, and H. Hidaka, "Thyroid hormones directly interact with vascular smooth muscle strips," *Molecular Pharmacology*, vol. 35, no. 6, pp. 760–765, 1989.

[32] K. Ojamaa, C. Balkman, and I. L. Klein, "Acute effects of triiodothyronine on arterial smooth muscle cells," *Annals of Thoracic Surgery*, vol. 56, Supplement 1, pp. S61–S67, 1993.

[33] C. Limas and C. J. Limas, "Influence of thyroid status on intracellular distribution of cardiac adrenoceptors," *Circulation Research*, vol. 61, no. 6, pp. 824–828, 1987.

[34] F. B. Davis, P. J. Davis, and S. D. Blas, "Role of calmodulin in thyroid hormone stimulation in vitro of human erythrocyte Ca^{2+}-ATPase activity," *Journal of Clinical Investigation*, vol. 71, no. 3, pp. 579–586, 1983.

[35] A. Rudinger, K. M. Mylotte, and P. J. Davis, "Rabbit myocardial membrane Ca^{2+}-adenosine triphosphatase activity: stimulation in vitro by thyroid hormone," *Archives of Biochemistry and Biophysics*, vol. 229, no. 1, pp. 379–385, 1984.

[36] J. Jansen, E. C. H. Friesema, C. Milici, and T. J. Visser, "Thyroid hormone transporters in health and disease," *Thyroid*, vol. 15, no. 8, pp. 757–768, 2005.

[37] H. Heuer and T. J. Visser, "Minireview: pathophysiological importance of thyroid hormone transporters," *Endocrinology*, vol. 150, no. 3, pp. 1078–1083, 2009.

[38] R. A. Dickey and S. Feld, "Guest editorial: the thyroid-cholesterol connection: an association between varying degrees of hypothyroidism and hypercholesterolemia in women," *Journal of Women's Health*, vol. 9, no. 4, pp. 333–336, 2000.

[39] K. M. Kutty, D. G. Bryant, and N. R. Farid, "Serum lipids in hypothyroidism—a re-evaluation," *Journal of Clinical Endocrinology & Metabolism*, vol. 46, pp. 55–56, 1978.

[40] J. Elder, A. McLelland, D. S. O'Reilly, C. J. Packard, J. J. Series, and J. Shepherd, "The relationship between serum cholesterol and serum thyrotropin, thyroxine and tri-iodothyronine concentrations in suspected hypothyroidism," *Annals of Clinical Biochemistry*, vol. 27, no. 2, pp. 110–113, 1990.

[41] T. Kuusi, M. R. Taskinen, and E. A. Nikkila, "Lipoproteins, lipolytic enzymes, and hormonal status in hypothyroid women at different levels of substitution," *Journal of Clinical Endocrinology and Metabolism*, vol. 66, no. 1, pp. 51–56, 1988.

[42] C. J. Packard, J. Shepherd, G. M. Lindsay, A. Gaw, and M. R. Taskinen, "Thyroid replacement therapy and its influence on postheparin plasma lipases and apolipoprotein-B metabolism in hypothyroidism," *Journal of Clinical Endocrinology and Metabolism*, vol. 76, no. 5, pp. 1209–1216, 1993.

[43] G. C. Ness, L. C. Pendleton, Y. C. Li, and J. Y. L. Chiang, "Effect of thyroid hormone on hepatic cholesterol 7α hydroxylase, LDL receptor, HMG-CoA reductase, farnesyl pyrophosphate synthetase and apolipoprotein A-I mRNA levels in hypophysectomized rats," *Biochemical and Biophysical Research Communications*, vol. 172, no. 3, pp. 1150–1156, 1990.

[44] L. Scarabottolo, E. Trezzi, P. Roma, and A. L. Catapano, "Experimental hypothyroidism modulates the expression of the low density lipoprotein receptor by the liver," *Atherosclerosis*, vol. 59, no. 3, pp. 329–333, 1986.

[45] R. Day, R. L. Gebhard, H. L. Schwartz et al., "Time course of hepatic 3-hydroxy-3-methylglutaryl coenzyme A reductase

activity and messenger ribonucleic acid, biliary lipid secretion, and hepatic cholesterol content in methimazole-treated hypothyroid and hypophysectomized rats after triiodothyronine administration: possible linkage of cholesterol synthesis to biliary secretion," *Endocrinology*, vol. 125, no. 1, pp. 459–468, 1989.

[46] E. C. S. Ellis, "Suppression of bile acid synthesis by thyroid hormone in primary human hepatocytes," *World Journal of Gastroenterology*, vol. 12, no. 29, pp. 4640–4645, 2006.

[47] O. Strand, "Influence of propylthiouracil and D- and L-thiiodothyronine on excretion of bile acids in bile fistula rats," *Proceedings of the Society for Experimental Biology and Medicine*, vol. 109, pp. 668–672, 1962.

[48] R. L. Gebhard and W. F. Prigge, "Thyroid hormone differentially augments biliary sterol secretion in the rat. II. The chronic bile fistula model," *Journal of Lipid Research*, vol. 33, no. 10, pp. 1467–1473, 1992.

[49] M. Cakir, E. Kayacetin, H. Toy, and S. Bozkurt, "Gallbladder motor function in patients with different thyroid hormone status," *Experimental and Clinical Endocrinology and Diabetes*, vol. 117, no. 8, pp. 395–399, 2009.

[50] F. Bergman and W. van der Linden, "Further studies on the influence of thyroxine on gallstone formation in hamsters," *Acta Chirurgica Scandinavica*, vol. 131, no. 4, pp. 319–328, 1966.

[51] W. Van Steenbergen, J. Fevery, R. De Vos, R. Leyten, K. P. M. Heirwegh, and J. De Groote, "Thyroid hormones and the hepatic handling of bilirubin. I. Effects of hypothyroidism and hyperthyroidism on the hepatic transport of bilirubin mono- and diconjugates in the Wistar rat," *Hepatology*, vol. 9, no. 2, pp. 314–321, 1989.

[52] H. Johansson, "Gastrointestinal motility function related to thyroid activity. An experimental study in the rat," *Acta Chirurgica Scandinavica*, vol. 359, pp. 1–88, 1966.

[53] W. R. Middleton, "Thyroid hormones and the gut," *Gut*, vol. 12, no. 2, pp. 172–177, 1971.

[54] R. L. Duret and P. A. Bastenie, "Intestinal disorders in hypothyroidism—clinical and manometric study," *The American Journal of Digestive Diseases*, vol. 16, no. 8, pp. 723–727, 1971.

[55] K. Kowalewski and A. Kolodej, "Myoelectrical and mechanical activity of stomach and intestine in hypothyroid dogs," *American Journal of Digestive Diseases*, vol. 22, no. 3, pp. 235–240, 1977.

[56] L. J. Miller, C. A. Gorman, and V. L. W. Go, "Gut-thyroid interrelationships," *Gastroenterology*, vol. 75, no. 5, pp. 901–911, 1978.

[57] R. B. Shafer, R. A. Prentiss, and J. H. Bond, "Gastrointestinal transit in thyroid disease," *Gastroenterology*, vol. 86, no. 5, pp. 852–858, 1984.

[58] S. Goto, D. F. Billmire, and J. L. Grosfeld, "Hypothyroidism impairs colonic motility and function. An experimental study in the rat," *European Journal of Pediatric Surgery*, vol. 2, no. 1, pp. 16–21, 1992.

[59] G. L. Eastwood, L. E. Braverman, E. M. White, and T. J. Vander Salm, "Reversal of lower esophageal sphincter hypotension and esophageal aperistalsis after treatment for hypothyroidism," *Journal of Clinical Gastroenterology*, vol. 4, no. 4, pp. 307–310, 1982.

[60] K. O. Adeniyi, O. O. Ogunkeye, S. S. Senok, and F. V. Udoh, "Influence of the thyroid state on the intrinsic contractile properties of the bladder muscle," *Acta Physiologica Hungarica*, vol. 82, no. 1, pp. 69–74, 1994.

[61] K. Ojamaa, J. D. Klemperer, and I. Klein, "Acute effects of thyroid hormone on vascular smooth muscle," *Thyroid*, vol. 6, no. 5, pp. 505–512, 1996.

[62] J. Zwaveling, M. Pfaffendorf, and P. A. Van Zwieten, "The direct effects of thyroid hormones on rat mesenteric resistance arteries," *Fundamental and Clinical Pharmacology*, vol. 11, no. 1, pp. 41–46, 1997.

[63] W. H. Dillmann, "Biochemical basis of thyroid hormone action in the heart," *American Journal of Medicine*, vol. 88, no. 6, pp. 626–630, 1990.

[64] G. A. Brent, "Mechanisms of disease: the molecular basis of thyroid hormone action," *The New England Journal of Medicine*, vol. 331, no. 13, pp. 847–853, 1994.

[65] K. W. Park, H. B. Dai, K. Ojamaa, E. Lowenstein, I. Klein, and F. W. Sellke, "The direct vasomotor effect of thyroid hormones on rat muscle resistance arteries," *Anesthesia and Analgesia*, vol. 85, no. 4, pp. 734–738, 1997.

[66] P. Sandblom, W. L. Voegtlen, and I. C. Ivy, "The effects of CCK on the choledochoduodenal mechanism (sphincter of Oddi)," *American Journal of Physiology*, vol. 113, pp. 175–180, 1935.

[67] J. Sand, H. Tainio, and I. Nordback, "Peptidergic innervation of human sphincter of Oddi," *Digestive Diseases and Sciences*, vol. 39, no. 2, pp. 293–300, 1994.

[68] J. Sand, P. Arvola, V. Jäntti et al., "The inhibitory role of nitric oxide in the control of porcine and human sphincter of Oddi activity," *Gut*, vol. 41, no. 3, pp. 375–380, 1997.

[69] J. Sand, I. Nordback, P. Arvola, I. Pörsti, A. Kalloo, and P. Pasricha, "Effects of botulinum toxin A on the sphincter of Oddi: an in vivo and in vitro study," *Gut*, vol. 42, no. 4, pp. 507–510, 1998.

[70] J. Sand, P. Arvola, I. Pörsti et al., "Histamine in the control of porcine and human sphincter of Oddi activity," *Neurogastroenterology and Motility*, vol. 12, no. 6, pp. 573–579, 2000.

[71] J. Sand, P. Arvola, and I. Nordback, "Calcium channel antagonists and inhibition of human sphincter of Oddi contractions," *Scandinavian Journal of Gastroenterology*, vol. 40, no. 12, pp. 1394–1397, 2005.

[72] V. P. Fomin, B. E. Cox, and R. Ann Word, "Effect of progesterone on intracellular Ca^{2+} homeostasis in human myometrial smooth muscle cells," *American Journal of Physiology*, vol. 276, no. 2, part 1, pp. C379–C385, 1999.

[73] M. Wakasugi, T. Noguchi, Y. I. Kazama, Y. Kanemaru, and T. Onaya, "The effects of sex hormones on the synthesis of prostacyclin (PGI2) by vascular tissues," *Prostaglandins*, vol. 37, no. 4, pp. 401–410, 1989.

[74] D. J. Beech, "Actions of neurotransmitters and other messengers on Ca^{2+} channels and K^{+} channels in smooth muscle cells," *Pharmacology and Therapeutics*, vol. 73, no. 2, pp. 91–119, 1997.

[75] A. R. Shepard and N. L. Eberhardt, "Molecular mechanisms of thyroid hormone action," *Clinics in Laboratory Medicine*, vol. 13, no. 3, pp. 531–541, 1993.

[76] B. G. Allen and M. P. Walsh, "The biochemical basis of the regulation of smooth-muscle contraction," *Trends in Biochemical Sciences*, vol. 19, no. 9, pp. 362–368, 1994.

2

Preoperative Gadoxetic Acid-Enhanced MRI and Simultaneous Treatment of Early Hepatocellular Carcinoma Prolonged Recurrence-Free Survival of Progressed Hepatocellular Carcinoma Patients after Hepatic Resection

Masanori Matsuda,[1] Tomoaki Ichikawa,[2] Hidetake Amemiya,[1] Akira Maki,[1] Mitsuaki Watanabe,[1] Hiromichi Kawaida,[1] Hiroshi Kono,[1] Katsuhiro Sano,[2] Utaroh Motosugi,[2] and Hideki Fujii[1]

[1] *First Department of Surgery, Yamanashi University School of Medicine, 1110 Shimokato, Chuo City, Yamanashi 409-3898, Japan*
[2] *Department of Radiology, Yamanashi University School of Medicine, 1110 Shimokato, Chuo City, Yamanashi 409-3898, Japan*

Correspondence should be addressed to Masanori Matsuda; masam@yamanashi.ac.jp

Academic Editor: Guy Maddern

Background/Purpose. The purpose of this study was to clarify whether preoperative gadoxetic acid-enhanced magnetic resonance imaging (EOB-MRI) and simultaneous treatment of suspected early hepatocellular carcinoma (eHCC) at the time of resection for progressed HCC affected patient prognosis following hepatic resection. *Methods*. A total of 147 consecutive patients who underwent their first curative hepatic resection for progressed HCC were enrolled. Of these, 77 patients underwent EOB-MRI (EOB-MRI (+)) before hepatic resection and the remaining 70 patients did not (EOB-MRI (−)). Suspected eHCCs detected by preoperative imaging were resected or ablated at the time of resection for progressed HCC. *Results*. The number of patients who underwent treatment for eHCCs was significantly higher in the EOB-MRI (+) than in the EOB-MRI (−) (17 versus 6; $P = 0.04$). Recurrence-free survival (1-, 3-, and 5-year; 81.4, 62.6, 48.7% versus 82.1, 41.5, 25.5%, resp., $P < 0.01$), but not overall survival (1-, 3-, and 5-year; 98.7, 90.7, 80.8% versus 97.0, 86.3, 72.4%, resp., $P = 0.38$), was significantly better in the EOB-MRI (+). Univariate and multivariate analyses showed that preoperative EOB-MRI was one of the independent factors significantly correlated with better recurrence-free survival. *Conclusions*. Preoperative EOB-MRI and simultaneous treatment of eHCC prolonged recurrence-free survival after hepatic resection.

1. Introduction

Hepatocellular carcinoma (HCC) is one of the most malignant tumors worldwide. Hepatic resection is still the most effective treatment for HCC; however, the recurrence rate is very high even after curative resection. The postoperative 5-year recurrence rate was shown to be higher than 70%, with 80% to 95% of recurrence being confined to the liver [1–4]. Intrahepatic recurrence has been classified as either metachronous multicentric-occurrence HCC (MC) or intrahepatic metastasis (IM) [5, 6]. Anatomic hepatic resection has been shown to be effective for micro IM within resected sections or segments with progressed HCC [7–9] but is ineffective for MC in the remnant liver. Recent studies have shown that hypovascular early HCC (eHCC), which is not an indication for resection, progresses to conventional hypervascular HCC. Hypovascular eHCC is thought to be one of the causes of multicentric recurrence of hypervascular HCC after hepatic resection. However, the effects of simultaneous treatment of suspected eHCC at the time of hepatic resection for progressed HCC on postoperative recurrence have never been evaluated.

A new magnetic resonance imaging (MRI) contrast medium, gadoxetic acid, or gadolinium ethoxybenzyl diethylenetriamine pentaacetic acid (Gd-EOB-DTPA) (Primovist, Bayer Healthcare, Osaka, Japan), which has the properties of both an extracellular gadolinium chelate and liver-specific (hepatocyte-targeting) contrast material, has become available [10–13]. Our previous study revealed that Gd-EOB-DTPA-enhanced MRI (EOB-MRI) was the most useful imaging technique for evaluating small HCC, including eHCC [13].

The purpose of this study was to clarify whether preoperative EOB-MRI and simultaneous treatment of suspected eHCC at the time of resection for progressed HCC affected the overall and recurrence-free survival of patients after initial hepatic resection for HCC.

2. Materials and Methods

2.1. Patients. A total of 147 consecutive progressed HCC patients without extrahepatic metastasis who underwent their first curative hepatic resection for HCC at the First Department of Surgery (Yamanashi University Hospital, Yamanashi, Japan) between 1 January 2005 and 31 December 2010 were retrospectively enrolled in this study. No postoperative death or in-hospital death was reported among these patients.

This study protocol followed the ethical guidelines of the Declaration of Helsinki amended in 2008, and written informed consent was obtained from each patient.

2.2. Preoperative Imaging Diagnosis. Preoperative imaging studies, including chest radiography, abdominal ultrasonography (AUS), computed tomography (CT), MRI, hepatic arteriography, CT during arterial portography (CTAP), and CT during hepatic arteriography (CTHA), were performed. One patient did not undergo contrast-enhanced CT, CTHA, or CTAP because of an allergy to the iodinated contrast material. In addition, CTHA and CTAP were not performed in one patient with mild renal dysfunction. EOB-MRI was introduced into our institute in January 2008. Since then, EOB-MRI has been performed before hepatic resection for HCC as essential imaging diagnostics. In this study, 77 patients underwent EOB-MRI (EOB-MRI (+) group) and the remaining 70 patients underwent conventional MRI (EOB-MRI (−) group) before hepatic resection for HCC. Hypovascular hepatic nodules showing low attenuation on unenhanced CT and CTAP and those showing low signal intensity on hepatocyte-phase images of EOB-MRI were diagnosed as suspected eHCCs [13, 14].

2.3. Indication of Hepatic Resection. Liver function reserve was assessed by liver biochemistry, Child-Pugh grading [15], and the indocyanine green retention rate at 15 min (ICGR15). Only patients with Child-Pugh class A and ICGR15 below 20% were offered major hepatic resection, which is defined as resection of two or more segments of the liver according to Couinaud's classification [16]. Patients with Child-Pugh class A and ICGR15 more than 20% and selected class B patients underwent minor hepatic resection, which is defined as resection of one segment or less of the liver. Suspected eHCCs detected by preoperative imaging diagnosis with or without EOB-MRI, and being more than 5 mm in diameter, were simultaneously resected or ablated at the time of resection for progressed HCC.

2.4. Pathological Diagnosis. All surgically resected specimens were fixed in 10% buffered formaldehyde. Sections of resected tumors and noncancerous livers were embedded in paraffin, sliced into 3 to 5 μm thick sections, and were then stained with hematoxylin-eosin for histological analyses. All suspected eHCCs were diagnosed strictly according to the pathological criteria proposed by the International Consensus Group for Hepatocellular Neoplasia (ICGHN) [17] by pathologists.

2.5. Postoperative Follow-Up. After the initial operation, patients were followed up at 2-week intervals for the first 2 months and monthly thereafter. Serum levels of α-fetoprotein (AFP), a *Lens culinaris* agglutinin reactive fraction of AFP (AFP-L3), and des-γ-carboxy prothrombin (DCP) were measured serially at least every 2 months. Imaging diagnosis, using CT or MRI, was performed at least every 4 months. When intrahepatic recurrence was suspected, the patient was hospitalized for diagnosis and treatment. Diagnosis of recurrence was made when intrahepatic hypervascular HCC was found by contrast-enhanced CT, MRI, or CTHA.

2.6. Treatment Strategy for Intrahepatic Recurrence of HCC. If intrahepatic recurrence was ≤3 nodules and all tumors were potentially resectable in terms of anatomical location and liver function, recurrence was managed using repeat hepatic resection. Recurrence was managed using radiofrequency ablation (RFA) if intrahepatic recurrence was solitary and completely ablative and hepatic function of the patient was not suitable for repeat hepatic resection or if the patient refused hepatic resection. Multiple intrahepatic recurrence (>3 nodules) was treated using transcatheter arterial chemoembolization (TACE) [18].

2.7. Statistical Analysis. Continuous data are expressed as the median (range) and were compared using the Mann-Whitney *U* test. Categorical variables were compared using the Chi-square test with Yates' correction or Fisher's exact test where appropriate. Survival was calculated by the Kaplan-Meier method and compared by means of the log-rank test. Univariate and multivariate analyses were performed using the Cox proportional hazards model to identify prognostic factors. Only differences with probability values below 0.05 were considered significant.

3. Results

3.1. Comparison of Background Factors between the Two Groups. A comparison of background factors between the EOB-MRI (+) and EOB-MRI (−) groups was performed (Table 1). The DCP value of patients in the EOB-MRI (−) group was significantly higher than that in the EOB-MRI (+) group (median: 57 mAU/mL; range: 12–30805 mAU/mL;

Table 1: Comparison of background factors between the EOB-MRI (+) and EOB-MRI (−) groups.

Factor	EOB-MRI (+) (n = 77)	EOB-MRI (−) (n = 70)	P value
Sex (male/female)	57/20	53/17	0.85
Age (years)*	68 (16–86)	69 (35–85)	0.71
History of blood transfusions (present/absent)	22/55	16/54	0.46
History of schistosomiasis japonica (present/absent)	10/67	12/58	0.50
Alcoholism (present/absent)	36/41	32/38	>0.999
Smoking (present/absent)	51/26	44/26	0.73
Diabetes mellitus (present/absent)	18/59	26/44	0.08
Esophageal varix (present/absent)	17/60	12/58	0.54
Albumin (g/dL)*	4.0 (3.1–4.8)	3.9 (3.2–4.7)	0.23
Total Bilirubin (mg/dL)	0.7 (0.3–1.6)	0.7 (0.2–1.4)	0.91
Alanine aminotransferase (IU/L)*	37 (9–168)	37 (10–286)	0.73
Platelets ($\times 10^4/\mu$L)*	12.4 (3.2–35.6)	13.7 (5.7–32.8)	0.12
Indocyanine green retention rate at 15 minutes (%)*	15.3 (5.4–30.6)	12.6 (5.5–38.0)	0.35
Prothrombin time (%)*	83.2 (54.6–113.5)	78.7 (61.7–100)	0.13
Child-Pugh score (A/B)	73/4	62/8	0.23
Alpha-fetoprotein (ng/mL)*	10.7 (9–17521)	14.3 (1.7–128900)	0.19
Alpha-fetoprotein L3 (%)*	1.2 (0–80.4)	2.1 (0–77.7)	0.33
Des-γ-carboxy prothrombin (mAU/mL)*	29.0 (9–17521)	57.0 (12–30805)	0.02
Hepatitis B surface antigen (positive/negative)	16/61	16/54	0.84
Hepatitis C antibodies (positive/negative)	45/32	41/29	>0.999
Tumor size in greatest dimension (cm)*	2.6 (0.9–10.7)	3.0 (1.0–9.0)	0.14
Number of tumors (solitary/multiple)	62/15	48/22	0.13
Fibrous capsule formation (present/absent)	55/22	58/12	0.12
Vascular invasion (present/absent)	14/63	18/52	0.32
Pathological diagnosis (well or moderate/poor)	61/16	57/13	0.84
Liver cirrhosis (present/absent)	41/36	36/34	0.87
AJCC Stage (I/II or III)	51/26	39/31	0.24
Hepatic resection (major/minor)	26/51	21/49	0.73
Treatment for eHCC	17/60	6/64	0.04

*Median (range).

versus 29.0 mAU/mL; 9–17521 mAU/mL; $P = 0.02$). The number of patients who underwent treatment for eHCCs at the time of hepatic resection was significantly higher in the EOB-MRI (+) group than in the EOB-MRI (−) group (17 versus 6; $P = 0.04$). No significant differences were observed in the other background factors between groups.

3.2. Simultaneous Treatment of Suspected eHCCs at the Time of Resection and Histological Evaluation of the Tumors. In the EOB-MRI (−) group, 8 suspected eHCCs from 6 patients were resected at the time of the operation. Histologically, 6 out of 8 resected tumors were eHCC and two were dysplastic nodules (DNs). On the other hand, 24 suspected eHCCs from 17 patients were treated in the EOB-MRI (+) group (23 were resected and one was ablated by microwaves without biopsy) at the time of the operation. Histological examination revealed that 21 out of 23 resected tumors were eHCC, one was DN, and one was accessory liver. In the EOB-MRI (+) group, 8 out of 21 eHCCs (38.1%) were detected at only hepatocyte phase of EOB-MRI.

3.3. Comparison of Overall and Recurrence-Free Survival after Hepatic Resection between the Two Groups. The 1-, 3-, and 5-year overall survival rates of 77 HCC patients in the EOB-MRI (+) group were 98.7, 90.7, and 80.8%, respectively, whereas the corresponding survival rates of 70 HCC patients in the EOB-MRI (−) group were 97.0, 86.3, and 72.4%, respectively (Figure 1). No significant differences were observed in the overall survival curves between the two groups ($P = 0.38$). On the other hand, the 1-, 3-, and 5-year recurrence-free survival rates of 77 HCC patients in the EOB-MRI (+) group were 81.4, 62.6, and 48.7%, respectively, whereas those of 70 HCC patients in the EOB-MRI (−) group were 82.1, 41.5, and 25.5%, respectively (Figure 2). Recurrence-free survival after hepatic resection was significantly better in the EOB-MRI (+) group than in the EOB-MRI (−) group ($P < 0.01$).

3.4. Univariate Analysis of Prognostic Factors for Overall and Recurrence-Free Survival after Hepatic Resection for HCC. Tables 2 and 3 summarize the results of univariate analysis of the 20 clinical and laboratory factors and 7 pathological and

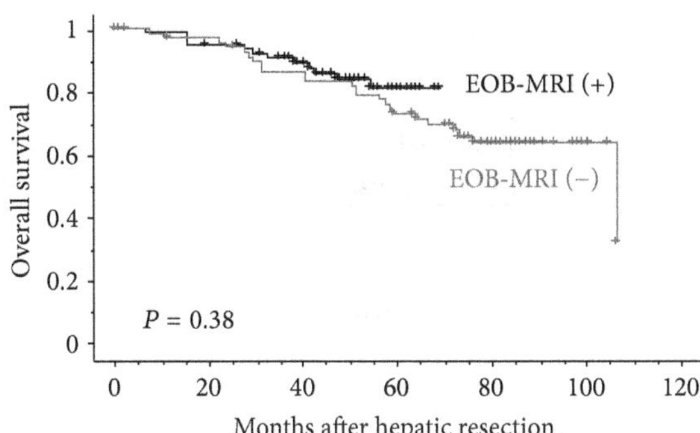

Figure 1: Overall survival curves of patients stratified according to the presence or absence of preoperative EOB-MRI after hepatic resection for progressed HCC.

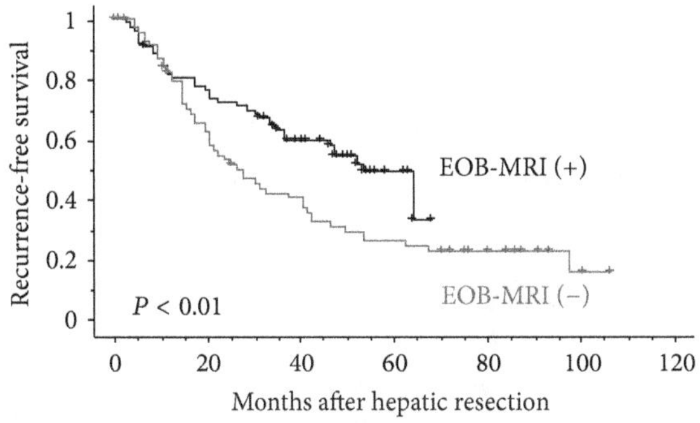

Figure 2: Recurrence-free survival curves of patients stratified according to the presence or absence of preoperative EOB-MRI after hepatic resection for progressed HCC.

tumor-related factors, respectively, for overall survival and recurrence-free survival among the 147 patients with HCC following curative hepatic resection.

In clinical and laboratory factors, the presence of an esophageal varix ($P = 0.02$), platelet count $10 \times 10^4/\mu L$ or less ($P < 0.01$), Child-Pugh class B ($P < 0.01$), and a DCP value more than 40 mAU/mL ($P = 0.03$) were correlated with significantly worse overall survival (Table 2). Other clinical and laboratory factors did not show any significant influence on overall survival after hepatic resection for HCC. In pathological and tumor-related factors, the presence of liver cirrhosis ($P = 0.01$) was correlated with significantly worse overall survival (Table 3).

In clinical and laboratory factors, preoperative EOB-MRI significantly reduced the risk of recurrence ($P < 0.01$). On the other hand, a serum albumin level of 3.5 g/dL or less ($P < 0.01$), platelet count $10 \times 10^4/\mu L$ or less ($P = 0.04$), Child-Pugh class B ($P < 0.01$), and being positive for hepatitis C antibodies ($P < 0.05$) were correlated with significantly worse recurrence-free survival (Table 2). In pathological and tumor-related factors, multiple progressed HCCs ($P < 0.01$) were correlated with significantly worse recurrence-free survival by univariate analysis (Table 3).

3.5. Multivariate Analysis of Prognostic Factors for Overall and Recurrence-Free Survival after Hepatic Resection for HCC. According to multivariate analysis for factors that could influence overall survival, a platelet count $10 \times 10^4/\mu L$ or less (HR 4.41, 95% CI 2.04–9.52, $P < 0.01$) and DCP value more than 40 mAU/mL (HR 3.55, 95% CI 1.72–7.34, $P < 0.01$) were selected as independent predictors of adverse overall survival of patients with HCC after hepatic resection (Table 4). On the other hand, preoperative EOB-MRI (HR 0.56, 95% CI 0.36–0.86, $P < 0.01$) and multiple progressed HCCs (HR 2.10, 95% CI 1.29–3.40, $P < 0.01$) were identified as independent factors significantly correlated with recurrence-free survival after hepatic resection (Table 4).

4. Discussion

The findings of this retrospective study showed that preoperative EOB-MRI and simultaneous treatment of eHCC prolonged recurrence-free survival but not overall survival of progressed HCC patients following hepatic resection. Univariate and multivariate analyses showed that preoperative EOB-MRI was one of the independent factors significantly correlated with recurrence-free survival after hepatic resection. To the best of our knowledge, this is the first study to show that simultaneous treatment of eHCC based on the preoperative imaging study including EOB-MRI prolonged recurrence-free survival after hepatic resection for HCC.

A new MR imaging contrast medium, gadoxetic acid, or Gd-EOB-DTPA, which has the properties of both an extracellular gadolinium chelate and liver-specific contrast material, has become available. Injection of a bolus of Gd-EOB-DTPA allows for the assessment of tumor vascularity using arterial phase imaging and enables hepatocyte-phase imaging approximately 20 minutes after its administration, with approximately 50% of the contrast material being taken up by hepatocytes [10–13]. EOB-MRI including a gradient dual-echo sequence and diffusion-weighted imaging has been recommended for the pretherapeutic evaluation of patients with HCC [19]. Our previous study showed that EOB-MRI was the most useful imaging technique for evaluating small HCC, including eHCC [13]. Hypovascular nodules that appear hypointense on hepatocyte-phase EOB-MRI may progress to conventional hypervascular hepatocellular carcinoma [20]. We previously showed that nodules more than 10 mm in diameter and containing fat were at a higher risk of developing hypervascularization [14]. Moreover, a maximum diameter more than 10 mm [21] or 15 mm or greater [22], increased growth rate, hyperintensity on T1-weighted images [23], hyperintensity on T2-weighted images, and a tumor volume doubling time of less than 542 days [24] were reported to be risk factors of hypervascularization in hypovascular nodules that appeared hypointense on hepatocyte-phase EOB-MRI.

TABLE 2: Univariate analysis of clinical and laboratory factors for overall and recurrence-free survival after hepatic resection for HCC.

Variable	Number of patients	Overall survival			Recurrence-free survival		
		HR	95% CI	P value	HR	95% CI	P value
Sex							
Male	110	1			1		
Female	37	0.81	0.37–1.79	0.61	0.66	0.39–1.16	0.13
Age (years)							
≦70	85	1			1		
>70	62	1.01	0.97–1.04	0.78	1.33	0.86–2.03	0.2
EOB-MRI							
Absent	70	1			1		
Present	77	0.72	0.34–1.15	0.38	0.57	0.37–0.87	<0.01
History of blood transfusion							
Absent	109	1			1		
Present	38	1.4	0.69–2.87	0.35	1.18	0.73–1.90	0.48
Alcoholism							
Absent	79	1			1		
Present	68	1.4	0.72–2.72	0.32	1.34	0.88–2.05	0.17
Smoking							
Absent	52	1			1		
Present	95	1.66	0.80–3.45	0.17	1.24	0.79–1.94	0.34
Diabetes mellitus							
Absent	103	1			1		
Present	44	1.5	0.76–2.93	0.24	1.32	0.85–2.07	0.22
Esophageal varix							
Absent	118	1			1		
Present	29	2.39	1.17–4.91	0.02	1.24	0.73–2.11	0.44
Albumin (g/dL)							
≦3.5	19	1			1		
>3.5	128	0.5	0.23–1.10	0.08	0.49	0.28–0.84	<0.01
Total bilirubin (mg/dL)							
≦1.0	133	1			1		
>1.0	14	0.42	0.10–1.78	0.24	0.71	0.34–1.49	0.36
Alanine aminotransferase (IU/L)							
≦30	59	1			1		
>30	88	1.44	0.71–2.95	0.31	1.5	0.96–2.34	0.08
Platelets ($\times 10^4/\mu$L)							
≦10	33	1			1		
>10	114	0.27	0.27–0.52	<0.01	0.6	0.37–0.97	0.04
Indocyanine green retention rate at 15 minutes (%)							
≦15	77	1			1		
>15	70	1.78	0.90–3.50	0.1	1.13	0.74–1.71	0.58
Prothrombin time (%)							
≦80	71	1			1		
>80	76	0.59	0.30–1.17	0.13	0.71	0.47–1.10	0.11
Child-Pugh classification							
A	137	1			1		
B	10	3.68	1.51–8.93	<0.01	2.65	1.32–5.32	<0.01
Alpha-fetoprotein (ng/mL)							
≦100	117	1			1		
>100	30	0.71	0.29–1.71	0.44	0.71	0.41–1.24	0.23

TABLE 2: Continued.

Variable	Number of patients	Overall survival			Recurrence-free survival		
		HR	95% CI	*P* value	HR	95% CI	*P* value
AFP-L3 (%)							
≦10	110	1			1		
>10	36	0.97	0.46–2.08	0.94	0.79	0.47–1.31	0.36
Des-γ-carboxy prothrombin (mAU/mL)							
≦40	76	1			1		
>40	68*	2.14	1.08–4.22	0.03	1.4	0.91–2.14	0.12
Hepatitis B surface antigen							
Negative	115	1			1		
Positive	32	0.97	0.44–2.14	0.94	0.62	0.35–1.10	0.09
Hepatitis C antibody							
Negative	61	1			1		
Positive	86	1.42	0.71–2.86	0.33	1.56	1.01–2.42	<0.05

*Three patients were excluded because of warfarin administration.

TABLE 3: Univariate analysis of pathological and tumor-related factors for overall and recurrence-free survival after hepatic resection for HCC.

Variable	Number of patients	Overall survival			Recurrence-free survival		
		HR	95% CI	*P* value	HR	95% CI	*P* value
Diameter of main tumor (cm)							
≦2.0	39	1			1		
>2.0	108	1.11	0.50–2.46	0.79	1.39	0.84–2.30	0.19
Number of advanced HCCs							
Solitary	110	1			1		
Multiple	37	1.26	0.60–2.62	0.54	1.96	1.22–3.14	<0.01
Fibrous capsule formation							
Absent	34	1			1		
Present	113	1.18	0.51–2.70	0.7	1.26	0.57–2.12	0.39
Vessel invasion							
Absent	115	1			1		
Present	32	0.95	0.43–2.10	0.9	1.03	0.62–1.71	0.91
Pathological diagnosis							
Well or moderate	118	1			1		
Poor	29	1.68	0.78–3.62	0.18	1.02	0.59–1.75	0.95
AJCC stage							
I	90	1			1		
II or III	57	1.29	0.67–2.49	0.45	1.29	0.83–1.98	0.25
Liver cirrhosis							
Absent	70	1			1		
Present	77	2.58	1.23–5.38	0.01	1.23	0.81–1.89	0.34

We showed that preoperative EOB-MRI and simultaneous treatment of eHCC at the time of resection for progressed HCC prolonged recurrence-free survival after hepatic resection. The recurrence-free survival curves of the two groups overlapped within one year after hepatic resection and after that the incidence of recurrence in the EOB-MRI (+) group became significantly lower than that in the EOB-MRI (−) group. We speculate that recurrence within one year of hepatic resection is mainly due to enlargement of preoperatively undetectable intrahepatic micro IM of resected progressed HCC, while recurrence after one year was MC that progressed from eHCC to hypervascular HCC or was *de novo* hypervascular HCC. We estimate that simultaneous treatment of eHCC at the time of resection for progressed HCC reduced MC by removing eHCC that may have progressed to hypervascular HCC.

One of the reasons why preoperative EOB-MRI and simultaneous treatment of eHCC at the time of resection prolonged recurrence-free survival but not overall survival after hepatic resection for HCC was early diagnosis and prompt treatment of recurrent HCC detected by our postoperative close follow-up.

TABLE 4: Multivariate analysis of prognostic factors for overall and recurrence-free survival after hepatic resection for HCC.

Variable	HR	95% CI	P value
Overall survival			
Esophageal varix (present)	1.49	0.65–3.38	0.34
Platelets ($\leqq 10 \times 10^4/\mu$L)	4.41	2.04–9.52	<0.01
Child-Pugh classification (B)	1.48	0.53–4.13	0.45
Des-γ-carboxy prothrombin (>40 mAU/mL)	3.55	1.72–7.34	<0.01
Liver cirrhosis (present)	1.92	0.89–4.15	0.1
Recurrence-free survival			
EOB-MRI (present)	0.56	0.36–0.86	<0.01
Albumin ($\leqq$3.5 g/dL)	1.68	0.87–3.26	0.12
Platelets ($\leqq 10 \times 10^4/\mu$L)	1.66	0.99–2.79	0.054
Child-Pugh classification (B)	1.52	0.61–3.79	0.36
Hepatitis C antibody (positive)	1.33	0.94–2.34	0.09
Number of advanced HCCs (multiple)	2.1	1.29–3.40	<0.01

Reducing postoperative recurrence after hepatic resection of HCC may not only diminish the burden on patients, but also preserve liver function.

5. Conclusions

The present study showed for the first time that preoperative EOB-MRI and simultaneous treatment of eHCC prolonged recurrence-free survival of progressed HCC patients following hepatic resection. However, because our data were based on a retrospective study and limited number of patients, further prospective studies are required to fully evaluate the significance of preoperative EOB-MRI and simultaneous treatment of eHCC.

References

[1] R. T.-P. Poon, S.-T. Fan, C.-M. Lo et al., "Improving survival results after resection of hepatocellular carcinoma: a prospective study of 377 patients over 10 years," *Annals of Surgery*, vol. 234, no. 1, pp. 63–70, 2001.

[2] M. Minagawa, M. Makuuchi, T. Takayama, and N. Kokudo, "Selection criteria for repeat hepatectomy in patients with recurrent hepatocellular carcinoma," *Annals of Surgery*, vol. 238, no. 5, pp. 703–710, 2003.

[3] H. Imamura, Y. Matsuyama, E. Tanaka et al., "Risk factors contributing to early and late phase intrahepatic recurrence of hepatocellular carcinoma after hepatectomy," *Journal of Hepatology*, vol. 38, no. 2, pp. 200–207, 2003.

[4] T. Takayama, "Surgical treatment for hepatocellular carcinoma," *Japanese Journal of Clinical Oncology*, vol. 41, no. 4, Article ID hyr016, pp. 447–454, 2011.

[5] M. Matsuda, H. Fujii, H. Kono, and Y. Matsumoto, "Surgical treatment of recurrent hepatocellular carcinoma based on the mode of recurrence: repeat hepatic resection or ablation are good choices for patients with recurrent multicentric cancer," *Journal of Hepato-Biliary-Pancreatic Surgery*, vol. 8, no. 4, pp. 353–359, 2001.

[6] Y. Matsumoto, H. Fujii, M. Matsuda, and H. Kono, "Multicentric occurrence of hepatocellular carcinoma: diagnosis and clinical significance," *Journal of Hepato-Biliary-Pancreatic Surgery*, vol. 8, no. 5, pp. 435–440, 2001.

[7] H. Imamura, Y. Matsuyama, Y. Miyagawa et al., "Prognostic significance of anatomical resection and des-γ-carboxy prothrombin in patients with hepatocellular carcinoma," *British Journal of Surgery*, vol. 86, no. 8, pp. 1032–1038, 1999.

[8] K. Hasegawa, N. Kokudo, H. Imamura et al., "Prognostic impact of anatomic resection for hepatocellular carcinoma," *Annals of Surgery*, vol. 242, no. 2, pp. 252–259, 2005.

[9] S. Eguchi, T. Kanematsu, S. Arii et al., "Comparison of the outcomes between an anatomical subsegmentectomy and a non-anatomical minor hepatectomy for single hepatocellular carcinomas based on a Japanese nationwide survey," *Surgery*, vol. 143, no. 4, pp. 469–475, 2008.

[10] S. A. Sung, M.-J. Kim, S. L. Joon, H.-S. Hong, E. C. Yong, and J.-Y. Choi, "Added value of gadoxetic acid-enhanced hepatobiliary phase MR imaging in the diagnosis of hepatocellular carcinoma," *Radiology*, vol. 255, no. 2, pp. 459–466, 2010.

[11] A. Kitao, Y. Zen, O. Matsui et al., "Hepatocellular carcinoma: signal intensity at gadoxetic acid-enhanced MR imaging—correlation with molecular transporters and histopathologic features," *Radiology*, vol. 256, no. 3, pp. 817–826, 2010.

[12] T. Tsuboyama, H. Onishi, T. Kim et al., "Hepatocellular carcinoma: hepatocyte-selective enhancement at gadoxetic acid-enhanced MR imaging—correlation with expression of sinusoidal and canalicular transporters and bile accumulation," *Radiology*, vol. 255, no. 3, pp. 824–833, 2010.

[13] K. Sano, T. Ichikawa, U. Motosugi et al., "Imaging study of early hepatocellular carcinoma: usefulness of gadoxetic acid-enhanced MR imaging," *Radiology*, vol. 261, no. 3, pp. 834–844, 2011.

[14] U. Motosugi, T. Ichikawa, K. Sano et al., "Outcome of hypovascular hepatic nodules revealing no gadoxetic acid uptake in patients with chronic liver disease," *Journal of Magnetic Resonance Imaging*, vol. 34, no. 1, pp. 88–94, 2011.

[15] R. N. H. Pugh, I. M. Murray Lyon, and J. L. Dawson, "Transection of the oesophagus for bleeding oesophageal varices," *British Journal of Surgery*, vol. 60, no. 8, pp. 646–649, 1973.

[16] C. Couinaud, *Le Foie. Etudes Anatomiques Et Chirurgicales*, Masson, Paris, France, 1957.

[17] International Consensus Group for Hepatocellular Neoplasia, "Pathologic diagnosis of early hepatocellular carcinoma: a report of the international consensus group for hepatocellular neoplasia," *Hepatology*, vol. 49, pp. 658–664, 2009.

[18] M. Matsuda, M. Asakawa, H. Amemiya, and H. Fujii, "*Lens culinaris* agglutinin-reactive fraction of AFP is a useful prognostic biomarker for survival after repeat hepatic resection for HCC," *Journal of Gastroenterology and Hepatology*, vol. 26, no. 4, pp. 731–738, 2011.

[19] Y. Ooka, F. Kanai, S. Okabe et al., "Gadoxetic acid-enhanced MRI compared with CT during angiography in the diagnosis of hepatocellular carcinoma," *Magnetic Resonance Imaging*, vol. 31, pp. 748–754, 2013.

[20] S. Kobayashi, O. Matsui, T. Gabata et al., "Relationship between signal intensity on hepatobiliary phase of gadolinium ethoxybenzyl diethylenetriamine pentaacetic acid (Gd-EOB-DTPA)-enhanced MR imaging and prognosis of borderline lesions of hepatocellular carcinoma," *European Journal of Radiology*, vol. 81, pp. 3002–3009, 2012.

[21] M. Takechi, T. Tsuda, S. Yoshioka et al., "Risk of hypervascularization in small hypovascular hepatic nodules showing hypointense in the hepatobiliary phase of gadoxetic acid-enhanced MRI in patients with chronic liver disease," *Japanese Journal of Radiology*, vol. 30, pp. 743–751, 2012.

[22] T. Kumada, H. Toyoda, T. Tada et al., "Evolution of hypointense hepatocellular nodules observed only in the hepatobiliary phase of gadoxetate disodium-enhanced MRI," *American Journal of Roentgenology*, vol. 197, no. 1, pp. 58–63, 2011.

[23] A. Higaki, K. Ito, T. Tamada et al., "High-risk nodules detected in the hepatobiliary phase of Gd-EOB-DTPA-enhanced MR imaging in cirrhosis or chronic hepatitis: incidence and predictive factors for hypervascular transformation, preliminary results," *Journal of Magnetic Resonance Imaging*, vol. 37, no. 6, pp. 1377–1383, 2013.

[24] T. Hyodo, T. Murakami, Y. Imai et al., "Hypovascular nodules in patients with chronic liver disease: risk factors for development of hypervascular hepatocellular carcinoma," *Radiology*, vol. 266, pp. 480–490, 2013.

3

Bleeding in Hepatic Surgery: Sorting through Methods to Prevent It

Fabrizio Romano, Mattia Garancini, Fabio Uggeri, Luca Degrate, Luca Nespoli, Luca Gianotti, Angelo Nespoli, and Franco Uggeri

Unit of Hepatobiliary and Pancreatic Surgery, Department of Surgery, San Gerardo Hospital, University of Milan-Bicocca, Via Donizetti 106, 20052 Monza, Italy

Correspondence should be addressed to Fabrizio Romano, fabrizio.romano@unimib.it

Academic Editor: Andrea Lauterio

Liver resections are demanding operations which can have life threatening complications although they are performed by experienced liver surgeons. The parameter "Blood Loss" has a central role in liver surgery, and different strategies to minimize it are a key to improve results. Moreover, recently, new technologies are applied in the field of liver surgery, having one goal: safer and easier liver operations. The aim of this paper is to review the different principal solutions to the problem of blood loss in hepatic surgery, focusing on technical aspects of new devices.

1. Introduction

Liver resection is considered the treatment of choice for liver tumours. Despite standardized techniques and technological advancing for liver resections, an intraoperative haemorrhage rate ranging from 700 to 1200 mL is reported with a postoperative morbidity rate ranging from 23% to 46% and a surgical death rate ranging from 4% to 5% [1–6].

The parameter "*Blood loss*" has a central role in liver surgery and different strategies to minimize it are a key to improve these results. Bleeding has to be considered a major concern for the hepatic surgeon because of several reasons. At first, it is certainly the major intraoperative surgical complication and cause of death and historically one of the major postoperative complication together with bile leaks and hepatic failure [5–9].

Besides, a high intraoperative blood loss is associated with a higher rate of postoperative complication and shorter long-term survival [10–13]. Furthermore, it is associated with an extensive use of vessel occlusion techniques, directly correlated with higher risk of postoperative hepatic failure. Last, a higher value of intraoperative blood loss is associated with a higher rate of perioperative transfusions; and host immunosuppression associated with transfusions with a dose-related relationship is correlated with a higher rate of complication (in particular infections) and recurrence of malignancies in neoplastic patients [11, 12, 14–21]. In order to reduce transfusions, hepatic surgeon has also not to misinterpret postoperative fluctuations of blood parameter: Torzilli et al. demonstrated that haemoglobin rate and haematocrit after liver resection show a steady and significant decrease until the third postoperative day and then an increase, so this situation has to be explained as physiological and does not justifies blood administration [22].

2. How Can We Reduce Bleeding in Live Surgery?

This study is based on the literature information and our own experience.

The aim of the study is to investigate the principal solutions to the problem of high blood loss in hepatic resection.

2.1. The Role of the Surgeon. Most blood loss during liver resection occurs during parenchymal transection. Hepatic surgeon has different ways to control bleeding.

2.1.1. Vessel Occlusion Techniques. Those techniques are based on the idea that to limit the blood flow through the liver during parenchymal transection can reduce the haemorrhage. Although various forms and modified techniques of vascular control have been practiced, there are basically two main strategies; inflow vascular occlusion and total vascular exclusion [23, 24]. Inflow vascular occlusions are techniques that limit anterograde blood flow with the clamping of all the triad of the hepato-duodenal ligament (*Pringle's manoeuvre*), only of the vascular pedicles (selective clamping of the portal vein and the hepatic artery or *bismuth technique*) or *intravascular portal clamping*. During Pringle's maneuvre, the hepatoduodenal ligament is encircled with a tape, and then a vascular clamp or tourniquet is applied until the pulse in the hepatic artery disappears distally. The PM has relatively little general haemodynamic effect and no specific anaesthetic management is required. However, bleeding can still occur from the backflow from the hepatic veins and from the liver transection plane during unclamping. The other concern is the ischaemic-reperfusion injury to the liver parenchyma, especially in patients with underlying liver diseases [25]. The continuous Pringle manoeuvre (CPM) can be safely applied to the normal liver under normothermic conditions for up to 60 minutes and up to 30 minutes in pathological (fatty or cirrhotic) livers, although much longer durations of continuous clamping 127 minutes in normal livers and 100 minutes in pathological livers have been reported to be safe [26, 27]. One way to extend the duration of clamping and to reduce ischaemia to the remnant liver is by the intermittent Pringle manoeuvre (IPM). It involves periods of inflow clamping that last for 15–20 minutes followed by periods of unclamping for five minutes (mode 15/5 or 20/5), or five minutes clamping followed by one minute unclamping (mode 5/1) [28, 29]. IPM permits a doubling of the ischaemia time, when compared with CPM, and the total clamping time can be extended to 120 minutes in normal livers and 60 minutes in pathological livers. The disadvantage of IPM is that bleeding occurs from the liver transaction surface during the unclamping period and, thus, the overall transection time is prolonged as more time is spent in achieving haemostasis. Belghiti et al. [28] revealed that there was no significant difference in total blood loss or volume of blood transfusion between CPM and IPM (mode 15/5). However, they noticed that pathological livers tolerated CPM poorly.

A newer perspective on inflow occlusion comes from the concept of ischaemic preconditioning (IP). It refers to an endogenous self-protective mechanism by which a short period of ischaemia followed by a brief period of reperfusion produces a state of protection against subsequent sustained ischaemia-reperfusion injury [30, 31]. The IP is performed with ten minutes of ischaemia followed by ten minutes of reperfusion before liver transaction with CPM [32]. Hemihepatic clamping (half-Pringle manoeuvre) interrupts the arterial and portal inflow selectively to the right or left liver lobe that is to be resected [33, 34]. It can be performed with or without prior hilar dissection. It can also be combined with simultaneous occlusion of the ipsilateral major hepatic vein. The advantage of this technique is that it avoids ischaemia in the remnant liver, avoids splanchnic congestion, and allows clear demarcation of the resection margin. The disadvantage is that bleeding from the parenchymal cut surface can occur from the nonoccluded liver lobe.

Segmental vascular clamping entails the occlusion of the ipsilateral hepatic artery branch and balloon occlusion of the portal branch of a particular segment. The portal branch is identified by intraoperative ultrasound and puncture with a cholangiography needle through which a guide wire and balloon catheter are passed [35, 36].

Total vascular exclusion (TVE) combines total inflow and outflow vascular occlusion of the liver, isolating it completely from the systemic circulation. It is done with complete mobilisation of the liver, encircling of the suprahepatic and infrahepatic IVC, application of the Pringle manoeuvre, and then clamping the infrahepatic IVC followed by clamping of the suprahepatic IVC. TVE is associated with significant haemodynamic changes and warrants close invasive and anaesthetic monitoring. Occlusion of the IVC leads to marked reduction of venous return and cardiac output, with a compensatory 80% increase in systemic vascular resistance and 50% increase in heart rate and, thus, not every patient can tolerate it. TVE can be applied to a normal liver for up to 60 minutes and for 30 minutes in a diseased liver. The ischaemic time can be extended when combined with hypothermic perfusion of the liver [37, 38]. Apart from the unpredictable haemodynamic intolerance, postoperative abdominal collections or abscesses and pulmonary complications are more common in TVE, when compared with CPM.

Inflow occlusion with extraparenchymal control of hepatic veins is a modified way of performing TVE. The main and any accessory right hepatic vein, the common trunk of the middle and left hepatic veins, or the separate trunks of the middle and left hepatic veins (15% of cases) are first dissected-free and looped. It has been reported that the trunks of the major hepatic veins can be safely looped in 90% of patients [39, 40]. The loops can then be tightened or the vessels can be clamped after inflow occlusion is applied, so that the liver lobe is isolated from the systemic circulation without interrupting the caval flow. It can be applied in a continuous or intermittent manner. The maximal ischaemia time is up to 58 minutes under continuous occlusion. This technique is more demanding than TVE, but it can avoid the haemodynamic drawbacks of TVE while at the same time provide almost a bloodless field for liver transection.

2.1.2. Instruments and Technique for Resections. Although a large part of improvements of these last decades in liver surgery can be correlated to a better knowledge of the surgical hepatic anatomy (Couinaud's segmentation of liver [41]), better monitoring during anaesthesia, and introduction of intraoperative ultrasonography and of other imaging techniques, the choice of surgical technique for sectioning the liver has surely important repercussions on the intervention's outcome.

There are two techniques we could define traditionally: the *finger fracture method* and the *clamp crushing method.* These are the oldest techniques for hepatic transection and are still employed especially by long-experienced surgeons. The use of traditional techniques to isolate bile ducts and vascular pedicles from the surrounding parenchyma provides for employment of clips or sutures for sealing bile ducts and vascular vessels and for other haemostasis techniques to stop haemorrhage from the resection's surface. There are several studies that sustain that traditional methods are still competitive with a new technique based on utilization of special devices [1, 42, 43].

Introduction of new devices for liver dissection surely have an important role, in particular for reduction of intraoperative blood loss. Actually the most important devices useful for liver resection are presented a technical point of view and analysed to find the advantages (A) and the disadvantages (D) correlated to their employment.

Harmonic Scalpel, HS (Johnson and Johnson Medical, Ethicon, Cincinnati, OH, USA), also known as "Ultrasonically Activated Scalpel" or "Ultrasonic Coagulation Shears," this instrument was introduced in the early 1990s. The ultrasound scissors system includes a generator with a foot switch, the reusable handle for the scalpel, and the cutting device with scissors. The scissors are composed by a moveable blade and by a fixed longitudinal blade that vibrates with an ultrasonic frequency of 55,5 kHz (55.500 vibrations per second). HS can simultaneously cut and coagulate causing protein denaturation by destroying the hydrogen bonds in proteins and by generation of heat in vibrating tissue. This generated heat denatures proteins and forms a sticky coagulum that covers the edges of dissection. Although the heat produces no smoke and thermal injury is limited, the depth of marginal necrosis is greater than that incurred by either the water jet or CUSA. The lateral spread of the energy is 500 micrometers.

A: HS is the only instrument that can simultaneously cut and coagulate (it can coagulate vessel until 2-3 mm of diameter [44]); it is useful on cirrhotic liver [45]; no electricity passes through the patient and there is no smoke production (especially useful in laparoscopic surgery); it can be used in laparoscopic and laparotomic surgery. D: the instrument results in a continuous bleeding risk related to the blind tissue penetration to coagulate vessels hidden into the hepatic parenchyma. Studies demonstrate that HS is not capable of reducing blood loss and operating time compared to traditional techniques [46, 47], cannot coagulate vessel over 2-3 mm of diameter which have to be clipped, and is legated or sealed with other instruments; HS is not easy to use as a blunt dissector and has substantially demonstrated its usefulness only during the resection of the superficial part of liver (2-3 cm) free from large vessels and bile ducts; besides some studies have demonstrated that HS increases the rate of postoperative bile leaks [48, 49], raising the concern that HS may not be effective in sealing bile ducts. The use of HS in liver cirrhosis is controversial. The greatest concern with the use of the harmonic scalpel is the risk of shearing [50]. Slight errors of movement can shear parenchyma without completely coagulating vessels and/or ducts. Moreover, it is expensive (the generator costs US$20.000 and the handle US$250).

2.1.3. Cavitron Ultrasonic Surgical Aspirator, CUSA (Valleylab). The use in liver surgery of this instrument, also known as ultrasonic dissector, was described for the first time in the literature in 1979 by Hodgson [51]. CUSA is a surgical system in which a pencil-grip surgical hand piece contains a transducer that oscillates longitudinally at 23 kHz and to which a hollow conical titanium tip is attached. The vibrating tip of the instrument causes explosion of cells with a high water content (just like hepatocytes) and fragmentation of parenchyma sparing blood and bile vessel because of their walls prevalently composed by connective cells poor of water but rich of intracellular bonds. The device is equipped by a saline solution irrigation system that cools the hand piece and washes the transection plane and by a constant suction system that removes fragmented bits of tissue and permits excellent visualization. A: CUSA is capable of dissecting, offering excellent visualization useful in particular during nonanatomical resections and approaching the deeper portion of the transaction plane [52, 53]. (1) The instrument allows surgeons to see clearly blood and biliary vessels as they dissect through the liver [54], (2) use of the instrument allows them to avoid prolonged extrahepatic vascular control, and (3) the operation actually takes less time because the vessels are continuously controlled during the dissection and there is little need for a prolonged search for bleeding or biliary vessels after the specimen has been removed.

A previous retrospective study from Fan showed that the ultrasonic dissector resulted in lower blood loss, lower morbidity, and lower mortality compared with the clamp crushing technique [55]. Furthermore, ultrasonic dissection resulted in a wider tumor-free margin because of a more precise transection plane.

D: CUSA cannot coagulate or realize haemostasis and even if some studies sustain it to be capable of reducing intraoperative blood loss, operating time, and duration of vessel occlusion [56], important studies demonstrate that CUSA cannot offer these advantages if compared with traditional techniques; a prospective trial by Rau et al. showed no statistical difference in the reduction of blood loss with the use of CUSA as compared to conventional methods [57]; another trial by Takayama et al. [53], in fact, noted a greater median blood loss. CUSA causes more frequent tumour exposure at the surgical margin than traditional techniques [1] and it is less useful for cirrhotic livers because the associated fibrosis prevents easy removal of hepatocytes [58]; besides, some authors found using CUSA method (compared to clamp crushing method) an increase of venous air embolism without evidence of hemodynamic compromise but with increased risk of paradoxical embolism in cirrhotic patients [59]. Moreover, CUSA should be used in association with other devices which are able to perform hemostasis. The instrument seems cumbersome and complicated to inexperienced operating room personnel. Therefore, it is easy for the instrument to malfunction. The fact that the instrument works by removing a margin of liver tissue makes it, by nature, less attractive for harvesting liver for living-donor transplantation.

2.1.4. Tissuelink Monopolar Floating Ball, TMFB (Floating Ball, TissueLink Medical, Dover, NH, USA). This new instrument was put on the market in 2002 and it is a linear device that employs radiofrequency (RF) energy focused at the tip to coagulate target tissue. The tip is provided with a low volume (4–6 mL/min) saline solution irrigation that makes easier the conduction of RF in surrounding tissue and cools the tip itself avoiding formation of chars. TMFB can seal vascular and bile structures up to 3 mm in diameter by collagen fusion. These qualities make this device an excellent instrument for achieving haemostasis and in particular for precoagulating (with a painting movement) parenchyma and vessels prior to transection, preventing blood loss.

Otherwise, continuously heating tissue underneath a cool layer, however, causes a buildup of steam that can result in tissue destruction. The latter phenomenon is known as steam popping [60].

There are two models on the market, the DS3.0 with blunt tip that simply coagulates and the DS3.5-C Dissecting Sealer that is provided with sharp tip that can also dissect. A: the instrument is, in a sense, "friendlier" to most surgeons. In other words, surgeons, who are usually adept at using cautery, can easily understand this mechanism of action and use it accordingly. TMFB can coagulate (and the Dissecting Sealer can also cut) tissues and seals blood and bile ducts up to 3 mm in diameter, is able to reduce blood loss and the recourse to vessel occlusion techniques if compared to traditional techniques [61–63], offers good results also in cirrhotic livers and cystopericystectomy [64], and has a saline irrigation that avoids production of smoke, chars, and sticky coagulum to which the device could stick causing new bleeding when it is moved away. TMFB, used on the cut liver surface after dissection, destroys eventual additional cancer cells at the margin of resection; in order to assure sterile margins, extra tissue destruction at the margins of resection may be desirable for tumor excisions. Otherwise, this could be a disadvantage in case of living-donor liver transplantation. It is available for both laparotomic and laparoscopic surgery and it is quite cheap and compatible with most electrosurgical generator currently available.

D: TMFB is not able to coagulate vessel over 2-3 mm of diameter which has to be clipped, legated, or sealed with other instruments [65]. Moreover, studies do not demonstrate its efficacy to reduce operating time if compared with traditional techniques [66].

2.1.5. The Aquamantys System. The Aquamantys System employs transcollation technology to simultaneously deliver RF (radiofrequency) energy and saline for haemostatic sealing and coagulation of soft tissue and bone at the surgical site. Transcollation technology is used in a wide variety of surgical procedures, including orthopaedic joint replacement, spinal surgery, orthopaedic trauma, and surgical oncology. Transcollation technology simultaneously integrates RF (radiofrequency) energy and saline to deliver controlled thermal energy to the tissue. This allows the tissue temperature to stay at or below 100°C, the boiling point of water. Unlike conventional electrosurgical devices which operate at high temperatures, transcollation technology does not result in smoke or char formation when put in contact with tissue. Blood vessels contain Type I and Type III collagen within their walls. Heating these collagen fibers causes radial compression, resulting in a decrease in vessel lumen diameter. Using the Aquamantys generator with patented bipolar and monopolar sealers, surgeons can achieve broad tissue-surface haemostasis by applying transcollation technology in a painting motion, or it can be used to spot-treat bleeding vessels. This is capable of sealing structures 3–6 mm in diameter without producing high temperature or excessive charring and eschar. Structures more than 6 mm in diameter should be divided in conventional manner with clips or ties. Constant suction is required to clear the saline used for irrigation.

A: its use is "friendlier" to most surgeons, easy to learn most surgeons are comfortable after 5-6 procedures. It seals blood and bile ducts up to 6 mm in diameter and is able to reduce blood loss and the recourse to vessel occlusion techniques. Moreover, it offers good results also in cirrhotic livers [67] and destroys eventual additional cancer cells at the margin of resection.

D: it is expensive and pace of liver transaction could be low.

2.1.6. Bipolar Vessel Sealing Device, BVSD (LigaSure, Valleylab Inc., Boulder, CO, USA). The use in liver surgery of this instrument was described for the first time in the literature in 2001 by Horgan [68]. The LigaSure System includes a generator with a foot switch and a clamp-form hand piece that can be used for parenchymal fragmentation and isolation of blood and bile structures just like in clamp crushing technique before application of energy; it employs RF to realize permanent occlusion of vessels or tissue bundle. The LigaSure generator has a Valleylab's Instant Response technology, a feedback-controlled response system that diagnoses the tissue type in the instrument jaws and delivers the appropriate amount of energy to effectively seal the vessel: when the seal cycle is complete, a generator tone is sound, and the output to the handset is automatically discontinued. BVSD is capable of obliterating the lumen of veins and arteries up to 7 mm in diameter by the fusion of elastin and collagen proteins of the vessel walls and that makes BVSB the only safe and real alternative to sutures and clips for sealing vessel [69–71].

A: BVSD coagulates sealing vessels up to 7 mm in diameter with minimal charring, thermal spread, or smoke; it is capable of reducing blood loss and the recourse to vessel occlusion techniques if compared to traditional techniques [8, 72, 73]. A recently published randomized controlled trial demonstrated that the use of LigaSure in combination with a clamp crushing technique resulted in lower blood loss and faster transaction speed in minor liver resections compared with the conventional technique of electric cautery or ligature for controlling vessels in the transection plane [74]. Otherwise, a more recent randomized trial from the same team was not able to show a real difference between the traditional techniques and the LigaSure vessel sealing system [75]. The instrument is available for both laparotomic and laparoscopic surgery [76]. Furthermore, the use of LigaSure System is not correlated with an increase of the rate of postoperative bile leaks and in some studies bile leakage was nihil [77] and that proves its effectiveness in obliterating also bile vessel. D: after the application the coagulated tissue often sticks to the instrument's jaws causing new bleeding when the device is moved away; BVSD seems to be less effective in presence of cirrhosis for two reasons: first the portal hypertension correlated with cirrhosis causes thinning of the dilated portal vein's walls and makes their obliteration less effective; second cirrhosis makes crushing technique difficult and the hepatic tissue between the blades may disperse the power applied causing vessel to bleed; moreover, it seems to be ineffective in cystopericystectomy [78] (even if some surgeons sustain its effectiveness in this surgery [79]).

2.1.7. Water Jet Scalpel: WJS. The WJS was introduced in 1982 by Papachristou [80]. The device consists of a pressure generating pump and a flexible hose connected to the hand piece. The liquid (saline solution) flows at a steady stream and is projected through the nozzle at the tip of the hand piece. The jet hits the liver at the desired line of transection and washes away the parenchyma, leaving the intrahepatic ducts and vessel undamaged, then the vascular and bile structures can be legated and the transection plane coagulated. The tip is reinforced by a suction tube which removes excess fluid, besides splashing is avoided by covering the area of dissection with a transparent sheet or a Petri dish. Compared to the CUSA, the water jet leaves a smoother cut surface and little hepatic degeneration or necrosis at the borders.

A: WJS can dissect, offering excellent visualization, and is effective also in the cirrhotic liver. In the only available prospective randomized trial of water jet in the literature, in which 31 patients underwent liver resection using water jet and another 30 patients underwent liver resection using CUSA, water jet transection reduced blood loss, blood transfusion, and transection time compared with CUSA [81]. Water jet techniques are quite good for dissecting out major hepatic veins when tumors are in proximity. This allows for delineation of hepatic veins, particularly at the junction with the inferior vena cava, and prevents positive margin.

D: WJS cannot coagulate or realize haemostasis and some studies demonstrate that it cannot achieve a reduction of intraoperative blood loss and operating time if compared with traditional techniques [82, 83]; using this technique is possible in cancerous seeding of the healthy abdominal organs and infection of the operators by hepatic viruses; moreover, in the literature some cases of gas embolism are described using this device [84]. Furthermore, the instrument may be more effective than the CUSA with respect to operating in the presence of cirrhosis. Papachristou and Barters [80] initially reported that the water jet was likely to be ineffective when there is increased fibrotic tissue. Later papers, however, describe successful resections with cirrhosis by using higher jet pressures. Une et al. [81] report that one does not need to use higher water jet pressures to dissect cirrhotic tissue effectively; instead, the same pressures as for normal parenchyma just need to be applied longer. The major concern of surgeons using the water jet is the associated splash. The latter effect is caused by solution bouncing off tissues. Besides, the obvious infectious concerns of the possibility of contaminating operating room personnel, the splash, bring up the notion of the possibility of cancerous seeding. This possibility must be considered in operations for malignancy and one needs to take additional care not to be exposed to the gross tumor during the dissection.

2.1.8. Staplers. Staplers can be used in liver surgery for control of inflow and outflow vessels, or to divide liver parenchyma [85, 86]. The stapler is rarely used as the principal instrument in hepatic resection. The device can add speed to the operation in open or laparoscopic surgery. Its primary use is for achieving control of hepatic vasculature, particularly the hepatic veins. Biliary radicals can be incorporated efficiently into the staple line. Division of the hepatic veins with a stapler as opposed to direct ligation proffers several advantages. First, it eliminates the risk of dissecting the hepatic veins and minimizes the risk of slipped ligature. Furthermore, the stapler simultaneously divides multiple venous branches, especially on the right side, that are too short to allow for a safe, rapid and more traditional ligation.

It is particularly useful in dividing the major trunk of hepatic veins or the middle hepatic vein deep in the transaction. Vascular staplers also can be used to divide the hepatic duct pedicle in the right or left hepatectomy [7]. The procedure starts by dividing the liver capsule by diathermy, the use of a stapler for transection of the liver parenchyma, followed by fracturing the liver tissue with a vascular clamp in a stepwise manner and subsequently divided with an ENDOGia vascular stapler. In a large series of 300 stapler hepatectomies, including 193 major hepatectomies, mortality of 4% and morbidity of 33% were reported which is comparable with conventional liver resection techniques. Vascular control was necessary in only 10% of the series, with an overall median blood loss of 700 mL [87]. Although the technique appears attractive, the financial cost is a serious drawback. One problem associated with the use of a stapler for liver transection is the increased risk of bile leak, since the stapler is not very effective in sealing small bile ducts [88]. Moreover, the surgeon must also be selective in the use of a stapler for the treatment of tumors particularly near the hilum in order to obtain sufficient margin. In case of stapler malfunction, the surgeon should be ready with a backup technique to achieve vein control in case of a sudden hemorrhage.

2.1.9. Habib's Technique. This technique, invented by Habib in 2002, is also known as bloodless hepatectomy technique [10, 89]. Resection is conducted using cooled tip radiofrequency probe that contains a 3 cm exposed tip to coagulate liver resection margins. Once a 2 cm wide coagulative necrosis zone is created by multiple applications of the probes in adjacent zones and at different depths, the division of the parenchyma with a surgical scalpel is possible. Both the remnant liver and the removed specimen have on the margin of resection a portion of necrotic coagulated liver 1 cm thick.

A: Habib's technique allows hepatic resections with marginal blood loss, without any vessel occlusion technique or intra- or postoperative transfusions. In a preliminary study of 15 cases of mainly segmental or wedge resection reported by Weber et al., the mean blood loss was only 30 ± 10 mL, and no complications such as bile leakage were observed [89]. Another group also reported low blood loss using this technique in liver resection [90]. Haemostasis is obtained only by RF thermal energy: no additional devices like stitches, knots, clips, or fibrin glue are needed [10, 89, 91, 92]; it is effective also in the cirrhotic liver and the 1 cm thick of burned coagulated surface assures margins free from tumour. The technique has the advantage of simplicity compared with the aforementioned transection techniques.

D: Habib's technique cannot be applied near the hilum or the cava vein for fear of damaging this structures and because the blood flow of large vessels subtracts RF energy and involves an incomplete coagulative necrosis [93, 94] (up to now the technique has been experienced only for segmental resection); the 1-cm-thick of burned coagulated layer in the surface involves the loss of part of healthy parenchyma and a higher rate of postoperative abdominal abscesses [92, 95]. Moreover, one potential disadvantage of this technique is the sacrifice of parenchymal tissue in the liver remnant, with a 1 cm wide necrotic tissue at the transection margin, which may be critical in cirrhotic patients who require major liver resection.

2.1.10. Chang's Needle Technique. This technique presented by Chang in 2001 [96] is based on the utilization of a special instrument equipped with an 18 cm straight inner needle with a hook near its top; Chang needle can be applied repeatedly to make overlapping interlocking mattress sutures with N° 1 silks along the inner side of the division line. After this phase, liver parenchyma can be divided directly by scissors, electrocautery or traditional resection methods applying new suture only for tubular structures of significant size.

A: Chang's needle technique can be safely used without vascular occlusion, without any other hemostatic technique thus obtaining a reduction in blood trasfusion rates. This method seems to be capable of reducing both intraoperative blood loss and resection time; besides it is surely cheap and is reported to be simple too [43].

D: it cannot be applied if the lesion is too close to inferior cava vein [97].

2.1.11. Gyrus PlasmaKinetic Pulsed Bipolar Coagulation Device. Gyrus (Gyrus Medical Inc., Maple Groves, MN, USA) is a bipolar cautery device which seals the hepatic parenchyma using a combination of pressure and energy that results in the fusion of collagen and elastin in the walls of the hepatic vasculature and bile ducts [98]. The device can reliably seal vessels up to 7 mm in diameter minimizing the amount of blood loss during the transection of the liver. Thermal spread and sticking to tissues is reduced by a cooling period after each pulse as the impedance of the coagulated tissue increased. This instrument has been widely used in previous gynaecological procedures and its use in liver surgery is relatively new. It could be used in a similar manner to the clamp-crush technique to transect hepatic parenchyma. After incising the hepatic capsule with Bovie, the instrument is inserted into the liver in an open manner and bipolar energy is applied as the forceps are slowly closed over the parenchyma. In a recent series, median blood loss rate is compared favourably with those in several large series using the traditional clamp-crush technique [99]. Moreover, blood loss and transfusion rates were comparable with those cited in recent report of alternative parenchymal transaction, as showed by results of Tan et al. [100]. In this study, Gyrus is compared favourably with Harmonic scalpel in terms of bile leakage and the author underlined the concorrential cost of the device. Moreover, it seems to be useful even in case of cirrhotic patients. Corvera et al. [98] have also reported the use of the Gyrus device in cirrhotic livers comparing it to the clamp and crush technique. They evaluated five patients in each group showing similar results between the two groups in terms of operating time, blood loss, and major postoperative complications.

2.1.12. Haemostasis Techniques. Coagulation of vessels over 1 mm of diameter can be achieved by positioning clips or sutures before division, or using devices like LigaSure, TMFB, or HS for their target vessels or staplers for the largest veins. Clips and sutures are used especially during transaction through traditional techniques.

During and after liver's transaction, haemostasis of the vascular structures under 1 mm of diameter is another important concern of the surgeon: firstly because the continuous bleeding from the little vessels in the parenchyma represents a considerable part of intraoperative blood loss, and secondly because it makes hard for the surgeon to visualize the surgical field. The stop of tearing small vessels that causes oozing from the cut surface can be achieved with normal monopolar or bipolar electrocoagulator, better if equipped with saline irrigation that makes them less traumatic and avoids formation of sticky coagulum. An alternative is represented by employment of Argon Beam Coagulator or TMFB that probably is the best device for stopping tearing of small vessels on the cut surface of the liver.

After the resection, another two precautions can be taken: application of mattress sutures for providing a mechanical compression of the bare surface and application of biological glue for realizing complete haemostasis through a chemical/biological action.

2.1.13. Choice of Surgical Strategy. The choice of surgical strategy is based on the preoperative evaluation and on the now indispensable intraoperative ultrasonography (IOUS); in fact several studies have demonstrated that the IOUS is capable of changing surgical strategy in over 40% of cases finding new lesions or diagnosing as inoperable lesions those which were thought as operable at the previous evaluation [101–104]. The kind of surgical strategy chosen for the intervention on the base of the effects strongly influences the operative outcome and the amount of operative blood loss. The most considerable aspect is the amplitude of the resection: a large resection like a right hemihepatectomy (or another typical resection) involves a higher bleeding and a risk of complications. From this point of view, the choice of segmental or wedge limited resections, when they are possible in respect of radical oncology standards, has to be considered as the best option [105, 106]. Usual surgical margins for removal of liver tumours are 1 cm of healthy parenchyma surrounding the lesion. Kokudo et al. in 2002 demonstrated that for colorectal metastases the surgical margin can be, in particular situations, lowered to 2 mm with increase of the pathology recurrence rate from O% for 5 mm margin to 6% for 2 mm margin [107].

This finding, combined with a contrast-enhanced IOUS during the resection, could be a rationale incentive for practising limited resections [108–110], and the possibility of an accurate investigation of the remnant liver through the IOUS.

2.1.14. Drug Administration for Reducing Intraoperative Blood Loss. Liver resection may cause a variable degree of hyperfibrinolytic states; this phenomenon occurs in the days immediately after hepatectomy and is more pronounced in patients with a diseased liver or in patients who have undergone to a wider hepatectomy extent [111–116]. So some authors propose the utilization of drugs with antifibrinolytic effect like Aprotinin that is reported to be capable of reducing intraoperative blood loss (especially during liver resection time) and transfusions [117–119]. Other authors propose utilization of the cheaper Tranexamic acid reporting similar results [120]. Although a theoretical risk of thromboembolic complications is present, no adverse drug effects like deep venous thrombosis, pulmonary embolism, or other circulatory disturbances were detected in both these studies.

3. Comparison of Different Liver Transection Techniques

The choice of transection techniques is currently a matter of preference for surgeons, as there are few data from prospective randomized trials that compared different techniques. It has been shown in small prospective randomized trials that clamp crushing or water jet may be preferable to CUSA in terms of quality of transection or speed of transaction [1, 121]. However, the results of these trials remain to be validated by larger-scale trials. CUSA dissection is still a widely used technique worldwide. Recently, a randomized trial compared four methods of liver transection, namely, clamp crushing, CUSA, Hydrojet, and dissecting sealer, with 25 patients in each group [122]. In that study, clamp crushing was associated with the fastest transection speed, lowest blood loss, and lowest blood transfusion requirement. Furthermore, clamp crushing was the most cost-effective technique. However, in that study, clamp crushing was performed with the Pringle maneuvre, whereas the other techniques were performed without the Pringle maneuvre. This might have resulted in bias in favor of clamp crushing. Another recent comparative study between clamp crushing technique (CRUSH), ultrasonic dissection (CUSA), or bipolar device (LigaSure) failed to show any difference between the three techniques in terms of intraoperative blood loss, blood transfusion, postoperative complications, and mortality [73]. Further prospective randomized studies are needed to determine which transection technique is the best. Moreover, a recent review of the Cochrane conclude that clamp-crush technique is advocated as the method of choice in liver parenchymal transection because it avoids special equipment, whereas the newer methods do not seem to offer any benefit in decreasing the morbidity or transfusion requirement. Otherwise in the comparison of different techniques, apart from the efficacy in transaction with low blood loss, the relative speed of transection and the potential complications are other parameters to be considered [121]. Furthermore, the use of special instruments for transection is costly, especially when two instruments are used in combination for transection and hemostasis. It is difficult to compare the relative cost of different transection instruments because some are reusable whereas others are designed for single use, and the cost of the same instrument varies substantially in different countries. Nonetheless, the cost of these various techniques should play a part in the surgeon's decision as to whether to use them or not.

3.1. The Role of the Anaesthetist. Patients who are subjected to liver surgery are usually pre- and intra-operationally treated with infusion of liquids, plasma expanders, and blood products: normally hepatic resections are in fact conduced in condition of euvolaemia or hypervolaemia to protect patients from the risk of consistent haemorrhage and haemodynamic's instability.

Despite this idea, several studies have demonstrated that a condition of low central venous pressure (LCVP) can reduce bleeding, recourse to vessel occlusion techniques, and transfusions during resection [111–113]. It has been scientifically demonstrated that intraoperative blood loss is correlated with inferior retrohepatic vena cava pressure [114].

Mendelez obtained very low blood loss results in major hepatic resections and managed to keep the CVP under

5 mmHg: this is possible with abstention from practising any infusion but intraoperative liquid infusion at the low speed of 75 mL/h and without any drug administration but employing hypotensive effects of normal anaesthetics (like Isoflurane, Morphine and Fentanyl). It is obvious that LCVP technique needs a strict monitoring of several parameters: in particular, systolic arterial pressure has constantly to be kept over 90 mmHg and diuresis over 25 mL/h. After the specimen is removed and after the realization of complete haemostasis starts, the infusion of liquids, and, if necessary, of plasma expanders and blood products until euvolaemia is obtained and haemoglobin value is over 8–10 g/dL [115].

LCVP has to be abandoned in case of uncontrollable haemorrhage (over 25% of total blood volume) or application of total vascular exclusion technique. Mendelez using LCVP reports a 0,4% rate of gas embolism [116]. This illustrates the importance of collaboration between surgeons and anaesthetists for a successful hepatectomy.

4. Conclusions

Improvement in the techniques of liver transection is one of the most important factors for improved safety of hepatectomy in recent years. The use of intraoperative ultrasound aids delineation of the proper transection plane and allows to transect tumor close to main vessels without bleeding. Clamp-crushing and ultrasonic dissection are currently the two most popular techniques of liver transection. The role of new instruments such as ultrasonic shear and RFA devices in liver transection remains unclear, with few data available in the literature.

The role of vascular exclusion including Pringle's maneuvre seems to be decreasing with improved transection technique. However, it remains a useful technique in reducing bleeding from inflow vessels, especially for surgeons with less experience in liver resection, and recent results show safety of this technique even for prolonged total time of ischemia. Maintenance of low central venous pressure remains an important adjunctive measure to reduce blood loss in liver transection.

As clear data for comparison of various liver transection techniques are lacking, currently the choice of technique is often based on the individual surgeon's preference. However, certain general recommendations can be made based on existing data and the author's experience. Clamp-crushing is a low-cost technique but it requires substantial experience to be used effectively for liver transection, especially in the cirrhotic liver. CUSA can be used in both cirrhotic and noncirrhotic liver, is associated with low blood loss, and has a well-established safety record, with low risk of bile leak. It is particularly useful in major hepatic resections when dissection of the major branches of the hepatic veins is required, or in cases where the tumor is in close proximity to a major hepatic vein, as it allows clear dissection of the hepatic vein from the tumor. The main disadvantage of the CUSA technique is slow transection.

Newer instruments such as the Harmonic scalpel, LigaSure, and TissueLink Dissector enhance the capability of hemostasis and allow faster transection. However, they lack the preciseness of CUSA in dissection of major hepatic veins, and HS more than others may be associated with increased risk of bile leak. Moreover, they are particularly useful in laparoscopic liver resection. They can also be used in combination with CUSA for sealing of vessels, but this increases the cost substantially. RFA-assisted transection is probably the most speedy liver transaction technique. However, the risk of thermal injury to major bile duct is a serious concern and its use is probably restricted to minor resection. Gyrus and Aquamantys are relatively new instruments and the literature does not allow to draw any conclusion about their efficacy and safety.

The experience of the surgeon in practising hepatic surgery, whatever is the method to perform it, is still a factor of primary importance. In spite of that, the advent of new diagnostic instruments, new devices for resection and coagulation, a better knowledge of the liver's anatomy and pathology, and a closer collaboration with the anaesthetist make the hepatic surgery a kind of surgery more defined and rational. From this point of view, new studies based on the use of different surgical strategies, association of different devices, and employment of different diagnostic and anaesthetic techniques are desirable.

References

[1] L. Aldrighetti, C. Pulitanò, M. Arru, M. Catena, R. Finazzi, and G. Ferla, ""Technological" approach versus clamp crushing technique for hepatic parenchymal transection: a comparative study," *Journal of Gastrointestinal Surgery*, vol. 10, no. 7, pp. 974–979, 2006.

[2] M. Rees, G. Plant, J. Wells, and S. Bygrave, "One hundred and fifty hepatic resections: evolution of technique towards bloodless surgery," *British Journal of Surgery*, vol. 83, no. 11, pp. 1526–1529, 1996.

[3] R. Doci, L. Gennari, P. Bignami et al., "Morbidity and mortality after hepatic resection of metastases from colorectal cancer," *British Journal of Surgery*, vol. 82, no. 3, pp. 377–381, 1995.

[4] J. Belghiti, K. Hiramatsu, S. Benoist, P. P. Massault, A. Sauvanet, and O. Farges, "Seven hundred forty-seven hepatectomies in the 1990s: an update to evaluate the actual risk of liver resection," *Journal of the American College of Surgeons*, vol. 191, no. 1, pp. 38–46, 2000.

[5] G. Gozzetti, A. Mazziotti, G. L. Grazi et al., "Liver resection without blood transfusion," *British Journal of Surgery*, vol. 82, no. 8, pp. 1105–1110, 1995.

[6] J. D. Cunningham, Y. Fong, C. Shriver, J. Melendez, W. L. Marx, and L. H. Blumgart, "One hundred consecutive hepatic resections: blood loss, transfusion, and operative technique," *Archives of Surgery*, vol. 129, no. 10, pp. 1050–1056, 1994.

[7] B. Descottes, F. Lachachi, S. Durand-Fontanier et al., "Right hepatectomies without vascular clamping: report of 87 cases," *Journal of Hepato-Biliary-Pancreatic Surgery*, vol. 10, no. 1, pp. 90–94, 2003.

[8] F. Romano, C. Franciosi, R. Caprotti, F. Uggeri, and F. Uggeri, "Hepatic surgery using the LigaSure vessel sealing system," *World Journal of Surgery*, vol. 29, no. 1, pp. 110–112, 2005.

[9] W. R. Jarnagin, M. Gonen, Y. Fong et al., "Improvement in perioperative outcome after hepatic resection: analysis of 1,803 consecutive cases over the past decade," *Annals of Surgery*, vol. 236, no. 4, pp. 397–407, 2002.

[10] G. Navarra, D. Spalding, D. Zacharoulis et al., "Bloodless hepatectomy technique," *HPB*, vol. 4, no. 2, pp. 95–97, 2002.

[11] C. B. Rosen, D. M. Nagomey, H. F. 1'aswell, S. I-Iegelson, D. Ilstrup, and J. A. Van Heerden, "Perioperative blood trasfusion and determinants of survival after liver resection for metastatic colorectal carcinama," *Annals of Surgery*, vol. 216, pp. 493–505, 1992.

[12] K. R. Stephenson, S. M. Steinberg, K. S. Hughes, J. T. Vetto, P. H. Sugarbaker, and A. E. Chang, "Perioperative blood transfusions are associated with decreased time to recurrence and decreased survival after resection of colorectal liver metastases," *Annals of Surgery*, vol. 208, no. 6, pp. 679–687, 1988.

[13] G. Torzilli, M. Makuuchi, Y. Midorikawa et al., "Liver resection without total vascular exclusion: hazardous or beneficial? An analysis of our experience," *Annals of Surgery*, vol. 233, no. 2, pp. 167–175, 2001.

[14] D. A. Kooby, J. Stockman, L. Ben-Porat et al., "Influence of transfusions on perioperative and long-term outcome in patients following hepatic resection for colorectal metastases," *Annals of Surgery*, vol. 237, no. 6, pp. 860–870, 2003.

[15] J. Fujimoto, E. Okamoto, N. Yamanaka, T. Tanaka, and W. Tanaka, "Adverse effect of perioperative blood transfusions on survival after hepatic resection for hepatocellular carcinoma," *Hepato-Gastroenterology*, vol. 44, no. 17, pp. 1390–1396, 1997.

[16] M. Ghio, P. Contini, C. Mazzei et al., "Soluble HLA class I, HLA class II, and Fas ligand in blood components: a possible key to explain the immunomodulatory effects of allogeneic blood transfusions," *Blood*, vol. 93, no. 5, pp. 1770–1777, 1999.

[17] B. D. Tait, A. J. F. d'Apice, L. Morrow, and L. Kennedy, "Changes in suppressor cell activity in renal dialysis patients after blood transfusion," *Transplantation Proceedings*, vol. 16, no. 4, pp. 995–997, 1984.

[18] J. Kaplan and S. Sarnaik, "Transfusion-induced immunologic abnormalities not related to AIDS virus," *The New England Journal of Medicine*, vol. 313, no. 19, p. 1227, 1985.

[19] P. K. Donnelly, B. K. Shenton, A. M. Alomran, D. M. Francis, G. Proud, and R. M. Taylor, "A new mechanism of humoral immunodepression in chronic renal failure and its importance to dialysis and transplantation," *Proceedings of the European Dialysis and Transplant Association. European Dialysis and Transplant Association*, vol. 20, pp. 297–304, 1983.

[20] V. Lenhard, D. Gemsa, and G. Opelz, "Transfusion-induced release of prostaglandin E2 and its role in the activation of T suppressor cells," *Transplantation Proceedings*, vol. 17, no. 6, pp. 2380–2382, 1985.

[21] R. J. Lawrence, A. J. Cooper, M. Loizidou, P. Alexander, and I. Taylor, "Blood transfusion and recurrence of colorectal cancer: role of platelet derived growth factors," *British Journal of Surgery*, vol. 77, no. 10, pp. 1106–1109, 1990.

[22] G. Torzilli, A. Gambetti, D. Del Fabbro et al., "Techniques for hepatectomies without blood transfusion, focusing on interpretation of postoperative anemia," *Archives of Surgery*, vol. 139, no. 10, pp. 1061–1065, 2004.

[23] E. K. Abdalla, R. Noun, and J. Belghiti, "Hepatic vascular occlusion: which technique?" *Surgical Clinics of North America*, vol. 84, no. 2, pp. 563–585, 2004.

[24] V. Smyrniotis, C. Farantos, G. Kostopanagiotou, and N. Arkadopoulos, "Vascular control during hepatectomy: review of methods and results," *World Journal of Surgery*, vol. 29, no. 11, pp. 1384–1396, 2005.

[25] Y. I. Kim, "Ischemia-reperfusion injury of the human liver during hepatic resection," *Journal of Hepato-Biliary-Pancreatic Surgery*, vol. 10, no. 3, pp. 195–199, 2003.

[26] V. E. Smyrniotis, G. G. Kostopanagiotou, J. C. Contis et al., "Selective hepatic vascular exclusion versus Pringle maneuver in major liver resections: prospective study," *World Journal of Surgery*, vol. 27, no. 7, pp. 765–769, 2003.

[27] D. J. Muilenburg, A. Singh, G. Torzilli, and V. P. Khatri, "Surgery in the Patient with Liver Disease," *Anesthesiology Clinics*, vol. 27, no. 4, pp. 721–737, 2009.

[28] J. Belghiti, R. Noun, R. Malafosse et al., "Continuous versus intermittent portal triad clamping for liver resection: a controlled study," *Annals of Surgery*, vol. 229, no. 3, pp. 369–375, 1999.

[29] L. Capussotti, A. Muratore, A. Ferrero, P. Massucco, D. Ribero, and R. Polastri, "Randomized clinical trial of liver resection with and without hepatic pedicle clamping," *British Journal of Surgery*, vol. 93, no. 6, pp. 685–689, 2006.

[30] P. A. Clavien, S. Yadav, D. Sindram, and R. C. Bentley, "Protective effects of ischemic preconditioning for liver resection performed under inflow occlusion in humans," *Annals of Surgery*, vol. 232, no. 2, pp. 155–162, 2000.

[31] G. Nuzzo, F. Giuliante, M. Vellone et al., "Pedicle clamping with ischemic preconditioning in liver resection," *Liver Transplantation*, vol. 10, no. 2, pp. S53–S57, 2004.

[32] P. A. Clavien, M. Selzner, H. A. Rüdiger et al., "A prospective randomized study in 100 consecutive patients undergoing major liver resection with versus without ischemic preconditioning," *Annals of Surgery*, vol. 238, no. 6, pp. 843–852, 2003.

[33] M. Makuuchi, T. Mori, and P. Gunven, "Safety of hemihepatic vascular occlusion during resection of the liver," *Surgery Gynecology and Obstetrics*, vol. 164, no. 2, pp. 155–158, 1987.

[34] P. G. Horgan and E. Leen, "A simple technique for vascular control during hepatectomy: the half-Pringle," *American Journal of Surgery*, vol. 182, no. 3, pp. 265–267, 2001.

[35] D. Castaing, O. J. Garden, and H. Bismuth, "Segmental liver resection using ultrasound-guided selective portal venous occlusion," *Annals of Surgery*, vol. 210, no. 1, pp. 20–23, 1989.

[36] N. Goseki, S. Kato, S. Takamatsu et al., "Hepatic resection under the intermittent selective portal branch occlusion by balloon catheter," *Journal of the American College of Surgeons*, vol. 179, no. 6, pp. 673–678, 1994.

[37] C. Huguet, P. Addario-Chieco, A. Gavelli, E. Arrigo, J. Harb, and R. R. Clement, "Technique of hepatic vascular exclusion for extensive liver resection," *American Journal of Surgery*, vol. 163, no. 6, pp. 602–605, 1992.

[38] D. Eyraud, O. Richard, D. C. Borie et al., "Hemodynamic and hormonal responses to the sudden interruption of caval flow: insights from a prospective study of hepatic vascular exclusion during major liver resections," *Anesthesia and Analgesia*, vol. 95, no. 5, pp. 1173–1178, 2002.

[39] G. Torzilli, M. Makuuchi, Y. Midorikawa et al., "Liver resection without total vascular exclusion: hazardous or beneficial? An analysis of our experience," *Annals of Surgery*, vol. 233, no. 2, pp. 167–175, 2001.

[40] D. Elias, P. Dubé, S. Bonvalot, B. Debanne, B. Plaud, and P. Lasser, "Intermittent complete vascular exclusion of the liver during hepatectomy: technique and indications," *Hepato-Gastroenterology*, vol. 45, no. 20, pp. 389–395, 1998.

[41] C. Couinaud, *Le Foie: Etudes Anatomique et Chirurgicales*, Masson, Paris, France, 1957.

[42] W. C. Meyers, S. Shekherdimian, S. M. Owen, B. H. Ringe, and A. D. Brooks, "Sorting through methods of dividing the liver," *European Surgery*, vol. 36, no. 5, pp. 289–295, 2004.

[43] Y. C. Chang, N. Nagasue, C. S. Chen, and X. Z. Lin, "Simplified hepatic resections with the use of a Chang's needle," *Annals of Surgery*, vol. 243, no. 2, pp. 169–172, 2006.

[44] S. Schmidbauer, K. K. Hallfeldt, G. Sitzmann, T. Kantelhardt, and A. Trupka, "Experience with ultrasound scissors and blades (UltraCision) in open and laparoscopic liver resection," *Annals of Surgery*, vol. 235, no. 1, pp. 27–30, 2002.

[45] H. Sugo, Y. Mikami, F. Matsumoto et al., "Hepatic resection using the harmonic scalpel," *Surgery Today*, vol. 30, no. 10, pp. 959–962, 2000.

[46] J. Kim, S. A. Ahmad, A. M. Lowy et al., "Increased biliary fistulas after liver resection with the harmonic scalpel," *American Surgeon*, vol. 69, no. 9, pp. 815–819, 2003.

[47] T. Okamoto, Y. Nakasato, S. Yanagisawa, H. Kashiwagi, Y. Yamazaki, and T. Aoki, "Hepatectomy using the coagulating shears type of ultrasonically activated scalpel," *Digestive Surgery*, vol. 18, no. 6, pp. 427–430, 2001.

[48] S. T. Fan, E. C. S. Lai, C. M. Lo, K. M. Chu, C. L. Liu, and J. Wong, "Hepatectomy with an ultrasonic dissector for hepatocellular carcinoma," *British Journal of Surgery*, vol. 83, no. 1, pp. 117–120, 1996.

[49] H. Nakayama, H. Masuda, M. Shibata, S. Amano, and M. Fukuzawa, "Incidence of bile leakage after three types of hepatic parenchymal transection," *Hepato-Gastroenterology*, vol. 50, no. 53, pp. 1517–1520, 2003.

[50] W. Schweiger, A. El-Shabrawi, G. Werkgartner et al., "Impact of parenchymal transection by Ultracision® harmonic scalpel in elective liver surgery," *European Surgery*, vol. 36, no. 5, pp. 285–288, 2004.

[51] W. J. B. Hodgson and A. Aufses Jr., "Surgical ultrasonic dissection of liver," *Surgical Rounds*, vol. 2, article 68, 1979.

[52] F. Fasulo, A. Giori, S. Fissi, F. Bozzetti, R. Doci, and L. Gennari, "Cavitron ultrasonic surgical aspirator (CUSA) in liver resection," *International Surgery*, vol. 77, no. 1, pp. 64–66, 1992.

[53] T. Takayama, M. Makuuchi, K. Kubota et al., "Randomized comparison of ultrasonic vs clamp transection of the liver," *Archives of Surgery*, vol. 136, no. 8, pp. 922–928, 2001.

[54] E. Felekouras, E. Prassas, M. Kontos et al., "Liver tissue dissection: ultrasonic or RFA energy?" *World Journal of Surgery*, vol. 30, no. 12, pp. 2210–2216, 2006.

[55] S. T. Fan, E. C. S. Lai, C. M. Lo, K. M. Chu, C. L. Liu, and J. Wong, "Hepatectomy with an ultrasonic dissector for hepatocellular carcinoma," *British Journal of Surgery*, vol. 83, no. 1, pp. 117–120, 1996.

[56] Y. Yamamoto, I. Ikai, M. Kume et al., "New simple technique for hepatic parenchymal resection using a Cavitron Ultrasonic Surgical Aspirator® and bipolar cautery equipped with a channel for water dripping," *World Journal of Surgery*, vol. 23, no. 10, pp. 1032–1037, 1999.

[57] H. G. Rau, M. W. Wichmann, S. Schinkel et al., "Surgical techniques in hepatic resections: ultrasonic aspirator versus jet-cutter. A prospective randomized clinical trial," *Zentralblatt fur Chirurgie*, vol. 126, no. 8, pp. 586–590, 2001.

[58] W. R. Wrightson, M. J. Edwards, and K. M. McMasters, "The role of the ultrasonically activated shears and vascular cutting stapler in hepatic resection," *American Surgeon*, vol. 66, no. 11, pp. 1037–1040, 2000.

[59] B. N. Koo, H. K. Kil, J. S. Choi, J. Y. Kim, D. H. Chun, and Y. W. Hong, "Hepatic resection by the Cavitron Ultrasonic Surgical Aspirator increases the incidence and severity of venous air embolism," *Anesthesia and Analgesia*, vol. 101, no. 4, pp. 966–970, 2005.

[60] S. A. Topp, M. McClurken, D. Lipson et al., "Saline-linked surface radiofrequency ablation: factors affecting steam popping and depth of injury in the pig liver," *Annals of Surgery*, vol. 239, no. 4, pp. 518–527, 2004.

[61] Y. Sakamoto, J. Yamamoto, N. Kokudo et al., "Bloodless liver resection using the monopolar floating ball plus LigaSure diathermy: preliminary results of 16 liver resections," *World Journal of Surgery*, vol. 28, no. 2, pp. 166–172, 2004.

[62] I. Di Carlo, F. Barbagallo, A. Toro, M. Sofia, T. Guastella, and F. Latteri, "Hepatic resections using a water-cooled, high-density, monopolar device: a new technology for safer surgery," *Journal of Gastrointestinal Surgery*, vol. 8, no. 5, pp. 596–600, 2004.

[63] T. A. Aloia, D. Zorzi, E. K. Abdalla, and J. N. Vauthey, "Two-surgeon technique for hepatic parenchymal transection of the noncirrhotic liver using saline-linked cautery and ultrasonic dissection," *Annals of Surgery*, vol. 242, no. 2, pp. 172–177, 2005.

[64] G. Torzilli, M. Donadon, M. Marconi et al., "Monopolar floating ball versus bipolar forceps for hepatic resection: A prospective randomized clinical trial," *Journal of Gastrointestinal Surgery*, vol. 12, no. 11, pp. 1961–1966, 2008.

[65] J. Arita, K. Hasegawa, N. Kokudo, K. Sano, Y. Sugawara, and M. Makuuchi, "Randomized clinical trial of the effect of a saline-linked radiofrequency coagulator on blood loss during hepatic resection," *British Journal of Surgery*, vol. 92, no. 8, pp. 954–959, 2005.

[66] L. Sandonato, M. Soresi, C. Cipolla et al., "Minor hepatic resectio for hepatocellular carcinoma in cirrhotic patients: kelly clamp crushing resection versus heat coagulative necrosis with bipolar radiofrequency devices," *The American Journal of Surgery*, pp. 1490–1495, 2011.

[67] D. A. Geller, A. Tsung, V. Maheshwari, L. A. Rutstein, J. J. Fung, and J. W. Marsh, "Hepatic resection in 170 patients using saline-cooled radiofrequency coagulation," *HPB*, vol. 7, no. 3, pp. 208–213, 2005.

[68] P. G. Horgan, "A novel technique for parenchymal division during hepatectomy," *American Journal of Surgery*, vol. 181, no. 3, pp. 236–237, 2001.

[69] S. M. Strasberg, J. A. Drebin, and D. Linehan, "Use of a bipolar vessel-sealing device for parenchymal transection during liver surgery," *Journal of Gastrointestinal Surgery*, vol. 6, no. 4, pp. 569–574, 2002.

[70] A. Nanashima, S. Tobinaga, T. Abo, T. Nonaka, T. Sawai, and T. Nagayasu, "Usefulness of the combination procedure of crash clamping and vessel sealing for hepatic resection," *Journal of Surgical Oncology*, vol. 102, no. 2, pp. 179–183, 2010.

[71] K. Tepetes, G. Christodoulidis, E. M. Spyridakis, and C. Chatzitheofilou, "Tissue preserving hepatectomy by a vessel sealing device," *Journal of Surgical Oncology*, vol. 97, no. 2, pp. 165–168, 2008.

[72] L. Patrlj, S. Tuorto, and Y. Fong, "Combined blunt-clamp dissection and LigaSure ligation for hepatic parenchyma dissection: postcoagulation technique," *Journal of the American College of Surgeons*, vol. 210, no. 1, pp. 39–44, 2010.

[73] K. Doklestić, A. Karamarković, B. Stefanović et al., "The efficacy of three transection techniques of the liver resection: a randomized clinical trial," *Hepatogastroenterology*, vol. 59, pp. 117–121, 2011.

[74] A. Saiura, J. Yamamoto, R. Koga et al., "Usefulness of LigaSure for liver resection: analysis by randomized clinical trial," *American Journal of Surgery*, vol. 192, no. 1, pp. 41–45, 2006.

[75] M. Ikeda, K. Hasegawa, K. Sano et al., "The vessel sealing system (LigaSure) in hepatic resection: a randomized controlled trial," *Annals of Surgery*, vol. 250, no. 2, pp. 199–203, 2009.

[76] D. P. Slakey, "Laparoscopic liver resection using a bipolar vessel-sealing device: LigaSure," *HPB*, vol. 10, no. 4, pp. 253–255, 2008.

[77] S. Evrard, Y. Bécouarn, R. Brunet, M. Fonck, C. Larrue, and S. Mathoulin-Pélissier, "Could bipolar vessel sealers prevent bile leaks after hepatectomy?" *Langenbeck's Archives of Surgery*, vol. 392, no. 1, pp. 41–44, 2007.

[78] H. Andoh, T. Sato, O. Yasui, S. Shibata, and T. Kurokawa, "Laparoscopic right hemihepatectomy for a case of polycystic liver disease with right predominance," *Journal of Hepato-Biliary-Pancreatic Surgery*, vol. 11, no. 2, pp. 116–118, 2004.

[79] M. Garancini, L. Gianotti, I. Mattavelli et al., "Bipolar vessel sealing system vs clamp crushing technique for liver parenchyma transection," *Hepato-Gastroenterology*, vol. 58, no. 105, pp. 127–132, 2011.

[80] D. N. Papachristou and R. Barters, "Resection of the liver with a water jet," *British Journal of Surgery*, vol. 69, no. 2, pp. 93–94, 1982.

[81] Y. Une, J. Uchino, T. Shimatura, T. Kamiyama, and I. Saiki, "Water jet scalpel for liver resection in hepatocellular carcinoma with or without cirrhosis," *International Surgery*, vol. 81, no. 1, pp. 45–48, 1996.

[82] R. Izumi, K. Yabushita, K. Shimizu et al., "Hepatic resection using a water jet dissector," *Surgery Today*, vol. 23, no. 1, pp. 31–35, 1993.

[83] H. G. Rau, M. W. Wichmann, S. Schinkel et al., "Surgical techniques in hepatic resections: ultrasonic aspirator versus jet-cutter. A prospective randomized clinical trial," *Zentralblatt fur Chirurgie*, vol. 126, no. 8, pp. 586–590, 2001.

[84] H. G. Rau, A. P. Duessel, and S. Wurzbacher, "The use of water-jet dissection in open and laparoscopic liver resection," *HPB*, vol. 10, no. 4, pp. 275–280, 2008.

[85] Y. Fong and L. H. Blumgart, "Useful stapling techniques in liver surgery," *Journal of the American College of Surgeons*, vol. 185, no. 1, pp. 93–100, 1997.

[86] H. Kaneko, Y. Otsuka, S. Takagi, M. Tsuchiya, A. Tamura, and T. Shiba, "Hepatic resection using stapling devices," *American Journal of Surgery*, vol. 187, no. 2, pp. 280–284, 2004.

[87] P. Schemmer, H. Friess, U. Hinz et al., "Stapler hepatectomy is a safe dissection technique: analysis of 300 patients," *World Journal of Surgery*, vol. 30, no. 3, pp. 419–430, 2006.

[88] W. X. Wang and S. T. Fan, "Use of the endo-GIA vascular stapler for hepatic resection," *Asian Journal of Surgery*, vol. 26, no. 4, pp. 193–196, 2003.

[89] J. C. Weber, G. Navarra, L. R. Jiao, J. P. Nicholls, S. L. Jensen, and N. A. Habib, "New technique for liver resection using heat coagulative necrosis," *Annals of Surgery*, vol. 236, no. 5, pp. 560–563, 2002.

[90] M. Stella, A. Percivale, M. Pasqualini et al., "Radiofrequency-assisted liver resection," *Journal of Gastrointestinal Surgery*, vol. 7, no. 6, pp. 797–801, 2003.

[91] K. S. Haghighi, F. Wang, J. King, S. Daniel, and D. L. Morris, "In-line radiofrequency ablation to minimize blood loss in hepatic parenchymal transection," *American Journal of Surgery*, vol. 190, no. 1, pp. 43–47, 2005.

[92] M. Pai, A. E. Frampton, S. Mikhail et al., "Radiofrequency assisted liver resection: analysis of 604 consecutive cases," *European Journal of Surgical Oncology*, vol. 38, pp. 274–280, 2012.

[93] M. Pai, L. R. Jiao, S. Khorsandi, R. Canelo, D. R. C. Spalding, and N. A. Habib, "Liver resection with bipolar radiofrequency device: Habibtrade mark 4X," *HPB*, vol. 10, no. 4, pp. 256–260, 2008.

[94] A. Ayav, L. Jiao, R. Dickinson et al., "Liver resection with a new multiprobe bipolar radiofrequency device," *Archives of Surgery*, vol. 143, no. 4, pp. 396–401, 2008.

[95] A. Ayav, P. Bachellier, N. A. Habib et al., "Impact of radiofrequency assisted hepatectomy for reduction of transfusion requirements," *American Journal of Surgery*, vol. 193, no. 2, pp. 143–148, 2007.

[96] Y. C. Chang, N. Nagasue, X. Z. Lin, and C. S. Chen, "Easier hepatic resections with a straight needle," *American Journal of Surgery*, vol. 182, no. 3, pp. 260–264, 2001.

[97] Y. C. Chang and N. Nagasue, "Blocking intrahepatic inflow and backflow using Chang's needle during hepatic resection: Chang's maneuver," *HPB*, vol. 10, no. 4, pp. 244–248, 2008.

[98] C. U. Corvera, S. A. Dada, J. G. Kirkland, R. D. Garrett, L. W. Way, and L. Stewart, "Bipolar pulse coagulation for resection of the cirrhotic liver," *Journal of Surgical Research*, vol. 136, no. 2, pp. 182–186, 2006.

[99] M. R. Porembka, M. B. M. Doyle, N. A. Hamilton et al., "Utility of the Gyrus open forceps in hepatic parenchymal transection," *HPB*, vol. 11, no. 3, pp. 258–263, 2009.

[100] J. Tan, A. Hunt, R. Wijesuriya, L. Delriviere, and A. Mitchell, "Gyrus PlasmaKinetic bipolar coagulation device for liver resection," *ANZ Journal of Surgery*, vol. 80, no. 3, pp. 182–185, 2010.

[101] P. J. Shukla, D. Pandey, P. P. Rao et al., "Impact of intra-operative ultrasonography in liver surgery," *Indian Journal of Gastroenterology*, vol. 24, no. 2, pp. 62–65, 2005.

[102] H. Bismuth, D. Castaing, and O. J. Garden, "The use of operative ultrasound in surgery of primary liver tumors," *World Journal of Surgery*, vol. 11, no. 5, pp. 610–614, 1987.

[103] E. D. Staren, M. Gambla, D. J. Deziel et al., "Intraoperative ultrasound in the management of liver neoplasms," *American Surgeon*, vol. 63, no. 7, pp. 591–597, 1997.

[104] G. A. Parker, W. Lawrence, J. S. Horsley et al., "Intraoperative ultrasound of the liver affects operative decision making," *Annals of Surgery*, vol. 209, no. 5, pp. 569–577, 1989.

[105] R. P. DeMatteo, C. Palese, W. R. Jarnagin, R. L. Sun, L. H. Blumgart, and Y. Fong, "Anatomic segmental hepatic resection is superior to wedge resection as an oncologic operation for colorectal liver metastases," *Journal of Gastrointestinal Surgery*, vol. 4, no. 2, pp. 178–184, 2000.

[106] N. Kokudo, K. Tada, M. Seki et al., "Anatomical major resection versus nonanatomical limited resection for liver metastases from colorectal carcinoma," *American Journal of Surgery*, vol. 181, no. 2, pp. 153–159, 2001.

[107] N. Kokudo, Y. Miki, S. Sugai et al., "Genetic and histological assessment of surgical margins in resected liver metastases from colorectal carcinoma: minimum surgical margins for successful resection," *Archives of Surgery*, vol. 137, no. 7, pp. 833–840, 2002.

[108] G. Torzilli, D. Del Fabbro, N. Olivari, F. Calliada, M. Montorsi, and M. Makuuchi, "Contrast-enhanced ultrasonography during liver surgery," *British Journal of Surgery*, vol. 91, no. 9, pp. 1165–1167, 2004.

[109] G. Torzilli, N. Olivari, E. Moroni et al., "Contrast-enhanced intraoperative ultrasonography in surgery for hepatocellular carcinoma in cirrhosis," *Liver Transplantation*, vol. 10, no. 2, pp. S34–S38, 2004.

[110] G. Torzilli, D. Del Fabbro, A. Palmisano et al., "Contrast-enhanced intraoperative ultrasonography during hepatectomies for colorectal cancer liver metastases," *Journal of Gastrointestinal Surgery*, vol. 9, no. 8, pp. 1148–1154, 2005.

[111] J. A. Melendez, V. Arslan, M. E. Fischer et al., "Perioperative outcomes of major hepatic resections under low central venous pressure anesthesia: blood loss, blood transfusion, and the risk of postoperative renal dysfunction," *Journal of the American College of Surgeons*, vol. 187, no. 6, pp. 620–625, 1998.

[112] C. Terai, H. Anada, S. Matsushima, S. Shimizu, and Y. Okada, "Effects of mild Trendelenburg on central hemodynamics and internal jugular vein velocity, cross-sectional area, and flow," *American Journal of Emergency Medicine*, vol. 13, no. 3, pp. 255–258, 1995.

[113] R. L. Hughson, A. Maillet, G. Gauquelin, P. Arbeille, Y. Yamamoto, and C. Gharib, "Investigation of hormonal effects during 10-h head-down tilt on heart rate and blood pressure variability," *Journal of Applied Physiology*, vol. 78, no. 2, pp. 583–596, 1995.

[114] V. Smyrniotis, G. Kostopanagiotou, K. Theodoraki, D. Tsantoulas, and J. C. Contis, "The role of central venous pressure and type of vascular control in blood loss during major liver resections," *American Journal of Surgery*, vol. 187, no. 3, pp. 398–402, 2004.

[115] H. Chen, N. B. Merchant, and M. S. Didolkar, "Hepatic resection using intermittent vascular inflow occlusion and low central venous pressure anesthesia improves morbidity and mortality," *Journal of Gastrointestinal Surgery*, vol. 4, no. 2, pp. 162–167, 2000.

[116] M. Johnson, R. Mannar, and A. V. O. Wu, "Correlation between blood loss and inferior vena caval pressure during liver resection," *British Journal of Surgery*, vol. 85, no. 2, pp. 188–190, 1998.

[117] G. V. Paputheodoridis and A. K. Burroughs, "Hemostasis in hepatic and biliary disorders," in *Surgery of the Liver and Biliary Tract*, L. H. Blumgart and Y. Fong, Eds., pp. 199–213, Saunders, London, UK, 3rd edition, 2000.

[118] A. Oguro, H. Taniguchi, T. Daidoh, A. Itoh, N. Tsukuda, and T. Takahashi, "Factors relating to coagulation, fibrinolysis and hepatic drainage after liver resection," *HPB Surgery*, vol. 7, no. 1, pp. 43–49, 1993.

[119] C. Lentschener, D. Benhamou, F. J. Mercier et al., "Aprotinin reduces blood loss in patients undergoing elective liver resection," *Anesthesia and Analgesia*, vol. 84, no. 4, pp. 875–881, 1997.

[120] C. C. Wu, W. M. Ho, S. B. Cheng et al., "Perioperative parenteral tranexamic acid in liver tumor resection: a prospective randomized trial toward "blood transfusion"-free hepatectomy," *Annals of Surgery*, vol. 243, no. 2, pp. 173–180, 2006.

[121] K. S. Gurusamy, V. Pamecha, D. Sharma, and B. R. Davidson, "Techniques for liver parenchymal transection in liver resection," *Cochrane Database of Systematic Reviews*, no. 1, Article ID CD006880, 2009.

[122] M. Lesurtel, M. Selzner, H. Petrowsky et al., "How should transection of the liver be performed? A prospective randomized study in 100 consecutive patients: comparing four different transection strategies," *Annals of Surgery*, vol. 242, no. 6, pp. 814–823, 2005.

4

Metabolomic Analysis of Liver Tissue from the VX2 Rabbit Model of Secondary Liver Tumors

R. Ibarra,[1,2] J-E. Dazard,[3] Y. Sandlers,[2] F. Rehman,[1] R. Abbas,[1] R. Kombu,[2] G-F. Zhang,[2] H. Brunengraber,[1,2] and J. Sanabria[1,2,4]

[1] *Departments of Surgery, Case Western Reserve University, School of Medicine and University Hospitals, Case Medical Center, 11100 Euclid Avenue, Cleveland, OH 44106, USA*

[2] *Departments of Nutrition, Case Western Reserve University, School of Medicine and University Hospitals, Case Medical Center, 11100 Euclid Avenue, Cleveland, OH 44106, USA*

[3] *Center for Proteomics and Bioinformatics, Case Western Reserve University, School of Medicine and University Hospitals, Case Medical Center, Cleveland, OH 44106, USA*

[4] *Department of Surgery, Cancer Treatment Centers of America, Chicago, IL 60099, USA*

Correspondence should be addressed to J. Sanabria; juan.sanabria@case.edu

Academic Editor: Harald Schrem

Purpose. The incidence of liver neoplasms is rising in USA. The purpose of this study was to determine metabolic profiles of liver tissue during early cancer development. *Methods.* We used the rabbit VX2 model of liver tumors (LT) and a control group consisting of sham animals implanted with Gelfoam into their livers (LG). After two weeks from implantation, liver tissue from lobes with and without tumor was obtained from experimental animals (LT+/LT−) as well as liver tissue from controls (LG+/LG−). Peaks obtained by Gas Chromatography-Mass Spectrometry were subjected to identification. 56 metabolites were identified and their profiles compared between groups using principal component analysis (PCA) and a mixed-effect two-way ANOVA model. *Results.* Animals recovered from surgery uneventfully. Analyses identified a metabolite profile that significantly differs in experimental conditions after controlling the False Discovery Rate (FDR). 16 metabolites concentrations differed significantly when comparing samples from (LT+/LT−) to samples from (LG+/LG−) livers. A significant difference was also shown in 20 metabolites when comparing samples from (LT+) liver lobes to samples from (LT−) liver lobes. *Conclusion.* Normal liver tissue harboring malignancy had a distinct metabolic signature. The role of metabolic profiles on liver biopsies for the detection of early liver cancer remains to be determined.

1. Introduction

The incidence of liver tumors is rising in the USA, and it represents the second most common malignancy of the GI tract [1]. Therapy relies on early tumor detection but up to 80% of patients are not eligible for surgery at the time of diagnosis due to advanced stage of disease or to a medical condition that prohibits surgery. Available tumor markers for liver cancer screening, that is, AFP, CA19.9 and CEA, lack high levels of sensitivity and specificity [2] making the early diagnosis of liver neoplasm a difficult challenge for the clinician. Serum metabolites related to oxidative stress are thought to be potential biomarkers for early detection of liver cancer [3–5].

Metabolomics is defined as the systematic quantitative measurement of time-related pluriparametric metabolic responses of multicellular systems to pathophysiological stimuli or genetic modification [4, 5]. It has been used to describe metabolic changes of all low-molecular-weight compounds present in biological samples of several malignant processes [6–12]. Metabolic profiling of urine samples by GC/MS techniques and on plasma by ^{1}H nuclear magnetic resonance (NMR) from patients with primary liver tumors had shown changes mainly related to the glycolytic pathway and lipid metabolism [13–20]. Metabolite profile within the liver tumor significantly differ from the ones seen within the distant noninvolved liver tissue from the same individual [21, 22]. It was hypothesized metabolic profiling from liver tissue obtained by a biopsy may provide us with distinct signatures for the detection of early malignancy, at a stage not detectable by standard imaging modalities. The aim of the present study was to define the metabolic changes that occur in the liver during the early development of hepatic malignancies. For this purpose, we made use of the extensively studied VX2 rabbit model of secondary liver tumors developed by Shope and Hurst in 1933 [23–28]. We described a statistically significant distinct metabolic profile of liver tissue harboring early malignancy.

Table 1

	Site effect	
	Distant (−)	Adjacent (+)
Treatment effect		
Tumor-implant *Treated Group* (LT)	(LT−)	(LT+)
	Rabbit #1	Rabbit #1
	Rabbit #2	Rabbit #2
	⋮	⋮
	rabbit #5	rabbit #5
Gelfoam-implant *Control Group* (LG)	(LG−)	(LG+)
	Rabbit #6	Rabbit #6
	Rabbit #7	Rabbit #7

2. Materials and Methods

2.1. Animal Model. A syngenic graft tumor was obtained by injection of a VX2 cell line in the thigh muscle (*Vastus medialis*) of a New Zealand white male rabbit as described by Rous et al., 1952 [29]. The VX2 cell line was obtained from Dr. Exner laboratory (Case Western Reserve University School of Medicine, Cleveland, OH). Tumor was left to grow within the hosted muscle for 1 month; then it was harvested and minced into cubes of 1 mm^3. Growths were stored at −80°C in Fetal Bovine Serum (Cambrex, East Rutherford, NJ) with 10% DMSO until implantation when tissue was thawed and washed 3 times in Hank's Buffered Salt Solution (HBSS). General chemicals and reagents were obtained from Sigma-Aldrich (St Louis, MO). All experiments were approved by the Institutional Animal Care and Use Committee (IACUC) of the Case Western Reserve University and were performed in accordance with their guidelines.

Adult New Zealand white male rabbits weighing 2.5–3 kg (Covance Princeton, NJ) were quarantined for 15 days in standard conditions with food (Rabbit Chow, NJ) and water *ad libitum* prior to any procedure. Preoperatively, rabbits were anesthetized with Xylazine (5 mg/kg), Ketamine (50 mg/kg), and Acetylpromazine (10 mg/kg) administered IM. Surgical site was shaved and swabbed with Betadine solution (Purdue Pharma, CT) and infiltrated subcutaneously (SC) with Marcaine 0.25% without epinephrine for local anesthesia. Antibiotic prophylaxis was given SC with Penicillin (50,000 units/kg) and Gentamicin (3 mg/kg) prior to the procedure and was continued once daily for 48 hours.

2.2. Experimental Design. Rabbits were first divided into two experimental groups, (i) the Treated Group ($n = 5$; 10 paired samples) underwent median laparotomy and surgical implantation of VX2 tumors in 2 separate sites (right medial and right posterior liver lobes). Each hepatotomy site was carefully closed and labeled with a 6 : 0 Prolene suture (Ethicon, NJ). The abdominal wall was closed in two layers. All experimental animals received equal tumor load (1 $mm^3 \times$ 2 implants). (ii) The Control Group ($n = 2$; 4 paired samples) consisted of animals implanted with Gelfoam (Ethicon, NJ) using the same surgical methodology. Two weeks after surgery all rabbits underwent a second laparotomy. Biopsies of healthy liver tissue were taken separately from the right lobe either adjacent to the tumor implant (LT+) or adjacent to the Gelfoam implant (LG+) and from the left lobe either distant from the tumor implant (LT−) or distant from the Gelfoam implant (LG−). Therefore, in this experimental design, tissue samples were obtained from 4 experimental subgroups (animals with tumor implants = LT+/LT−, and animals with Gelfoam implants = LG+/LG−) as explained in Table 1.

For the purpose of these studies, the tumor Treatment Effect and biopsy Site Effect are the main effects referring to the treated versus control and to the adjacent versus distant comparisons, respectively. In short, this experimental design is a two-way factorial design, where main effects (treatment, site) and interaction effect (treatment × site) can be analyzed statistically, with repeated measures on $n = 7$ units (rabbits), amounting to a total of $2n = 14$ paired observations as explained in Table 1.

2.3. Pathology Evaluation. Samples were immediately frozen on liquid nitrogen and labeled and stored at −80°C. The rest of the liver was surgically removed and perfused-fixed with 10% formaldehyde and 90% PBS at room temperature. All surgical procedures were performed under sterile conditions.

Postoperatively, 20 mL of normal saline (0.9% NS) was given for insensible water losses and Buprenorphine (0.1 mg/kg; Sigma, MO) was given SC twice daily for 48 hours for pain control. All animals were examined three times a day for 72 hours and twice a day afterwards until sacrificed 2 weeks after tumor implantation. In prior study tumor growth was recognized as early as 14 days after tumor grafting.

Liver tissue obtained from each experimental group was sliced and embedded in paraffin and stained with hematoxylin and eosin (H&E) for histological examination. Blinded slides were assessed by a pathologist for evidence of tumor development. Tumor size and volume were calculated from digital records using Digi3 Digital Binocular Microscope with DigiPro 3.0 software (LaboMed, CA).

2.4. Liver Tissue Preparation. Powdered frozen liver tissue (25 mg) was spiked with 5 nmol of heptadecanoic acid (C^{17}) as internal standard and extracted with 2 mL of

CH_3CN/methanol (1 : 1 precooled at −12°C and degassed with nitrogen flow) using a Polytron homogenizer. The slurry was centrifuged at 3,800 rpm for 30 minutes at 4°C and the supernatant was separated and dried with nitrogen gas flow. The residue was oximated with 30 μL of 15 mg/mL of methoxyamine hydrochloride in dry pyridine and incubated at 30°C for 90 minutes. Derivatization was finished with 70 μL of N-methyl-N-trimethyl-silyl-trifluoroacetamide with 1% trimethyl-chlorosilane (MSTFA + 1% TMSC) and the mixture was incubated again at 37°C for 40 min. Samples were then submitted for spectrometric analyses.

2.5. Gas Chromatography-Mass Spectrometry (GC-MS). GC-MS analyses were performed on an Agilent 6890 gas chromatograph interfaced to an Agilent 5973 mass spectrometer equipped with a Phenomenex ZB-5 MSi capillary column (30 m × 0.25 mm i.d., 0.25 μm film thicknesses). Injection volume was 1 μL in splitless mode. Injector temperature was set at 250°C and the transfer line at 275°C. The carrier gas was helium at a constant flow rate of 1 mL/min. The GC oven temperature was initially kept at 60°C for 1 min and increased at a rate of 10°C/min to a final temperature of 325°C held for 10 min. EI ion source temperature was set to 250°C and the MS quadrupole temperature to 150°C. Mass spectra were acquired in scan mode with a mass range of 45 to 800 m/z. Raw data were deconvoluted with the National Institute of Standards and Technology (NIST) Automated Mass Spectral Deconvolution and Identification Software (AMDIS). After spectral analysis and data processing of 113 signals, 56 signals could be identified in 80% of all samples. Identified signals were confirmed by our metabolomic library and the Fiehn library (Agilent Technologies Inc, Santa Clara, CA). For further quantification, the data was exported to the SpectConnect server (Massachusetts Institute of Technology, Cambridge, MA) [30]. The concentration of each metabolite was expressed as its relative peak area (divided by the area of the corresponding internal standard in the same chromatogram). All 56 identified metabolic compounds were further used for statistical analyses.

2.6. Statistical Analyses. All analyses were carried out using the R language and environment, a platform from the R project for statistical modeling, computing, and graphics (http://www.r-project.org/).

2.6.1. Preprocessing of Features. Features (metabolites) were first log-transformed and then variance-stabilized and normalized by our recently developed "*joint adaptive mean-variance regularization*" procedure as previously described [31, 32]. This helps remove sources of systematic variation in the measured intensities (bias and variance due to experimental artifacts) and to ensure that the usual assumption of normality and homoscedasticity are met for statistical inference purposes.

2.6.2. Principal Component Analysis. Principal component analysis (PCA) was carried out and results displayed as *scree plots* (determines the order and the number of principal components (PCs) accounting for the largest variance in the data) and as a 2D *biplot* (uses the first two PCs to display information about (i) the metabolites as indicated by their variance and covariances, and (ii) the relationship between samples as indicated by interindividual distances).

2.6.3. Statistical Inference of Differential Metabolite Concentrations for Label-Free GC-MS Analyses. Statistical modeling was performed using a linear mixed-effect model of analysis of variance (mixed two-way ANOVA), fitted univariately to each individual variable (single metabolite concentration). For statistical inference, we used empirical Bayes methods and posterior estimators derived from them (moderated F-, t-, and B statistics) that have proven to result in greater statistical power [31–35] and to be useful for ranking variables in terms of evidence for differential expression [32, 35–38]. Information was borrowed by constraining the within-block correlations to be equal between variables and by using empirical Bayes methods to moderate the standard deviations between them [39]. These methods are particularly appropriate when only few samples are available, as is always the case in high throughput datasets [35].

2.6.4. Reports for Label-Free GC-MS Analyses. Contrasts were built for each of the effects of interest, and coefficients were estimated accordingly. Variables were ranked in order of evidence of differential concentration. Corresponding P-values were adjusted for multiple testing using the positive FDR (denoted pFDR) [40], a recent extension of the False Discovery Rate (FDR) procedure of Benjamini-Hochberg [41] that is less conservative [40, 42]. Tables report top-to-bottom ranked metabolites (rows) from the model fit for each metabolite and contrast of interest. Each table consists of columns with the following information: the estimated $\log_2$-fold change or M log-ratio ($M = \log_2$ (FC)) for each individual metabolite in theeffect or contrast of interest. Moderated t- and B-statistics represent different measures of statistical significance. The moderated t-statistic corresponds to the usual t-statistic except that information has been borrowed across variables (metabolites), while the B-statistic is the empirical Bayes $\log_2$ of the posterior odds that the metabolite is differentially expressed. Finally raw and adjusted P-values are listed. Note that in every list all the metabolites are ranked by adjusted P-value and then by B-statistic.

2.6.5. Power Analysis and Sample Size Calculation. We used the method described in Liu and Hwang [43] and the pFDR as described above. After variance stabilization and normalization of the data as described above [31, 32], the usual distributional assumptions of test statistics become applicable [43]. Under the above assumption and assuming a balanced paired design, denote the experimental group sample size by n_g (individual rabbits per group), the common standard deviation (to all metabolites) by σ, and the effect size by Δ/σ. We calculated the group sample size n_g required to detect, for example, a minimum fold change FC (Δ) in the treatment effect (tumor versus control Gelfoam) with at most α% FDR as a function of power $1 - \beta$, the parameter π_0

(interpreted as the probability of non-differentially expressed metabolites), the common standard deviation σ, and for a fixed level α of pFDR. Based on the data, parameters estimates were $\widehat{\pi}_0 \approx 0.88 - 0.96$ and $\widehat{\sigma} \approx 0.95 - 1.05$, which is consistent with estimates found in other platforms in high dimensional data [43]. Under the above assumptions and estimations, for fixed $\widehat{\pi}_0 = 0.92$ and $\widehat{\sigma} = 1.00$, while controlling the FDR at less than 10%, a group sample size as low as $n_g = 5$ can detect a twofold change on the transformed scale with more than 90% power (Figure 1).

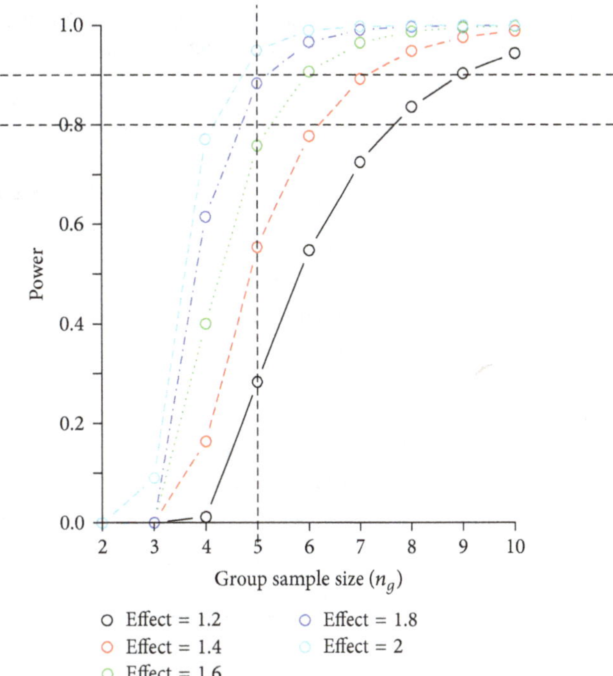

FIGURE 1: *Power analyses and sample size calculations.* The plots show statistical power curves ($1 - \beta$) for the main treatment effect (tumor versus control Gelfoam) as a function of group sample size (n_g). Results are reported for a range of fixed fold change, for the fixed estimated median standard deviation common to all metabolites $\widehat{\sigma} = 1.00$, and for fixed $\widehat{\pi}_0 = 0.92$, while controlling the False Discovery Rate at 10%. Results show that a group sample size of $n_g = 5$ in a balanced paired experimental design detects a twofold change in the effect of interest with more than 90% power.

3. Results

Tumor grew in all experimental animals (Figure 2). All tumors were similar in size, with a maximum diameter of 8.4 ± 5.96 mm and a tumor volume of 241.8 ± 78.6 mm^3. There was no evidence for tumor spread or distant metastasis by gross examination of the abdomen, chest, and brain. Animals from the control group presented normal livers without signs of the Gelfoam implant. All rabbits were clinically stable and no differences were noted regarding their food and water intake or their body weight.

Principal component analysis (PCA) showed that a minimum of two components explained at least 58% of the total variance of the data. Based on the metabolic concentration profiles, PCA was able to separate liver tissue samples of animals where tumor was implanted (LT+/LT−) from liver tissue samples of animals where Gelfoam was implanted (LG+/LG−) (Figure 3). Furthermore, PCA analysis shows that the liver tissue samples adjacent to the tumor could not be separated from the liver tissue samples distant from the tumor, whether this was observed in the treated samples (LT+/LT−) or in the Gelfoam control samples (LG+/LG−). This is indicative of an overall lack of site effect. In contrast, PCA analysis shows an overall strong treatment effect as evidenced by the clear separation of treated samples (LT+/LT−) from control samples (LG+/LG−). Also, this clear separation remained evident whether considering liver tissue samples adjacent to the tumor only (LT+ versus LG+) or liver tissue samples distant from the tumor (LT− versus LG−).

These results were further confirmed by ANOVA analyses: Table 2 lists the metabolic compounds whose concentrations were found statistically different in the treatment effect, that is, between the treated group (LT+/LT−) and the control group (LG+/LG−). A total of 16 identified compounds (10 downregulated, 6 upregulated) had False Discovery Rate-adjusted P-values (for multiplicity of testing) below the 10% FDR level. Interestingly, no statistically significant changes in metabolic compound concentrations were detected in the overall site effect, that is, between the experimental distant group (LT+ and LG+) and the adjacent group (LT− and LG−). To evaluate if this absence of significance could be due to a confounding effect of the Sham-treated samples over the tumor-treated samples, we analyzed the relative concentrations of metabolic compounds between adjacent versus distal (LT+ versus LT−) biopsy samples in the treated samples alone (Table 3). This comparison revealed a list of 20 identified compounds (14 down-regulated, 6 up-regulated)

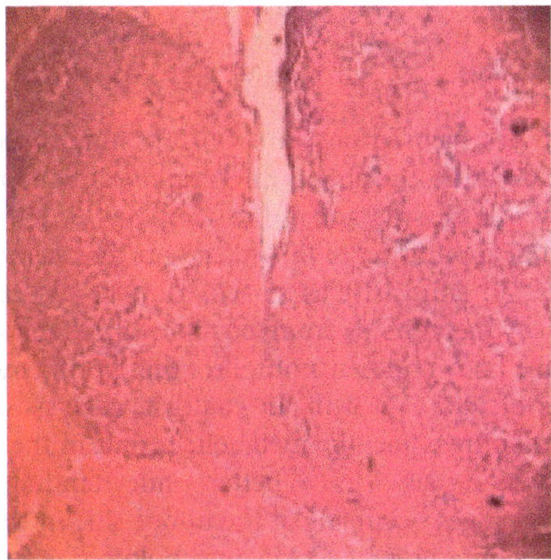

FIGURE 2: *Microscopic morphology of VX2 tumors.* All implanted tumor grafts showed macroscopic growth on liver sites. At histology, most tumors had a pseudocapsule formed by fibrotic tissue that surrounded the tumor which contained typical epithelial cells with malignant morphology without neoangiogenesis, tumor invasion, or lymphocyte infiltration at this stage of tumor growth (panel ×20).

TABLE 2: Table below shows the differentially expressed metabolites for the overall treatment effect (tumor-treated LT versus Sham-treated LG) with at most 10% FDR. Metabolites are ranked from top to bottom by (1) statistical significance (B) and (2) magnitude of change (M).

(a) 10 downregulated

	ID	Downregulated $M = \log_2(\text{FC})$	FDR Adj. P values	$B = \log_2(\text{Odds})$
1	Uracil	−5.9822	4.52E − 53	141.4358
2	Erythriol	−5.0750	9.78E − 41	101.6021
3	α-Hydroxyglutaric acid	−3.2867	2.28E − 19	42.2173
4	Salicylic acid	−2.8973	1.18E − 15	32.6557
5	Ethanolamine	−2.0405	1.38E − 08	15.8544
6	Glycolic acid	−1.1588	1.58E − 03	4.6512
7	Amino ethyl phosphate	−1.0952	2.72E − 03	4.0824
8	Citrate	−0.9941	6.46E − 03	3.2435
9	L-Serine	−0.6642	6.86E − 02	1.0709
10	D-ribose-5-phosphate	−0.6495	7.08E − 02	0.9943

(b) 6 up-regulated

	ID	Up-regulated $M = \log_2(\text{FC})$	FDR Adj. P-values	$B = \log_2(\text{Odds})$
1	Glucose	5.0586	1.08E − 40	100.9430
2	Glycerol	3.0981	1.55E − 17	37.4367
3	Threonic acid	2.3402	8.15E − 11	21.0678
4	Glycerol-3-P	1.6936	2.54E − 06	10.7094
5	O-acetylsalicylic acid	0.9825	6.62E − 03	3.1519
6	Inositol	0.7428	4.27E − 02	1.5101

that had a FDR-adjusted P-values below the 10% FDR level. Graphical illustration of Tables 2 and 3 results are displayed in a space of statistical significance known as volcano plots (Figures 4(a) and 4(b), resp.).

4. Discussion

Recent studies focused on primary liver tumors that have aimed to describe metabolic fingerprints of tumor development. While plasma and urine samples [13, 15, 16] give the potential application of this technique for diagnosis and followup in a noninvasive approach, they are susceptible to variations of metabolites from possible simultaneous processes in the body and may not reflect the specific metabolic alterations of tumor growth. In contrast, analysis of tissue samples will only reflect the metabolic profile of the affected organ, providing us with a better understanding of the metabolic changes occurring at the tumor site. In this study we used a nontargeted GC-MS metabolomic approach to profile the changes present in the tumor periphery as well as the metabolic response of healthy nonadjacent liver tissue in the VX2 rabbit model of secondary liver tumors. Principal component analysis performed on metabolic profiles in liver tissue differentiated animals with tumor from Sham animals as early as 14 days after tumor grafting. We profiled 56 metabolites and most of our findings resemble previously described changes for HCC [17, 21, 22] and other tumors [6, 10, 44]. Changes are mostly related to the metabolism of carbohydrates, lipids, and amino acids and related to inflammation and oxidative stress. Relevant metabolites (Table 4) in liver metabolism and their profile under the influence of a growing tumor are discussed.

4.1. Carbohydrates. The high concentrations of glucose observed in samples from the experimental group when compared to Shams seems opposite of what has been described in the literature. In the tumor mass, an upregulation of glycolysis should use glucose as its principal substrate lowering its concentration. Yang et al. analyzed tumor tissue samples from 17 patients with HCC and compared them with the noninvolved adjacent liver tissue as a control [22]. They found a significantly lower concentration of glucose in the tumor samples, and this concentration was even lower in high grade tumors when compared to low grade tumors. Differences may be due to different sampling design; (i) in our study the tissue samples did not include the tumor mass and (ii) in the human study a group of healthy humans was not included as a control. In addition, the glucose uptake of cancer cells is about 30 times higher due to the increase expression of glucose transporters and hexokinase [45]. Our results showed an increase in the amount of glucose available for the hepatocytes in the healthy noninvolved liver

TABLE 3: Table below shows the differentially expressed metabolites for the site effect (distant versus adjacent biopsy) in the treatment group alone (LT− versus LT+) with at most 10% FDR. Metabolites are ranked from top to bottom by (1) statistical significance (B) and (2) magnitude of change (M).

(a) 14 downregulated

	ID	Down-regulated $M = \log_2(\text{FC})$	FDR Adj. P values	$B = \log_2(\text{Odds})$
1	Uracil	−3.00112	$3.83E - 35$	83.65428
2	Erythriol	−2.70968	$9.69E - 30$	68.06919
3	α-Hydroxyglutaric acid	−1.626	$2.75E - 12$	24.07396
4	Salicylic acid	−1.43637	$4.63E - 10$	18.63641
5	Ethanolamine	−1.11231	$1.17E - 06$	10.90255
6	Amino ethyl phosphate	−0.64698	0.004687	3.236894
7	D-Ribose-5-phosphate	−0.556	0.013184	2.212044
8	Citrate	−0.54086	0.014689	2.056548
9	β-Alanine	−0.48647	0.025933	1.533321
10	Glycolic acid	−0.41113	0.050703	0.900165
11	Glycine	−0.39026	0.058594	0.743548
12	L-Alanine	−0.33772	0.085378	0.385349
13	L-Serine	−0.33726	0.085378	0.382457
14	Aminomalonic acid	−0.31862	0.095196	0.267971

(b) 6 up-regulated

	ID	Up-regulated $M = \log_2(\text{FC})$	FDR Adj. P-values	$B = \log_2(\text{Odds})$
1	Glucose	2.477314	$1.30E - 25$	56.78349
2	Glycerol	1.546767	$2.37E - 11$	21.72003
3	Threonic acid	1.349669	$4.13E - 09$	16.37445
4	Glycerol-3-P	0.733706	0.001424	4.35813
5	Inositol	0.56952	0.012116	2.354559
6	O-acetylsalicylic acid	0.447728	0.037053	1.194456

that can be used by the highly active glycolytic metabolism induced by the tumor. The glycolytic disturbances found in this tumor model were accentuated in the healthy tissue close to the tumor when compared with the lobe without tumor, a finding probably due to the presence of a highly active tumor grown in need of energy substrates promoting a "stealing phenomenon" from the surrounding parenchyma and perhaps a relative state of starvation in distant but normal liver tissue.

Although the concentration of lactate was not significantly higher in samples of liver tissue adjacent to the tumor when compared to tissue samples distant from the tumor from the same animal group, a trend was noted. The classic finding in cancer, described by Warburg in 1930 [19], represents an increase in the rate of glycolysis with the final reduction of pyruvate into lactate by the enzyme lactate dehydrogenase (LDH) in order to regenerate the nicotinamide adenine dinucleotide (NAD+) necessary for the glycolytic pathway under an impaired oxidation of pyruvate in the mitochondria [18]. This effect is largely attributed to the activation of hypoxia-inducible factor-1b (HIF-1b) in tumor cells, which increases the expression of glucose transporters and glycolytic enzymes, resulting in an upregulation of glycolysis [4, 6, 7, 46]. A recent study of metabolites in plasma and urine from a rat model of diethylnitrosamine-induced HCC found a similar increase in lactate production in the presence of tumor and its level was related to HCC invasion and metastasis [45]. The acidic environment that surrounds the cancer cells has been recently related to a "reversed Warburg effect" in which lactate increases the metastatic potential of the tumor cell and 3-hydroxybutyrate (a ketone body) promotes tumor growth [47–49]. The lack of significance may be due to sample timing where the tumor has not reached enough size to influence surrounding liver tissue towards a more anaerobic metabolism or to a sample site where cells analyzed were not malignant and their anaerobic metabolism, which is enhanced in tumorigenic cells as mean of survival is not manifested in normal cells with established blood supply. Disturbances of the normal oxidative process is manifested as well by a significantly lower concentration of citrate and α-hydroxyglutaric acid from liver tissue adjacent to the tumor (LT+) when compared to liver

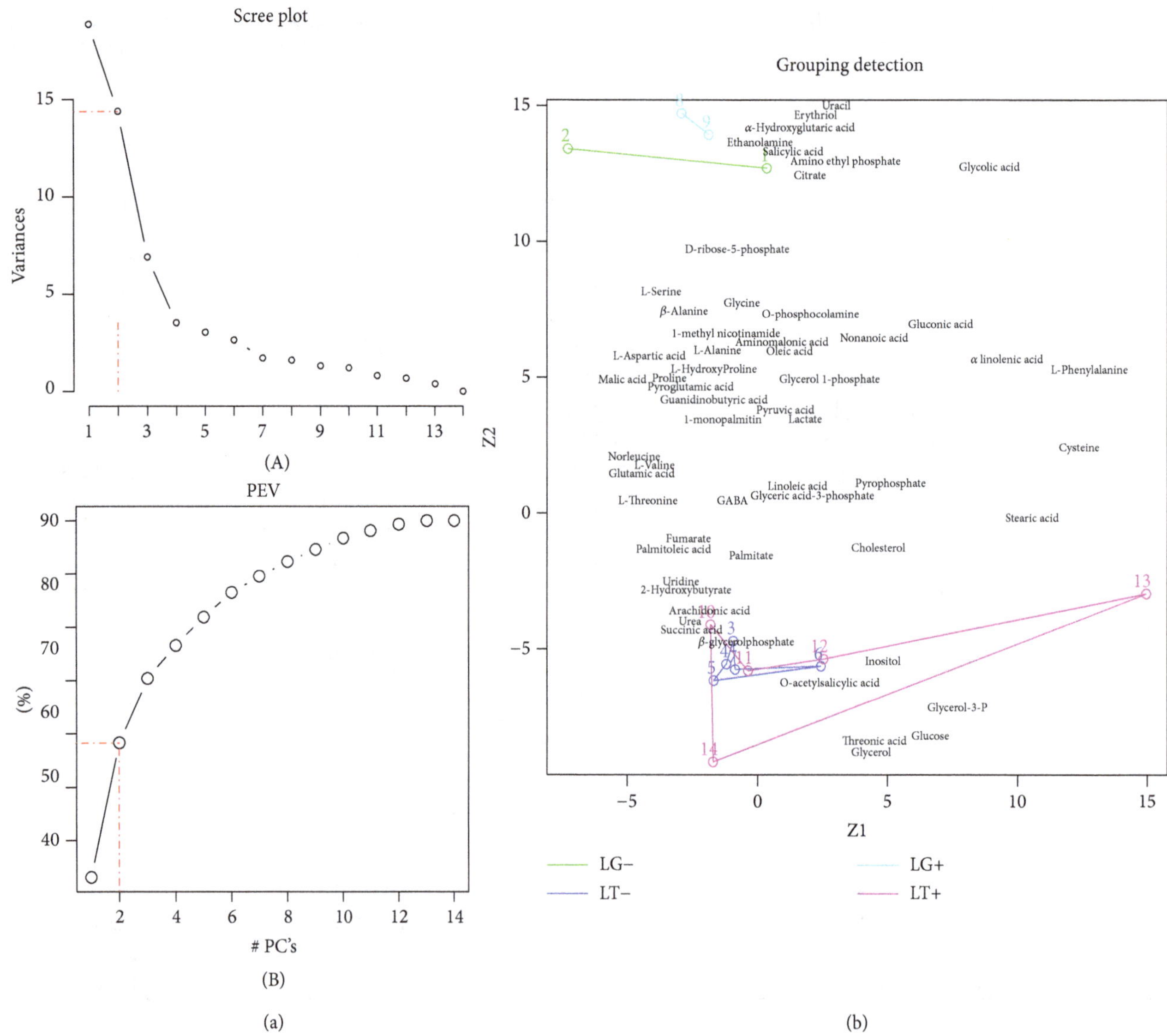

Figure 3: *Principal component analysis (PCA).* (a) PCA scree plots showing how much of variance is accounted for by each principal component (A) and that a minimum of two principal components ([Z1, Z2]) is enough to explain ~58% of the total variance (percentage of explained variance-PEV) in the data (B). (b) PCA biplot of samples and metabolites in the [Z1, Z2] principal component space. Note how the control group samples (LG+ and LG−) overlap with each other, as well as the treated group samples (LT+ and LT−) with each other. In addition, note the clear separation between the distant group samples (LT+ and LG+) and between the adjacent group samples (LT− and LG−).

tissue distant to the tumor (LT−); nevertheless, the present studies cannot elucidate if these changes are due to increase consumption, decrease production, or both.

4.2. Lipids. Many studies have noted disturbances of lipid metabolism in cancer cells [7, 14, 17]. Yang reported decreased lipid concentrations in tissue samples from HCC compared to noninvolved liver tissue, suggesting an increased utilization as an energy substrate via β-oxidation and as a substrate for the synthesis of cell membranes due to the demand of proliferating cells [22]. The decrease in the levels of ethanolamine, the second most common head group for membrane phospholipids, suggests increased utilization due to cell proliferation. Increased activity of the enzyme ethanolamine kinase has been reported in cancer cells and it has been attributed to the synthesis of phosphoethanolamine, a component of cell membranes [50]. Furthermore, we observed an increase in the levels of glycerol and glycerol-3-P in all samples from the experimental group when compared to the Shams suggesting an increase in triglycerides catabolism. Glycerol-3-P can fuel up glycolysis via dihydroxyacetone phosphate (DHAP). The above described changes suggested disturbances of lipid metabolism in normal hepatocytes induced by the presence

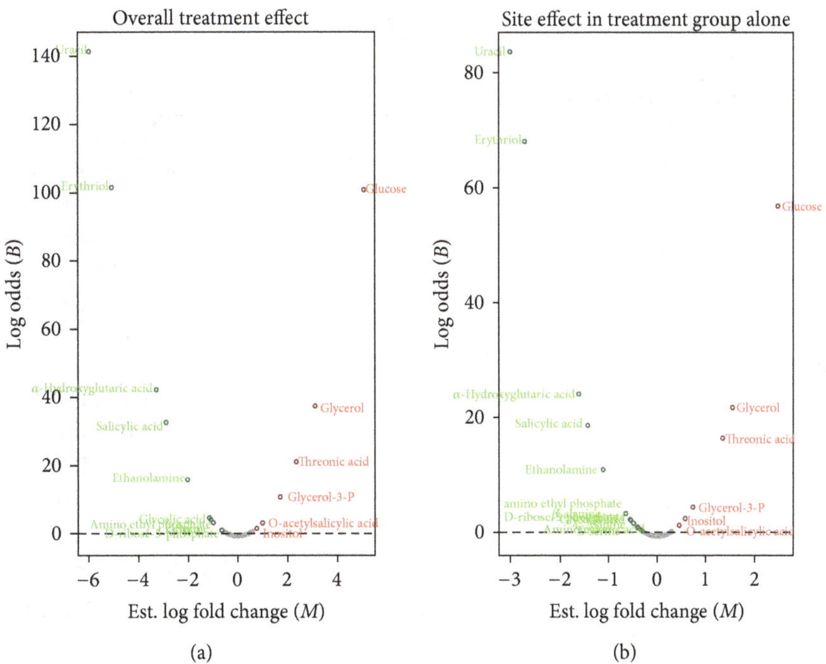

FIGURE 4: *t-test volcano plots.* (a) Overall treatment effect. (b) Site effect, conditioning on the Treated Group. The volcano plot is a scatter plot of all metabolite species arranged by an individual measure of magnitude of change of expression between experimental groups (horizontal axis) versus a corresponding measure of statistical significance (vertical axis). The horizontal axis represents the estimated log-fold-change of differential expression, denoted $\log_2(\mathrm{FC})$ or M. The vertical axis represents the log-odds of differential expression, denoted $\log_2(\mathrm{Odds})$ or B. The most significant metabolites are those that have the largest M in absolute value and the largest B. Metabolites (dots) whose relative concentrations are significantly downregulated (green) and upregulated (red) between experimental conditions are distributed in the upper left-hand side and upper right-hand side directions of the plot, respectively. The nonregulated metabolites are shown with grey dots. The horizontal dotted line represents a null log-odds of differential expression. FDR was controlled at 10%.

of nearby immortal cells. Metabolic changes are mainly characterized by an increased β-oxidation and by the provision of substrates for cell membrane synthesis.

4.3. Amino Acids. Studies describe significant disturbances in the metabolism of several aminoacids, such as alanine, glycine, and glutamate [13, 21, 22]. In this study the concentration of L-serine, L-alanine, and glycine were significantly downregulated, while the concentration of glutamate was unchanged, which may be due to a balance between increase consumption for protein synthesis proposed by some and increase production through accelerated protein breakdown by others [8]. The levels of cysteine, a precursor of glutathione, were noted to have a trend to be decreased in the (LT+) tissue when compared to the noninvolved liver lobe (LT−). This difference may be explained by an increase synthesis of glutathione by the surrounding hepatocytes (LT+) to cope with oxidative stress. To support this finding, aminomalonic acid, a dicarboxylic acid derived from cysteine via β-elimination of the sulfur residue, was found to be significantly lower in (LT+) samples when compared to the (LT−) samples.

The levels of β-alanine (an amino acid that differs from α-alanine) were found to be decreased in samples from (LT+) tissue. β-alanine is a product of the degradation of dihydrouracil, which is an intermediate in the catabolism of uracil. The levels of uracil and the ribose ring D-ribose-5-P were also found to be decreased in the (LT+) samples. These findings suggest a status of accelerated cell proliferation, also found in plasma samples of patients with leukemia [44].

Two metabolites were noted to be regulated in liver tissue adjacent to tumor implantation (LT+). Although their concentration did not reach statistical difference when compared to liver tissue distant from tumor implantation (LT−), their relative different concentrations may have biological implications. 1-Methylnicotinamide (MNA) is a product of the catabolism of nicotinamide via enzymatic methylation by the enzyme nicotinamide N-methyltranferase (NNMT); this enzyme has been found to be upregulated in liver cirrhosis [51] and liver tumors [52]. In our study the levels of MNA were found to be higher in samples of tissue adjacent to the tumor (LT+) when compared to samples of tissue away from the tumor (LT−). It has also been shown that the increased catabolism of NAD^+ will further stimulate the conversion of pyruvate to lactate to replenish the NAD^+ pool required for glycolysis. Furthermore, MNA has also been linked with hypermethylation of DNA reducing the expression of tumor suppressor genes, thus promoting tumor cell growth [53] and prostacyclin dependent anti-inflammatory and antithrombotic effects [54, 55]. The regulation of liver GABA_A receptors plays an important role in the regulation of hepatocyte regeneration proliferation and in the pathogenesis of HCC [56],

TABLE 4: Relevant metabolites and their relative variation between liver tissue samples from adjacent (LT+) and distant (LT−) to tumor implantation site.

Metabolites	Adjacent to tumor (LT+)	Distant to tumor (LT−)	Type related mechanism
Glucose	↑	—	Increase glucose uptake
Lactate	↑	—	Increased β-oxidation—increased glycolysis
Glycerol	↑	—	Lipid metabolism
Glycerol-3-phosphate	↑	—	Increased lipids catabolism
Threonic acid	↑	—	Vitamin C metabolite
Inositol	↑	—	Oxidative stress—glutathione synthesis
Ethanolamine	↓	—	Cell replication—membranes
L-serine/L-alanine/glycine	↓	—	Protein synthesis
β-alanine	↓	—	Cell replication—uracil catabolism
Aminomalonic acid	↓	—	Oxidative stress—cysteine metabolism
Citrate	↓	—	Citrate cycle—oxidative-redox mitochondrial status
D-Ribose-5-phosphate	↓	—	Purine synthesis
Uracil	↓	—	Cell replication
1-methyl nicotinamide	↑	—	Nicotinamide catabolism—NNMT activation
GABA	↓	—	Cell replication

↑: for relative increase; ↓: for relative decrease; —: for no relative change. LT+: healthy liver tissue adjacent to the tumor and LT−:healthy liver tissue distant from the tumor.

since their activation results in cell hyperpolarization inhibiting DNA synthesis. A transient hepatocyte depolarization has been reported after partial hepatectomy in rats [57]. An increase in DNA replication mediated by polyamines follows cell depolarization. Human HCC tissues have been found to be depolarized and have decreased $GABA_A$-$\beta3$ receptor expression when compared to adjacent nontumor tissue [58]. Moreover, the restoration of membrane potentials resulted in a decreased proliferative activity and slower growth rates in human HCC cell lines [59]. In the present study we noted a trend towards a decreased concentration of GABA in (LT+) samples suggesting a depolarized state that facilitates cell proliferation.

Precursors of proinflammatory mediators have roles in many cellular processes, including inflammation, proliferation, and apoptosis. Their specific role in cancer is under investigation [60]. Threonic acid (not to be confounded with the amino acid threonine) is a metabolite of ascorbic acid and it further enhances the cellular uptake of ascorbic acid. This metabolite was found to be different between all groups (LT+, LT−, and Shams). Its role in liver metabolism in relation to cancer or oxidative stress remains to be determined.

The findings of our study must be interpreted in light of some limitations. The metabolic and redox status of an animal with a tumor growth may be a function not only of the tumor biology and its mass but also, among other factors, their nutritional status. Although the number of Sham animals was low, the metabolites in the right and left lobes were identical and did not differ from the metabolic profile of healthy rabbits already known (Fiehn library at Agilent Technologies Inc, Santa Clara, CA). Furthermore, the process of obtaining samples for metabolic profiling is an invasive one. In spite of these boundaries, the present study showed that metabolic disturbances in animals with early liver tumor growth can be detected and perhaps metabolic signatures of liver tumor growth may overcome the limitations of current biomarkers used in the clinical setting.

Metabolic changes found in the very early growth of a secondary liver tumor resemble the ones previously described in HCC [14–16], suggesting that these biochemical alterations are not specific to the biology of the tumor but to the response of the surrounding healthy liver tissue in response to a malignant growth with rapid cell proliferation in need of energy substrates. Changes observed in the healthy tissue adjacent to the tumor share metabolic characteristics typically found in neoplastic tissue; they may point to metabolic alterations that precede the morphological changes in the tumor surroundings suggested by others [15]. Metabolic signatures in tissue from subjects with tumor development could prove to be useful in the early detection of liver malignancies.

5. Conclusions

Principal component analyses of the metabolic profile from liver tissue differentiated animals with tumor when compared to animals without tumor as early as 14 days after tumor grafting. Different metabolic patterns were seen in tissue samples from healthy liver close to the tumor, healthy liver away from the tumor, and healthy liver from Sham animals. Further studies to correlate the metabolic profiles of tumor tissue and serum are required and could become a promising clinical tool for the early detection of liver tumors and their recurrence.

Abbreviations

HCC: Hepatocellular carcinoma
AFP: α-Fetoprotein
CA19.9: Carbohydrate antigen 19.9

CEA: Carcinoembryonic antigen
GS-MS: Gas Chromatography-Mass Spectrometry
IM: Intramuscular
DMSO: Dimethylsulfoxide
HBSS: Hank's Buffered Salt Solution
PBS: Phosphate buffered saline
SC: Subcutaneous
NS: Normal saline
H&E: Hematoxylin and eosin
MSTFA: N-Methyl-N-trimethyl-silyl-trifluoroacetamide
TMSC: Trimethyl-chlorosilane
NIST: National Institute of Standards and Technology
AMDIS: Automated Mass Spectral Deconvolution and Identification Software
LDH: Lactate dehydrogenase
NAD^+: Nicotinamide adenine dinucleotide
HIF-1b: Hypoxia-inducible factor-1b
MNA: 1-Methylnicotinamide
NNMT: Nicotinamide N-methyltranferase
G3P: Glycerol-3-phosphate
DHAP: Dihydroxyacetone phosphate
IRP2: Iron regulatory protein 2
GABA: γ-Aminobutyric acid.

Disclosure

This work was presented in part at the International Hepato-Pancreato-Biliary Association (IHPBA) Buenos Aires, 2010.

Acknowledgments

This work was supported by the RoadMap grant initiative of NIDDK (5R33DK070291) and by Grant (1R01ES013925). Dr. RA Ibarra was supported by a Ruth L. Kirschstein National Research Service Award NIH/NIDDK (T32-DK007319). Dr. J-E Dazard was supported by the Case Comprehensive Cancer Center, NIH-NCI (P30-CA043703). Dr. G Jacobs, Department of Pathology, CWRU.

References

[1] World Health Organization, "Cancer," Fact Sheet 297, 2009, http://www.who.int/mediacentre/factsheets/fs297/en/.

[2] M. Sherman, K. M. Peltekian, and C. Lee, "Screening for hepatocellular carcinoma in chronic carriers of hepatitis B virus: incidence and prevalence of hepatocellular carcinoma in a North American urban population," *Hepatology*, vol. 22, no. 2, pp. 432–438, 1995.

[3] R. Abbas, R. S. Kombu, R. A. Ibarra, K. K. Goyal, H. Brunengraber, and J. R. Sanabria, "The dynamics of glutathione species and ophthalmate concentrations in plasma from the VX2 rabbit model of secondary liver tumors," *HPB Surgery*, vol. 2011, Article ID 709052, 8 pages, 2011.

[4] N. Vinayavekhin, E. A. Homan, and A. Saghatelian, "Exploring disease through metabolomics," *ACS Chemical Biology*, vol. 5, no. 1, pp. 91–103, 2010.

[5] D. Ryan and K. Robards, "Metabolomics: the greatest omics of them all?" *Analytical Chemistry*, vol. 78, no. 23, pp. 7954–7958, 2006.

[6] J. L. Griffin and R. A. Kauppinen, "Tumour metabolomics in animal models of human cancer," *Journal of Proteome Research*, vol. 6, no. 2, pp. 498–505, 2007.

[7] J. L. Griffin and J. P. Shockcor, "Metabolic profiles of cancer cells," *Nature Reviews Cancer*, vol. 4, no. 7, pp. 551–561, 2004.

[8] C. Yang, A. D. Richardson, J. W. Smith, and A. Osterman, "Comparative metabolomics of breast cancer," *Pacific Symposium on Biocomputing. Pacific Symposium on Biocomputing*, pp. 181–192, 2007.

[9] P. Gao, C. Lu, F. Zhang et al., "Integrated GC-MS and LC-MS plasma metabonomics analysis of ankylosing spondylitis," *Analyst*, vol. 133, no. 9, pp. 1214–1220, 2008.

[10] S. Tiziani, V. Lopes, and U. L. Günther, "Early stage diagnosis of oral cancer using 1H NMR-Based metabolomics1,2," *Neoplasia*, vol. 11, no. 3, pp. 269–276, 2009.

[11] K. Odunsi, R. M. Wollman, C. B. Ambrosone et al., "Detection of epithelial ovarian cancer using 1H-NMR-based metabonomics," *International Journal of Cancer*, vol. 113, no. 5, pp. 782–788, 2005.

[12] J. E. Ippolito, J. Xu, S. Jain et al., "An integrated functional genomics and metabolomics approach for defining poor prognosis in human neuroendocrine cancers," *Proceedings of the National Academy of Sciences of the United States of America*, vol. 102, no. 28, pp. 9901–9906, 2005.

[13] H. Wu, R. Xue, L. Dong et al., "Metabolomic profiling of human urine in hepatocellular carcinoma patients using gas chromatography/mass spectrometry," *Analytica Chimica Acta*, vol. 648, no. 1, pp. 98–104, 2009.

[14] H. Gao, Q. Lu, X. Liu et al., "Application of 1H NMR-based metabonomics in the study of metabolic profiling of human hepatocellular carcinoma and liver cirrhosis," *Cancer Science*, vol. 100, no. 4, pp. 782–785, 2009.

[15] J. Yang, G. Xu, Y. Zheng et al., "Diagnosis of liver cancer using HPLC-based metabonomics avoiding false-positive result from hepatitis and hepatocirrhosis diseases," *Journal of Chromatography B*, vol. 813, no. 1-2, pp. 59–65, 2004.

[16] J. Chen, W. Wang, S. Lv et al., "Metabonomics study of liver cancer based on ultra performance liquid chromatography coupled to mass spectrometry with HILIC and RPLC separations," *Analytica Chimica Acta*, vol. 650, no. 1, pp. 3–9, 2009.

[17] R. Xue, Z. Lin, C. Deng et al., "A serum metabolomic investigation on hepatocellular carcinoma patients by chemical derivatization followed by gas chromatography/mass spectrometry," *Rapid Communications in Mass Spectrometry*, vol. 22, no. 19, pp. 3061–3068, 2008.

[18] Á. D. Ortega, M. Sánchez-Aragó, D. Giner-Sánchez, L. Sánchez-Cenizo, I. Willers, and J. M. Cuezva, "Glucose avidity of carcinomas," *Cancer Letters*, vol. 276, no. 2, pp. 125–135, 2009.

[19] O. Warburg, "On the origin of cancer cells," *Science*, vol. 123, no. 3191, pp. 309–314, 1956.

[20] H. R. Christofk, M. G. Vander Heiden, M. H. Harris et al., "The M2 splice isoform of pyruvate kinase is important for cancer metabolism and tumour growth," *Nature*, vol. 452, no. 7184, pp. 230–233, 2008.

[21] A. D. Southam, J. M. Easton, G. D. Stentiford, C. Ludwig, T. N. Arvanitis, and M. R. Viant, "Metabolic changes in flatfish hepatic tumours revealed by NMR-based metabolomics and metabolic correlation networks," *Journal of Proteome Research*, vol. 7, no. 12, pp. 5277–5285, 2008.

[22] Y. Yang, C. Li, X. Nie et al., "Metabonomic studies of human hepatocellular carcinoma using high-resolution magic-angle spinning 1H NMR spectroscopy in conjunction with multivariate data analysis," *Journal of Proteome Research*, vol. 6, no. 7, pp. 2605–2614, 2007.

[23] R. E. Shope and E. W. Hurst, "Infectious papillomatosis of rabbits: with a note on the histopathology," *The Journal of Experimental Medicine*, vol. 58, pp. 607–624, 1933.

[24] J. H. Chen, Y. C. Lin, Y. S. Huang, T. J. Chen, W. Y. Lin, and K. W. Han, "Induction of VX2 carcinoma in rabbit liver: comparison of two inoculation methods," *Laboratory Animals*, vol. 38, no. 1, pp. 79–84, 2004.

[25] B. Liang, C.-S. Zheng, G.-S. Feng et al., "Correlation of hypoxia-inducible factor 1α with angiogenesis in liver tumors after transcatheter arterial embolization in an animal model," *CardioVascular and Interventional Radiology*, vol. 33, no. 4, pp. 806–812, 2010.

[26] B. D. Weinberg, E. Blanco, S. F. Lempka, J. M. Anderson, A. A. Exner, and J. Gao, "Combined radiofrequency ablation and doxorubicin-eluting polymer implants for liver cancer treatment," *Journal of Biomedical Materials Research A*, vol. 81, no. 1, pp. 205–213, 2007.

[27] M. Vali, J. A. Vossen, M. Buijs et al., "Targeting of VX2 rabbit liver tumor by selective delivery of 3-bromopyruvate: a biodistribution and survival study," *Journal of Pharmacology and Experimental Therapeutics*, vol. 327, no. 1, pp. 32–37, 2008.

[28] J. Deng, S. Virmani, G.-Y. Yang et al., "Intraprocedural diffusion-weighted PROPELLER MRI to guide percutaneous biopsy needle placement within rabbit VX2 liver tumors," *Journal of Magnetic Resonance Imaging*, vol. 30, no. 2, pp. 366–373, 2009.

[29] P. Rous, J. G. Kidd, and W. E. Smith, "Experiments on the cause of the rabbit carcinomas derived from virus-induced papillomas. II. Loss by the Vx2 carcinoma of the power to immunize hosts against the papilloma virus," *The Journal of Experimental Medicine*, vol. 96, pp. 159–174, 1952.

[30] M. P. Styczynski, J. F. Moxley, L. V. Tong, J. L. Walther, K. L. Jensen, and G. N. Stephanopoulos, "Systematic identification of conserved metabolites in GC/MS data for metabolomics and biomarker discovery," *Analytical Chemistry*, vol. 79, no. 3, pp. 966–973, 2007.

[31] J.-E. Dazard and J. Sunil Rao, "Joint adaptive meanvariance regularization and variance stabilization of high dimensional data," *Computational Statistics and Data Analysis*, vol. 56, no. 7, pp. 2317–2333, 2012.

[32] J.-E. Dazard, H. Xu, and A. Santana, "MVR R package: mean variance regularization," Comprehensive R Archive Network, 2011.

[33] B. Efron, "Robbins, empirical Bayes and microarrays," *The Annals of Statistics*, vol. 31, no. 2, pp. 366–378, 2003.

[34] B. Efron, R. Tibshirani, J. D. Storey, and V. Tusher, "Empirical bayes analysis of a microarray experiment," *Journal of the American Statistical Association*, vol. 96, no. 456, pp. 1151–1160, 2001.

[35] I. Lönnstedt, R. Rimini, and P. Nilsson, "Empirical bayes microarray ANOVA and grouping cell lines by equal expression levels," *Statistical Applications in Genetics and Molecular Biology*, vol. 4, article 7, 2005.

[36] M. A. Newton, C. M. Kendziorski, C. S. Richmond, F. R. Blattner, and K. W. Tsui, "On differential variability of expression ratios: improving statistical inference about gene expression changes from microarray data," *Journal of Computational Biology*, vol. 8, no. 1, pp. 37–52, 2001.

[37] G. K. Smyth, "Linear models and empirical bayes methods for assessing differential expression in microarray experiments," *Statistical Applications in Genetics and Molecular Biology*, vol. 3, no. 1, article 3, 2004.

[38] C. M. Kendziorski, M. A. Newton, H. Lan, and M. N. Gould, "On parametric empirical Bayes methods for comparing multiple groups using replicated gene expression profiles," *Statistics in Medicine*, vol. 22, no. 24, pp. 3899–3914, 2003.

[39] M. A. Newton, A. Noueiry, D. Sarkar, and P. Ahlquist, "Detecting differential gene expression with a semiparametric hierarchical mixture method," *Biostatistics*, vol. 5, no. 2, pp. 155–176, 2004.

[40] J. D. Storey, "The positive false discovery rate: a Bayesian interpretation and the q-value," *The Annals of Statistics*, vol. 31, no. 6, pp. 2013–2035, 2003.

[41] Y. Benjamini and Y. Hochberg, "Controlling the false discovery rate: a practical and powerful approach to multiple testing," *Journal of the Royal Statistical Society*, vol. 57, pp. 289–300, 1995.

[42] J. D. Storey, "A direct approach to false discovery rates," *Journal of the Royal Statistical Society B*, vol. 64, no. 3, pp. 479–498, 2002.

[43] P. Liu and J. T. G. Hwang, "Quick calculation for sample size while controlling false discovery rate with application to microarray analysis," *Bioinformatics*, vol. 23, no. 6, pp. 739–746, 2007.

[44] D. A. MacIntyre, B. Jiménez, E. J. Lewintre et al., "Serum metabolome analysis by 1H-NMR reveals differences between chronic lymphocytic leukaemia molecular subgroups," *Leukemia*, vol. 24, no. 4, pp. 788–797, 2010.

[45] J. R. Griffiths, P. M. J. McSheehy, S. P. Robinson et al., "Metabolic changes detected by in vivo magnetic resonance studies of HEPA-1 wild-type tumors and tumors deficient in hypoxia-inducible factor-1β (HIF-1β): evidence of an anabolic role for the HIF-1 pathway," *Cancer Research*, vol. 62, no. 3, pp. 688–695, 2002.

[46] Z.-F. Li, J. Wang, C. Huang et al., "Gas chromatography/time-of-flight mass spectrometry-based metabonomics of hepatocarcinoma in rats with lung metastasis: elucidation of the metabolic characteristics of hepatocarcinoma at formation and metastasis," *Rapid Communications in Mass Spectrometry*, vol. 24, no. 18, pp. 2765–2775, 2010.

[47] S. Pavlides, D. Whitaker-Menezes, R. Castello-Cros et al., "The reverse Warburg effect: aerobic glycolysis in cancer associated fibroblasts and the tumor stroma," *Cell Cycle*, vol. 8, no. 23, pp. 3984–4001, 2009.

[48] G. Bonuccelli, A. Tsirigos, D. Whitaker-Menezes et al., "Ketones and lactate "fuel" tumor growth and metastasis: evidence that epithelial cancer cells use oxidative mitochondrial metabolism," *Cell Cycle*, vol. 9, no. 17, pp. 3506–3514, 2010.

[49] W. E. Gall, K. Beebe, K. A. Lawton et al., "α-hydroxybutyrate is an early biomarker of insulin resistance and glucose intolerance in a nondiabetic population," *PLoS ONE*, vol. 5, no. 5, Article ID e10883, 2010.

[50] R. Biedroń, M. Ciszek, M. Tokarczyk et al., "1-Methylnicotinamide and nicotinamide: two related anti-inflammatory

agents that differentially affect the functions of activated macrophages," *Archivum Immunologiae et Therapiae Experimentalis*, vol. 56, no. 2, pp. 127–134, 2008.

[51] A. Momchilova, T. Markovska, and R. Pankov, "Ha-ras-transformation alters the metabolism of phosphatidylethanolamine and phosphatidylcholine in NIH 3T3 fibroblasts," *Cell Biology International*, vol. 23, no. 9, pp. 603–610, 1999.

[52] R. Pumpo, G. Sarnelli, A. Spinella, G. Budillon, and R. Cuomo, "The metabolism of nicotinamide in human liver cirrhosis: a study on N-methylnicotinamide and 2-pyridone-5-carboxamide production," *American Journal of Gastroenterology*, vol. 96, no. 4, pp. 1183–1187, 2001.

[53] B. R. Clark, J. T. Murai, and A. Pomeranz, "Altered distribution and excretion of N1 methylnicotinamide in rats with Walker 256 carcinosarcoma," *Cancer Research*, vol. 35, no. 7, pp. 1727–1733, 1975.

[54] J. R. Kuykendall, R. Cox, and D. Kinder, "1-Methylnicotinamide stimulates cell growth and inhibits hemoglobin synthesis in differentiating murine erythroleukemia cells," *Toxicology in Vitro*, vol. 21, no. 8, pp. 1656–1662, 2007.

[55] S. Chlopicki, J. Swies, A. Mogielnicki et al., "1-Methylnicotinamide (MNA), a primary metabolite of nicotinamide, exerts anti-thrombotic activity mediated by a cyclooxygenase-2/prostacyclin pathway," *British Journal of Pharmacology*, vol. 152, no. 2, pp. 230–239, 2007.

[56] G. Y. Minuk, "Gaba and hepatocellular carcinoma," *Molecular and Cellular Biochemistry*, vol. 207, no. 1-2, pp. 105–108, 2000.

[57] X. K. Zhang, T. Gauthier, F. J. Burczynski, G. Q. Wang, Y. Gong, and G. Y. Minuk, "Changes in liver membrane potentials after partial hepatectomy in rats," *Hepatology*, vol. 23, no. 3, pp. 549–551, 1996.

[58] G. Y. Minuk, M. Zhang, Y. Gong et al., "Decreased hepatocyte membrane potential differences and GABAA-$\beta 3$ expression in human hepatocellular carcinoma," *Hepatology*, vol. 45, no. 3, pp. 735–745, 2007.

[59] D. Sun, Y. Gong, H. Kojima et al., "Increasing cell membrane potential and GABAergic activity inhibits malignant hepatocyte growth," *American Journal of Physiology—Gastrointestinal and Liver Physiology*, vol. 285, no. 1, pp. G12–G19, 2003.

[60] M. Nakanishi and D. W. Rosenberg, "Roles of cPLA2α and arachidonic acid in cancer," *Biochimica et Biophysica Acta*, vol. 1761, no. 11, pp. 1335–1343, 2006.

5

Surgical Options for Initially Unresectable Colorectal Liver Metastases

Irinel Popescu and Sorin Tiberiu Alexandrescu

Dan Setlacec Center of General Surgery and Liver Transplantation, Fundeni Clinical Institute, Carol Davila University of Medicine and Pharmacy, Fundeni Street No. 258, 022328 Bucharest, Romania

Correspondence should be addressed to Irinel Popescu, irinel.popescu@icfundeni.ro

Academic Editor: Luciano De Carlis

Although the frontiers of liver resection for colorectal liver metastases have broadened in recent decades, approximately 75% of these patients present with unresectable metastases at the time of their diagnosis. In the past, these patients underwent only palliative treatment, without the chance of a cure. In the previous two decades, several therapeutic strategies have been developed that render resectable those metastases that were initially unresectable, thus offering the chance of long-term survival and even a cure to these patients. The oncosurgical modalities that are available include liver resection following portal vein ligation/embolization, "two-stage" liver resection, one-stage ultrasonically guided liver resection, hepatectomy following conversion chemotherapy, and liver resection combined with thermal ablation. Moreover, in recent years, certain authors have recommended the revisiting of the concept of liver transplantation in highly selected patients with unresectable colorectal liver metastases and favorable prognostic factors. By employing such therapies, the number of patients with colorectal liver metastases who undergo a potentially curative treatment could increase to 40%. The safety profile of these approaches is acceptable (morbidity rates as high as 45%, mortality rates of less than 5%). Furthermore, the 5-year survival rates (approximately 30%) are significantly increased over those that were achieved with palliative treatment.

1. Introduction

The current treatment for patients with liver metastases from colorectal cancer is multimodal, including liver resection, chemotherapy, targeted therapies (monoclonal antibodies), interventional radiology, and radiotherapy. The complete resection of liver metastases results in 5-year overall survival rates that range from 21% to 58% [1–3], which are significantly higher than those rates that are achieved by nonsurgical therapies (5-year survival rates less than 5%) [4]. Thus, the only potentially curative therapy in patients with colorectal liver metastases (CRLM) includes complete resection of the liver metastases.

At present, CRLMs are considered resectable when the following criteria are met [5, 6]:

(a) the complete resection of all known disease can be achieved,

(b) at least two contiguous liver segments can be preserved, with adequate vascular inflow and outflow, with biliary drainage,

(c) the remnant liver volume is adequate to avoid postoperative liver failure.

In patients with a healthy liver, the volume of the future liver remnant (FLR) should represent more than 25% of the total liver volume (TLV) to avoid postoperative liver failure [7–9]. However, in patients with chronic liver disease or chemotherapy-induced liver injury, a minimum of 40% of the TLV should be preserved [9–12].

Therefore, although the frontiers of liver resection have broadened over the previous two decades [13], approximately three quarters of patients with CRLM are not eligible for an initially curative liver resection (R0) after a preoperative evaluation [14].

The most common causes of the initial unresectability are the following.

(1) A single, very large liver metastasis, the resection of which would not spare a sufficient volume of liver parenchyma to avoid postoperative liver failure.

(2) Multiple bilobar liver metastases, the complete resection of which would not preserve a sufficient volume of functional liver parenchyma.

(3) CRLM involving or located in close proximity to either the bifurcation of the portal vein or the confluence of the three hepatic veins with the inferior vena cava (IVC). In this case, the resection of the liver metastasis would not allow for the preservation of a minimum of two adjacent liver segments with adequate vascular inflow and outflow.

Until 20 years ago, the only available treatment for these patients was palliative chemotherapy, the goals of which were to increase progression-free and overall survival; however, there was no prospect of a cure. Although survival rates increased with the advent of new chemotherapeutics (such as Oxaliplatin and Irinotecan) and targeted therapies (e.g., Bevacizumab, Cetuximab, and Panitumumab), the current survival rates for these cases are still modest compared to those that can be achieved by liver resection. Therefore, several therapeutic strategies were introduced to achieve a complete resection in these patients [15].

2. Therapeutic Options

In Figure 1, we schematically present those situations in which metastases are considered unresectable and the therapeutic options that are available for conversion to resectability.

2.1. Liver Resection Following Portal Vein Embolization/Ligation. In certain instances, although a minimum of two adjacent segments with appropriate vascular inflow and outflow, and biliary drainage can be preserved following the complete resection of CRLM, the volume of the remaining liver parenchyma may be insufficient to avoid postoperative liver failure. Such situations are generally encountered in patients who (1) require a right trisectionectomy, or (2) when a right hemihepatectomy must be performed, but the volume of the left hemiliver is prohibitively small (Figures 1(a) and 1(b)). To avoid postoperative liver failure in these patients, it is advisable to attempt to increase the volume of the FLR prior to the liver resection.

This goal may be achieved by initially performing portal vein embolization (PVE) or ligation (PVL). If the volume of the FLR following a PVE/PVL increases sufficiently to prevent the risk of postoperative liver failure, liver resection should be performed 4–8 weeks later.

This therapeutic strategy is based on the observation that increasing the volume of the FLR improves the function of the residual liver parenchyma following the hepatectomy [16, 17].

The reports of Kinoshita and Makuuchi revealed that the ligation or embolization of the right portal vein induces a process of atrophy-hypertrophy of the liver (increasing the safety of liver resection) in patients with hepatocellular carcinoma or hilar cholangiocarcinoma [18, 19]. Therefore, other authors applied the same procedure in patients with CRLM whose FLR was insufficient to avoid postoperative liver failure [10, 20–22]. The rationale for such an approach is that the embolization or ligation of the right portal branch abolishes the portal inflow into the right hemiliver, leading to its atrophy; alternatively, the portal inflow into the left hemiliver increases, causing hypertrophy of the FLR.

This approach permits the performance of the scheduled hepatectomy (while concomitantly reducing the risk of fatal liver failure) in more than 50% of patients who were otherwise unresectable due to a small FLR.

Concerns regarding the comparative effectiveness of PVE versus PVL have been raised by certain authors. In an animal model, Furrer et al. revealed that the hypertrophy of the left hemiliver significantly increased following PVL versus PVE. These authors hypothesized that the entrapment of a greater number of macrophages in the embolized liver (due to the foreign-body reaction that is induced by the material used for embolization) explains this result [23]. Their conclusion that PVL is superior to PVE in inducing a regenerative response of the remnant liver is in contrast to that of Wilms et al., who stated that although PVL and PVE both induce liver hypertrophy, PVE is the most effective technique to increase the FLR [24]. These authors stated that PVE-induced vascular occlusion is more durable than that induced by PVL. Furthermore, the cause of the inferior regeneration in the ligation group was reported to be the formation of collaterals between the occluded and nonoccluded portions of the liver. To avoid this undesirable situation, certain authors recommended the transection and ethanol injection into the ligated portal branch [20]. Lastly, in addition to these experimental studies, a retrospective study of 35 patients revealed that PVL and PVE are similar in terms of both increasing the FLR and the conversion to resectability rate [25].

PVE- or PVL-induced liver hypertrophy involves both segments 2-3 and segment 4. Most patients that are subjected to PVL/PVE require a right trisectionectomy. In such patients, the principal objective of this maneuver is to increase the volume of segments 2-3 and not the volume of segment 4 (which is resected). To primarily increase the volume of the left lateral section, certain authors state that the optimum approach is to concomitantly occlude the right portal vein and the portal branches to segment 4 (right trisection portal vein embolization-R3PE) [26]. In 2000, Nagino et al. presented results that support this hypothesis, demonstrating that the volume gain of the left lateral section was higher in patients with R3PE relative to patients who received right portal vein embolization [26]. To date, we have performed R3PL in one patient, and the results were outstanding: the percent of FLR gain was 16.22%, whereas

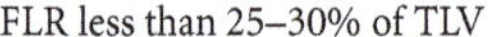

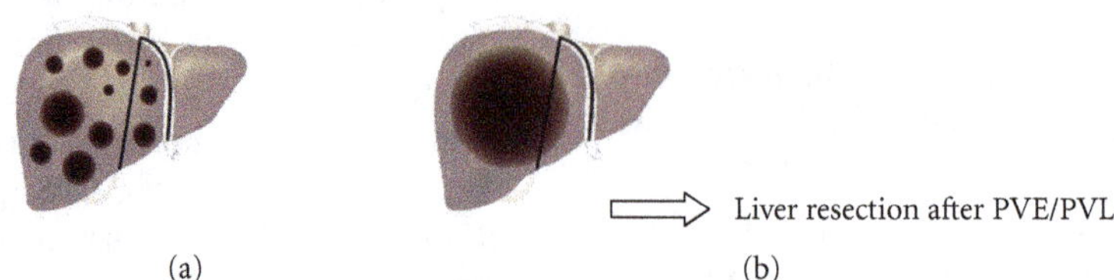

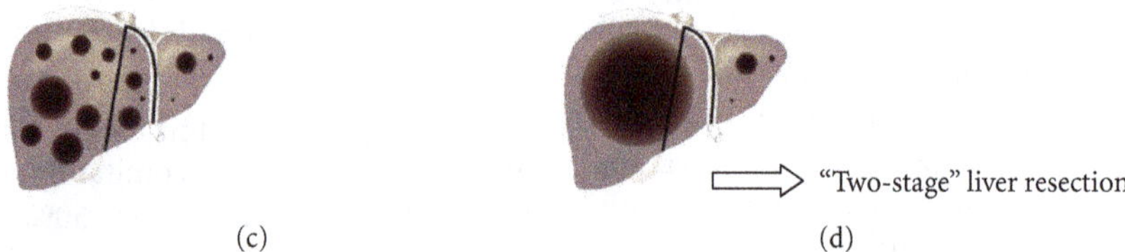

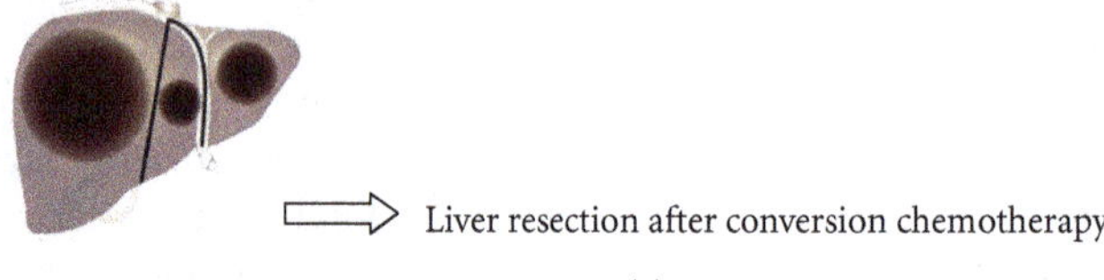

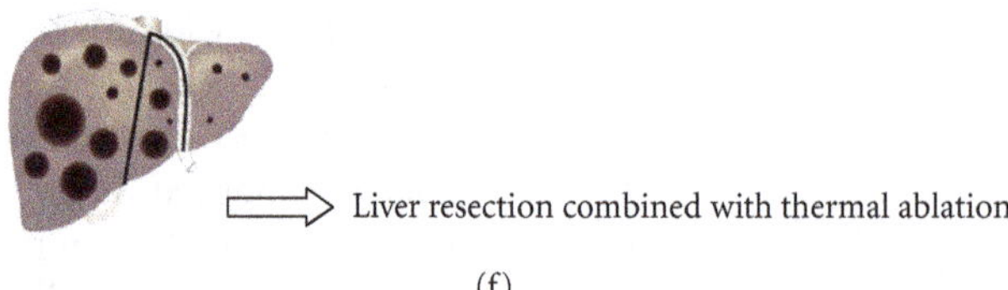

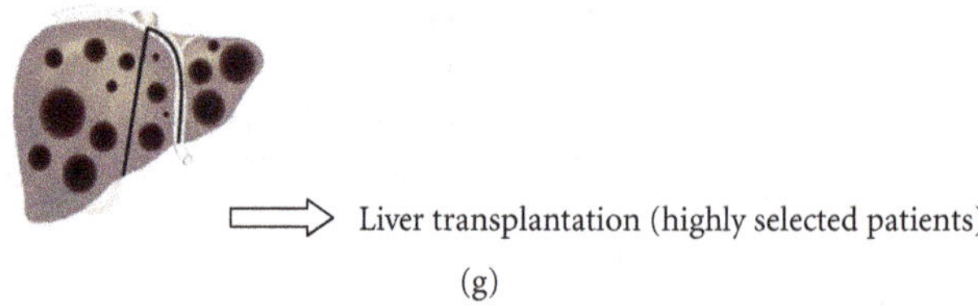

FIGURE 1: Strategies used for potentially curative treatment of the initially unresectable CRLM, depending on the location, number, and size of the lesions.

this metric was 10.8% in the patients who received a right portal branch ligation [27]. However, another study that was published in 2005 failed to confirm these results, revealing that the mean volume of segments 2-3 following embolization and the rate of the segments 2-3 volume increase were similar between the patients who received a R3PE and those that received a standard right portal vein embolization [7]. Therefore, definitive conclusions cannot be drawn regarding the usefulness of the embolization of the portal branches to segment 4, and further studies are required to clarify this subject. Most centers now prefer to routinely perform only right portal branch embolization/ligation in such patients.

To achieve a more marked and rapid hypertrophy of the FLR following portal vein ligation, Schnitzbauer et al. [28] and de Santibanes et al. [29] recently recommended the association of right portal vein ligation with "in situ liver transection/splitting". Using this approach, the authors achieved a significant and more rapid hypertrophy of the FLR, enabling subsequent curative liver resection during the same hospitalization. The authors concluded that this technique induces the rapid and more robust growth of the FLR [28] than is reported with portal vein occlusion alone. Moreover, this approach allows for the performance of a staged liver resection during a single hospital stay [29].

Two formulas can be used to calculate the percent of the FLR gain following PVE/PVL:

(a) (Volume of the FLR following PVE − Volume of the FLR prior to PVE) × 100/Volume of the FLR prior to PVE [30],

(b) %FLR following PVE −%FLR prior to PVE [12].

In a series of 30 patients, the percent of the FLR gain (calculated using the first formula) was 42% [10], whereas the FLR gain ranged from 9.7% to 13% in different series using the second formula [21, 27, 30]. In most patients, these percentages are generally sufficient to allow for a safe resection of liver metastases.

When PVE is planned, Bevacizumab should be used with caution given that Aussilhou et al. revealed the detrimental effect of this medication on the FLR gain; this effect is especially strong in patients who are older than 60 years and received more than six cycles [31]. However, other authors have demonstrated that this monoclonal antibody does not impair liver regeneration following PVE [32].

The most severe complications of right PVE are liver hematoma, liver abscess, thrombosis of the left portal vein, portal hypertension, and cholangitis. In a meta-analysis that was performed by Aboulkhir et al., the morbidity rate following PVE was 2.2%, and the mortality was zero [30].

The resectability rate following PVE/PVL in different centers ranges from 60% to 88% [10, 21, 22]. The primary reason of failure to perform the curative hepatectomy is not insufficient hypertrophy of the FLR but rather the progression of the disease. In our series, 5 of 13 patients (38%) exhibited disease progression following PVL, precluding a curative liver resection. The other 8 patients underwent successful complete resection of the initially unresectable CRLM. The resectability rate was therefore 62% [27].

The morbidity and mortality rates that were observed following curative hepatectomy were less than 35% and 4%, respectively, in most series [10, 22].

The 5-year survival rate of these patients was approximately 38% [10, 21].

It must be noted that in patients with liver metastases in the FLR, this approach is not recommended, due to the risk of rapid growth of these metastases. Such approach may jeopardize the chances of a subsequent potentially curative liver resection. Such patients should undergo a "two-stage" liver resection (see below) to clear the remnant liver prior to the PVE [33].

2.2. Two-Stage Liver Resection. The term "two-stage" liver resection has been used by a small number of authors to define a strategy that consists of a single liver resection that is performed following PVL and which does not include a sequential liver resection [20]. Herein, we shall use the nomenclature of "two-stage" liver resection for those procedures that consist of two consecutive hepatectomies.

This therapeutic strategy is used in patients with multiple bilobar CRLM, whose resection will not spare a sufficient amount of liver parenchyma to avoid postoperative liver failure. These patients usually require a right hepatectomy or a right trisectionectomy along with wedge resections of the metastases that are located in the left hemiliver or in the left lateral section (Figures 1(c) and 1(d)).

To avoid such extensive resections, which are accompanied by a high risk of postoperative fatal liver failure, it is recommended that a complete resection of the liver metastases be achieved in a two-stage surgical procedure. In the first stage, a limited resection of the metastases from the left hemiliver or the left lateral section (future liver remnant) is performed. In stage two (following the regeneration of the FLR), the bulk of the metastatic burden is resected by a right hepatectomy or trisectionectomy. FLR regeneration is essential to minimize the risks of hepatic failure following the second operation. Thus, PVE/PVL may be suitable in patients with small FLR to increase the safety of the second hepatectomy. To facilitate the second operation and to avoid disease progression between the first and the second intervention, it may be useful to deliver systemic or locoregional chemotherapy to shrink the metastatic bulk. To minimize the inhibitory effects of the chemotherapeutic drugs on liver regeneration, the chemotherapy should be begun three weeks following the first hepatectomy. This sequence is necessary, as liver regeneration is essential to the feasibility of the second resection [34].

Such a therapeutic approach is especially useful in patients with synchronous bilobar CRLM [35] given that (1) it avoids the cumulative risks of a simultaneous primary tumor resection and major hepatectomy, and (2) it allows for the evaluation of the chemosensitivity of the liver metastases and the guiding of the adjuvant therapy following the second operation. The resection of the primary tumor is performed in the first stage, along with a limited resection of the metastases from the future liver remnant (generally from the left hemiliver or the left lateral section). Occasionally, a right portal vein ligation is also performed during the first operation. Short-course chemotherapy (systemic or locoregional) should begin three weeks later. If the residual lesions will be stable or responsive to chemotherapy, the second liver resection should be performed.

The results of such an approach were first published by the Paul Brousse group in 2000. This group reported a resectability rate of 81% [34]. In other series, the resectability rate ranged from 66% to 75% [27, 33].

Among the published series, the morbidity rates following the first resection were less than 31%, and the mortality rates were zero [33, 34].

The morbidity rate following the second liver resection ranges from 45% to 56% [27, 33, 34]. Despite these relative high morbidity rates, the mortality was zero in most series [27, 33]. Nonetheless, a mortality rate of 15% following the second operation was reported by Adam et al. [34]. The authors explained that this result was a consequence of the combination of (1) the diminished tolerance of such patients to perioperative complications due to their advanced neoplastic disease and (2) the effects of the adjuvant procedures that were used to facilitate liver resection (chemotherapy, PVE).

The 3-year survival rates of these patients ranged from 35% to 54% [27, 33, 34], with a median survival of 44 months from the diagnosis of liver metastases [34].

In selected patients with multiple bilobar colorectal liver metastases, a "two-stage" liver resection could be avoided, by performing ultrasonically-guided hepatectomy.

2.3. One-Stage Ultrasonically Guided Liver Resection. The implementation of ultrasonography in liver surgery dramatically alters the approach to liver metastases, permitting a more accurate diagnosis and challenging the traditional paradigms of liver resection.

Intraoperative ultrasound (IOUS) allows for the detection of additional CRLM that were not revealed by preoperative imaging methods and is the most accurate technique for detecting liver tumors [36, 37]. However, standard IOUS may miss lesions that are smaller than 1 cm, especially in patients who are undergoing preoperative chemotherapy, whose CRLM exhibit a similar echo-pattern to that of the surrounding liver parenchyma. The use of contrast-enhanced IOUS (CE-IOUS) was demonstrated to improve the detection of CRLM and is the most sensitive and specific method for the diagnosis of CRLM [38].

In the mid 1980s, IOUS was first used to guide the puncture and balloon occlusion of the portal branch that feeds the portion of the liver to be resected, allowing for limited anatomical liver resections instead of major hepatectomies [39–41]. This technique decreased the risk of postoperative liver failure and was recommended principally in patients who have HCCs on liver cirrhosis.

In addition, IOUS offers a better estimation of the spatial relationships between the liver tumors and the intrahepatic vessels, permitting the resection of liver masses with the preservation of intrahepatic vascular structures even when the tumors are located in close proximity to major intrahepatic vessels. Furthermore, even when major hepatic vein(s) must be resected, color Doppler IOUS findings provide reliable information that may lead to the preservation of a portion of the liver parenchyma that is drained by those vein(s), avoiding major hepatectomies [42–45]. Thus, a novel liver resection technique was developed in recent years that is referred to as "ultrasonically guided hepatectomy". This technique opened the door to new procedures that allow for radical but conservative liver resections, reducing the requirement for major hepatic resections [46–48].

Because many patients exhibit colorectal liver metastases that are considered unresectable due to the insufficient remnant liver parenchyma following major hepatectomies, the use of this surgical technique (which spares a significant amount of functional liver parenchyma) allows for the complete resection of the metastases, reducing the risk of developing postoperative liver failure. Thus, this technique was used more frequently in patients with CRLM.

Moreover, ultrasonically guided liver resection decreases the requirement for major hepatectomies, obviating the requirement for portal vein occlusion prior to the liver resection and/or the necessity of a "two-stage" liver resection in selected patients.

In patients with CRLM that are located in close proximity to major hepatic veins or near the first-degree portal branches, a major hepatectomy is still the main surgical option at most centers. If the remnant liver volume following a major hepatectomy is critically small, a liver resection following portal vein occlusion, either by PVE or PVL, is generally recommended. In such instances, the patient is exposed to an interventional radiology procedure or a laparotomy prior to the curative liver resection. Each of these procedures presents additional risks of morbidity [30]. The development of the ultrasonically guided hepatectomy in recent years permits a more limited liver resection of poorly located CRLM, avoiding the necessity of a prehepatectomy PVE/PVL. In a series of 22 patients who presented poorly located liver tumors and who were scheduled for initial ultrasonically guided liver resection, a limited resection with or without hepatic vein preservation was achieved in 91% cases, providing lower morbidity rates than major resections following PVE and no mortality [43]. The rate of local recurrence (at the transection surface) was zero at a mean follow-up period of 23 months. Because this approach avoids portal vein occlusion (and its associated morbidity), the comfort of the patient is also improved. Moreover, the resectability rate following portal vein occlusion does not exceed 60–88%, due to either insufficient hypertrophy of the remnant liver or disease progression in the interval between the portal vein occlusion and the liver regeneration [21, 22, 49]. When an initial ultrasonically guided hepatectomy is performed, the risk of disease progression is avoided, and the hypertrophy of the FLR is no longer necessary. Thus, the resectability rate that is achieved by the ultrasonically guided approach appears to be higher than those that are achieved by PVE/PVL, broadening the indications for curative surgery in cases of CRLM [43].

In patients with multiple bilobar CRLM, the ultrasonically guided technique may also represent an effective alternative to the "two-stage" hepatectomy, permitting a curative and conservative liver resection [44]. The advantages of this approach over the "two-stage" liver resection are the comfort of the patient, a lower morbidity rate [44], and an increased possibility of repeat resections if the patient develops recurrent metastases [50–52]. Furthermore, the recurrence rate following one-stage ultrasonically guided liver resection was similar to that reported after "two-stage liver resection".

Due to the aforementioned benefits, the one-stage ultrasonically guided liver resection should be part of the armamentarium of the liver surgeon, especially in the context of patients with complex tumoral presentations.

2.4. Liver Resection Following Conversion Chemotherapy. This therapeutic strategy was first presented by the Paul Brousse group in 1996 [53] and is recommended in patients with a small number of large CRLM, the resection of which would not spare a sufficient amount of functional liver to prevent postoperative liver failure (Figure 1(e)). The goal of this approach is to "downsize" the liver metastases to an extent that allows for their complete resection. Therefore, a chance of a potentially curative liver resection is available to patients who otherwise may have only benefited from palliative treatment.

Until 20 years ago, the only efficient chemotherapeutic regimen that was used in patients with unresectable

CRLM consisted of 5-Fluorouracil (5-FU) and Folinic acid. Although this chemotherapy increases the overall survival rates and the progression-free survival rates of these patients, the response rates were less than 23%, and only anecdotal cases of liver metastases that shrink sufficiently to allow for a subsequent curative hepatectomy were reported [54–56].

The advent of new chemotherapeutic agents such as Oxaliplatin and Irinotecan led to significantly better results. The response rates that have been achieved by FOLFOX and FOLFIRI regimens range from 40% to 56% [57–59]. A strong correlation was observed between the response rates and the resection rates of patients with initially unresectable CLRM [60]. Therefore, more patients became resectable following so-called conversion chemotherapy. Folprecht et al. thus concluded that resectability should be considered a new endpoint for preoperative chemotherapy, focusing on the curative potential of this oncosurgical treatment [60].

The Paul-Brousse group published their updated results in 2004, reporting a 12.5% rate of conversion to resectability in 1104 patients with initially unresectable CRLM (following an average of 10 courses of chemotherapy) [14]. Apart from these very large series of patients, other centers have subsequently reported similar results in smaller numbers of selected patients who presented with initially unresectable CRLM that were rendered resectable by different chemotherapy regimens [61–63].

In many reports, the morbidity rates following hepatectomy in patients with initially unresectable CRLM [14, 62, 64] ranges from 23% to 28%, which are similar to those rates that are observed in patients with initially resectable CRLM. However, certain authors have reported significantly higher incidences of postoperative complications in patients who receive resections following "downsizing" chemotherapy, raising concerns regarding the deleterious effects of the preoperative chemotherapy on the liver parenchyma (see below) [65, 66]. The postoperative mortality rates are reported to be less than 2% in most centers, which are similar to those rates that have been achieved in patients who did not receive preoperative chemotherapy [14, 53, 62, 66].

The 5-year survival rate of patients who were rendered resectable by chemotherapy was 33% in the Paul Brousse group, a rate that was higher than those that were achieved by new palliative chemotherapeutic regimens in similar patients [14]. Although this survival rate is significantly lower than what can be achieved in patients with initially resectable CRLM (*P* value = 0.01), the 5-year disease-free survival rate of 22% that was reported in initially unresectable patients appears to fully justify the efforts to render to resectability, these patients with otherwise dismal prognosis [14].

The addition of targeted therapies (e.g., Bevacizumab, Cetuximab, and Panitumumab) to chemotherapy regimens may be useful in further increasing the rate of conversion to resectability in initially unresectable lesions. This hypothesis was confirmed in a series of patients whose liver metastases were refractory to previous rounds of conventional chemotherapy. The advent of Cetuximab to the next-line chemotherapy rendered 7% of these patients resectable, with morbidity and mortality rates of 50% and 3.7%, respectively, and a median survival of 20 months [67]. This study, similar to those of Zorzi et al., demonstrated that monoclonal antibodies in combination with conventional chemotherapy have no detrimental effects on the safety of liver resection [32]. Furthermore, Gruenberger et al. revealed that Bevacizumab has little detrimental impact on liver regeneration following hepatectomy [68]. However, it should be noted that the use of vascular endothelial growth factor inhibitors (e.g., Bevacizumab) prior to major surgery increases the risks of bleeding and wound healing complications [69]. This therapy should be discontinued 5–8 weeks prior to the surgical intervention [68, 70].

Several issues should be kept in mind when deciding to take this therapeutic approach.

(i) The response to chemotherapy cannot be assumed to persist. Metastases occasionally shrink and become resectable following several cycles of chemotherapy. However, if the chemotherapy is continued, the metastases may regrow and again become unresectable, closing the "window of opportunity" for a potentially curative hepatectomy [71]. Therefore, if the systemic disease is controlled, the liver resection should be scheduled as soon as the metastases become resectable.

(ii) If the chemotherapy is continued beyond the point when the metastases become resectable, it is possible the liver metastases will become smaller and will no longer be visible on imaging (CT/MR/PET scans). Such metastases are referred to as "vanishing metastases." Unfortunately, this "radiological complete response" or "clinical complete response" [72] does not indicate a cure, as a "pathologic complete response" is achieved in fewer than 20% of cases [73, 74]. In one-third of patients with radiological complete response, a laparotomy may reveal small metastases that were missed by the imaging methods or residual scars, the resection of which would reveal viable tumor cells. Alternatively, in patients without macroscopic residual tissue (on laparotomy) and negative (contrast-enhanced) intraoperative ultrasound, pathologic examination of the resected specimens, including liver segments where the metastases where initially located, revealed viable metastatic cells in 75% of cases [74, 75]. An indirect confirmation of the presence of viable tumor cells at the sites of the former metastases (which were invisible on laparotomy) is given by certain reports. In a series of patients with 31 CRLM that disappeared following chemotherapy and which were not observed on laparotomy, the resection of the initial metastases site was not performed. After a one-year follow-up, 23 (74%) metastases recurred in situ [74].

The survival benefit that is achieved by performing liver resection in patients with clinical complete response following chemotherapy was revealed by another study. Fourteen patients with radiological complete response following chemotherapy were not subjected to a liver resection, achieving a 5-year overall survival of 14% and a median survival of 30 months. In 25 patients who suffered from initially unresectable CRLM that were rendered to resectability by a FOLFOXIRI regimen and further resected, the 5-year survival rate was 43%, and the median survival was significantly higher (61 months, *P* value = 0.006) [62].

For these reasons, laparotomy is mandatory in patients with vanishing metastases, with the aim of resecting the macroscopic residual metastatic tissue or the sites of the initial CRLM ("blind resection").

The resection of the metastases sites is a very demanding operation, especially in patients with (initially) multiple metastases located deep in the liver. In such cases, computer-based virtual surgery planning is very useful, merging pre- and postchemotherapy computed tomography data. Recently, Oldhafer et al. presented such a surgical approach. Information that is processed using a computer is then intraoperatively transferred to the liver surface using an image-guided stereotactically navigated ultrasound dissector, enabling the surgeon to perform the resection [75].

In patients with initially multiple bilobar CRLM that become "invisible" following chemotherapy and that cannot be identified intraoperatively, it is frequently impossible to assume a complete resection of the metastatic sites. Thus, a small number of these "missing metastases" will remain. In such situations, Elias et al. recommended the placement of a chemotherapy catheter in the hepatic artery, allowing for a hepatic arterial infusion (HAI) with Oxaliplatin, along with systemic 5-FU and Folinic acid [76]. Using this approach, following a median follow-up period of 51 months, the missing metastases did not recur in 62% of the patients. The recurrence rate following HAI with Oxaliplatin was significantly lower than those that were noted in patients who were treated by systemic chemotherapy alone (*P* value = 0.01) [76].

Alternatively, it should be noted that a small number (4–15%) of CRLM that were treated by systemic chemotherapy prior to the liver resection achieved a complete pathologic response [72, 73, 77]. The complete pathologic response was observed both in patients with or without a radiologic complete response. The predictive factors for a complete pathologic response were age less than 60 years, maximum metastasis diameter of less than 3 cm, CEA levels at diagnosis below 30 ng/mL, an objective response following chemotherapy [72] and the use of hepatic arterial infusion chemotherapy [76]. The addition of Bevacizumab to the Oxaliplatin-based chemotherapeutic regimens did not appear to increase the incidence of the complete pathologic response (11.3% versus 11.6%; *P* value = 0.59) [78]. Patients with complete pathologic response achieved uncommonly high survival rates (76% at 5 years) [72].

(iii) Treatment with new chemotherapeutic drugs induces alterations of the nontumoral liver parenchyma, potentially impacting the results of the liver resection.

The initial belief was that use of Irinotecan may cause nonalcoholic fatty liver disease (NAFLD), which represents a spectrum of diseases. The mildest form of NAFLD is macrovesicular steatosis, and the most severe form is non-alcoholic steatohepatitis (NASH) [79]. Although a study that was published in 2003 revealed a correlation between prior treatment with chemotherapy and steatosis and highlighted the fact that morbidity rates following liver resections were significantly higher in patients with marked steatosis [80], more recent studies have reported differing results. In 2006, a multicenter trial revealed that Irinotecan was associated with steatohepatitis but not with steatosis [81]. Moreover, this latter study noted that the mortality rate was significantly higher in patients with steatohepatitis (14.7%) than in patients without steatohepatitis (1.6%, *P* value = 0.001).

The first study to reveal a correlation between Oxaliplatin and non-tumoral liver parenchyma injury was published in 2004 [82]. The results indicated that 78% of the patients who were preoperatively treated with Oxaliplatin exhibited sinusoidal alterations. These results were subsequently confirmed by other reports [83–85], which revealed that Oxaliplatin-based preoperative chemotherapy was associated with sinusoidal dilatation and congestion, peliosis, and venoocclusive disease. One of these studies reported that only long-course Oxaliplatin-based chemotherapy (6 or more cycles) is significantly associated with sinusoidal injury [85]. However, in a series that was presented by Vauthey et al., the risk of sinusoidal dilatation did not appear to increase with the duration of chemotherapy (although their patients received relatively short-course treatments) [81]. Interestingly, the addition of Bevacizumab to Oxaliplatin-based regimens appears to reduce the incidence and severity of hepatic injury [78]. The impact of these liver injuries on the clinical outcome of the patients who received resections following Oxaliplatin-based chemotherapy was assessed in several reports. None of these studies reported increased mortality rates following liver resection in patients with Oxaliplatin-related sinusoidal injury [79]. Two trials revealed that a limited course (fewer than 6 cycles) of Oxaliplatin-based therapy was not associated with increased morbidity rates following liver resection [81, 86]. However, Karoui et al. observed a statistically higher incidence of postoperative complications in patients who underwent a major hepatectomy following preoperative chemotherapy when compared with the patients who were subjected to a similar liver resection without preoperative chemotherapy [66]. Similarly, Nakano et al. observed that sinusoidal injury was significantly associated with increased morbidity and longer hospital stays in patients who underwent a major hepatectomy [85].

The above-mentioned pitfalls that are associated with preoperative chemotherapy justify the scheduling of the liver resection as soon as the metastases become resectable.

2.5. Liver Resection Combined with Thermal Ablation for Unresectable CRLM. This type of approach is especially recommended in patients with multiple bilobar CRLM who present with fewer than 3 liver metastases in the FLR, with each of these metastases being less than 3 cm in maximum diameter (Figure 1(f)). Another indication for this approach is when one or a small number of metastases are anatomically poorly located (e.g., in close proximity to the confluence of the three hepatic veins and the inferior vena cava or at the bifurcation of the portal vein) [87].

The operation consists of the resection of the main tumor bulk (generally by a right trisectionectomy) and thermal ablation of the unresected metastases from the remnant liver (frequently the left lateral section) [88].

This approach could be performed in a "two-stage" manner in patients with synchronous unresectable CRLM, as described by Lygidakis et al. [89]. In the first stage, the following procedures are performed: (1) the resection of the primary colorectal tumor, (2) the ligation and transection of the relevant (right or left) primary portal branch, (3) the ablation of the metastatic nodules in the contralateral hemiliver, and (4) the insertion of an arterial catheter into the hepatic artery for locoregional chemo(immuno)therapy. The second stage of the operation consists of the resection of the tumoral liver (usually by right hemihepatectomy or trisectionectomy).

Thermal ablation can be achieved using radiofrequencies, microwaves, lasers, or cryotherapy.

To increase the chances of a complete hyperthermic ablation, the Pringle maneuver can be performed during the ablation [88].

The morbidity and mortality rates (44% and 2.3%, resp.) [27, 90] of patients undergoing combined liver resection and thermal ablation of unresectable CRLM appear to be similar to those of patients with initially unresectable CRLM that are rendered resectable by other therapeutic strategies.

A retrospective study that was published in 2004 reported a significantly higher local recurrence rate following resection combined with RFA (5%) than was observed following complete resection of the CRLM (2%). However, the patients were not stratified according to the maximum diameter of the ablated CRLM in this study [90]. It was recently demonstrated that the best results achieved by thermoablation are observed in patients whose CRLM were less than 3 cm in maximum diameter. Thus, a significantly higher rate (P value = 0.0001) of sustained complete ablation was achieved in patients whose lesions were less than 3 cm (66.7%) than for the patients with metastases that were larger than 3 cm (33.3%) [91]. One retrospective study (including resectable and unresectable CRLM) revealed that the local recurrence rate following the radiofrequency ablation (RFA) of metastases that were less than 3 cm in maximum diameter was 1.3% after a follow-up period of 33 months [92]. Moreover, another retrospective study (including patients with single CRLM treated by RFA or liver resection) determined that the 5-year overall and local recurrence-free survival rates were similar for patients with CRLM that were smaller than 3 cm who were treated either with RFA or liver resection [87].

However, in patients with multiple bilobar CRLM who are treated with a combination of RFA and liver resection, the overall and disease-free survival rates were significantly lower than for patients who underwent a complete resection of CRLM but significantly higher than in the patients who were treated by chemotherapy alone [90]. Moreover, Rivoire et al. revealed in a study of 57 patients with initially unresectable CRLM that the overall survival rates were similar for patients who underwent a complete liver resection following conversion chemotherapy and those who received liver resection combined with cryotherapy [93].

These results justify liver resection combined with thermal ablation of initially unresectable CRLM in patients who fulfill the above-mentioned criteria.

However, due to the lower recurrence rates achieved by the ultrasonically guided liver resection technique, this approach may be more suitable than liver resection combined with thermal ablation.

2.6. Liver Transplantation—A Future Opportunity? Unfortunately, there are still many patients with multiple bilobar colorectal cancer liver metastases who are not amenable to complete resection by any of the above-mentioned therapeutic strategies. In such patients, the only chance of complete removal of the liver metastases is total hepatectomy followed by liver transplantation (Figure 1(g)).

This approach was used in the early period of liver transplantation, achieving 1- and 5-year overall survival rates of 62% and 18%, respectively [94].

Due to organ shortages, it was considered that the allocation of an organ to a patient with such a short life expectancy following the transplantation was not ethically acceptable.

Currently, unresectable CRLM are considered to be a contraindication to liver transplantation.

However, the above-mentioned survival rates appear to be higher than those that can be achieved by palliative treatment, suggesting that even using the therapeutic options that were available thirty years ago, liver transplantation offered a higher survival benefit than the best palliative treatment that is currently available. Furthermore, due to recent progress in the fields of posttransplant immunosuppression and medical oncology and due to the more refined methods that are used in selecting patients to receive tailored therapies (based on reliable pathologic and biologic markers), improved survival rates could be achieved for selected patients who undergo liver transplantation.

Moreover, the ethical issues could be challenged by the use of a living donor liver transplantation given that, in such instances, the willing donation is directed toward a certain patient and not to the community [95]. Meanwhile, it is also considered unethical to offer a marginal graft to a patient with a good chance of long-term survival following liver transplantation. Because the number of available marginal grafts has increased in recent years, it may be acceptable to allocate such organs in selected patients with CRLM, at least in the setting of controlled trials.

Although the available data do not support liver transplantation as a routine procedure in patients with CRLM, we believe that a discussion of the current advances in this field and of the recently published results is worthwhile and should encourage debate on this issue.

By reviewing the largest series of patients undergoing liver transplantation for unresectable CRLM [96], it was revealed that 66% of patients with histologically negative lymph nodes were genetically positive for micrometastases when mutant allele-specific amplification (MASA) method was used to search for micrometastases in DNA from the regional lymph nodes of the primary colorectal cancer [97]. Those patients who were both genetically and histologically negative exhibited a significantly longer overall survival (P value = 0.011) than the other patients. Thus, Kappel et al. concluded that the genetic detection of micrometastases by MASA may be a powerful prognostic indicator for selecting patients with colorectal liver metastases who could benefit from liver transplantation [97].

Over the previous two decades, certain further developments have emerged that may improve patient selection and the results of liver transplantation. For example, the advent of MDCT, gadolinium-enhanced MRI, and PET/CT scans has improved the detection of extrahepatic metastases, permitting the better selection of patients with colorectal cancer that had metastasized only to the liver. Recent studies have identified several biological parameters (such as the expression of p53, thymidylate synthase, Ki-67, K-ras, and human telomerase reverse transcriptase, as well as the type, density, and location of immune cells within the tumor) that may be more sensitive predictors of outcome in patients with CRLM than are the current histopathological methods that are used to stage colorectal cancer [98, 99]. Using a panel that incorporates these parameters, it may be possible to identify a highly selected group of patients who could greatly benefit from liver transplantation. Moreover, it has been hypothesized that the progress in posttransplant immunosuppressive therapy may decrease recurrence rates and improve the survival of patients who undergo liver transplantation for malignant disease, primarily due to the use of m-TOR inhibitors. Such immunosuppressive agents (sirolimus, temsirolimus) inhibit tumor growth and proliferation and exhibit antiangiogenic effects. These effects are in contrast to traditional immunosuppressive drugs, which appear to promote malignant cell proliferation [100, 101].

Over the past several years, taking into account the better expertise of transplant surgeons and the above-mentioned progress in both the selection of patients with CRLM and in the efficacy of posttransplant immunosuppressive regimens, certain authors have argued that the outcome of selected patients who undergo liver transplantation for unresectable liver metastases from colorectal cancer may be significantly improved [102]. For these reasons, certain authors have proposed a rational revisitation of the concept of liver transplantation in such patients. Thus, a pilot study (SECA-study) that aims to assess the survival and quality of life in patients receiving pretransplant chemotherapy, liver transplantation for unresectable CRLM, and posttransplant Sirolimus-based immunosuppressive regimen began in Norway in November 2006. The preliminary data of this study reveal a 94% survival rate after a median 25 months of postoperative follow-up and an excellent quality of life [102]. However, only 40% of these patients are disease-free after a median follow-up period of 25 months.

Favorable results were also recently reported in two patients with CRLM who were treated with liver resection followed by hepatic artery infusion chemotherapy and who underwent a liver transplantation for intraarterial chemotherapy-induced sclerosing cholangitis. The two patients were disease-free at 2 and 5 years following transplantation, respectively.

Based on these disparate results, definitive conclusions cannot be drawn; however, due to ethical considerations (i.e., organ shortage), liver transplantation with grafts from brain-dead donors cannot be accepted until 5-year survival rates exceed 50% [102].

However, if the results that are achieved by liver transplantation will become significantly higher than those can be achieved by nonsurgical therapies, it may eventually be difficult, in the future, to defend the prohibition of living-donor liver transplantation or liver transplantation with marginal grafts in highly selected patients with unresectable CRLM. Such a position would be difficult given that ethical considerations would no longer be valid in such situations.

3. Conclusions

Selected patients with initially unresectable CRLM may be rendered resectable following portal vein embolization or ligation, resulting in an important survival benefit or even a cure.

"Two-stage" hepatectomies (with/without PVE/PVL) may be performed safely, achieving complete resection of liver metastases and long-term survival.

The use of ultrasonographically guided hepatectomies decreases the requirement for major hepatectomies, portal vein occlusion and "two-stage" liver resections in patients with CRLM that are close to the hepatocaval confluence or in cases of multiple bilobar disease. This approach provides (1) an improved comfort and safety profile over "two-stage" liver resections and major hepatectomies following PVE/PVL and (2) a similar oncological benefit to other strategies.

Liver resection following conversion chemotherapy in previously unresectable patients may offer a considerable survival benefit. RFA could be combined with liver resection to increase the number of patients who are eligible for complete removal and ablation of CRLM.

In the future, highly selected patients with unresectable CRLM and favorable prognostic factors who receive liver transplantations with grafts from marginal donors or from living donors could achieve better survival rates than would be possible with palliative treatment. However, further studies and perioperative treatment improvements are required before this procedure achieves social acceptance.

Acknowledgments

This paper is partly supported by the Sectoral Operational Programme Human Resources Development (SOPHRD), financed from the European Social Fund, and by the Romanian Government under the Contract number POS-DRU/89/1.5/S/64153.

References

[1] M. A. Choti, J. V. Sitzmann, M. F. Tiburi et al., "Trends in long-term survival following liver resection for hepatic colorectal metastases," *Annals of Surgery*, vol. 235, no. 6, pp. 759–766, 2002.

[2] I. Popescu, M. Ionescu, S. Alexandrescu et al., "Surgical treatment of liver metastases from colorectal cancer," *Chirurgia*, vol. 101, no. 1, pp. 13–24, 2006.

[3] J. Scheele and A. Altendorf-Hofmann, "Resection of colorectal liver metastases," *Langenbeck's Archives of Surgery*, vol. 384, no. 4, pp. 313–327, 1999.

[4] M. Van den Eynde and A. Hendlisz, "Treatment of colorectal liver metastases: a review," *Reviews on Recent Clinical Trials*, vol. 4, no. 1, pp. 56–62, 2009.

[5] C. Charnsangavej, B. Clary, Y. Fong, A. Grothey, T. M. Pawlik, and M. A. Choti, "Selection of patients for resection of hepatic colorectal metastases: expert consensus statement," *Annals of Surgical Oncology*, vol. 13, no. 10, pp. 1261–1268, 2006.

[6] T. M. Pawlik, R. D. Schulick, and M. A. Choti, "Expanding criteria for resectability of colorectal liver metastases," *Oncologist*, vol. 13, no. 1, pp. 51–64, 2008.

[7] L. Capussotti, A. Muratore, A. Ferrero, G. C. Anselmetti, A. Corgnier, and D. Regge, "Extension of right portal vein embolization to segment IV portal branches," *Archives of Surgery*, vol. 140, no. 11, pp. 1100–1103, 2005.

[8] T. De Baere, A. Roche, D. Elias, P. Lasser, C. Lagrange, and V. Bousson, "Preoperative portal vein embolization for extension of hepatectomy indications," *Hepatology*, vol. 24, no. 6, pp. 1386–1391, 1996.

[9] E. K. Abdalla, M. E. Hicks, and J. N. Vauthey, "Portal vein embolization: rationale, technique and future prospects," *British Journal of Surgery*, vol. 88, no. 2, pp. 165–175, 2001.

[10] D. Azoulay, D. Castaing, A. Smail et al., "Resection of nonresectable liver metastases from colorectal cancer after percutaneous portal vein embolization," *Annals of Surgery*, vol. 231, no. 4, pp. 480–486, 2000.

[11] R. Kianmanesh, O. Farges, E. K. Abdalla, A. Sauvanet, P. Ruszniewski, and J. Belghiti, "Right portal vein ligation: a new planned two-step all-surgical approach for complete resection of primary gastrointestinal tumors with multiple bilateral liver metastases," *Journal of the American College of Surgeons*, vol. 197, no. 1, pp. 164–170, 2003.

[12] K. Kubota, M. Makuuchi, K. Kusaka et al., "Measurement of liver volume and hepatic functional reserve as a guide to decision-making in resectional surgery for hepatic tumors," *Hepatology*, vol. 26, no. 5, pp. 1176–1181, 1997.

[13] M. Minagawa, M. Makuuchi, G. Torzilli et al., "Extension of the frontiers of surgical indications in the treatment of liver metastases from colorectal cancer: long-term results," *Annals of Surgery*, vol. 231, no. 4, pp. 487–499, 2000.

[14] R. Adam, V. Delvart, G. Pascal et al., "Rescue surgery for unresectable colorectal liver metastases downstaged by chemotherapy: a model to predict long-term survival," *Annals of Surgery*, vol. 240, no. 4, pp. 644–658, 2004.

[15] D. Jaeck, P. Bachellier, J. C. Weber, E. Oussoultzoglou, and M. Greget, "Progrs dans la chirurgie d'exrse des mtastases hpatiques des cancers colorectaux," *Bulletin de l'Academie Nationale de Medecine*, vol. 187, no. 5, pp. 863–876, 2003.

[16] M. Ijichi, M. Makuuchi, H. Imamura, and T. Takayama, "Portal embolization relieves persistent jaundice after complete biliary drainage," *Surgery*, vol. 130, no. 1, pp. 116–118, 2001.

[17] K. Uesaka, Y. Nimura, and M. Nagino, "Changes in hepatic lobar function after right portal vein embolization: an appraisal by biliary indocyanine green excretion," *Annals of Surgery*, vol. 223, no. 1, pp. 77–83, 1996.

[18] H. Kinoshita, K. Sakai, and K. Hirohashi, "Preoperative portal vein embolization for hepatocellular carcinoma," *World Journal of Surgery*, vol. 10, no. 5, pp. 803–808, 1986.

[19] M. Makuuchi, B. L. Thai, K. Takayasu et al., "Preoperative portal embolization to increase safety of major hepatectomy for hilar bile duct carcinoma: a preliminary report," *Surgery*, vol. 107, no. 5, pp. 521–527, 1990.

[20] N. J. Lygidakis, L. Vlachos, S. Raptis et al., "New frontiers in liver surgery. Two-stage liver surgery for the management of advanced metastatic liver disease," *Hepato-Gastroenterology*, vol. 46, no. 28, pp. 2216–2228, 1999.

[21] D. Elias, J. F. Ouellet, T. De Baère, P. Lasser, and A. Roche, "Preoperative selective portal vein embolization before hepatectomy for liver metastases: long-term results and impact on survival," *Surgery*, vol. 131, no. 3, pp. 294–299, 2002.

[22] D. Jaeck, P. Bachellier, H. Nakano et al., "One or two-stage hepatectomy combined with portal vein embolization for initially nonresectable colorectal liver metastases," *American Journal of Surgery*, vol. 185, no. 3, pp. 221–229, 2003.

[23] K. Furrer, Y. Tian, T. Pfammatter et al., "Selective portal vein embolization and ligation trigger different regenerative responses in the rat liver," *Hepatology*, vol. 47, no. 5, pp. 1615–1623, 2008.

[24] C. Wilms, L. Mueller, C. Lenk et al., "Comparative study of portal vein embolization versus portal vein ligation for induction of hypertrophy of the future liver remnant using a mini-pig model," *Annals of Surgery*, vol. 247, no. 5, pp. 825–834, 2008.

[25] B. Aussilhou, M. Lesurtel, A. Sauvanet et al., "Right portal vein ligation is as efficient as portal vein embolization to induce hypertrophy of the left liver remnant," *Journal of Gastrointestinal Surgery*, vol. 12, no. 2, pp. 297–303, 2008.

[26] M. Nagino, J. Kamiya, M. Kanai et al., "Right trisegment portal vein embolization for biliary tract carcinoma: technique and clinical utility," *Surgery*, vol. 127, no. 2, pp. 155–160, 2000.

[27] I. Popescu, S. Alexandrescu, A. Croitoru, and M. Boros, "Strategies to convert to resectability the initially unresectable colorectal liver metastases," *Hepato-Gastroenterology*, vol. 56, no. 91-92, pp. 739–744, 2009.

[28] A. A. Schnitzbauer, S. A. Lang, H. Goessmann, S. Nadalin, J. Baumgart, S. A. Farkas et al., "Right portal vein ligation combined with in situ splitting induces rapid left lateral liver lobe hypertrophy enabling 2-staged extended right hepatic resection in small-for-size settings," *Annals of Surgery*, vol. 255, no. 3, pp. 405–414, 2012.

[29] S. E. De, F. A. Alvarez, and V. Ardiles, "How to avoid postoperative liver failure: a novel method," *World Journal of Surgery*, vol. 36, no. 1, pp. 125–128, 2012.

[30] A. Abulkhir, P. Limongelli, A. J. Healey et al., "Preoperative portal vein embolization for major liver resection: a meta-analysis," *Annals of Surgery*, vol. 247, no. 1, pp. 49–57, 2008.

[31] B. Aussilhou, S. Dokmak, S. Faivre, V. Paradis, V. Vilgrain, and J. Belghiti, "Preoperative liver hypertrophy induced by portal flow occlusion before major hepatic resection for colorectal metastases can be impaired by bevacizumab," *Annals of Surgical Oncology*, vol. 16, no. 6, pp. 1553–1559, 2009.

[32] D. Zorzi, Y. S. Chun, D. C. Madoff, E. K. Abdalla, and J. N. Vauthey, "Chemotherapy with bevacizumab does not affect liver regeneration after portal vein embolization in the treatment of colorectal liver metastases," *Annals of Surgical Oncology*, vol. 15, no. 10, pp. 2765–2772, 2008.

[33] D. Jaeck, E. Oussoultzoglou, E. Rosso et al., "A two-stage hepatectomy procedure combined with portal vein embolization to achieve curative resection for initially unresectable multiple and bilobar colorectal liver metastases," *Annals of Surgery*, vol. 240, no. 6, pp. 1037–1051, 2004.

[34] R. Adam, A. Laurent, D. Azoulay et al., "Two-stage hepatectomy: a planned strategy to treat irresectable liver tumors," *Annals of Surgery*, vol. 232, no. 6, pp. 777–785, 2000.

[35] N. J. Lygidakis, A. D. Bhagat, P. Vrachnos, and L. Grigorakos, "Challenges in everyday surgical practice: synchronous

bilobar hepatic colorectal metastases—newer multimodality approach," *Hepato-Gastroenterology*, vol. 54, no. 76, pp. 1020–1024, 2007.

[36] D. V. Sahani, S. P. Kalva, K. K. Tanabe et al., "Intraoperative US in patients undergoing surgery for liver neoplasms: comparison with MR imaging," *Radiology*, vol. 232, no. 3, pp. 810–814, 2004.

[37] G. Torzilli and M. Makuuchi, "Intraoperative ultrasonography in liver cancer," *Surgical Oncology Clinics of North America*, vol. 12, no. 1, pp. 91–103, 2003.

[38] M. Donadon, F. Botea, D. Del Fabbro, A. Palmisano, M. Montorsi, and G. Torzilli, "The surgical policy predicts the impact of contrast enhanced intraoperative ultrasound for colorectal liver metastases," *European Journal of Radiology*, vol. 67, no. 1, pp. 177–178, 2008.

[39] M. Makuuchi, H. Hasegawa, and S. Yamazaki, "Ultrasonically guided subsegmentectomy," *Surgery Gynecology and Obstetrics*, vol. 161, no. 4, pp. 346–350, 1985.

[40] D. Castaing, O. J. Garden, and H. Bismuth, "Segmental liver resection using ultrasound-guided selective portal venous occlusion," *Annals of Surgery*, vol. 210, no. 1, pp. 20–23, 1989.

[41] Y. Shimamura, P. Gunven, and Y. Takenaka, "Selective portal branch occlusion by balloon catheter during liver resection," *Surgery*, vol. 100, no. 5, pp. 938–941, 1986.

[42] A. Muratore, P. Conti, M. Amisano, H. Bouzari, and L. Capussotti, "Bisegmentectomy 7-8 as alternative to more extensive liver resections," *Journal of the American College of Surgeons*, vol. 200, no. 2, pp. 224–228, 2005.

[43] G. Torzilli, M. Montorsi, F. D. Del, A. Palmisano, M. Donadon, and M. Makuuchi, "Ultrasonographically guided surgical approach to liver tumours involving the hepatic veins close to the caval confluence," *British Journal of Surgery*, vol. 93, no. 10, pp. 1238–1246, 2006.

[44] G. Torzilli, F. Procopio, F. Botea, M. Marconi, F. D. Del, M. Donadon et al., "One-stage ultrasonographically guided hepatectomy for multiple bilobar colorectal metastases: a feasible and effective alternative to the 2-stage approach," *Surgery*, vol. 146, no. 1, pp. 60–71, 2009.

[45] K. Sano, M. Makuuchi, K. Miki et al., "Evaluation of hepatic venous congestion: proposed indication criteria for hepatic vein reconstruction," *Annals of Surgery*, vol. 236, no. 2, pp. 241–247, 2002.

[46] T. Takayama and M. Makuuchi, "Intraoperative ultrasonography and other techniques for segmental resections," *Surgical Oncology Clinics of North America*, vol. 5, no. 2, pp. 261–269, 1996.

[47] G. Torzilli, A. Palmisano, D. Del Fabbro, M. Donadon, and M. Montorsi, "Technical tricks for radical but conservative liver resection: the ultrasound guidance," *Minerva Chirurgica*, vol. 60, no. 3, pp. 159–165, 2005.

[48] G. Torzilli, M. Montorsi, M. Donadon et al., ""Radical but conservative" is the main goal for ultrasonography-guided liver resection: prospective validation of this approach," *Journal of the American College of Surgeons*, vol. 201, no. 4, pp. 517–528, 2005.

[49] D. Azoulay, D. Castaing, A. Smail et al., "Resection of nonresectable liver metastases from colorectal cancer after percutaneous portal vein embolization," *Annals of Surgery*, vol. 231, no. 4, pp. 480–486, 2000.

[50] A. Muratore, R. Polastri, H. Bouzari, V. Vergara, A. Ferrero, and L. Capussotti, "Repeat hepatectomy for colorectal liver metastases: a worthwhile operation?" *Journal of Surgical Oncology*, vol. 76, no. 2, pp. 127–132, 2001.

[51] S. Suzuki, T. Sakaguchi, Y. Yokoi et al., "Impact of repeat hepatectomy on recurrent colorectal liver metastases," *Surgery*, vol. 129, no. 4, pp. 421–428, 2001.

[52] J. Yamamoto, T. Kosuge, K. Shimada, S. Yamasaki, Y. Moriya, and K. Sugihara, "Repeat liver resection for recurrent colorectal liver metastases," *American Journal of Surgery*, vol. 178, no. 4, pp. 275–281, 1999.

[53] H. Bismuth, R. Adam, F. Lévi et al., "Resection of nonresectable liver metastases from colorectal cancer after neoadjuvant chemotherapy," *Annals of Surgery*, vol. 224, no. 4, pp. 509–522, 1996.

[54] W. C. Fowler, B. L. Eisenberg, and J. P. Hoffman, "Hepatic resection following systemic chemotherapy for metastatic colorectal carcinoma," *Journal of Surgical Oncology*, vol. 51, no. 2, pp. 122–125, 1992.

[55] "Modulation of fluorouracil by leucovorin in patients with advanced colorectal cancer: evidence in terms of response rate," *Journal of Clinical Oncology*, vol. 10, no. 6, pp. 896–903, 1992.

[56] A. Wein, C. Riedel, F. Köckerling et al., "Impact of surgery on survival in palliative patients with metastatic colorectal cancer after first line treatment with weekly 24-hour infusion of high-dose 5-fluorouracil and folinic acid," *Annals of Oncology*, vol. 12, no. 12, pp. 1721–1727, 2001.

[57] J. Y. Douillard, A. Sobrero, C. Carnaghi et al., "Metastatic colorectal cancer: integrating irinotecan into combination and sequential chemotherapy," *Annals of Oncology*, vol. 14, Supplement 2, pp. ii7–ii12, 2003.

[58] R. M. Goldberg, D. J. Sargent, R. F. Morton et al., "A randomized controlled trial of fluorouracil plus leucovorin, irinotecan, and oxaliplatin combinations in patients with previously untreated metastatic colorectal cancer," *Journal of Clinical Oncology*, vol. 22, no. 1, pp. 23–30, 2004.

[59] C. Tournigand, T. André, E. Achille et al., "FOLFIRI followed by FOLFOX6 or the reverse sequence in advanced colorectal cancer: a randomized GERCOR study," *Journal of Clinical Oncology*, vol. 22, no. 2, pp. 229–237, 2004.

[60] G. Folprecht, A. Grothey, S. Alberts, H. R. Raab, and C. H. Köhne, "Neoadjuvant treatment of unresectable colorectal liver metastases: correlation between tumour response and resection rates," *Annals of Oncology*, vol. 16, no. 8, pp. 1311–1319, 2005.

[61] T. Delaunoit, S. R. Alberts, D. J. Sergent et al., "Chemotherapy permits resection of metastatic colorectal cancer: experience from intergroup N9741," *Annals of Oncology*, vol. 16, no. 3, pp. 425–429, 2005.

[62] G. Masi, F. Loupakis, L. Pollina et al., "Long-term outcome of initially unresectable metastatic colorectal cancer patients treated with 5-fluorouracil/leucovorin, oxaliplatin, and irinotecan (FOLFOXIRI) followed by radical surgery of metastases," *Annals of Surgery*, vol. 249, no. 3, pp. 420–425, 2009.

[63] C. Pozzo, M. Basso, A. Cassano et al., "Neoadjuvant treatment of unresectable liver disease with irinotecan and 5-fluorouracil plus folinic acid in colorectal cancer patients," *Annals of Oncology*, vol. 15, no. 6, pp. 933–939, 2004.

[64] R. Adam, E. Avisar, A. Ariche et al., "Five-year survival following hepatic resection after neoadjuvant therapy for nonresectable colorectal [liver] metastases," *Annals of Surgical Oncology*, vol. 8, no. 4, pp. 347–353, 2001.

[65] D. Elias, P. Lasser, P. Rougier, M. Ducreux, C. Bognel, and A. Roche, "Frequency, technical aspects, results, and indications of major hepatectomy after prolonged intra-arterial hepatic chemotherapy for initially unresectable hepatic tumors,"

Journal of the American College of Surgeons, vol. 180, no. 2, pp. 213–219, 1995.

[66] M. Karoui, C. Penna, M. Amin-Hashem et al., "Influence of preoperative chemotherapy on the risk of major hepatectomy for colorectal liver metastases," *Annals of Surgery*, vol. 243, no. 1, pp. 1–7, 2006.

[67] R. Adam, T. Aloia, F. Lévi et al., "Hepatic resection after rescue cetuximab treatment for colorectal liver metastases previously refractory to conventional systemic therapy," *Journal of Clinical Oncology*, vol. 25, no. 29, pp. 4593–4602, 2007.

[68] B. Gruenberger, D. Tamandl, J. Schueller et al., "Bevacizumab, capecitabine, and oxaliplatin as neoadjuvant therapy for patients with potentially curable metastatic colorectal cancer," *Journal of Clinical Oncology*, vol. 26, no. 11, pp. 1830–1835, 2008.

[69] F. A. Scappaticci, L. Fehrenbacher, T. Cartwright et al., "Surgical wound healing complications in metastatic colorectal cancer patients treated with bevacizumab," *Journal of Surgical Oncology*, vol. 91, no. 3, pp. 173–180, 2005.

[70] M. D'Angelica, P. Kornprat, M. Gonen et al., "Lack of evidence for increased operative morbidity after hepatectomy with perioperative use of bevacizumab: a matched case-control study," *Annals of Surgical Oncology*, vol. 14, no. 2, pp. 759–765, 2007.

[71] G. Mentha, A. D. Roth, S. Terraz et al., "'Liver first' approach in the treatment of colorectal cancer with synchronous liver metastases," *Digestive Surgery*, vol. 25, no. 6, pp. 430–435, 2009.

[72] R. Adam, D. A. Wicherts, R. J. De Haas et al., "Complete pathologic response after preoperative chemotherapy for colorectal liver metastases: myth or reality?" *Journal of Clinical Oncology*, vol. 26, no. 10, pp. 1635–1641, 2008.

[73] M. C. B. Tan, D. C. Linehan, W. G. Hawkins, B. A. Siegel, and S. M. Strasberg, "Chemotherapy-induced normalization of FDG uptake by colorectal liver metastases does not usually indicate complete pathologic response," *Journal of Gastrointestinal Surgery*, vol. 11, no. 9, pp. 1112–1119, 2007.

[74] S. Benoist, A. Brouquet, C. Penna et al., "Complete response of colorectal liver metastases after chemotherapy: does it mean cure?" *Journal of Clinical Oncology*, vol. 24, no. 24, pp. 3939–3945, 2006.

[75] K. J. Oldhafer, G. A. Stavrou, G. Prause, H. O. Peitgen, T. C. Lueth, and S. Weber, "How to operate a liver tumor you cannot see," *Langenbeck's Archives of Surgery*, vol. 394, no. 3, pp. 489–494, 2009.

[76] D. Elias, D. Goere, V. Boige et al., "Outcome of posthepatectomy-missing colorectal liver metastases after complete response to chemotherapy: impact of adjuvant intra-arterial hepatic oxaliplatin," *Annals of Surgical Oncology*, vol. 14, no. 11, pp. 3188–3194, 2007.

[77] D. G. Blazer, Y. Kishi, D. M. Maru et al., "Pathologic response to preoperative chemotherapy: a new outcome end point after resection of hepatic colorectal metastases," *Journal of Clinical Oncology*, vol. 26, no. 33, pp. 5344–5351, 2008.

[78] D. Ribero, H. Wang, M. Donadon et al., "Bevacizumab improves pathologic response and protects against hepatic injury in patients treated with oxaliplatin-based chemotherapy for colorectal liver metastases," *Cancer*, vol. 110, no. 12, pp. 2761–2767, 2007.

[79] E. K. Abdalla and J. N. Vauthey, "Chemotherapy prior to hepatic resection for colorectal liver metastases: helpful until harmful?" *Digestive Surgery*, vol. 25, no. 6, pp. 421–429, 2009.

[80] D. A. Kooby, Y. Fong, A. Suriawinata et al., "Impact of steatosis on perioperative outcome following hepatic resection," *Journal of Gastrointestinal Surgery*, vol. 7, no. 8, pp. 1034–1044, 2003.

[81] J. N. Vauthey, T. M. Pawlik, D. Ribero et al., "Chemotherapy regimen predicts steatohepatitis and an increase in 90-day mortality after surgery for hepatic colorectal metastases," *Journal of Clinical Oncology*, vol. 24, no. 13, pp. 2065–2072, 2006.

[82] L. Rubbia-Brandt, V. Audard, P. Sartoretti et al., "Severe hepatic sinusoidal obstruction associated with oxaliplatin-based chemotherapy in patients with metastatic colorectal cancer," *Annals of Oncology*, vol. 15, no. 3, pp. 460–466, 2004.

[83] T. Aloia, M. Sebagh, M. Plasse et al., "Liver histology and surgical outcomes after preoperative chemotherapy with fluorouracil plus oxaliplatin in colorectal cancer liver metastases," *Journal of Clinical Oncology*, vol. 24, no. 31, pp. 4983–4990, 2006.

[84] N. N. Mehta, R. Ravikumar, C. A. Coldham et al., "Effect of preoperative chemotherapy on liver resection for colorectal liver metastases," *European Journal of Surgical Oncology*, vol. 34, no. 7, pp. 782–786, 2008.

[85] H. Nakano, E. Oussoultzoglou, E. Rosso et al., "Sinusoidal injury increases morbidity after major hepatectomy in patients with colorectal liver metastases receiving preoperative chemotherapy," *Annals of Surgery*, vol. 247, no. 1, pp. 118–124, 2008.

[86] B. Nordlinger, H. Sorbye, B. Glimelius et al., "Perioperative chemotherapy with FOLFOX4 and surgery versus surgery alone for resectable liver metastases from colorectal cancer (EORTC Intergroup trial 40983): a randomised controlled trial," *The Lancet*, vol. 371, no. 9617, pp. 1007–1016, 2008.

[87] H. Hur, Y. T. Ko, B. S. Min et al., "Comparative study of resection and radiofrequency ablation in the treatment of solitary colorectal liver metastases," *American Journal of Surgery*, vol. 197, no. 6, pp. 728–736, 2009.

[88] D. Elias, A. Goharin, A. El Otmany et al., "Usefulness of intratoperative radiofrequency thermoablation of liver tumours associated or not with hepatectomy," *European Journal of Surgical Oncology*, vol. 26, no. 8, pp. 763–769, 2000.

[89] N. J. Lygidakis, G. Singh, E. Bardaxoglou et al., "Two-stage liver surgery for advanced liver metastasis synchronous with colorectal tumor," *Hepato-Gastroenterology*, vol. 51, no. 56, pp. 413–418, 2004.

[90] E. K. Abdalla, J. N. Vauthey, L. M. Ellis et al., "Recurrence and outcomes following hepatic resection, radiofrequency ablation, and combined resection/ablation for colorectal liver metastases," *Annals of Surgery*, vol. 239, no. 6, pp. 818–827, 2004.

[91] A. Veltri, P. Sacchetto, I. Tosetti, E. Pagano, C. Fava, and G. Gandini, "Radiofrequency ablation of colorectal liver metastases: small size favorably predicts technique effectiveness and survival," *CardioVascular and Interventional Radiology*, vol. 31, no. 5, pp. 948–956, 2008.

[92] P. Abitabile, U. Hartl, J. Lange, and C. A. Maurer, "Radiofrequency ablation permits an effective treatment for colorectal liver metastasis," *European Journal of Surgical Oncology*, vol. 33, no. 1, pp. 67–71, 2007.

[93] M. Rivoire, F. De Cian, P. Meeus, S. Ńgrier, H. Sebban, and P. Kaemmerlen, "Combination of neoadjuvant chemotherapy with cryotherapy and surgical resection for the treatment of unresectable liver metastases from colorectal carcinoma: long-term results," *Cancer*, vol. 95, no. 11, pp. 2283–2292, 2002.

[94] E. Hoti and R. Adam, "Liver transplantation for primary and metastatic liver cancers," *Transplant International*, vol. 21, no. 12, pp. 1107–1117, 2008.

[95] B. Kocman, D. Mikulic, S. Jadrijevic, M. Poljak, I. Kocman, S. Gasparov et al., "Long-term survival after living-donor liver transplantation for unresectable colorectal metastases to the liver: case report," *Transplantation Proceedings*, vol. 43, no. 10, pp. 4013–4015, 2011.

[96] F. Mühlbacher and F. Piza, "Orthotopic liver transplantation for secondary malignancies of the liver," *Transplantation Proceedings*, vol. 19, no. 1, Part 3, pp. 2396–2398, 1987.

[97] S. Kappel, D. Kandioler, R. Steininger et al., "Genetic detection of lymph node micrometastases: a selection criterion for liver transplantation in patients with liver metastases after colorectal cancer," *Transplantation*, vol. 81, no. 1, pp. 64–70, 2006.

[98] J. Galon, A. Costes, F. Sanchez-Cabo et al., "Type, density, and location of immune cells within human colorectal tumors predict clinical outcome," *Science*, vol. 313, no. 5795, pp. 1960–1964, 2006.

[99] T. M. Pawlik and M. A. Choti, "Shifting from clinical to biologic indicators of prognosis after resection of hepatic colorectal metastases," *Current Oncology Reports*, vol. 9, no. 3, pp. 193–201, 2007.

[100] M. Guba, P. Von Breitenbuch, M. Steinbauer et al., "Rapamycin inhibits primary and metastatic tumor growth by antiangiogenesis: involvement of vascular endothelial growth factor," *Nature Medicine*, vol. 8, no. 2, pp. 128–135, 2002.

[101] J. J. Fung, D. Kelly, Z. Kadry, K. Patel-Tom, and B. Eghtesad, "Immunosuppression in liver transplantation beyond calcineurin inhibitors," *Liver Transplantation*, vol. 11, no. 3, pp. 267–280, 2005.

[102] A. Foss, R. Adam, and S. Dueland, "Liver transplantation for colorectal liver metastases: revisiting the concept," *Transplant International*, vol. 23, no. 7, pp. 679–685, 2010.

6

MDCT Imaging Findings of Liver Cirrhosis: Spectrum of Hepatic and Extrahepatic Abdominal Complications

Guillermo P. Sangster, Carlos H. Previgliano, Mathieu Nader, Elisa Chwoschtschinsky, and Maureen G. Heldmann

Department of Radiology, LSU Health Shreveport, 1501 Kings Highway, Shreveport, LA 71103, USA

Correspondence should be addressed to Carlos H. Previgliano; cprevi@lsuhsc.edu

Academic Editor: Vito R. Cicinnati

Hepatic cirrhosis is the clinical and pathologic result of a multifactorial chronic liver injury. It is well known that cirrhosis is the origin of multiple extrahepatic abdominal complications and a markedly increased risk of hepatocellular carcinoma (HCC). This tumor is the sixth most common malignancy worldwide and the third most common cause of cancer related death. With the rising incidence of HCC worldwide, awareness of the evolution of cirrhotic nodules into malignancy is critical for an early detection and treatment. Adequate imaging protocol selection with dynamic multiphase Multidetector Computed Tomography (MDCT) and reformatted images is crucial to differentiate and categorize the hepatic nodular dysplasia. Knowledge of the typical and less common extrahepatic abdominal manifestations is essential for accurately assessing patients with known or suspected hepatic disease. The objective of this paper is to illustrate the imaging spectrum of intra- and extrahepatic abdominal manifestations of hepatic cirrhosis seen on MDCT.

1. Introduction

Hepatic cirrhosis is the clinical and pathologic result of a multifactorial chronic liver injury characterized by extensive fibrosis and nodular regeneration replacing the normal liver parenchyma [1]. It is well known that cirrhosis is associated with a markedly increased risk of hepatocellular carcinoma (HCC), the sixth most common malignancy worldwide and third most common cause of cancer related death. The detection of hepatic malignancy in cirrhotic patients is a diagnostic challenge due to distortion of the hepatic architecture [2]. In this article we discuss and illustrate the wide spectrum of intra- and extrahepatic findings on Computed Tomography (CT) in patients with cirrhosis.

2. Hepatic Manifestations

Common pathologic features of cirrhosis include hepatic fibrosis, nodular distortion of hepatic architecture, and perfusion abnormalities. Thefibrotic changes appear as bridging bands or focal confluent fibrosis. Bridging bands usually have variable thickness and may mimic a tumor capsule due to delayed contrast enhancement. Focal confluent fibrosis is defined as a peripheral wedge-shaped hypoattenuated area on unenhanced and venous phase CT. On delayed phase, enhancement of the lesion may occur [3]. Overlying capsular retraction with volume loss in areas of focal confluent fibrosis is an important feature to differentiate this entity from malignant conditions [4] (Figure 1).

Morphologic changes of the liver vary with the stage of cirrhosis. More than 60% of patients with early cirrhosis have hepatomegaly. Additional early detectable morphologic changes of the liver include widening of the porta hepatis, enlargement of the interlobar fissure, and expansion of pericholecystic space [5]. During advanced stages shrinkage of the liver is seen, especially in alcohol-induced cirrhosis. The medial segment (IV) of the left lobe shrinks with concomitant hypertrophy of the lateral segments (II, III), giving a "tongue-like" appearance. These changes lead to a nodular contour and heterogeneity of the liver, which is classically associated with cirrhosis.

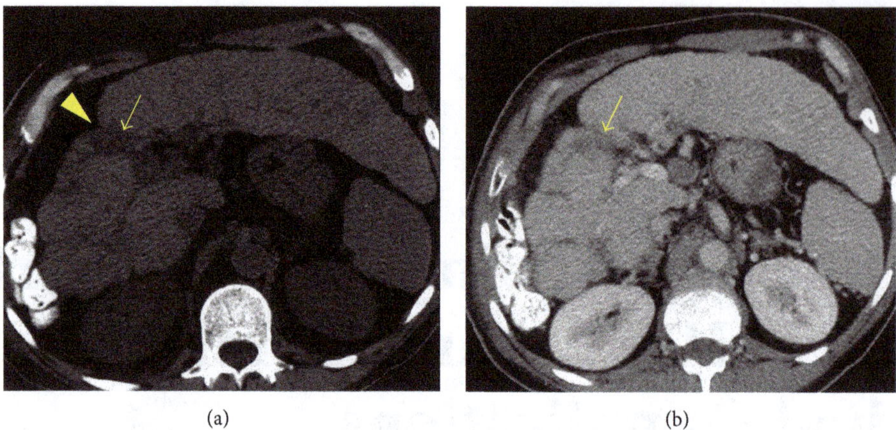

FIGURE 1: Confluent fibrosis in a 55-year-old male with alcoholic cirrhosis. (a) An unenhanced axial CT image shows a v-shaped area of subtle hypoattenuation (arrow) in hepatic segment 5. Note the retraction of the hepatic contour (arrowhead). (b) A portal venous phase axial image obtained at the same level as image (a) reveals an area of decreased portal venous flow (arrow).

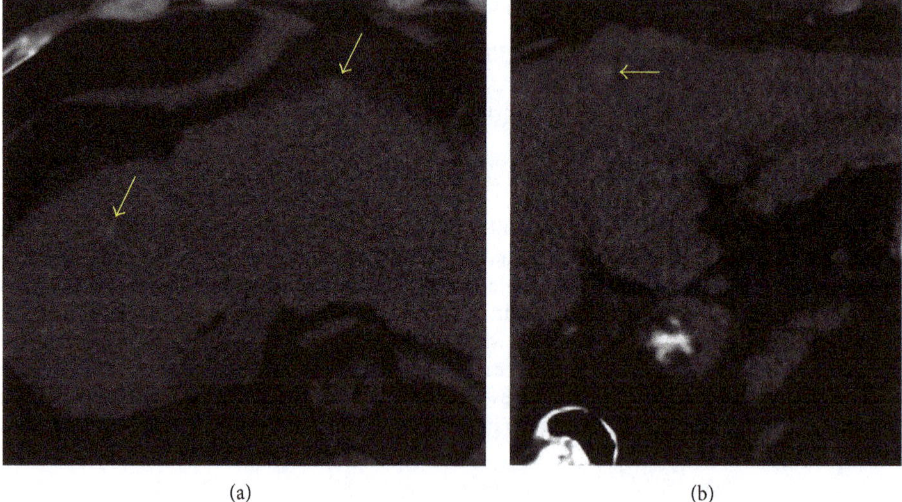

FIGURE 2: Siderotic regenerative nodules in a patient with cirrhosis. Unenhanced axial (a) and coronal (b) CT images show multiple subcentimeter high attenuation hepatic nodules (arrows). Note the nodular hepatic surface in this patient with micronodular cirrhosis.

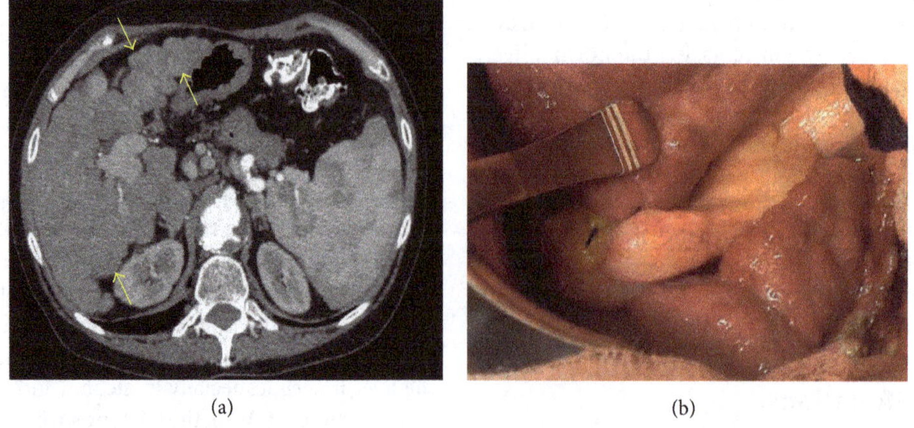

FIGURE 3: Macronodular regenerative nodules, due to alcohol-induced cirrhosis. (a) Arterial phase CT shows multiple nodular isodense lesions deforming the liver margin (arrows). The contour bulge caused by the nodular regeneration may help to detect the lesions. (b) Intraoperative photograph of macronodular cirrhosis.

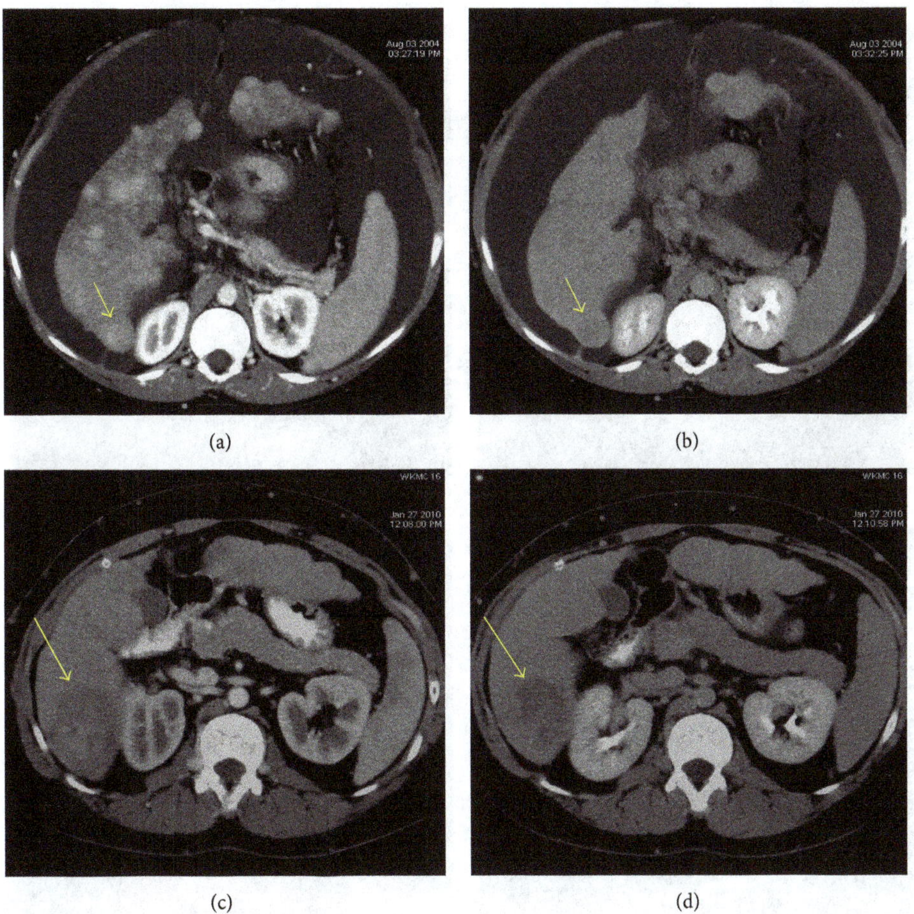

FIGURE 4: Dysplastic nodule in hepatic cirrhosis. Axial ((a), (b)) CT images during arterial and excretory phases show a dominant heterogeneous slightly hyperdense lesion in the segment VI compatible with dysplastic nodule (arrows); this lesion demonstrates a larger size compared with the remaining nodular hepatic lesions raising the possibility of DN in a patient with normal alpha feto protein value. Six-year imaging followup ((c), (d)) showing malignant transformation of this lesion (long arrows).

Hepatic steatosis is a nonspecific reversible response of hepatocytes to chronic injury, commonly seen in alcohol-induced cirrhosis. A diffuse uniform fatty infiltration involving the entire liver is the most common pattern. When hepatosteatosis occurs, the average liver attenuation is at least 10 Hounsfield Units (HU) less than the splenic parenchyma on unenhanced CT [6]. The identification of normal course vascular structures in areas of fatty infiltration is crucial to differentiate this abnormality from hepatic tumors.

Evolving hepatic nodular lesions are another important feature of cirrhosis. In attempt to standardize the terminology, an international working party has suggested terms and definitions of nodular lesions in cirrhotic patients. These are categorized as regenerative nodules, dysplastic nodules, and HCC [7].

A regenerative nodule (RN) is a well-defined area of liver parenchyma that has enlarged in response to necrosis and altered circulation. Based on gross morphologic features, the nodular regeneration can be classified as micronodular (<3 mm in diameter) or macronodular (>3 mm in diameter). Unless a regenerative nodule contains iron, it is rarely seen on a noncontrast CT [8]. If iron deposition is present (siderotic nodule), the nodule appears hyperdense to the surrounding liver on a non-contrast CT (Figure 2). Micronodular changes are rarely identified on CT, despite being present in all cirrhotic livers [8]. Regenerative nodules do not enhance in the arterial phase (Figure 3) and are isodense to the remaining parenchyma on the venous phase, making them indistinguishable from the hepatic background. The accuracy of non-contrast CT in detecting a RN is approximately 25% [8]. A combination of micro- and macronodular regeneration is the most common morphologic presentation seen in cirrhotic patients.

A dysplastic nodule (DN) is defined as a nodular region of dysplastic hepatocytes without histologic features of malignancy. DNs commonly measure 5–10 mm and most of them are undetectable by CT since, even after the administration of contrast, the majority is isoattenuating. Dysplastic nodules can be further characterized as low grade or high grade, according to the degree of dysplasia [7]. Tumor angiogenesis appears to be a mandatory step in the evolution of dysplastic nodules to HCC. During this process, there is a progressive increase in the arterial supply and a concomitant decrease in the portal venous supply to these lesions [9]. The major

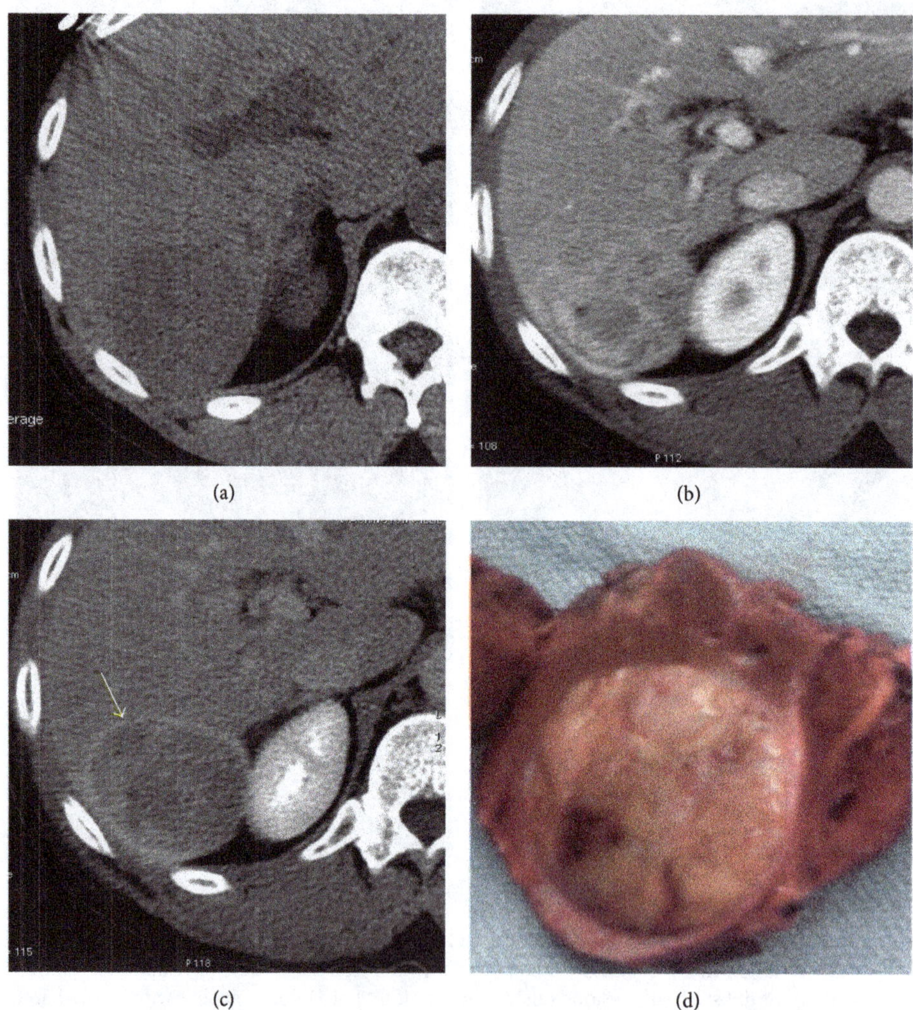

FIGURE 5: Solitary HCC. Axial CT images of the right hepatic lobe during precontrast (a), postcontrast venous (b), and delayed (c) phases show a well-defined heterogeneous solid enhancing mass occupying hepatic segment 7. Note the delayed enhancement of the lesion capsule ((c), arrow). (d) Photograph of the surgical specimen.

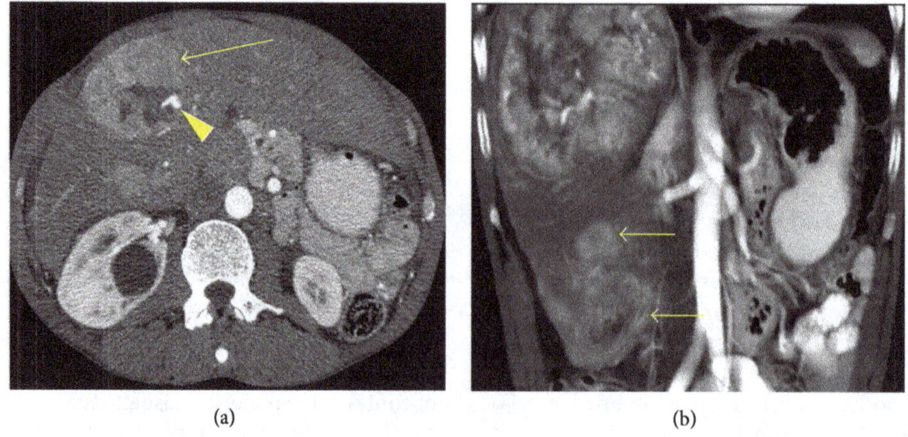

FIGURE 6: Multicentric HCC with a variegated appearance. (a) Arterial phase contrast-enhanced axial CT image shows a large heterogeneous mass that enhances intensely with multiple adjacent nodular areas with different attenuation patterns (long arrow). Intralesional arterioportal shunting is noted (arrowhead). (b) Coronal maximum intensity projection (MIP) reconstruction demonstrates additional smaller satellite hypervascular lesions (short arrows).

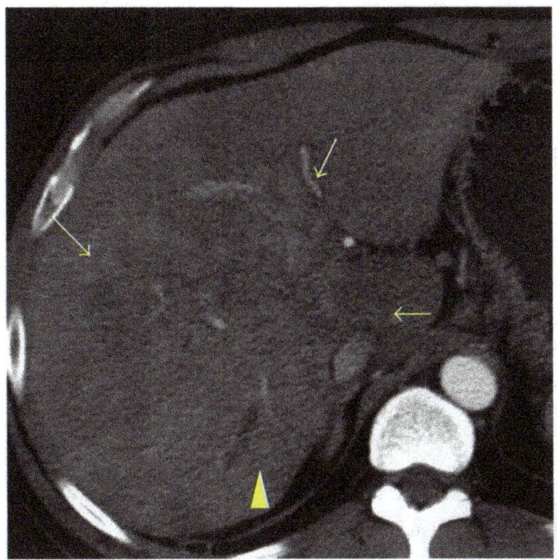

FIGURE 7: Diffuse hepatocellular carcinoma. Arterial-phase contrast enhanced axial CT scan demonstrates a large ill-defined heterogeneous mass occupying the right hepatic lobe (arrows). Focal intrahepatic biliary dilatation is seen (arrowhead).

shift in angiogenesis typically occurs during the transition from low-grade DNs to high-grade DNs [10]. New vessels composed of nontriadal arteries become dominant and the absence of portal tracts is noted. The increasingly dedifferentiated nodule appears more markedly enhanced on postcontrast early arterial phase image, occasionally mimicking an HCC (Figure 4). Several reports have described the detectability of dysplastic nodules on dynamic CT scans. In a large series of liver transplantation specimens, small DNs (<5 mm) were never identified at preoperative imaging [9]. The detection rate for dysplastic nodules smaller than 2 cm has been reported, in pretransplant three-phase helical CT study, to be 39% [11].

HCC is a malignant neoplasm composed of cells with hepatocellular differentiation and is almost exclusively seen in patients with cirrhosis. The development of HCC in the cirrhotic liver is described either as de novo hepatocarcinogenesis or as a multistep progression, from low-grade dysplastic nodules to high-grade dysplastic nodule, then to dysplastic nodule with microscopic foci of HCC, then to small HCC, and finally to overt carcinoma [12].

HCC is classified histologically as trabecular, pseudoglandular, compact, and scirrhous, with the trabecular pattern being the most common. The fibrolamellar type of HCC has distinct clinical, histologic, and prognostic features and is commonly seen in young patients with no history of cirrhosis or chronic liver disease. The lesion appearance varies greatly according to size [13]. Small lesions enhance homogeneously, while large lesions are heterogeneous with a characteristic mosaic pattern, due to intralesional necrosis. Approximately 80%–90% of HCCs are highly vascular lesions demonstrating intense contrast enhancement during the arterial phase. In the venous phase, HCC demonstrates washout and becomes isodense with the liver parenchyma, thereby making its detection difficult [14]. About 10%–20% of HCCs are hypovascular

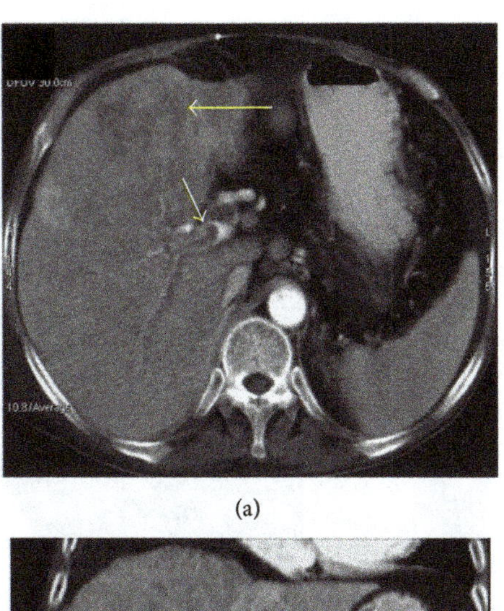

(a)

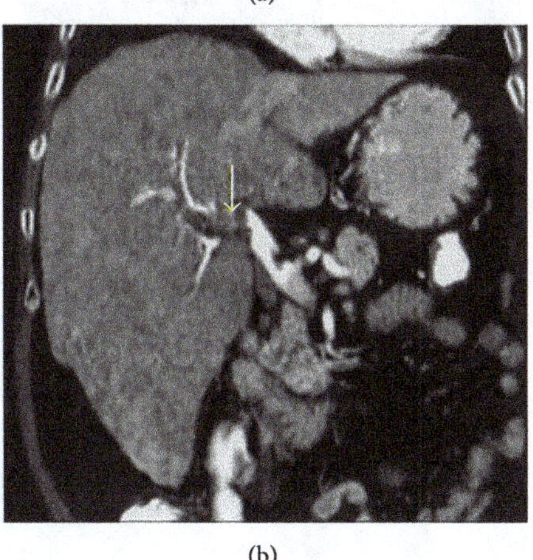

(b)

FIGURE 8: Portal vein thrombosis in a patient with HCC complicating hepatic cirrhosis. (a) Arterial phase contrast enhanced axial CT image shows a large filling defect in the portal vein indicating endoluminal thrombus (short arrow). A small peripheral HCC is noted in the hepatic segment 4 (long arrow). (b) a Coronal MIP reconstruction best depicts the filling defects in the main portal vein (arrow).

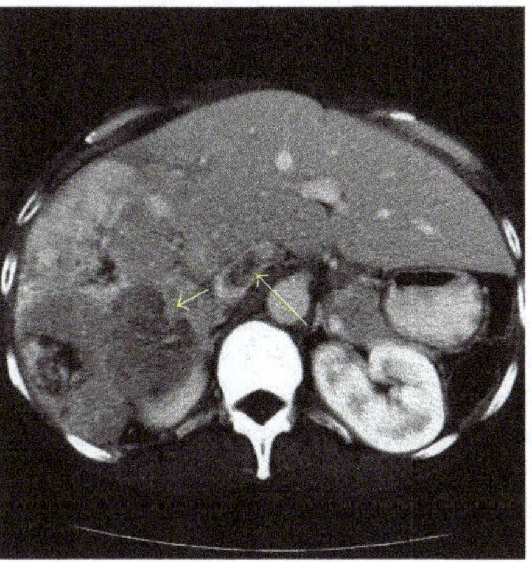

FIGURE 9: HCC invading the inferior vena cava. Contrast enhanced axial CT scan shows a central filling defect in the inferior vena cava (long arrow). Large peripheral enhancing hepatocellular carcinoma compressing the right kidney is also shown (short arrow).

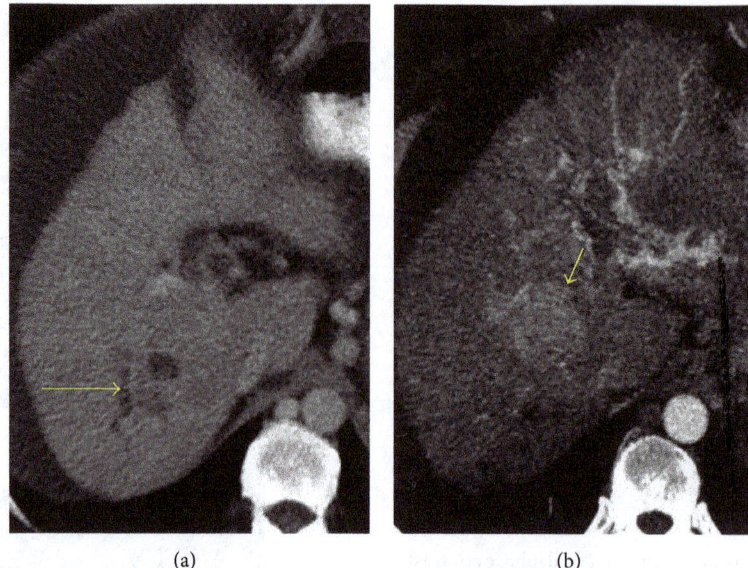

Figure 10: HCC only detected in the arterial phase. (a) A portal venous phase axial image shows intrahepatic biliary dilatation (long arrow) but fails to depict the HCC. (b) Arterial phase axial MIP reconstruction clearly delineates the hypervascular mass (short arrow).

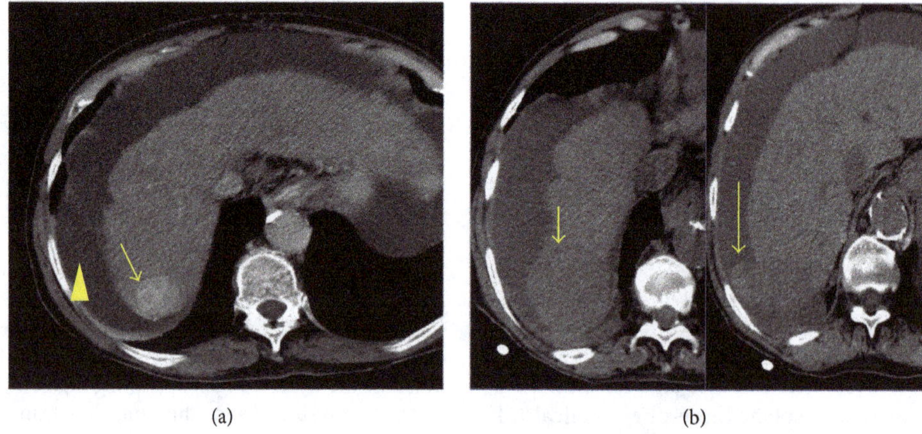

Figure 11: Ruptured HCC. (a) Contrast-enhanced CT shows a focus of HCC in the right lobe of the liver (long arrow). Low density fluid in the perihepatic space is also seen (arrowhead). (b) Three months later, the patient complained of increased abdominal pain. A nonenhanced CT obtained at the same level as (a) demonstrates an abnormally shaped right hepatic lobe (short arrow) associated with high density ascitic fluid consistent with hemoperitoneum (long arrow). Ruptured HCC was confirmed at surgery.

and show contrast enhancement slightly less than that in the surrounding liver on arterial phase images, making the imaging differentiation with DNs difficult. The intranodular vascular changes of these lesions revealed by findings of CTAP (CT during arterial portography) and CTHA (CT during hepatic angiography) and correlated with histological analysis explain why high-grade DNs and early-stage-well-differentiated HCC are hypodense relative to the surrounding liver. Both lesions have decreased portal tracts (including normal hepatic arteries), without increased abnormal arteries. And, when the increased abnormal arterial supply compensated for the decreased normal hepatic arterial supply, they are isodense [15]. Understanding this blood supply pattern is important for early detection, characterization, and treatment for early-stage HCC [15].

Most HCCs have a fibrous capsule that is usually hypodense on hepatic arterial phase and enhance on delayed phase. HCC may present as a solitary mass (Figure 5), a dominant mass with daughter lesions (multicentric type) (Figure 6), or as a diffusely infiltrating neoplasm (Figure 7). Less frequently, it is multifocal with small foci usually less than 2 cm in both hepatic lobes, which may mimic liver metastasis [1]. HCC is very locally invasive and may extend to the bile ducts, portal vein (Figure 8), inferior vena cava (IVC) (Figure 9), and hepatic veins. Distant metastasis from HCC may be seen in the lungs, adrenals, adjacent lymph nodes, and bones. CT is accurate in staging HCC by detecting the number of lesions and involved segments, regional adenopathy, vascular tumor invasion, and metastases [14].

The use of MDCT with dynamic contrast-enhanced triple-phase technique and reformatted images is essential to detect small HCC lesions; however, it remains the most challenging area in imaging cirrhotic liver. This technique demonstrates up to 30% more tumor nodules and in

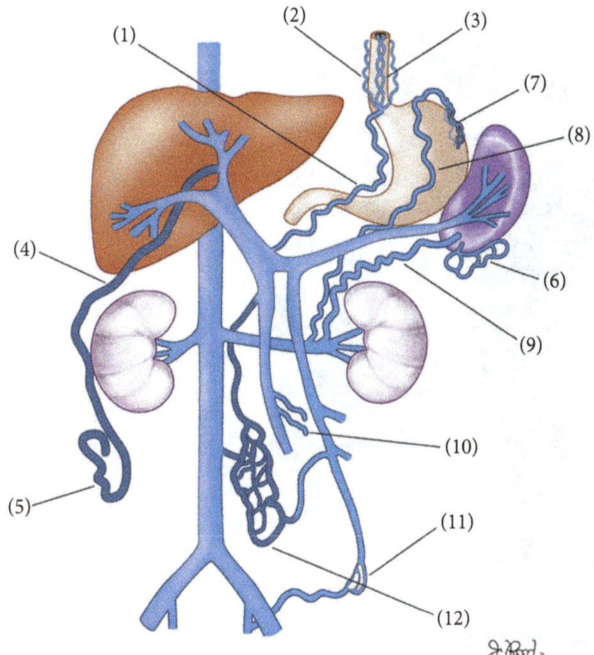

(1) Coronary
(2) Paraesophageal
(3) Esophageal
(4) Paraumbilical
(5) Caput medusae
(6) Perisplenic
(7) Retrogastric
(8) Gastrorenal shunt
(9) Splenorenal shunt
(10) Mesenteric
(11) Hemorrhoidal
(12) Retroperitoneal paravertebral

FIGURE 12: Portosystemic collateral vessels in portal hypertension.

approximately 10% of cases of HCC will be the only phase to demonstrate the lesion [16] (Figure 10). Despite optimal arterial phase imaging, a large number of small (<1.5 cm) HCCs remain isodense relative to the background and go undetected on CT. Reported sensitivity for dynamic triple-phase contrast enhanced CT ranges from 50% to 96% and the specificity from 75% to 96%. It is well known that to obtain the best conspicuity of lesions, thinner slices (collimation, 1.5 mm; image reconstruction interval, 3 mm) and late arterial phase images (30–35 seconds after injection of contrast medium) should be acquired [17]. On the basis of explanted livers, it has been reported that the detection of hepatocellular carcinomas smaller than 2 cm, using three-phase helical dynamic CT, was 60% and the detection of those larger than 2 cm was 82% [11]. The reported sensitivity using previous state-of-the-art MR imaging technique and correlation with explanted liver pathologic results is also disappointing in detecting small HCCs and dysplastic nodules smaller than 2.0 cm [18].

Considering that in this country 60%–90% of HCCs occur in cirrhotic livers [19] and early-stage detection is difficult, the American Association for the Study of Liver Diseases (AASLD) includes a recommendation for periodic imaging surveillance in patients with liver cirrhosis and stated that the diagnosis of HCC can be made safe if a mass larger than 1.0 cm shows typical features of HCC (arterial hypervascularity and venous or delayed phase washout) at contrast material enhanced CT or MRI, obviating the need for biopsy if these features are present [20]. In our institution, surveillance guidelines are those based on the updated AASLD report. Four-phase MDCT is usually the preferred technique in our practice and contrast-enhanced MRI is used for problem solving cases or in those patients with any contraindication for contrast-enhanced CT.

Arterioportal shunting is a well-known phenomenon that occurs in patients with cirrhosis and HCC. The typical imaging presentation is a wedge-shaped area of high attenuation seen on the arterial phase that becomes isodense to the liver parenchyma during the portal venous phase. The classic imaging finding is the presence of contrast material in distal portal branches, with minimal or no contrast in the proximal portal vein or superior mesenteric vein during the arterial phase [6]. Spontaneous rupture of HCC is an unusual complication identified in approximately 8% of the cases (Figure 11).

3. Extrahepatic Abdominal Manifestations

Extrahepatic abnormalities associated with cirrhosis include portal hypertension, ascites, splenomegaly, diffuse intra and retroperitoneal edema, small bowel, and gallbladder wall thickening.

A variety of morphologic alterations are seen in cirrhotic patients due to portal hypertension. Portal hypertension is defined as a portal pressure greater than 5–10 mm Hg. Portosystemic collaterals develop spontaneously, as blood flow is shunted away from the liver to low pressure systemic vessels (hepatofugal flow) [21] (Figure 12). Gastrointestinal variceal bleeding is the most common clinical presentation in patients with altered flow dynamics.

Varices appear as well-defined tubular or serpentine homogeneous structures. On unenhanced CT, varices may mimic adenopathy, masses, or nonopacified bowel loops. The administration of intravenous contrast is vital to delineate dilated venous structures.

The left gastric venous collaterals (coronary varices) are seen in approximately 80% of cirrhotic patients. These vessels are located in the lesser omentum, between the medial wall of the upper gastric body and the posterior margin of the left lobe. A 5-6 mm left gastric vein on CT is an indicator of portal hypertension.

Esophageal varices are located in the wall of the lower esophagus and appear as intraluminal protrusions with scalloped borders (Figure 13). Paraesophageal varices are found around the esophageal wall and arise from the posterior branch of the left gastric vein, whereas the esophageal varices arise from the anterior branch.

Paraumbilical venous collaterals vessels are found in 43% of patients with portal hypertension. They appear as circular or tubular enhancing structures in the falciform ligament and are supplied by the left portal vein. "Caput medusae" refers to collateral vessels that radiate from the umbilicus and are situated in the subcutaneous fat. These vessels are supplied by paraumbilical and omental veins (Figure 14).

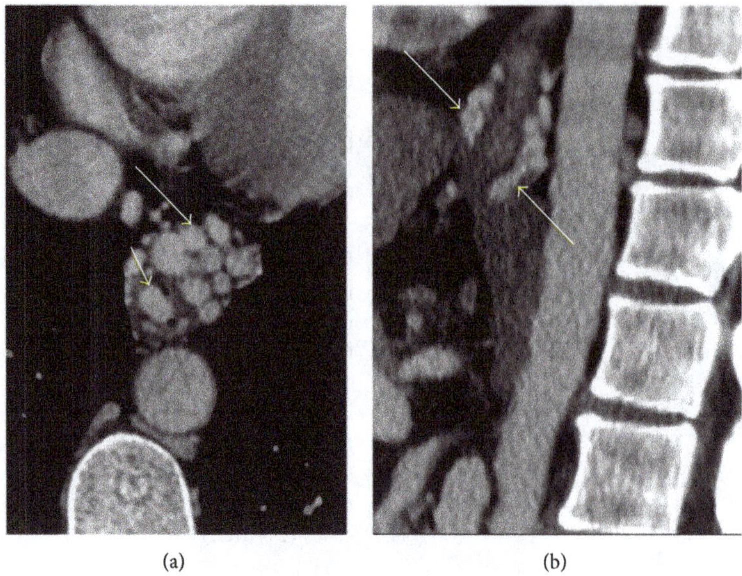

(a) (b)

FIGURE 13: Esophageal and paraesophageal varices. Arterial phase axial (a) and sagittal (b) MIP reconstructions demonstrate multiple intramural (short arrow) and paraesophageal (long arrows) serpiginous tubular structures consistent with varices.

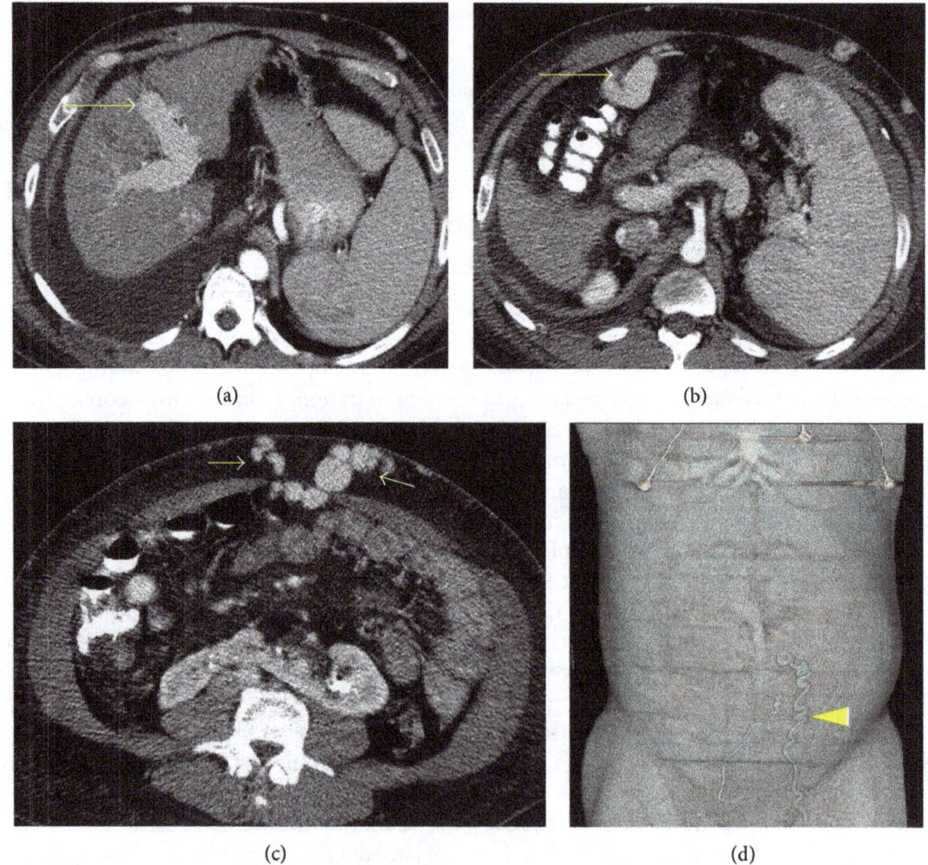

(a) (b) (c) (d)

FIGURE 14: Paraumbilical varices. Contrast-enhanced axial images ((a)–(c)) demonstrate a paraumbilical varix originating from the left portal vein (long arrows) and extending to the abdominal wall (short arrows). A volume rendered reconstruction (d) demonstrates the caput medusae in the abdominal wall (arrow).

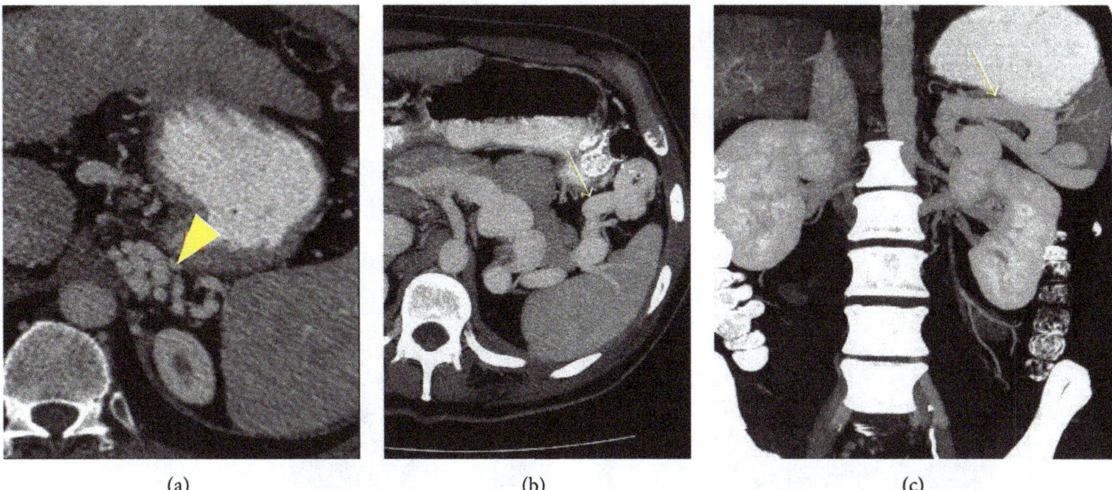

FIGURE 15: A cirrhotic patient with retrogastric varices and a splenorenal shunt. Axial contrast-enhanced images ((a), (b)) and a coronal MIP reconstruction (c) demonstrate retrogastric varices ((a), arrowhead) draining into a patent gastrorenal shunt (arrows).

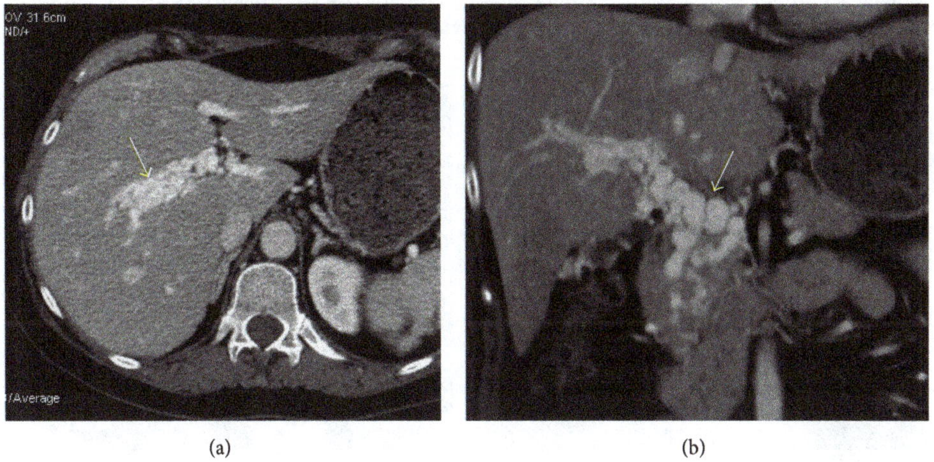

FIGURE 16: Chronic portal venous thrombosis with cavernous transformation of the portal vein. Axial (a) and coronal (b) contrast-enhanced CT images demonstrate multifocal serpiginous tubular structures in the hepatic hilum consistent with portoportal collateral vessels (arrows).

Another group of varices are seen in the anteroinferior aspect of the spleen. These varices are easily identified by their axial orientation and position in the perisplenic fat.

The retrogastric varices are seen in the posteromedial aspect of the gastric fundus near the cardia and may be difficult to diagnose. They are fed by the left gastric or the gastroepiploic vein.

Portosystemic shunts commonly involve the gastrorenal and the splenorenal systems. Retrogastric varices drain into the left renal vein through the gastrorenal shunt, whereas perisplenic varices drain directly into the left renal vein via the splenorenal shunt (Figure 15).

Portal vein thrombosis may occur in patients with cirrhosis and portal hypertension. After administration of contrast, the portal vein shows a central hypodensity corresponding to the intraluminal thrombus. In this situation, the hepatic arterial flow to the liver is increased, developing scattered peripheral transient high attenuation areas known as transient hepatic attenuation differences. In subacute and chronic portal thrombosis, a cavernous transformation of the portal vein may manifest as multiple tubular collaterals in the porta hepatis (Figure 16). When the portal vein is occupied by tumor thrombus, intraluminal enhancement may be seen.

Portal hypertension is considered the most common cause of splenomegaly in the United States (Figure 17). Foci of hemosiderin deposition in the spleen are seen in about 9%–12% of patients with portal hypertension [22]. These foci are called Gamna-Gandy bodies, and their CT imaging pattern varies from hypo- to hyperdense spots, depending on the presence of secondary calcium deposition (Figure 18).

Mesenteric edema is defined as increased attenuation of the adipose tissue that surrounds the mesenteric vessels or their branches. Mesenteric edema in patients with cirrhosis has a multifactorial pathogenesis. Inflammation, hemorrhage, neoplastic infiltration, and hypoproteinemia due to hepatic insufficiency are the most frequent conditions identified. The frequency of mesenteric edema in patients with cirrhosis is 86%, and it is usually associated with

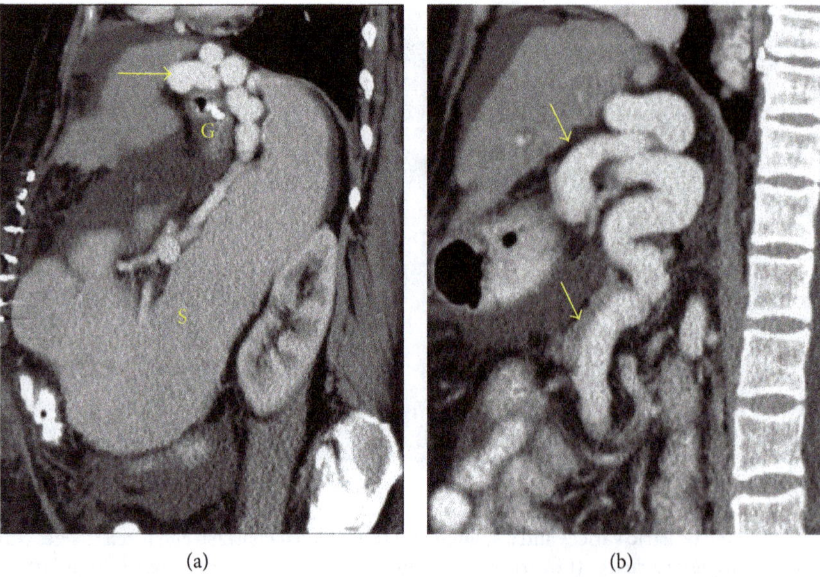

Figure 17: Splenomegaly in a cirrhotic patient with portal hypertension. Sagittal contrast-enhanced CT images ((a)-(b)) show an enlarged spleen (S) associated with retrogastric varices (long arrow) and splenorenal shunt (short arrows). G: gastric fundus.

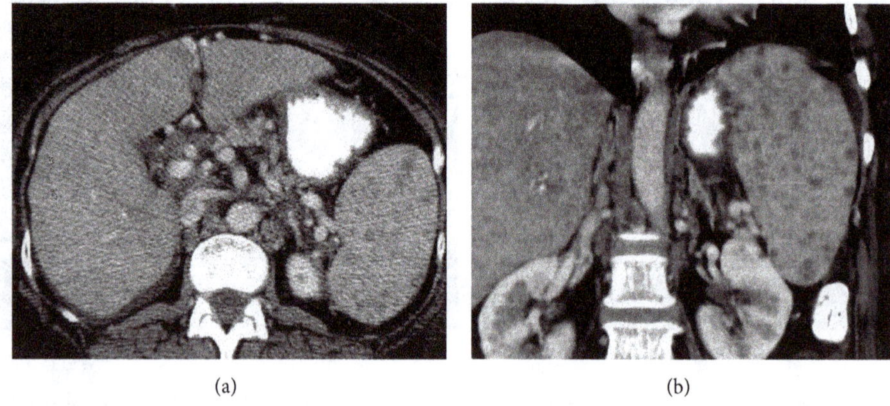

Figure 18: Gamna-Gandy bodies in a patient with portal hypertension. Axial (a) and coronal (b) contrast-enhanced CT images demonstrate an enlarged spleen with multiple low density foci representing hemosiderin deposition.

omental and retroperitoneal edema. Most of the patients with mesenteric, omental, or retroperitoneal edema demonstrate a patchy, infiltrative pattern of fat stranding. The presence of retroperitoneal edema without mesenteric edema is uncommon. In some instances, focal edema may simulate a soft tissue mass. The severity of mesenteric edema parallels other manifestations of fluid overload in patients with cirrhosis such as subcutaneous edema, pleural effusion, and ascites [16].

Gastrointestinal wall thickening occurs in 64% of cirrhotic patients, usually as a result of submucosal edema. The jejunum and the ascending colon are the most common sites of involvement (Figure 19). In almost all cases, the pattern of wall thickening is concentric with homogeneous enhancement after administration of intravenous contrast. Thickening of the colonic haustra has been described in patients with cirrhosis [17].

Hepatic cirrhosis may cause diffuse gallbladder wall thickening. The exact pathophysiologic mechanism leading to edema of the gallbladder wall is uncertain, but it is likely due to elevated portal venous pressure, decreased intravascular osmotic pressure, hypoproteinemia, or a combination of these factors [18]. Recognition of this abnormality is essential to avoid erroneous interpretations and unnecessary cholecystectomy.

Ascites is defined as the pathologic accumulation of fluid in the peritoneal cavity. It is the most common complication of cirrhosis [19]. Within 10 years of the diagnosis of compensated cirrhosis, about 50% of patients will have developed ascites [20]. The development of ascites is the final consequence of anatomic and pathophysiologic abnormalities occurring in patients with cirrhosis. The formation of ascites is governed by the same principles as edema formation at other sites: net capillary permeability and the

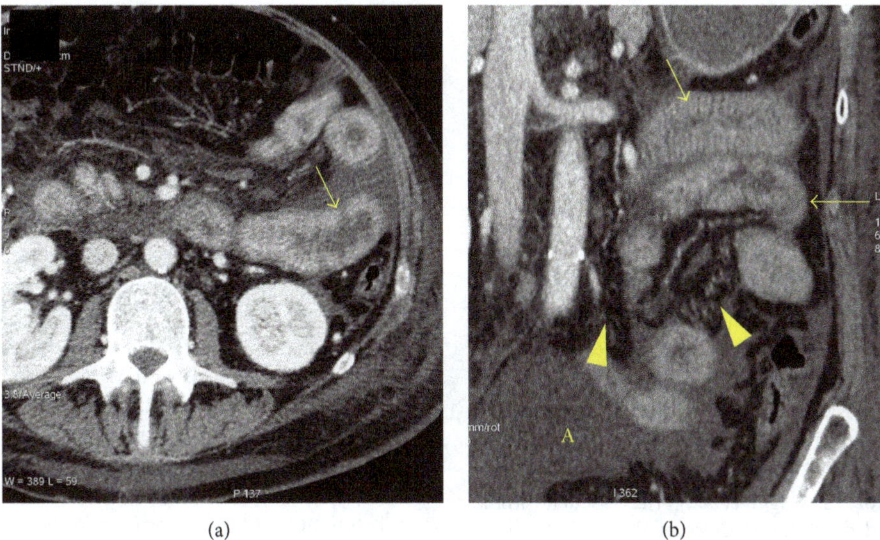

(a) (b)

FIGURE 19: Small bowel wall thickening in a patient with hypoproteinemia due to hepatic cirrhosis. Axial (a) and coronal (b) contrast-enhanced CT images show diffuse thickening of the bowel wall and folds (arrows). Ascites (A) and mesenteric edema (arrowheads) are noted.

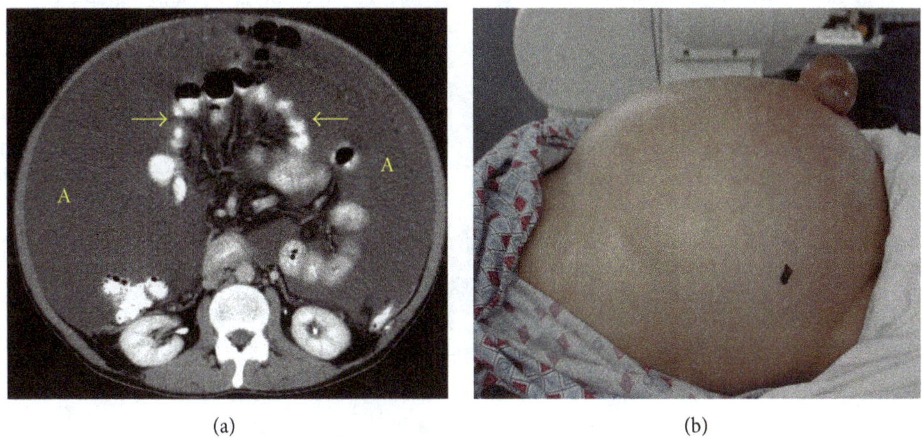

(a) (b)

FIGURE 20: Tension ascites in a cirrhotic patient. (a) An axial contrast-enhanced CT demonstrates a large intraperitoneal low density fluid collection (A). Central displacement of the bowel and mesenteric structures (arrows) commonly seen in patients with benign intraperitoneal fluid (transudate). (b) Photograph of the patient's abdomen before decompressive paracentesis.

hydraulic/oncotic pressure gradients. Patients with cirrhosis but without portal hypertension do not develop ascites. Typical ascitic fluid in cirrhotic patients is a yellow-amber transudate with a total protein concentration of less than 2.5 g/dL and with relatively few cells (Figure 20).

4. Summary

Hepatic cirrhosis is a multifactorial condition with increasing incidence worldwide. HCC, its most lethal complication, is seen in 11% of cases after 5 years of hepatitis related cirrhosis. A triple phase evaluation of the liver with CT is essential to detect small HCCs. The recognition of the extrahepatic abdominal complications is vital for adequate clinical assessment and treatment.

References

[1] J. J. Brown, M. J. Naylor, and N. Yagan, "Imaging of hepatic cirrhosis," *Radiology*, vol. 202, no. 1, pp. 1–16, 1997.

[2] G. Brancatelli, R. L. Baron, M. S. Peterson, and W. Marsh, "Helical CT screening for hepatocellular carcinoma in patients with cirrhosis: frequency and causes of false-positive interpretation," *American Journal of Roentgenology*, vol. 180, no. 4, pp. 1007–1014, 2003.

[3] Y. Itai, S. Murata, and Y. Kurosaki, "Straight border sign of the liver: spectrum of CT appearances and causes," *Radiographics*, vol. 15, no. 5, pp. 1089–1102, 1995.

[4] K. Ohtomo, R. L. Baron, G. D. Dodd III et al., "Confluent hepatic fibrosis in advanced cirrhosis: appearance at CT," *Radiology*, vol. 188, no. 1, pp. 31–35, 1993.

[5] A. A. Gupta, D. C. Kim, G. A. Krinsky, and V. S. Lee, "CT and MRI of cirrhosis and its mimics," *American Journal of Roentgenology*, vol. 183, no. 6, pp. 1595–1601, 2004.

[6] P. J. Mergo, P. R. Ros, P. C. Buetow, and J. L. Buck, "Diffuse disease of the liver: radiologic-pathologic correlation," *Radiographics*, vol. 14, no. 6, pp. 1291–1307, 1994.

[7] I. R. Wanless, F. Callea, J. R. Craig et al., "Terminology of nodular hepatocellular lesions," *Hepatology*, vol. 22, no. 3, pp. 983–993, 1995.

[8] G. D. Dodd III, R. L. Baron, J. H. Oliver III, and M. P. Federle, "Spectrum of imaging findings of the liver in end-stage cirrhosis: part II, focal abnormalities," *American Journal of Roentgenology*, vol. 173, no. 5, pp. 1185–1192, 1999.

[9] O. Matsui, M. Kadoya, T. Kameyama et al., "Benign and malignant nodules in cirrhotic livers: distinction based on blood supply," *Radiology*, vol. 178, no. 2, pp. 493–497, 1991.

[10] M. Roncalli, E. Roz, G. Coggi et al., "The vascular profile of regenerative and dysplastic nodules of the cirrhotic liver: implications for diagnosis and classification," *Hepatology*, vol. 30, no. 5, pp. 1174–1178, 1999.

[11] J. H. Lim, C. K. Kim, W. J. Lee et al., "Detection of hepatocellular carcinomas and dysplastic nodules in cirrhotic livers: accuracy of helical CT in transplant patients," *American Journal of Roentgenology*, vol. 175, no. 3, pp. 693–698, 2000.

[12] W. B. Coleman, "Mechanisms of human hepatocarcinogenesis," *Current Molecular Medicine*, vol. 3, no. 6, pp. 573–588, 2003.

[13] R. L. Baron and M. S. Peterson, "From the RSNA refresher courses: screening the cirrhotic liver for hepatocellular carcinoma with CT and MR imaging: opportunities and pitfalls," *Radiographics*, vol. 21, pp. S117–S132, 2001.

[14] R. L. Baron, J. H. Oliver III, G. D. Dodd III, M. Nalesnik, B. L. Holbert, and B. Carr, "Hepatocellular carcinoma: evaluation with biphasic, contrast-enhanced, helical CT," *Radiology*, vol. 199, no. 2, pp. 505–511, 1996.

[15] O. Matsui, "Imaging of multistep human hepatocarcinogenesis by CT during intra-arterial contrast injection," *Intervirology*, vol. 47, no. 3-5, pp. 271–276, 2004.

[16] J. H. Oliver III and R. L. Baron, "Helical biphasic contrast-enhanced CT of the liver: technique, indications, interpretation, and pitfalls," *Radiology*, vol. 201, no. 1, pp. 1–14, 1996.

[17] A. Ronzoni, D. Artioli, R. Scardina et al., "Role of MDCT in the diagnosis of hepatocellular carcinoma in patients with cirrhosis undergoing orthotopic liver transplantation," *American Journal of Roentgenology*, vol. 189, no. 4, pp. 792–798, 2007.

[18] G. A. Krinsky, V. S. Lee, N. D. Theise et al., "Hepatocellular carcinoma and dysplastic nodules in patients with cirrhosis: prospective diagnosis with MR imaging and explantation correlation," *Radiology*, vol. 219, no. 2, pp. 445–454, 2001.

[19] R. D. Redvanly, R. C. Nelson, A. C. Stieber, and G. D. Dodd III, "Imaging in the preoperative evaluation of adult liver-transplant candidates: goals, merits of various procedures, and recommendations," *American Journal of Roentgenology*, vol. 164, no. 3, pp. 611–617, 1995.

[20] J. Bruix and M. Sherman, "Management of hepatocellular carcinoma: an update," *Hepatology*, vol. 53, no. 3, pp. 1020–1022, 2011.

[21] R. H. Wachsberg, P. Bahramipour, C. T. Sofocleous, and A. Barone, "Hepatofugal flow in the portal venous system: pathophysiology, imaging findings, and diagnostic pitfalls," *Radiographics*, vol. 22, no. 1, pp. 123–140, 2002.

[22] K. M. Elsayes, V. R. Narra, G. Mukundan, J. S. Lewis Jr., C. O. Menias, and J. P. Heiken, "MR imaging of the spleen: spectrum of abnormalities," *Radiographics*, vol. 25, no. 4, pp. 967–982, 2005.

7

Effect of the Human Amniotic Membrane on Liver Regeneration in Rats

Mesut Sipahi,[1] Sevinç Şahin,[2] Ergin Arslan,[1] Hasan Börekci,[1] Bayram Metin,[3] and Nuh Zafer Cantürk[4]

[1]*Department of General Surgery, School of Medicine, Bozok University, 66100 Yozgat, Turkey*
[2]*Department of Pathology, School of Medicine, Bozok University, 66100 Yozgat, Turkey*
[3]*Department of Thoracic Surgery, School of Medicine, Bozok University, 66100 Yozgat, Turkey*
[4]*Department of General Surgery, School of Medicine, Kocaeli University, 41000 Kocaeli, Turkey*

Correspondence should be addressed to Mesut Sipahi; sipahi@dr.com

Academic Editor: Richard Charnley

Introduction. Operations are performed for broader liver surgery indications for a better understanding of hepatic anatomy/physiology and developments in operation technology. Surgery can cure some patients with liver metastasis of some tumors. Nevertheless, postoperative liver failure is the most feared complication causing mortality in patients who have undergone excision of a large liver mass. The human amniotic membrane has regenerative effects. Thus, we investigated the effects of the human amniotic membrane on regeneration of the resected liver. *Methods.* Twenty female Wistar albino rats were divided into control and experimental groups and underwent a 70% hepatectomy. The human amniotic membrane was placed over the residual liver in the experimental group. Relative liver weight, histopathological features, and biochemical parameters were assessed on postoperative day 3. *Results.* Total protein and albumin levels were significantly lower in the experimental group than in the control group. No difference in relative liver weight was observed between the groups. Hepatocyte mitotic count was significantly higher in the experimental group than in the control group. Hepatic steatosis was detected in the experimental group. *Conclusion.* Applying the amniotic membrane to residual liver adversely affected liver regeneration. However, mesenchymal stem cell research has the potential to accelerate liver regeneration investigations.

1. Introduction

The liver is a vital metabolic organ and is the first of many locations for the development of cancer metastases due to dual feeding by the hepatic artery and portal vein. Hepatic resection is a safe method for some benign and malignant diseases, and the mortality rate of liver resection has decreased to <5% due to advances in technology, surgical techniques, and a better understanding of hepatic physiology and anatomy [1]. In particular, liver resection for colorectal cancer metastasis affects survival positively. In fact, some patients have a potentially curative treatment [2]. However, liver failure is one of the most common complications of liver resection surgery and the main cause of morbidity and mortality [3–5]. Factors predictive of liver failure include patient, surgical, and postoperative factors. Diabetes mellitus, obesity, steatohepatitis, hepatitis B and C, malnutrition, renal failure, hyperbilirubinemia, thrombocytopenia, pulmonary disease, liver cirrhosis, and age >65 years which are factors predictive of postoperative liver failure. Postoperative factors include hemorrhage and intra-abdominal infections. Operative factors include a blood loss >1200 mL during surgery, blood transfusion requirement, resection of the vena cava or other vessels, operative time >240 min, resected liver volume >50%, right lobe resection with major hepatectomy, a skeletonized hepatoduodenal ligament, and remnant liver <25% of the liver mass [4]. Portal vein embolization and two-stage hepatectomy methods are currently applied successfully to prevent postoperative liver failure [6]. However, estimated postresection liver volume is one of the most important factors limiting resection. A rapid regeneration method after hepatectomy could expand the indications for liver resection in selected patients.

The human amniotic membrane (HAM) is currently used to treat corneal wounds in patients with burns injuries and intestinal anastomosis, as it has a positive healing effect [7, 8]. The HAM also has hypoimmunogenic properties and has been used as a xenograft without tissue rejection [7, 9]. Because of this feature in many animal experiments study, human amniotic membrane was successfully used as xenograft and allograft [7, 8, 10]. In the present study, we investigated the effects of overlaying the HAM on remnant liver and on its regeneration after liver resection.

2. Materials and Methods

This study was performed at the Kocaeli University Experimental Animal Research Center with approval (number = 7/2 – 2013) from the Kocaeli University Institutional Ethics Committee.

2.1. Animals. Twenty female Wistar rats (weight range, 212–275 g; same age) were used in this study. Standard rat chow and tap water were provided to the rats. The rats were maintained under a 12-h light:dark photoperiod and normal laboratory conditions. All surgical procedures were performed in the afternoon to prevent an influence of the circadian rhythm. The rats were divided randomly into control ($n = 10$) and experimental groups ($n = 10$).

2.2. HAM Preparation. Written consent was obtained from pregnant women who were negative for hepatitis B and C as well as human immunodeficiency virus. The placenta was transported quickly after cesarean section to the laboratory in a sterile box with saline. A 20 mL sterile syringe was immersed in the saline and used to separate the membrane with air. The HAM was dissected while immersed in Dakin's solution for 15 min to clean off the blood and other contaminants. Mechanical cleaning was performed using saline. The HAM was incubated with saline containing 50 mg/mL penicillin, 50 mg/mL streptomycin, 100 μg/mL neomycin, and 2.5 mg/mL amphotericin B for 10 min. The HAM was sectioned into 1.5- × 3-cm pieces and maintained between wet sterile cloths impregnated with saline.

2.3. Surgical Procedures. The rats were fasted for 6 h before surgery. Anesthesia was induced by intraperitoneal administration of 50 mg/kg ketamine (Ketalar; Parke Davis, İstanbul, Turkey) and 5 mg/kg xylazine hydrochloride (Rompun; Bayer AG, Leverkusen, Germany). The rats were provided water. The abdominal area was disinfected with 10% povidone-iodine solution, and a midline abdominal incision was made under sterile conditions. The left lateral and medial lobes of the liver were cut, and a 70% hepatectomy was performed based on the method described by Higgis [11, 12]. The abdominal incision was closed using continuous 3/0 Prolene sutures. After the hepatectomy, the 1.5- × 3-cm sections of HAM were overlaid onto the remnant liver in the experiential group. All other procedures were performed exactly the same between the two groups. Resected liver weight was recorded as the excision weight (mg). The rats were offered food and water postoperatively. Approximately 72 h later, the rats were anesthetized using the same method, and their weights (g) were measured. The abdominal and chest cavities were opened via a midline thoracoabdominal incision. Blood (2 mL) was drawn from the heart prior to excision of the remnant liver. The remnant liver weight (mg) was measured, and a specimen was maintained in 10% formaldehyde for pathological examination. The blood samples were centrifuged for 5 min at 3500 rpm, and the serum fraction was transferred to a separate tube for biochemical analyses.

2.4. Relative Liver Weight. Preoperative liver weight was considered to be 3.4% of the preoperative body weight and calculated [13]. Residual liver weight was calculated as the excised liver weight subtracted from the preoperative liver weight. Regenerative liver weights were calculated by subtracting the residual liver weight from the remnant liver weight during necropsy. Relative liver weight was calculated as the regenerative liver weight divided by the preoperative liver weight multiplied by 100. Relative liver weight was standardized as such [14].

2.5. Biochemical Analyses. Blood samples were collected from the heart, and the serum was separated by centrifugation (3000 rpm at 4°C for 15 min) and stored at −80°C for biochemical analyses. Serum total protein (T Prot) g/dL, total bilirubin (T Bil) mg/dL, direct bilirubin (D Bil) mg/dL, indirect bilirubin (I Bil) mg/dL, and albumin (Alb) g/dL levels were determined using an automated Architect C-4000 analyzer (Abbott Laboratories, Abbott Park, IL, USA). Aspartate aminotransferase (AST) IU/L, alanine aminotransferase (ALT) IU/L, and lactate dehydrogenase (LDH) IU/L levels were measured using an Architect C-8000 autoanalyzer (Abbott Laboratories) at Bozok University, School of Medicine, Central Laboratory, Yozgat, Turkey.

2.6. Histopathological Analyses. All specimens were transported to the pathology laboratory in 10% neutral formalin. Approximately 1-mm^2 tissue pieces were sampled from each case. All samples were processed in an automated system (Excelsior ES; Thermo Scientific, Rockford, IL, USA), and paraffin blocks were prepared using the HistoStar embedding station (Thermo Scientific). Two tissue sections 3–6-μm-thick were obtained from each case using a microtome (Shandon-Finesse ME+; Thermo Scientific). One was stained with hematoxylin and eosin (H&E) using an automated slide staining machine (Varistain Gemini; Thermo Scientific), and the other one was stained using a Ki-67 antibody (7 mL-RTU, mouse anti-human monoclonal antibody clone K2; Leica Biosystems, Danvers, MA, USA) in an automated immunohistochemical staining system (Leica-Bond Max, Leica Biosystems). The H&E- and Ki-67-stained slides were evaluated under a light microscope (BX53F; Olympus, Tokyo, Japan) by a pathologist. Nuclear staining for Ki-67 was considered as positive. The number of Ki-67-stained cells was

TABLE 1: The results of the biochemical analysis.

n	T Prot (g/dL)	Alb (g/dL)	T bil (mg/dL)	D Bil (mg/dL)	AST (IU/L)	ALT (IU/L)	LDH (IU/L)
				Study group			
1	6,4	3,1	0,1	0,1	163	76	74
2	6,3	3,2	0,2	0,1	171	96	217
3	5,9	3	0,2	0,1	234	99	349
4	5,3	2,5	0,1	0,1	241	89	212
5	6,5	3,2	0,2	0,2	221	136	144
6	6	3	0,1	0,1	162	76	580
7	5,5	2,8	0,1	0,1	433	100	196
8	5,9	2,8	0,1	0,1	192	77	625
9	6	3	0,2	0,1	159	88	176
				Control group			
1	7,3	3,3	0,2	0,1	326	123	654
2	7,3	3,5	0,2	0,1	141	103	324
3	6,8	3,2	0,2	0,1	171	114	140
4	6,7	3,2	0,2	0,1	196	103	543
5	6,8	3,2	0,1	0,1	155	118	503
6	6,9	3,2	0,2	0,1	222	110	400
7	7,5	3,3	0,2	0,1	161	78	254
8	6,3	3	0,2	0,1	182	103	190

counted in three different areas containing most of the Ki-67 positive cells using a ×100 objective with immersion oil. Then, the arithmetic mean of the number of Ki-67-positive cells was calculated. All H&E sections were evaluated for mitotic figures in 10 high power fields (×40 objective) and for histopathological changes.

2.7. Statistical Analyses. The SPSS for Windows 18.0 (SPSS Inc., Chicago, IL, USA) software package was used for statistical analyses. Means, standard deviations, ranges, and percentages were calculated. The Mann-Whitney U test was used for normally distributed data of weight loss, mitotic count, and levels of AST, LDH, total and direct bilirubin, and C-reactive protein. Ki-67 expression, relative liver weight, ALT, and total protein values were in the normal range. Student's t-test was used to examine these parameters. A P value < 0.05 was considered significant.

3. Results

Two rats in the control group died during the surgical procedure due to vena cava injuries. Direct bilirubin value was >7 mg/dL due to an iatrogenic bile duct obstruction in one rat in the experimental group, and the rat was excluded. Thus, nine rats were included in the experimental group and eight in the control group.

Mean preoperative body weights in the experimental and control group were 246.33 and 256.63 g, and postoperative weights were 221.11 and 221.00 g, respectively. Weight loss was calculated to be 31.38 g. No difference was detected between the groups in terms of weight loss ($P = 0.277$).

The control group had normal appearance of the resected livers. But, in the study group, they were like fatty liver disease

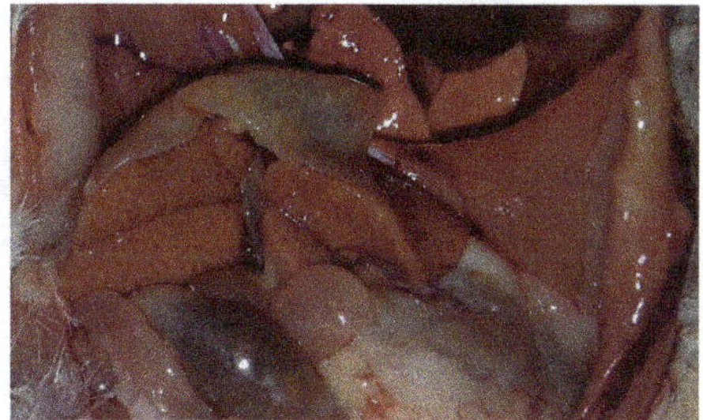

FIGURE 1: Resected liver in study group.

(Figure 1). The mean resected liver weight was 5.41 ± 0.36 g in the experimental group and 5.82 ± 0.43 g in the control group. Excision percentages were calculated according to the preoperative liver weight. Consequently, a mean of 64.83% of the liver tissue was excised in the experimental group and 66.76% in the control group ($P = 0.103$). The results of the biochemical analysis are shown in Table 1. Serum total protein and albumin levels were higher in the control group than in the experimental group ($P < 0.01$). No significant differences were observed in the AST, ALT, LDH, and total and direct bilirubin levels between the groups. The mean Ki-67 level in the postoperative remnant liver tissue was 54.67 ± 8.99 in the experimental group and 51.75±9.00 in the control group ($P = 0.515$) (Figure 2). Relative liver weight tended to be higher in the experimental group (29.61 ± 5.60 g) than in the control group (27.34 ± 3.77 g) ($P = 0.348$). In contrast, the mitotic index in the remnant liver tissue was 4.22 ± 2.91 in the experimental group and 0.50 ± 1.07 in the control group ($P < 0.01$) (Table 2, Figure 3). Histopathologically, there was no specific change, tumor cell, and significant difference in inflammatory cells in the liver of study and

TABLE 2: Ki-67 levels and evaluation of liver weights.

n	Ki-67 level	Resected liver weigh (g)	Residual liver weigh (g)	Relative liver weight (g)
		Study group		
1	57	4,89	2,32	37,82
2	61	5,84	3,51	31,97
3	57	4,92	2,97	23,9
4	62	5,54	3,27	25,87
5	55	5,49	3,18	31,67
6	49	5,32	2,84	24,19
7	58	5,68	2,55	37,77
8	60	5,24	2,58	23,99
9	33	5,86	3,39	29,31
		Control group		
1	48	5,1	2,72	26,59
2	53	5,97	2,81	34,49
3	47	5,56	3,18	25,62
4	60	6,06	2,99	27,99
5	42	6,32	2,76	28,38
6	41	5,59	2,88	21,94
7	67	5,69	2,95	24,24
8	56	6,36	2,89	29,43

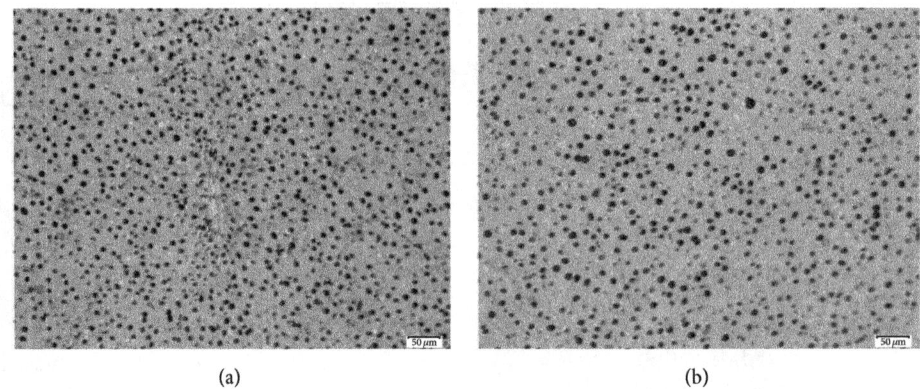

(a) (b)

FIGURE 2: (a) Microscopic photo illustrating high Ki-67 positivity of a case of control group (Avidin-biotin-peroxidase method, ×200). (b) Microscopic photo illustrating high Ki-67 positivity of an amniotic membrane used case (Avidin-biotin-peroxidase method, ×200).

control groups. However, macrovesicular steatosis with large and small droplets was detected in all postoperative remnant liver tissues. Steatosis comprised 70% to 95% of those tissues. Thus, severe hepatic macrovesicular steatosis was observed in residual liver tissue from the experimental group compared with the control group (Figure 4).

4. Discussion

The liver is capable of regenerating and can reach its previous size and function quickly. Thus, hepatic resections are often completed easily without complications, although posthepatectomy liver failure may arise in cases of massive hepatic resection [15]. The liver regeneration process in rats and mice is completed within 5–7 days after surgery [16]. The incidence rate of liver failure is reported to be 10% in patients undergoing major liver resection [17]. Posthepatectomized liver failure is a major cause of mortality and morbidity in patients undergoing liver resection [4]. According to Shoup et al., posthepatectomy liver failure results in a threefold increased risk of death in patients with a postresection volume <25% of the preoperative liver volume [18]. Methods such as portal vein embolization and two-stage hepatectomy have been used successfully to increase residual volume [6]. Techniques that enable rapid regeneration of residual liver volume can be effective for preventing posthepatectomy failure and expand resection indications.

Liver regeneration is regulated by complex mechanisms. Intercellular communication, growth factors, and cytokines, particularly hepatocyte growth factor, transforming growth factor-α, epidermal growth factor, tumor necrosis factor, and interleukin-6, play important roles in liver regeneration. Some studies have shown that these factors accelerate regeneration and growth of the liver mass [19, 20].

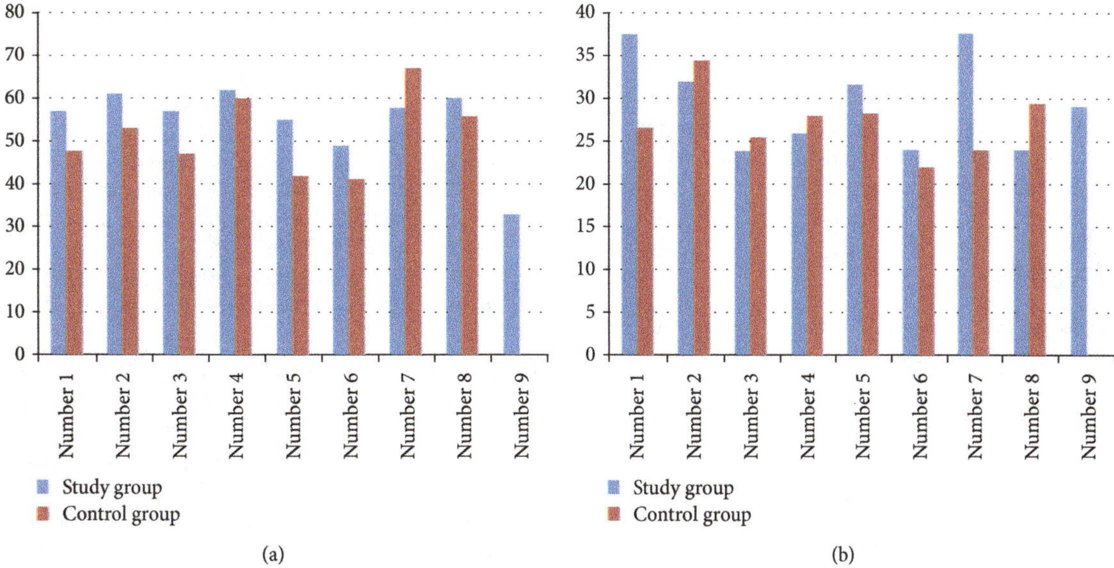

FIGURE 3: (a) Ki-67 levels. (b) Relative Liver weights (g).

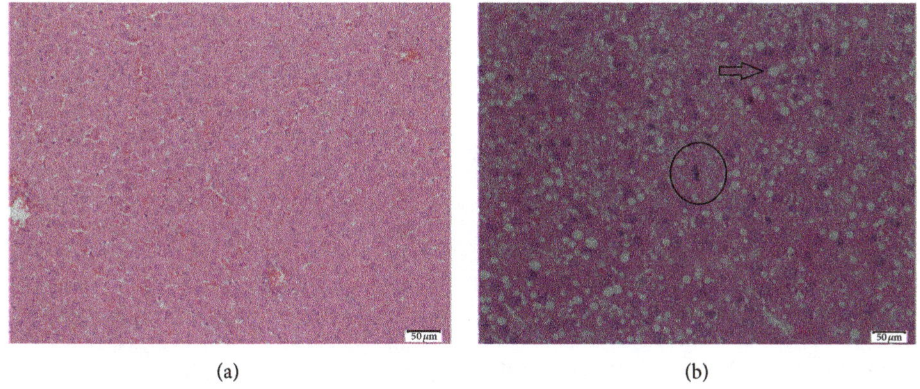

FIGURE 4: (a) The biopsy of a case of control group showing no considerable specific pathology (H&E, ×200). (b) The photomicrograph of an amniotic membrane used case showing extensive macrovesicular steatosis (*arrow*) and a mitotic figure (*circle*) (H&E, ×400).

HAM is a mesenchymal stem cell source that expresses these factors [7]. HAM has the potential for cells to differentiate into hepatocytes, cardiomyocytes, chondrocytes, pancreatic B-cells, and neuronal cells [9]. Laminin is a major component of the HAM that plays an important role in cell differentiation and shaping. [9]. Jia et al. resected 70% of the rat liver and showed a positive effect on liver regeneration by placing HAM on the abdominal wall muscles [10].

We found no difference in AST, ALT, LDH, or total and direct bilirubin levels between the groups in our study. Total protein and albumin levels were significantly lower in the experimental group than in the control group. No differences in relative liver weights or Ki-67 levels were detected between the groups on postoperative day 3. Severe hepatic steatosis was observed in the experimental group compared with the control group. Based on these findings, we concluded that applying the HAM was ineffective for enhancing liver regeneration and could lead to liver cirrhosis. Previous studies used the HAM as a xenograft without tissue rejection reactions in organs such as the intestines, skin, and cornea [7, 8, 21]. The HAM is hypoimmunogenic with no HLA class II antigens. It has low levels of HLA class IA and high levels of class IB and HLA-G [9, 22]. Jia et al. showed that placing HAM in the abdominal muscles increased the rate of liver regeneration [10]. We believe that our negative results were caused by immune response mechanisms, cytokines, and cell interactions. However, the evaluation parameters were inadequate in our study. The number of mitoses was higher in the experimental group than in the control group, which was a sign of increased liver regeneration induced by the HAM. However, the increase in mitosis was not reflected by an increase in relative liver weight. We do not have mitotic results from day 1 or 7. In the literature, we found no experiments using rat amniotic membrane. But we think that using allograft may be of different results. Thus, additional studies are needed using different methods.

5. Conclusion

Spreading the HAM on rat liver negatively affected liver regeneration. Nevertheless, stem cell research, such as studies using the HAM, continues to provide hope for postoperative liver regeneration. Further clinical and experimental studies are needed to understand the mechanisms.

Acknowledgment

This study was supported by the Bozok University BAP unit (Scientific Research Project Unit).

References

[1] M. Demiray, H. F. Kucuk, M. Yildirim, and N. O. Barisik, "No harmful effect of mycophenolate mofetil on liver regeneration: an experimental study," *Transplantation Proceedings*, vol. 44, no. 6, pp. 1743–1746, 2012.

[2] J.-N. Vauthey, T. M. Pawlik, D. Ribero et al., "Chemotherapy regimen predicts steatohepatitis and an increase in 90-day mortality after surgery for hepatic colorectal metastases," *Journal of Clinical Oncology*, vol. 24, no. 13, pp. 2065–2072, 2006.

[3] R. G. Dan, O. M. Creţu, O. Mazilu et al., "Postoperative morbidity and mortality after liver resection. Retrospective study on 133 patients," *Chirurgia*, vol. 107, no. 6, pp. 737–744, 2012.

[4] R. Kauffmann and Y. Fong, "Post-hepatectomy liver failure," *Hepatobiliary Surgery and Nutrition*, vol. 3, no. 5, pp. 238–246, 2014.

[5] F. Ayan, E. Aytaç, S. Saygili et al., "Effects of lycopene on oxidative stress and remnant liver histology after partial hepatectomy in rats," *The Turkish Journal of Gastroenterology*, vol. 22, no. 4, pp. 408–413, 2011.

[6] Y. Yokoyama, M. Nagino, and Y. Nimura, "Mechanisms of hepatic regeneration following portal vein embolization and partial hepatectomy: a review," *World Journal of Surgery*, vol. 31, no. 2, pp. 367–374, 2007.

[7] M. Uludag, B. Citgez, O. Ozkaya et al., "Effects of amniotic membrane on the healing of primary colonic anastomoses in the cecal ligation and puncture model of secondary peritonitis in rats," *International Journal of Colorectal Disease*, vol. 24, no. 5, pp. 559–567, 2009.

[8] A. A. Mohammadi, H. G. Johari, and S. Eskandari, "Effect of amniotic membrane on graft take in extremity burns," *Burns*, vol. 39, no. 6, pp. 1137–1141, 2013.

[9] A. Toda, M. Okabe, T. Yoshida, and T. Nikaido, "The potential of amniotic membrane/amnion-derived cells for regeneration of various tissues," *Journal of Pharmacological Sciences*, vol. 105, no. 3, pp. 215–228, 2007.

[10] X. Jia, Z. Haitao, L. Ji, and L. Ning, "Research on liver regeneration driven by the amniotic membrane," *Chinese Medical Journal*, vol. 127, no. 7, pp. 1382–1384, 2014.

[11] G. Higgins and R. Anderson, "Experimental pathology of the liver, I. Restoration of the liver of the white rat following partial surgical removal," *Archives of Pathology*, vol. 12, pp. 186–202, 1931.

[12] E. Steiger, H. M. Vars, and S. J. Dudrick, "A technique for long-term intravenous feeding in unrestrained rats," *Archives of Surgery*, vol. 104, no. 3, pp. 330–332, 1972.

[13] K. Kogure, Y.-Q. Zhang, H. Shibata, and I. Kojima, "Immediate onset of DNA synthesis in remnant rat liver after 90% hepatectomy by an administration of follistatin," *Journal of Hepatology*, vol. 29, no. 6, pp. 977–984, 1998.

[14] F. C. Fishback, "A morphologic study of regeneration of the liver after partial removal," *Archives of Pathology*, vol. 7, pp. 955–977, 1929.

[15] G. Garcea and G. J. Maddern, "Liver failure after major hepatic resection," *Journal of Hepato-Biliary-Pancreatic Surgery*, vol. 16, no. 2, pp. 145–155, 2009.

[16] G. K. Michalopoulos, "Liver regeneration," *Journal of Cellular Physiology*, vol. 213, no. 2, pp. 286–300, 2007.

[17] C. Paugam-Burtz, S. Janny, D. Delefosse et al., "Prospective validation of the 'fifty-fifty' criteria as an early and accurate predictor of death after liver resection in intensive care unit patients," *Annals of Surgery*, vol. 249, no. 1, pp. 124–128, 2009.

[18] M. Shoup, M. Gonen, M. D'Angelica et al., "Volumetric analysis predicts hepatic dysfunction in patients undergoing major liver resection," *Journal of Gastrointestinal Surgery*, vol. 7, no. 3, pp. 325–330, 2003.

[19] K. Takahashi, S. Murata, and N. Ohkohchi, "Novel therapy for liver regeneration by increasing the number of platelets," *Surgery Today*, vol. 43, no. 10, pp. 1081–1087, 2013.

[20] J. G. Tralhão, A. M. Abrantes, E. Hoti et al., "Hepatectomy and liver regeneration: from experimental research to clinical application," *ANZ Journal of Surgery*, vol. 84, no. 9, pp. 665–671, 2013.

[21] J. A. P. Gomes, A. Romano, M. S. Santos, and H. S. Dua, "Amniotic membrane use in ophthalmology," *Current Opinion in Ophthalmology*, vol. 16, no. 4, pp. 233–240, 2005.

[22] U. Manuelpillai, J. Tchongue, D. Lourensz et al., "Transplantation of human amnion epithelial cells reduces hepatic fibrosis in immunocompetent CCl_4-treated mice," *Cell Transplantation*, vol. 19, no. 9, pp. 1157–1168, 2010.

8

Comparison of Ranson, Glasgow, MOSS, SIRS, BISAP, APACHE-II, CTSI Scores, IL-6, CRP, and Procalcitonin in Predicting Severity, Organ Failure, Pancreatic Necrosis, and Mortality in Acute Pancreatitis

Ajay K. Khanna,[1] Susanta Meher,[1] Shashi Prakash,[1] Satyendra Kumar Tiwary,[1] Usha Singh,[2] Arvind Srivastava,[3] and V. K. Dixit[4]

[1] *Department of General Surgery, Institute of Medical Sciences, Banaras Hindu University, Varanasi, Ultra Pradesh 221005, India*
[2] *Department of Pathology, Institute of Medical Sciences, Banaras Hindu University, Varanasi, Ultra Pradesh 221005, India*
[3] *Department of Radiodiagnosis, Institute of Medical Sciences, Banaras Hindu University, Varanasi, Ultra Pradesh 221005, India*
[4] *Department of Gastroenterology, Institute of Medical Sciences, Banaras Hindu University, Varanasi, Ultra Pradesh 221005, India*

Correspondence should be addressed to Ajay K. Khanna; akhannabhu@gmail.com

Academic Editor: Attila Olah

Background. Multifactorial scorings, radiological scores, and biochemical markers may help in early prediction of severity, pancreatic necrosis, and mortality in patients with acute pancreatitis (AP). *Methods.* BISAP, APACHE-II, MOSS, and SIRS scores were calculated using data within 24 hrs of admission, whereas Ranson and Glasgow scores after 48 hrs of admission; CTSI was calculated on day 4 whereas IL-6 and CRP values at end of study. Predictive accuracy of scoring systems, sensitivity, specificity, and positive and negative predictive values of various markers in prediction of severe acute pancreatitis, organ failure, pancreatic necrosis, admission to intensive care units and mortality were calculated. *Results.* Of 72 patients, 31 patients had organ failure and local complication classified as severe acute pancreatitis, 17 had pancreatic necrosis, and 9 died (12.5%). Area under curves for Ranson, Glasgow, MOSS, SIRS, APACHE-II, BISAP, CTSI, IL-6, and CRP in predicting SAP were 0.85, 0.75, 0.73, 0.73, 0.88, 0.80, 0.90, and 0.91, respectively, for pancreatic necrosis 0.70, 0.64, 0.61, 0.61, 0.68, 0.61, 0.75, 0.86, and 0.90, respectively, and for mortality 0.84, 0.83, 0.77, 0.76, 0.86, 0.83, 0.57, 0.80, and 0.75, respectively. *Conclusion.* CRP and IL-6 have shown a promising result in early detection of severity and pancreatic necrosis whereas APACHE-II and Ranson score in predicting AP related mortality in this study.

1. Introduction

Acute pancreatitis (AP) is defined as an inflammatory process of the pancreas with possible peripancreatic tissue and multiorgan involvement inducing multiorgan dysfunction syndrome (MODS) with an increased mortality rate [1]. The incidence of acute pancreatitis per 100,000 population ranges from 5 to 80 cases per year, with the highest incidence rates being seen in Finland and the USA [2].

According to the Atlanta Classification, severe acute pancreatitis (SAP) is defined as an AP associated with local and/or systemic complications. Atlanta classification is a clinically based classification defining AP, severity, and complications. Development of organ dysfunction within 72 h of symptom onset is defined as an early severe acute pancreatitis (ESAP). Early severe acute pancreatitis is characterized by a short course, progressive MODS, early hypoxemia, increased incidence of necrosis, infection, and abdominal compartment syndrome (ACS) [3]. Multiorgan dysfunction syndrome, the extent of pancreatic necrosis, infection, and sepsis are the major determinants of mortality in AP [4]. Pancreatic necrosis is considered as a potential risk for infection, which represents the primary cause of late mortality. Occurrence of acute respiratory (ARF), cardiovascular (CVF), and renal failures (RF) can predict the fatal outcome in SAP [5]. A wide range of mortality (20%–60%) has been reported in

SAP. AP occurs when pancreatic enzymes are prematurely activated inside the pancreas leading to autodigestion of the gland and local inflammation [6]. These enzymes can also reach the bloodstream, stimulating the production of inflammatory cytokines and tumor necrosis factor-α (TNF-α) from leukocytes. The release of those substances triggers an inflammatory cascade, which leads to the SIRS [7]. Accurate diagnosis of SAP on admission to the hospital is of paramount importance and there is, therefore, agreement about the need for finding predictors of severe disease to identify patients who are at risk of morbidity and death.

Severe acute pancreatitis implies the presence of organ failure, local complications, or pancreatic necrosis and associated disruption of the pancreatic blood supply [8]. Several prognostic markers have been developed for severity stratification in acute pancreatitis. Multifactorial scoring systems incorporating clinical and biochemical criteria for severity assessment have been in use for some decades. These include the 11 criteria described by Ranson et al. in the 1970s [9], the Glasgow score (eight criteria), [10], MOSS score (12 criteria), BISAP score (5 criteria), and the acute physiology and chronic health evaluation (APACHE II) score (14 criteria) [11]. The sensitivity and specificity of these scoring systems for predicting severe acute pancreatitis range between 55% and 90%, depending on the cut-off number and the timing of scoring [12]. Limitations of these scoring systems have been either the inability to obtain a complete score until at least 48 hours into the illness (Ranson and Glasgow scores) or the complexity of the scoring system itself (APACHE II). The APACHE-II score has not been developed specifically for acute pancreatitis but has been proven to be an early and reliable tool.

Regarding imaging dynamic contrast-enhanced CT (DCT), it is the imaging modality of choice for staging acute pancreatitis and for detecting complications [13]. DCT has been shown to detect pancreatic parenchymal necrosis with a diagnostic sensitivity of 87% and an overall detection rate of 90% [13]. The morphologic severity of acute pancreatitis can be determined using a CT severity index (CTSI) that was developed by Balthazar and coworkers and then simplified and extended to monitor organ failure by Silverman, Banks, and colleagues in 2004 [13]. Comparison of the original CTSI with mortality showed a good correlation between higher CTSI values and mortality and morbidity, and this holds true for the modified CTSI. Furthermore, the modified CTSI correlates well with the length of hospital stay and the development of organ failure [13].

Among single biochemical markers, C-reactive protein (CRP) remains the most useful. Despite its delayed increase, peaking not earlier than 72 h after the onset of symptoms, it is accurate and widely available. As a single prognostic marker, an elevated C-reactive protein (CRP) concentration of greater than 150 mg/L indicates that acute pancreatitis has a complicated course with a sensitivity of 85% in the first 72 h after the onset of symptoms. Although detection of elevated CRP levels is sensitive for severe acute pancreatitis it is not specific for the disease, and other causes of inflammation such as cholangitis and pneumonia need to be ruled out before severity assessment by measurement of CRP [14]. Among them the proinflammatory cytokine interleukin 6 (IL-6) seems to be the most promising parameter for use in clinical routine. It has been proven to be significantly increased in severe acute pancreatitis in comparison with mild disease already on the day of admission to hospital [15], with a peak concentration on day 3 after the clinical onset of the disease, and therefore to be helpful for early severity stratification. Sensitivities of 69–100% with specificities in the range 70–86% for the detection of severe acute pancreatitis are reported [15]. As the concentrations increase earlier than those of acute-phase proteins, several clinical studies have addressed the usefulness of the early prediction of severe acute pancreatitis, resulting in promising results for interleukin 6. Procalcitonin (PCT) is another marker that has been evaluated as a prognostic indicator for pancreatitis. Procalcitonin, the biologically inactive propeptide of calcitonin, is a more rapid acute-phase reactant with the ability to indicate a status of bacterial or fungal infection and sepsis. Several studies have indicated its diagnostic value for the differentiation between mild and severe acute pancreatitis within the first 24 h of disease presentation [16], showing a sensitivity of 89% and a specificity of 82%, in a recent meta-analysis, but with a significant heterogeneity between individual studies [17].

2. Material and Methods

The aim of this prospective study was to study the various prognostic markers like Ranson, Glasgow, APACHE II, MOSS, SIRS, BISAP, CTSI, IL-6, CRP, and procalcitonin in cases of acute pancreatitis and to analyze the comparison between various prognostic markers in prediction of severe acute pancreatitis (SAP), organ failure (OF), pancreatic necrosis (PNec), length of hospital stay (LOHS), requirement of ICU admission (ICUA), and mortality in acute pancreatitis.

After approval by the Institutional Review Board, this prospective study included 72 patients who were clinically suspected to have acute pancreatitis in a single surgical unit in Department of General Surgery, IMS, BHU, in collaboration with the Department of Gastroenterology, Department of Pathology, Department of Radiology, and Causality services from July 2010 to July 2012. Informed and written consent was obtained from all patients. The diagnosis of acute pancreatitis (AP) was based on the presence of two of the following three features: (1) abdominal pain characteristic of AP, (2) serum amylase and/or lipase $\geq$3 times the upper limit of normal, and (3) characteristic finding of AP on abdominal CT Scan.

Demographic, radiographic, and laboratory data were collected from all these patients. In all these patients the following prognostic markers were used to know the severity of the disease (SAP), pancreatic necrosis (PNec), requirement of ICU admission, length of hospital stay (LOHS), and mortality: (1) Ranson score, (2) Glasgow score, (3) MOSS score, (4) SIRS score, (5) APACHE II score, (6) BISAP score, (7) CTSI score, (8) IL-6, (9) CRP, and (10) procalcitonin. BISAP score, APACHE II score, and multiple organ system score (MOSS) were calculated using data from the first

24 hours of admission and Ranson and Glasgow scores were calculated using data in first 24 hours and after 48 hours of admission. Presence of features of systemic inflammatory response syndrome (SIRS) was noted within the first 24 hours of admission. 2 mL of blood sample was collected on day 1 for IL-6. Serum was extracted after centrifugation in the Department of Pathology and stored at −72°C. Another 2 mL of blood sample was collected for procalcitonin card test. It is a semiquantitative method for rapid calculation of procalcitonin value using B.R.A.H.M.S. PCT-Q card. For this, serum was extracted from the blood sample after centrifugation. One drop of serum was put into the card and reading was taken after 30 minutes. Color of the test bar was matched with color given on the card. Value was noted according to the colour coding. Value ranging from <0.5 ng/mL up to >10 ng/mL. >0.5 ng/mL is taken as the cut-off value for detection of severity of acute pancreatitis according to the previous literature. This test was done in 42 cases only. On day 2 another 2 mL of blood sample was collected for C-reactive protein (CRP) and stored as serum at −72°C along with the samples of IL-6 to determine the value at the end of the study. CECT was performed in required cases on day 4 to look for pancreatic necrosis (PNec), local complications, and possible aetiology of AP. CTSI score was noted after CT scan.

Patients were classified as mild AP and severe AP, based on the presence of organ failure for more than 48 hrs and local complications. Organ failure included shock (systolic blood pressure < 90 mmHg), pulmonary insufficiency (arterial PO_2 < 60 mmHg at room air or the need for mechanical ventilation), or renal failure (serum creatinine level > 2 mg/dL after rehydration or hemodialysis). PNec was assessed by CECT; evidence of PNec on CT was defined as lack of enhancement of pancreatic parenchyma with contrast. At the end of the study, values of IL-6 and CRP were calculated using ELISA kit.

2.1. Statistics. Normally distributed continuous variables were expressed as means. At the selected cut-off scores, each predictive system was evaluated for significant relationship to the severity, organ failure, pancreatic necrosis, need for ICU admission, and mortality by two-by-two contingency tables. The diagnostic cut-off value was expressed as its sensitivity, specificity, positive predictive value, negative predictive value, accuracy, and the area under the curve (AUC) under the receiver-operator characteristic (ROC) curve. The predictive accuracy of each scoring system and biochemical marker was measured by the area under the receiver-operating curve (AUC). All statistical analysis was made with SPSS software version 16.

3. Observation and Results

3.1. Patient's Characteristics. Mean age of presentation was 40.5 years (range 18–76) with 51.4% males and 91.7% Hindu. The etiologies of AP included biliary (64%), alcoholic (13%), idiopathic (9%), hypertriglyceridemia (2%), post-ERCP (2%), and trauma (2%) (Table 1).

Table 1: Etiology of acute pancreatitis.

Etiology	No. of cases	Percentage
Biliary	44	61.1
Alcoholic	13	18.0
Idiopathic	9	12.5
Hypertriglyceridemia	2	2.8
Post-ERCP	2	2.8
Traumatic	2	2.8

ERCP: endoscopic retrograde cholangiopancreatography.

Thirty-one patients (43.1%) were diagnosed as having SAP (organ failure with local complications), twenty five patients (34.7%) developed persistent organ failure, and seventeen patients (23.6%) had evidence of pancreatic necrosis on CECT. The average length of hospital stay was 10 days. Nine patients (12.5%) needed ICU admission and nine patients (12.5%) died during hospitalization. 54 patients (75%) underwent CECT abdomen on day-4. IL-6 and CRP were done in 60 patients of whom 46.7% had IL-6 value of ≥50 pg/mL and 41.7% of cases had CRP value of ≥150 mg/L. Table 2 shows patient characteristics of the study cohort.

3.2. Comparison of Scoring Systems in Predicting SAP, Organ Failure, Pancreatic Necrosis, Length of Hospital Stay, ICU Admission, and Mortality. In prediction of SAP according to the AUC (with 95% CI) CRP (0.91 (0.83–0.99)) and IL-6 (0.90 (0.81–0.99)) had the highest accuracy, followed by APACHE II (0.88 (0.79–0.97)) and Ranson (0.85 (0.76–0.92)). Also for prediction of pancreatic necrosis according to AUC (with 95% CI) CRP (0.90 (0.82–0.97)) and IL-6 (0.86 (0.77–0.94)) had the highest accuracy as compared to other markers, followed by CTSI (0.75 (0.59–0.91)) and for prediction of mortality according to AUC (with 95% CI) accuracy was highest for APACHE II 0.86 (0.77–0.95) followed by Ranson score (0.84 (0.75–0.94)). AUCs for each scoring system in predicting SAP, PNEC, and mortality are shown in Table 3. Among the various markers CRP and IL-6 had the highest accuracy in predicting both SAP and PNEC but for mortality APACHE II and Ranson showed a little higher accuracy than the above two markers.

Among the multifactorial scoring systems, APACHE II and Ransons score had highest accuracy for predicting SAP and PNEC (Figures 1(a) and 1(c)). CTSI score as expected had the highest accuracy for prediction of pancreatic necrosis among the scoring systems (Figure 1(b)).

On the basis of the highest sensitivity and specificity values generated from the receiver-operating characteristic curves, the following cut-offs were selected for further analysis. Ranson ≥ 3, Glasgow ≥ 3, MOSS ≥ 5, BISAP ≥ 2, APACHE II ≥ 8, CTSI ≥ 5, procalcitonin ≥ 0.5 ng/mL, CRP ≥ 150 mg/L, and IL-6 ≥ 50 pg/mL. The observed incidence of severe disease, organ failure, pancreatic necrosis, need for ICU admission, average length of hospital stay, and mortality stratified by the various markers with their cut-offs is given in the Table 4. The number of patients with Ranson score ≥ 3 was 35, Glasgow ≥ 3 was 31, MOSS ≥ 5 was 42, APACHE II ≥ 8 was

Table 2: Patients characteristics.

Patients characteristics	No. of cases	Percentage
Sex		
Male	37	51.4
Female	35	48.6
Religion		
Hindu	66	91.7
Muslim	6	8.3
Age group		
11–20	9	12.5
21–30	17	23.6
31–40	12	16.7
41–50	16	22.2
51–60	5	6.9
61–70	13	18.1
Comorbidities		
Diabetes mellitus	3	4.2
Hypertension	1	1.4
Other	2	2.8
No comorbid condition	62	86.1
Both DM and hypertension	4	5.6
BMI		
<18.5	1	1.4
18.5–24.9	55	76.4
25–29.9	14	19.4
30–34.9	2	2.8
Presentations		
Pain abdomen	72	100
Radiating	62	86.1
Nonradiating	10	13.9
Peritonitis	62	86.1
Localized	36	58.1
Diffuse	26	41.9
Nausea	6	8.3
Vomiting	51	70.8
Distension abdomen	29	40.2
Nonpassage of flatus and stool	21	29.2
Breathlessness	22	30.6

32, SIRS was 39, BISAP ≥ 2 was 36, procalcitonin ≥ 0.5 ng/mL was 24, CRP ≥ 150 mg/L was 25, and IL-6 ≥ 50 pg/mL was 28.

IL-6, CRP, and procalcitonin have the highest sensitivity for prediction of SAP. The specificity, PPV, NPV, and accuracy of IL-6 and CRP are also very high for prediction of SAP. Regarding OF the sensitivity for prediction is very high for procalcitonin, IL-6, APACHE II, and Ransons score and CRP is more specific and more accurate in prediction of OF. CRP is highly sensitive and specific for prediction of PNec with a very high accuracy. IL-6 and CTSI scores are the next markers which had a very high sensitivity for prediction of PNec. There was a higher need of ICU admission in patients with SIRS and a high MOSS, APACHE and Ranson scores. Regarding mortality, multifactorial scoring systems (APACHE II, Ranson, SIRS, and Glasgow), procalcitonin, and IL-6 were more accurate in predicting mortality. IL-6 and APACHE II were more accurate in predicting mortality (Table 5).

Table 3: AUC (area under curve) of different prognostic markers in predicting SAP, PNEC, and mortality.

AUC (95% CI)	SAP	PNEC	Mortality
Ranson	0.85 (0.76–0.92)	0.70 (0.55–0.89)	0.84 (0.75–0.94)
Glasgow	0.75 (0.63–0.86)	0.64 (0.49–0.79)	0.83 (0.73–0.93)
MOSS	0.73 (0.61–0.85)	0.61 (0.46–0.77)	0.77 (0.62–0.92)
SIRS	0.73 (0.61–0.85)	0.61 (0.46–0.76)	0.76 (0.64–0.88)
APACHE II	0.88 (0.79–0.97)	0.68 (0.58–0.83)	0.86 (0.77–0.95)
BISAP	0.80 (0.71–0.91)	0.61 (0.47–0.72)	0.83 (0.69–0.97)
IL-6	0.90 (0.81–0.99)	0.86 (0.77–0.94)	0.80 (0.69–0.91)
CRP	0.91 (0.83–0.99)	0.90 (0.82–0.97)	0.75 (0.63–0.88)
CTSI	0.66 (0.53–0.79)	0.75 (0.59–0.91)	0.57 (0.35–0.78)

MOSS: multiple organ system score, APACHE II: acute physiology and chronic health evaluation II, SIRS: systemic inflammatory response syndrome, BISAP: bedside index for severe acute pancreatitis, IL-6: interleukin 6, CRP: C-reactive protein, and CTSI: CT severity index.

4. Discussion

In this study we have compared all the scoring systems, biochemical and radiological markers for prediction of morbidity and mortality in acute pancreatitis. We confirmed that single biochemical markers can be used as a reliable indicator for early stratification of severity of acute pancreatitis within 24 hours of admission.

The overall mortality in our cohort was 12.5% and 43.1% of patients had SAP. As expected the proportion of patients with severe disease and mortality in our cohort was higher as compared to previous studies [18]; this is probably because of a more number of referred cases admitted in our hospital.

Ranson's score is composed of 11 measures that are recorded as binary values on admission and at 48 hrs, and its primary aim was to evaluate the function of early operative intervention in patients with AP. A composite score of 3 or more is commonly used to classify a patient as having severe disease. Studies confirmed sensitivity from 40% to 90% [19]. Glasgow score proposed by Imrie for both alcohol and biliary acute pancreatitis seems to be more precise than that of Ranson, with a sensitivity for the assessment of severe acute pancreatitis of 56%–85% [20] using 8 laboratory factors within the first 48 h of treatment to calculate it [10], and more than three positive criteria indicate severe acute pancreatitis. Though fewer markers are taken into account, this score as well as the Ranson score predicts severe acute pancreatitis. Another commonly used severity index is the APACHE II index [21, 22]. This clinical tool measures the physiological response to injury and inflammation-driven stress and was initially designed to predict prolonged intensive care unit treatment and mortality. Papachristou et al. [18] found sensitivity, specificity, and accuracy of 84.2%, 89.8%, and 94% of Ranson criteria for prediction of SAP and 70.3%, 71.9% and 78% for APACHE II score. In our study we have

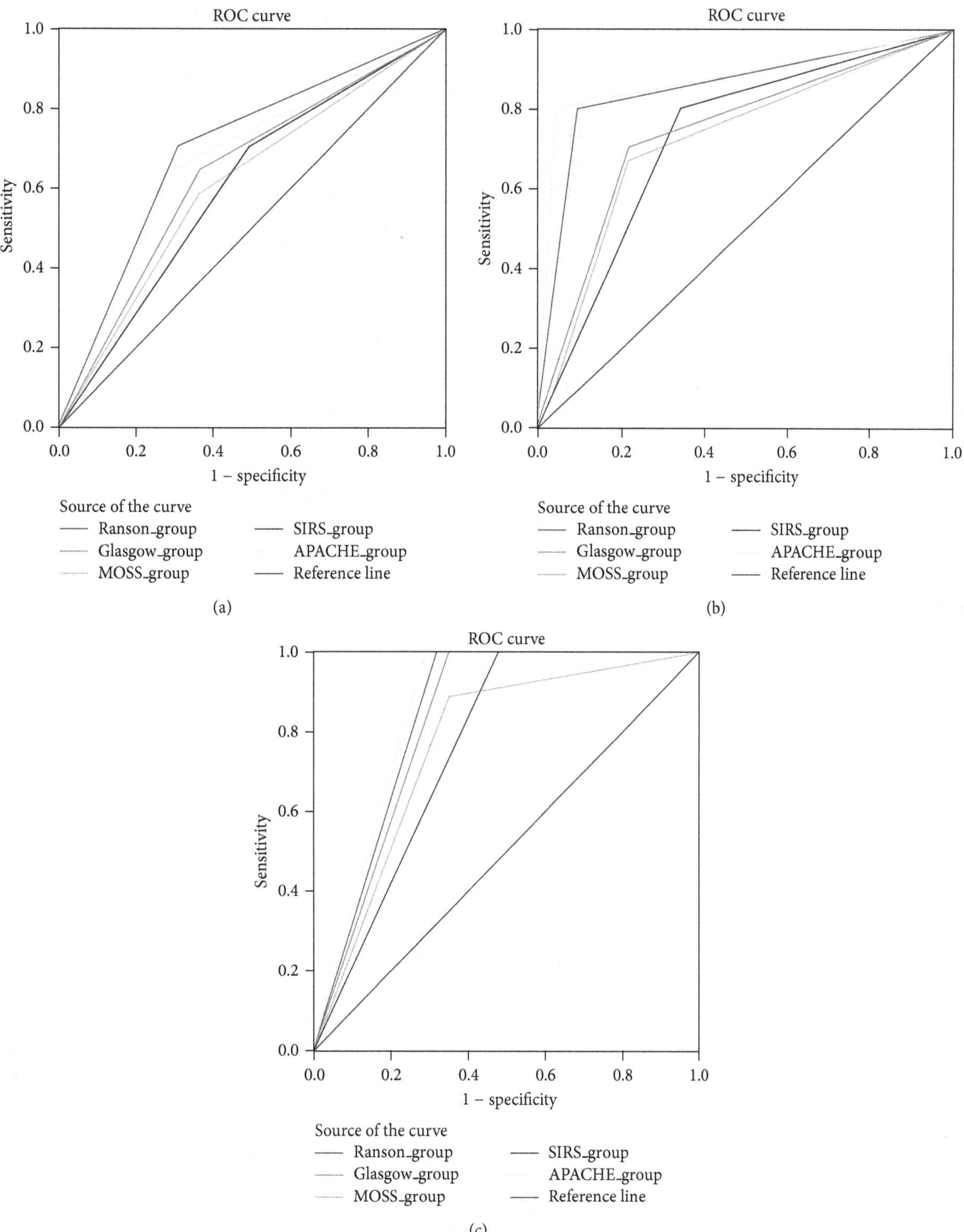

FIGURE 1: AUC comparison of various scoring systems in predicting SAP (a), pancreatic necrosis (b), and mortality (c). Diagonal segments are produced by ties.

found sensitivity, specificity, and accuracy of 83.9%, 78%, and 85% of Ranson criteria for prediction of SAP and 80.6%, 82.9%, and 88% for APACHE II score. Similar result has been found for prediction of pancreatic necrosis and mortality. For Glasgow score we found 71%, 78%, and 75% sensitivity, specificity and accuracy for prediction of SAP, respectively, which is in accordance with the study done by Blamey et al. [10].

BISAP and MOSS scores are newly developed prognostic scoring systems containing data that are frequently evaluated

Table 4: Incidence of SAP, OF, PNec, ICUA, and mortality stratified by Ranson, Glasgow, MOSS, APACHE II, SIRS, BISAP scores, Procalcitonin, IL-6, and CRP.

Markers	No. (%)	%SAP (*n*)	%OF (*n*)	%PNec (*n*)	%ICUA (*n*)	%MORT (*n*)	LOHS (days)
Ranson							
<3	37 (51.4)	13.5 (5)	5.4 (2)	13.5 (5)	2.7 (1)	0 (0)	8.24
≥3	35 (48.6)	74.3 (26)	65.7 (23)	34.3 (12)	22.9 (8)	25.7 (9)	12.08
Total	72 (100)	43.1 (31)	34.7 (25)	23.6 (17)	12.5 (9)	12.5 (9)	10.1
Glasgow							
<3	41 (56.9)	22.0 (9)	14.6 (6)	14.6 (6)	2.4 (1)	0 (0)	8.14
≥3	31 (43.1)	71.0 (22)	61.3 (19)	35.5 (11)	25.8 (8)	29.0 (9)	12.7
Total	72 (100)	43.1 (31)	34.7 (25)	23.6 (17)	12.5 (9)	12.5 (9)	10.1
MOSS							
<5	30 (41.7)	23.3 (7)	13.3 (4)	16.7 (5)	0 (0)	0 (0)	8.5
≥5	42 (58.3)	57.1 (24)	50.0 (21)	28.6 (12)	21.4 (9)	21.4 (9)	11.23
Total	72 (100)	43.1 (31)	34.7 (25)	23.6 (17)	12.5 (9)	12.5 (9)	10.1
APACHE II							
<8	40 (55.6)	15.0 (6)	2.5 (1)	15.0 (6)	2.5 (1)	0 (0)	8.22
≥8	32 (44.4)	78.1 (25)	75.0 (24)	34.4 (11)	25.0 (8)	28.1 (9)	12.48
Total	72 (100)	43.1 (31)	34.7 (25)	23.6 (17)	12.5 (9)	12.5 (9)	10.1
SIRS							
Absent	33 (45.8)	18.2 (6)	12.1 (4)	15.2 (5)	0 (0)	0 (0)	7.84
Present	39 (54.2)	64.1 (25)	53.8 (21)	30.8 (12)	23.1 (9)	23.1 (9)	12.02
Total	72 (100)	43.1 (31)	34.7 (25)	23.6 (17)	12.5 (9)	12.5 (9)	10.1
BISAP							
<2	36 (50)	22.2 (8)	13.9 (5)	19.4 (7)	5.6 (2)	2.7 (1)	7.5
≥2	36 (50)	63.9 (23)	55.6 (20)	27.8 (10)	19.4 (7)	22.8 (8)	10.2
Total	72 (100)	43.1 (31)	34.7 (25)	23.6 (17)	12.5 (9)	12.5 (9)	10.1
CTSI							
<5	23 (42.6)	39.1 (9)	34.8 (8)	17.4 (4)	13.0 (3)	8.7 (2)	8.6
≥5	31 (57.4)	54.8 (17)	41.9 (13)	38.7 (12)	12.9 (4)	16.1 (5)	11.22
Total	54 (100)	48.1 (26)	38.9 (21)	29.6 (16)	13.5 (7)	13.5 (7)	9.91
Procalcitonin							
<0.5 ng/mL	18 (42.9)	16.7 (3)	0 (0)	16.7 (3)	5.6 (1)	0 (0)	9.19
>0.5 ng/mL	24 (57.1)	79.7 (19)	70.8 (17)	45.8 (11)	20.8 (5)	29.2 (7)	11.5
Total	42 (100)	52.4 (22)	40.5 (17)	33.3 (14)	14.3 (6)	16.7 (7)	10.92
IL-6							
<50 pg/mL	32 (53.3)	6.2 (2)	3.1 (1)	3.1 (1)	3.1 (1)	0 (0)	7.68
≥50 pg/mL	28 (46.7)	96.4 (27)	78.6 (22)	57.1 (16)	25.0 (7)	32.1 (9)	13.7
Total	60 (100)	48.3 (29)	38.3 (23)	23.6 (17)	13.3 (8)	12.5 (9)	10.69
CRP							
<150 mg/L	35 (58.3)	11.4 (4)	11.4 (4)	0 (0)	5.7 (2)	8.6 (3)	8.54
≥150 mg/L	25 (41.7)	100 (25)	76.0 (19)	68.0 (17)	24.0 (6)	24.0 (6)	13.28
Total	60 (100)	48.3 (29)	38.3 (23)	23.6 (17)	13.3 (8)	12.5 (9)	10.91

SAP: severe acute pancreatitis, OF: organ failure, PNec: pancreatic necrosis, ICUA: intensive care unit admission, LOHS: length of hospital stay, MOSS: multiple organ system score, APACHE II: acute physiology and chronic health evaluation II, SIRS: systemic inflammatory response syndrome, BISAP: bedside index for severe acute pancreatitis, IL-6: interleukin 6, CRP: C-reactive protein, and CTSI: CT severity index.

at the time of admission which are accurate in predicting patient's outcome [23]. BISAP and MOSS scores have the advantage over Ranson and Glasgow scores of being calculated within 24 hrs of admission. BISAP score is higher in patients having SIRS, in older patients and in patients with altered mental status, whereas Ranson score seems to perform accurate prediction of persistent organ failure (sensitivity 92%, specificity 74.5%, PPV 65.7%, and NPV 94.6%). BISAP has the disadvantage that it cannot easily distinguish transient from persistent organ failure. SIRS is one of the leading events responsible for the mortality of AP. In our study we have a sensitivity of 80.6%, 84%, and 100% for prediction of SAP, OF, and mortality and an accuracy of 73%, 61%, and 76%, respectively.

TABLE 5: Sensitivity, specificity, PPV, NPV, and accuracy of different markers in predicting SAP, OF, PNec, need for ICU admission, and mortality.

	Sensitivity	Specificity	PPV	NPV	Accuracy	Kappa (95% CI)
			Severe acute pancreatitis			
Ranson	83.9	78.0	74.3	86.5	80.6	0.61 (0.40–0.75)
Glasgow	71.0	78.0	71.0	78.0	75.0	0.49 (0.27–0.66)
MOSS	77.4	56.1	57.1	76.7	65.3	0.32 (0.10–0.49)
APACHE II	80.6	82.9	78.2	85.0	81.9	0.63 (0.42–0.78)
SIRS	80.6	65.9	64.1	81.8	72.2	0.45 (0.23–0.61)
BISAP	74.2	68.3	63.4	77.8	70.8	0.42 (0.19–0.59)
CTSI	65.4	50.0	54.8	60.9	57.4	0.15 (−0.11–0.39)
IL-6	93.1	96.8	96.4	93.8	95.0	0.90 (0.73–1.0)
CRP	86.2	100	100	88.6	93.3	0.87 (0.70–0.87)
Procalcitonin	86.4	75.0	79.2	83.3	81	0.62 (0.33–0.79)
			Organ failure			
Ranson	92.0	74.5	65.7	94.6	80.6	0.61 (0.42–0.69)
Glasgow	76.0	74.5	61.3	85.4	75.0	0.48 (0.26–0.64)
MOSS	84.0	55.3	50.0	86.7	65.3	0.34 (0.14–0.46)
APACHE II	96.0	60.9	49.0	97.5	70.8	0.44 (0.30–0.48)
SIRS	84.0	61.7	53.8	87.9	69.4	0.40 (0.20–0.53)
BISAP	80.0	66.0	55.6	86.1	70.8	0.42 (0.20–0.56)
CTSI	65.2	45.5	45.5	65.2	53.6	0.10 (−0.15–0.32)
IL-6	95.7	33.3	78.6	75.0	78.1	0.35 (0.03–0.50)
CRP	82.6	83.8	76.0	88.6	83.3	0.65 (0.42–0.80)
Procalcitonin	100	72.0	70.8	100	83.3	0.68 (0.45–0.68)
			Pancreatic necrosis			
Ranson	70.6	58.2	34.3	86.5	61.1	0.21 (0.01–0.36)
Glasgow	64.7	63.6	35.5	85.4	63.9	0.22 (0.01–0.39)
MOSS	70.6	45.5	28.6	83.3	51.4	0.11 (−0.07–0.24)
APACHE II	64.7	61.8	34.4	85.0	62.5	0.20 (−0.004–0.37)
SIRS	70.6	50.9	30.8	84.8	55.6	0.15 (−0.04–0.29)
BISAP	58.8	52.7	27.8	80.6	54.2	0.08 (−0.11–0.25)
CTSI	87.5	55.3	45.2	91.3	57.4	0.20 (−0.31–0.36)
IL-6	94.1	72.1	57.1	96.9	78.3	0.55 (0.35–0.61)
CRP	100	81.4	68.0	100	86.7	0.71 (0.53–0.71)
Procalcitonin	78.6	53.6	45.8	83.3	61.9	0.27 (0.003–0.85)
			ICU admission			
Ranson	88.9	57.1	22.9	97.3	61.1	0.21 (0.45–0.25)
Glasgow	88.9	63.5	25.8	97.6	66.7	0.26 (0.09–0.31)
MOSS	100	47.6	21.4	100	54.2	0.19 (0.06–0.19)
APACHE II	88.9	61.9	25.0	97.5	65.3	0.24 (0.08–0.29)
SIRS	100	52.4	23.1	100	58.3	0.22 (0.09–0.21)
BISAP	77.8	54.0	19.4	94.4	56.9	0.14 (−0.01–0.20)
CTSI	87.5	55.3	45.2	91.3	64.8	0.001 (−0.15–0.12)
IL-6	87.5	59.6	25.0	96.9	63.3	0.23 (0.05–0.29)
CRP	75.0	63.5	24.0	94.3	65.0	0.20 (0.01–0.31)
Procalcitonin	83.3	47.2	20.8	94.4	52.4	0.14 (−0.06–0.21)
			Mortality			
Ranson	100	58.7	25.7	100	63.9	0.26 (0.12–0.26)
Glasgow	100	65.7	29.0	100	64.4	0.32 (0.16–0.32)
MOSS	100	47.6	21.4	100	54.2	0.19 (0.06–0.19)

TABLE 5: Continued.

	Sensitivity	Specificity	PPV	NPV	Accuracy	Kappa (95% CI)
APACHE II	100	63.5	28.1	100	68.1	0.30 (0.15–0.30)
SIRS	100	52.4	23.1	100	58.3	0.22 (0.09–0.21)
BISAP	88.9	55.6	22.2	97.2	59.7	0.19 (0.04–0.24)
CTSI	71.4	44.7	16.1	91.3	48.1	0.07 (−0.10–0.16)
IL-6	100	62.7	32.1	100	68.3	0.34 (0.16–0.34)
CRP	66.7	62.7	24.0	91.4	63.3	0.17 (−0.03–0.31)
Procalcitonin	100	51.4	29.2	100	59.5	0.26 (0.07–0.26)

SAP: severe acute pancreatitis, OF: organ failure, PNec: pancreatic necrosis, ICUA: intensive care unit admission, LOHS: length of hospital stay, MOSS: multiple organ system score, APACHE II: acute physiology and chronic health evaluation II, SIRS: systemic inflammatory response syndrome, BISAP: bedside index for severe acute pancreatitis, IL-6; interleukin 6, CRP: C-reactive protein, and CTSI: CT severity index.

Computed tomography severity index has shown a strong positive correlation with the development of complications and mortality in patients with AP [12, 24]. It was developed by Balthazar et al. to evaluate the degree of pancreatic edema, necrosis and the presence of peripancreatic fluid collections. In the CTSI pilot study, a score of 7–10 was able to predict 92% morbidity and 17% mortality rate in patients with AP, compared to the low morbidity (2%) and mortality (0%) associated with a CTSI score of 0-1 [25]. In our study we have found that CTSI had the highest sensitivity of 87.5% and 91.3% NPV among multifactorial scoring system in prediction of pancreatic necrosis as expected and the lowest sensitivity in prediction of organ failure (65.2%).

C-Reactive protein (CRP) is an acute phase reactant produced by the liver in response to interleukin-1, interleukin-6, and tumor necrosis factor-α and it is the most widely available, low-cost, and well-studied marker of severity in AP. A cut-off level of 150 mg/L within the first 48 hrs of symptom onset has sensitivity and specificity of 80–86% and 61–84%, respectively, for SAP and accuracy > 80% for necrotizing pancreatitis [26], CRP was done in 60 patients in our study; 58.3% of patients were having CRP value < 150 mg/L whereas 41.7% of cases had value of ≥150 mg/L. In patients having CRP level > 150 mg/L incidence of SAP, OF, PNEC, ICUA, MORT, and LOHS was found to be 100% (25), 76.0% (19), 68.0% (17), 24.0% (6), and 24.0% (6) with an average length of hospital stay of 13.8 days, respectively. In our study CRP had the highest sensitivity (100%), NPV (100%), and specificity (81.4%) for pancreatic necrosis, followed by sensitivity of 86.2% and specificity and PPV of 100% for prediction of SAP. As a whole CRP is a good marker for prediction of complications and mortality in acute pancreatitis. The AUC for prediction for PNec was higher for CRP 0.90 (0.82–0.77).

Activated leukocytes release proinflammatory cytokines that stimulate the liver to produce acute phase proteins. Since the concentration of cytokines increases before acute phase proteins, numerous clinical studies have been done to assess the usefulness of cytokines, such as interleukin-(IL-) 1, IL-6, IL-8, IL-10, and IL-18, in predicting severity early in the course of AP. Most trials have focused on the proinflammatory cytokines IL-6. Value of IL-6 is significantly elevated in SAP on the day of admission and tends to peak at 72 hrs after the clinical onset of disease, which makes IL-6 an excellent marker of early severity stratification. A 2009 meta-analysis, defining severity by the Atlanta Classification, revealed that the sensitivity and specificity ranges for IL-6 in the first three days of admission were 81–83.6% and 75.6–85.3%, respectively, with an IL-6 AUC of 0.75 on day one and 0.88 on the second day of admission [24]. In our study IL-6 was done in 60 patients. 53.3% of patients were having IL-6 value <50 pg/mL and 46.7% were having value of ≥50 pg/mL. In patients having IL-6 level >50 pg/mL incidence of SAP, OF, PNEC, ICUA, MORT, and average LOHS found was to be 96.4% (27), 78.6% (22), 57.1% (16), 25.0% (7), and 32.1% (9) with an average length of hospital stay of 13.7 days, respectively. IL-6 has the highest sensitivity for prediction of SAP (93.1%), organ failure (95.7%), pancreatic necrosis (94.1%), and mortality (100%). Regarding specificity it has the highest specificity (96.8%) for SAP. It has very high NPV (93.8%) and accuracy (95.0%) for prediction of SAP. It has very high NPV (100%) for mortality and NPV (96.9%) for prediction of pancreatic necrosis.

Procalcitonin (PCT) is a propeptide of the hormone calcitonin, which is released by hepatocytes, peripheral monocytes, and G-cells of the thyroid gland. PCT level can be measured by a semiquantitative strip test for fast results or by a fully automated assay to obtain a more accurate measurement. An increased PCT level has been found to be an early predictor of severity [27–29], pancreatic necrosis, and organ failure [30] in patients with AP. In a recent meta-analysis a subgroup of 8 studies using PCT cut-off values of 0.5 ng/mL as a discriminator found that the sensitivity and specificity of PCT for development of SAP were 73% and 87%, respectively, with an overall AUC of 0.88 [31]. In our study procalcitonin has 100% sensitivity for prediction of organ failure and mortality with a sensitivity of 86.4% for prediction of SAP.

At the end of the study we found that for prediction of SAP IL-6 had the highest sensitivity of 93.1%, followed by CRP (86.2%), procalcitonin (86.4%), and Ranson score (83.9%). CRP had the highest specificity of 100% with an accuracy of 95%, followed by IL-6 (96.4%) with an accuracy of 95%. Ranson and APACHE II scores come as the next best predictors of SAP. For prediction of organ failure procalcitonin had the highest sensitivity and NPV of 100%, followed by IL-6, Ranson, and APACHE II scores. Accuracy for prediction of organ failure is the highest for procalcitonin (83.3%) and APACHE II scores (83.3%). For prediction of pancreatic necrosis it is the CRP which has the maximum sensitivity and NPV of 100%, followed by IL-6 which has a sensitivity of 94.1% and NPV of 96.9%. Ranson and MOSS scores are the next best predictors of pancreatic necrosis. CTSI has a sensitivity of 87.5% for prediction of pancreatic necrosis. The AUC for pancreatic necrosis is the highest for CRP (0.90), followed by IL-6 (0.86), and Ranson score (0.70). Requirement of ICU admission was best predicted by MOSS score and SIRS with 100% sensitivity and NPV, followed by Ranson and Glasgow. Glasgow score has the highest accuracy for need of ICU requirement (66.7%). For the mortality predictors it is IL-6, procalcitonin, Ranson, Glasgow, APACHE II, MOSS, and SIRS which have 100% sensitivity and NPV; AUC for mortality prediction is the highest for Ranson (0.84) and APACHE II scores (0.86).

5. Conclusion

We conclude that determining the serum concentration of IL-6 on the first day and/or together with serum CRP concentration on the 2nd day of admission is helpful in earlier prediction and assessment of the severity of acute pancreatitis taking into consideration the disadvantages of multifactorial scoring systems. However, there is no ideal single method in assessing the severity of the disease. Individual preference and available institutional facilities influence the method chosen for prognostic assessment of acute pancreatitis.

Disclosure

The authors disclose that this work bears no financial assistance from any source which requires to be mentioned.

Authors' Contribution

Professor Ajay K. Khanna, Professor Usha Singh, Professor Arvind Srivastava, and Professor V. K. Dixit carried out the study design. Dr. Susanta Meher and Dr. Shashi Prakash were responsible for data acquisitation. Professor Ajay K. Khanna, Dr. Susanta Meher, Dr. Shashi Prakash, Dr. Satyendra Kumar Tiwary, Professor Usha Singh, Professor Arvind Srivastava, and Professor V. K. Dixit analysed and interpreted the data. Dr. Susanta Meher and Dr. Shashi Prakash drafted the paper. Professor Ajay K. Khanna and Dr. Satyendra Kumar Tiwary revised the paper. Dr. Susanta Meher provided the statistical advice.

References

[1] I. A. Al Mofleh, "Severe acute pancreatitis: pathogenetic aspects and prognostic factors," *World Journal of Gastroenterology*, vol. 14, no. 5, pp. 675–684, 2008.

[2] P. A. Banks, "Epidemiology, natural history, and predictors of disease outcome in acute and chronic pancreatitis," *Gastrointestinal Endoscopy*, vol. 56, no. 6, pp. S226–S230, 2002.

[3] H.-Q. Tao, J.-X. Zhang, and S.-C. Zou, "Clinical characteristics and management of patients with early acute severe pancreatitis: Experience from a medical center in China," *World Journal of Gastroenterology*, vol. 10, no. 6, pp. 919–921, 2004.

[4] A. Buter, C. W. Imrie, C. R. Carter, S. Evans, and C. J. McKay, "Dynamic nature of early organ dysfunction determines outcome in acute pancreatitis," *British Journal of Surgery*, vol. 89, no. 3, pp. 298–302, 2002.

[5] L. Kong, N. Santiago, T.-Q. Han, and S.-D. Zhang, "Clinical characteristics and prognostic factors of severe acute pancreatitis," *World Journal of Gastroenterology*, vol. 10, no. 22, pp. 3336–3338, 2004.

[6] T. Hirano and T. Manabe, "A possible mechanism for gallstone pancreatitis: repeated short-term pancreaticobiliary duct obstruction with exocrine stimulation in rats," *Proceedings of the Society for Experimental Biology and Medicine*, vol. 202, no. 2, pp. 246–252, 1993.

[7] J. Norman, "Role of cytokines in the pathogenesis of acute pancreatitis," *American Journal of Surgery*, vol. 175, no. 1, pp. 76–83, 1998.

[8] P. A. Banks, "Practice guidelines in acute pancreatitis," *American Journal of Gastroenterology*, vol. 92, no. 3, pp. 377–386, 1997.

[9] J. H. C. Ranson, K. M. Rifkind, D. F. Roses, S. D. Fink, K. Eng, and F. C. Spencer, "Prognostic signs and the role of operative management in acute pancreatitis," *Surgery Gynecology and Obstetrics*, vol. 139, no. 1, pp. 69–81, 1974.

[10] S. L. Blamey, C. W. Imrie, J. O'Neill, W. H. Gilmour, and D. C. Carter, "Prognostic factors in acute pancreatitis," *Gut*, vol. 25, no. 12, pp. 1340–1346, 1984.

[11] W. A. Knaus, E. A. Draper, D. P. Wagner, and J. E. Zimmerman, "APACHE II: a severity of disease classification system," *Critical Care Medicine*, vol. 13, no. 10, pp. 818–829, 1985.

[12] E. J. Balthazar, "Acute pancreatitis: assessment of severity with clinical and CT evaluation," *Radiology*, vol. 223, no. 3, pp. 603–613, 2002.

[13] E. J. Balthazar, P. C. Freeny, and E. van Sonnenberg, "Imaging and intervention in acute pancreatitis," *Radiology*, vol. 193, no. 2, pp. 297–306, 1994.

[14] M. Büchler, P. Malfertheiner, C. Schoetensack, W. Uhl, W. Scherbaum, and H. G. Beger, "Value of biochemical and imaging procedures for the diagnosis of acute pancreatitis-results of a prospective clinical study," *Zeitschrift fur Gastroenterologie*, vol. 24, pp. 100–109, 1986.

[15] G. Sathyanarayan, P. K. Garg, H. K. Prasad, and R. K. Tandon, "Elevated level of interleukin-6 predicts organ failure and severe disease in patients with acute pancreatitis," *Journal of Gastroenterology and Hepatology*, vol. 22, no. 4, pp. 550–554, 2007.

[16] M.-L. Kylänpää-Bäck, A. Takala, E. A. Kemppainen et al., "Procalcitonin, soluble interleukin-2 receptor, and soluble E-selectin in predicting the severity of acute pancreatitis," *Critical Care Medicine*, vol. 29, no. 1, pp. 63–69, 2001.

[17] S. Purkayastha, A. Chow, T. Athanasiou et al., "Does serum procalcitonin have a role in evaluating the severity of acute pancreatitis? A question revisited," *World Journal of Surgery*, vol. 30, no. 9, pp. 1713–1721, 2006.

[18] G. I. Papachristou, V. Muddana, D. Yadav et al., "Comparison of BISAP, Ranson's, APACHE-II, and CTSI scores in predicting

organ failure, complications, and mortality in acute pancreatitis," *American Journal of Gastroenterology*, vol. 105, no. 2, pp. 435–441, 2010.

[19] C. Wilson, A. Heads, A. Shenkin, and C. W. Imrie, "C-reactive protein, antiproteases and complement factors as objective markers of severity in acute pancreatitis," *British Journal of Surgery*, vol. 76, no. 2, pp. 177–181, 1989.

[20] N. J. M. London, J. P. Neoptolemos, J. Lavelle, I. Bailey, and D. James, "Contrast-enhanced abdominal computed tomography scanning and prediction of severity of acute pancreatitis: a prospective study," *British Journal of Surgery*, vol. 76, no. 3, pp. 268–272, 1989.

[21] Y. P. Yeung, B. Y. K. Lam, and A. W. C. Yip, "APACHE system is better than Ranson system in the prediction of severity of acute pancreatitis," *Hepatobiliary and Pancreatic Diseases International*, vol. 5, no. 2, pp. 294–299, 2006.

[22] M. Larvin and M. J. McMahon, "APACHE-II score for assessment and monitoring of acute pancreatitis," *The Lancet*, vol. 2, no. 8656, pp. 201–205, 1989.

[23] S. L. Taylor, D. L. Morgan, K. D. Denson, M. M. Lane, and L. R. Pennington, "A comparison of the ranson, glasgow, and APACHE II scoring systems to a multiple organ system score in predicting patient outcome in pancreatitis," *American Journal of Surgery*, vol. 189, no. 2, pp. 219–222, 2005.

[24] E. Aoun, J. Chen, D. Reighard, F. C. Gleeson, D. C. Whitcomb, and G. I. Papachristou, "Diagnostic accuracy of interleukin-6 and interleukin-8 in predicting severe acute pancreatitis: a meta-analysis," *Pancreatology*, vol. 9, no. 6, pp. 777–785, 2009.

[25] E. J. Balthazar, D. L. Robinson, A. J. Megibow, and J. H. C. Ranson, "Acute pancreatitis: value of CT in establishing prognosis," *Radiology*, vol. 174, no. 2, pp. 331–336, 1990.

[26] J. P. Neoptolemos, E. A. Kemppainen, J. M. Mayer et al., "Early prediction of severity in acute pancreatitis by urinary trypsinogen activation peptide: a multicentre study," *The Lancet*, vol. 355, no. 9219, pp. 1955–1960, 2000.

[27] I. S. Modrau, A. K. Floyd, and O. Thorlacius-Ussing, "The clinical value of procalcitonin in early assessment of acute pancreatitis," *American Journal of Gastroenterology*, vol. 100, no. 7, pp. 1593–1597, 2005.

[28] Y. Mandi, G. Farkas, T. Takacs, K. Boda, and J. Lonovics, "Diagnostic relevance of procalcitonin, IL-6, and sICAM-1 in the prediction of infected necrosis in acute pancreatitis," *International Journal of Pancreatology*, vol. 28, no. 1, pp. 41–49, 2000.

[29] N. Bülbüller, O. Doğru, R. Ayten, H. Akbulut, Y. S. Ilhan, and Z. Çetinkaya, "Procalcitonin is a predictive marker for severe acute pancreatitis," *Ulusal Travma ve Acil Cerrahi Dergisi*, vol. 12, no. 2, pp. 115–120, 2006.

[30] M.-L. Kylänpää-Bäck, A. Takala, E. Kemppainen, P. Puolakkainen, R. Haapiainen, and H. Repo, "Procalcitonin strip test in the early detection of severe acute pancreatitis," *British Journal of Surgery*, vol. 88, no. 2, pp. 222–227, 2001.

[31] R. Mofidi, S. A. Suttie, P. V. Patil, S. Ogston, and R. W. Parks, "The value of procalcitonin at predicting the severity of acute pancreatitis and development of infected pancreatic necrosis: systematic review," *Surgery*, vol. 146, no. 1, pp. 72–81, 2009.

9

Assessment of Liver Remnant Using ICG Clearance Intraoperatively during Vascular Exclusion: Early Experience with the ALIIVE Technique

Lawrence Lau,[1] Christopher Christophi,[1] Mehrdad Nikfarjam,[1] Graham Starkey,[1] Mark Goodwin,[2] Laurence Weinberg,[3] Loretta Ho,[3] and Vijayaragavan Muralidharan[1]

[1]*Department of Surgery, Austin Health, University of Melbourne, Melbourne, VIC 3084, Australia*
[2]*Department of Radiology, Austin Health, Melbourne, VIC 3084, Australia*
[3]*Department of Anaesthesia, Austin Health, University of Melbourne, Melbourne, VIC 3084, Australia*

Correspondence should be addressed to Lawrence Lau; thelau@gmail.com

Academic Editor: Attila Olah

Background. The most significant risk following major hepatectomy is postoperative liver insufficiency. Current preoperative assessment of the future liver remnant relies upon assumptions which may not be valid in the setting of advanced resection strategies. This paper reports the feasibility of the *ALIIVE* technique which assesses the liver remnant with ICG clearance intraoperatively during vascular exclusion. *Methods.* 10 patients undergoing planned major liver resection (hemihepatectomy or greater) were recruited. Routine preoperative assessment included CT and standardized volumetry. ICG clearance was measured noninvasively using a finger spectrophotometer at various time points including following parenchymal transection during inflow and outflow occlusion before vascular division, the ALIIVE step. *Results.* There were one case of mortality and three cases of posthepatectomy liver failure. The patient who died had the lowest ALIIVE ICG clearance (7.1%/min versus 14.4 ± 4.9). Routine preoperative CT and standardized volumetry did not predict outcome. *Discussion/Conclusion.* The novel ALIIVE technique is feasible and assesses actual future liver remnant function before the point of no return during major hepatectomy. This technique may be useful as a check step to offer a margin of safety to prevent posthepatectomy liver failure and death. Further confirmatory studies are required to determine a safety cutoff level.

1. Introduction

Surgical resection remains the foundation for curative treatment of liver malignancies. Resection strategies balance the goal of macroscopic tumour clearance and preserving adequate future liver remnant (FLR) [1]. Inadequate FLR leads to posthepatectomy liver failure (PHLF) as defined by deterioration in the ability of the liver to maintain its synthetic, excretory, and detoxifying functions [2]. This is the most common cause of mortality following hepatectomy [3]. Current assessments of FLR are based on computed tomography (CT) imaging and are contingent upon the predicted volume of liver remnant either as a percentage of the total preoperative liver volume (CT volumetry) or as a percentage of an ideal total liver volume as calculated by body surface area (standardized volumetry) [4]. Increasingly, advanced strategies, which enhance technical resectability, have gained prominence. These strategies include preoperative chemotherapy [5], combining local ablation with resection [6], portal vein embolisation [7, 8], 2-staged resection [9], and recently the associating liver partition and portal vein ligation for staged hepatectomy (ALPPS) technique [10]. While rapid liver hypertrophy induced by these advanced techniques has increased resectability, increase in parenchymal volume has not been shown to definitively correlate with increased functional liver capacity. In the climate of these advances, the applicability of current assessment is uncertain. The presence of patient-related factors such as age, diabetes, and obesity and parenchyma-related factors such as cirrhosis, cholestasis, steatosis, and chemotherapy injury further cloud idealized volumetry [11–14]. Functional FLR measurement using hepatobiliary scintigraphy has been shown to be a better predictor in those with parenchymal disease [15, 16]. However, both techniques suffer due to potential discrepancy between the planned and actual transection planes. Furthermore, the functional contribution of liver parenchyma that is poorly perfused or has poor venous drainage after transection is impossible to predict [17–19].

Indocyanine green (ICG) is tricarbocyanine dye taken up exclusively by hepatocytes and excreted into bile without enterohepatic recirculation [20, 21]. It is widely used to evaluate preoperative liver functional reserve [22–26] and as an early indicator of outcome following liver resection [22, 23, 25, 27] and orthotopic liver transplantation [28–34].

In this report, we describe a novel technique which may be used intraoperatively to assess true FLR. This study assesses the technical feasibility and early experience of the novel ALIIVE technique in the assessment of liver remnant using ICG clearance intraoperatively during vascular exclusion of the liver being resected. This technique may potentially be utilized as a final safety check step that evaluates the sufficiency of the actual future remnant before the irreversible step of vascular division. Potentially, if insufficient future liver remnant function was found at this step, the planned hepatectomy may be converted to an ALPPS procedure. Conversely, in the setting of a planned ALPPS procedure, if sufficient future liver remnant was confirmed during the ALIIVE check step, completion of the hepatectomy as a single-staged procedure may prevent reoperation and the morbidity associated with a two-staged procedure.

2. Methods

This prospective technical feasibility study was approved by Austin Health Human Research Ethics Committee (project number: HREC/13/Austin/150). Signed, written informed consent was obtained from each patient.

2.1. Patient Selection. From February 2014 to August 2014, consecutive patients planned for hemihepatectomy or greater at Austin Health in Melbourne, Australia, were recruited for this study. All patients were discussed at the Austin Health Hepatobiliary Multi-Disciplinary Team Meeting prior to planned resection.

2.2. Routine Future Liver Remnant Assessment. Routine preoperative FLR assessment was performed using two techniques.

2.2.1. CT Volumetry. Preoperative multiphase contrast-enhanced CT scans of the abdomen were obtained routinely as part of staging and planning for surgery with portal venous phase images reconstructed at 3 mm slice thickness. CT volumetry expresses the predicted FLR volume as a percentage of total liver volume based on the reconstructed images (%FLRV). Liver volumes were then calculated by a specialist hepatobiliary radiologist using VitreaWorkstation (Toshiba Medical, Tokyo, Japan) by manually drawing regions of interest around the areas of the liver to denote the volumes of the tumour (TV), FLR (FLRV), and total liver volume (TLV). Segments were demarcated according to the conventional Couinaud classification. The %FLRV is calculated by the following formula:

$$\%\text{FLRV} = \frac{\text{FLRV}}{\text{TLV} - \text{TV}} \times 100\%. \quad (1)$$

2.2.2. Standardized Volumetry. Similar to CT volumetry, reconstructed CT scans were used to calculate FLRV while standardized total liver volume (sTLV) was calculated based on patient body surface area (BSA) according to the following formula:

$$\text{sTLV} = -794.41 + 1267.28 \times \text{BSA}, \quad (2)$$

where

$$\text{BSA} = \sqrt{\frac{\text{height (cm)} \times \text{weight (kg)}}{3600}}. \quad (3)$$

Standardized future liver remnant (sFLR) is calculated as

$$\text{sFLR} = \frac{\text{FLRV}}{\text{sTLV}}. \quad (4)$$

A %FLRV or sFLR >20% and >30% in patients with normal and suspected diseased liver parenchyma (cholestasis, steatosis, and >6 cycles of preoperative chemotherapy) was considered sufficient [35–37].

2.3. ICG Clearance. ICG clearance was assessed using the LiMON module of the PulsioFlex monitor (Pulsion Medical Systems, Munich, Germany) to obtain the PDR (%/min). ICG clearance was performed during the following time points (Figure 1): (1) before anaesthesia (ICG1), (2) under anaesthesia following laparotomy ± subsegmental tumour clearance of FLR (ICG2), (3) during inflow occlusion (hepatic artery and portal vein) to the lobe for resection (ICG3), (4) following parenchymal transection and inflow occlusion (ICG4), and (5) during inflow and outflow occlusion following parenchymal transection of the lobe for resection (ICG5 a.k.a. the ALIIVE step). For each ICG measurement, a bolus of 25 mg of ICG was injected into a central venous catheter. The ICG elimination was detected by noninvasive pulse spectrophotometry and the ICG PDR was automatically calculated within six minutes. A delay of 30 minutes was required between measurements. Maximum allowable daily dose is 5 mg/kg.

2.4. Anaesthesia. General anaesthesia was managed by specialist anaesthetists using a protocol designed to standardise care. Prior to induction of anaesthesia all patients received intrathecal morphine (300 μg) inserted at the L3/4 intervertebral space. Induction of anaesthesia consisted of a balanced technique using propofol (1–3 mg/kg), fentanyl (1–3 μg/kg),

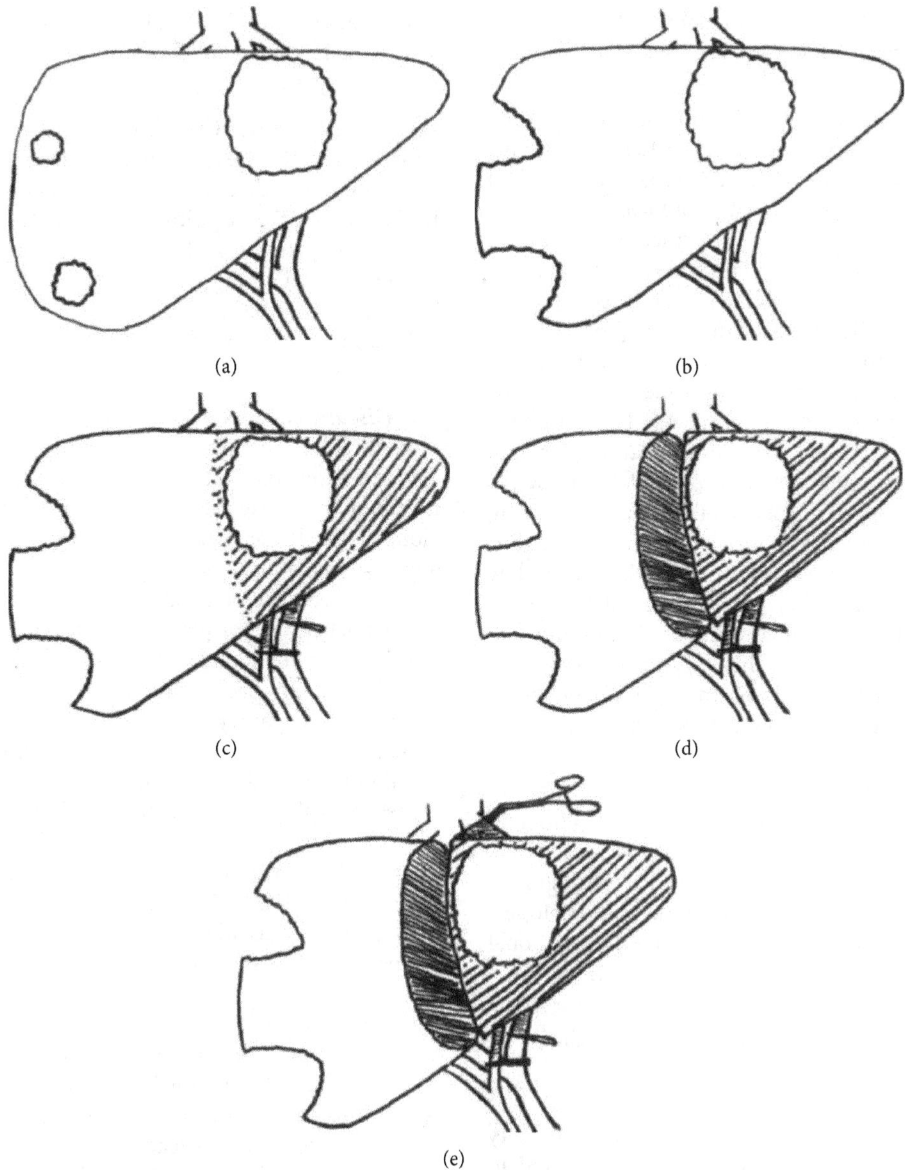

FIGURE 1: Schematic diagram of ICG clearance time points in a liver with a large left-sided tumour and two small superficial right-sided tumours: (a) ICG1: preoperative, (b) ICG2: under anaesthesia following clearance of future liver remnant, (c) ICG3: during inflow control to the side to be resected, (d) ICG4: during inflow control following parenchymal transection, and (e) ICG5: the ALIIVE step, during inflow and outflow control following parenchymal transection.

and a nondepolarising neuromuscular blocker. Maintenance of anaesthesia was achieved with sevoflurane or desflurane in a 50% oxygen : 50% air ratio titrated to a bispectral index (BIS) of 40 to 60. Intraoperative analgesia consisted of a remifentanil infusion (0.1 to 0.3 μg/kg/min) that was discontinued prior to surgical closure. Intraoperative monitoring consisted of continuous electrocardiography, pulse oximetry, invasive blood pressure, central venous pressure, urine output, and core body temperature. Flow based haemodynamic variables (cardiac index, stroke volume variation, and stroke volume) were evaluated continuously with the PulsioFlex monitor using a ProAQT sensor (Pulsion Medical Systems, Munich, Germany). During the hepatic parenchymal resection phase, fluid therapy was limited and an infusion of glyceryl trinitrate (GTN) was used where necessary to achieve a central venous pressure of less than 5 mmHg. After hepatic resection, the GTN was discontinued and patients were rendered euvolemic. Vasoactive drugs (e.g., phenylephrine, noradrenaline, and metaraminol) were used to maintain blood pressure within 20% of the preoperative value. Fluid intervention was confined to Plasmalyte solution (Baxter Healthcare, Toongabbie, NSW, Australia). The intraoperative transfusion trigger for packed red cell transfusion was a haemoglobin concentration of less than 70 g/L or less than

80 g/L in the setting of ongoing or uncontrolled bleeding, myocardial ischaemia, or a low cardiac output state.

2.5. Surgical Resection. Intraoperative ultrasound was used for intraoperative intrahepatic staging, to identify tumour margin and hepatic anatomy. If required, subsegmental resection was performed to clear the future liver remnant of tumour. Anatomical resection was performed in accordance with Couinaud's liver segmental classification. Portal and hepatic arterial inflow to the segments for resection were dissected extrahepatically and occluded with vascular bull-dog clamps to allow for ICG clearance assessment (ICG3). Liver parenchymal transection was performed using a combination of an ultrasonic surgical aspirator (CUSA, Radionics, Burlington, MA, USA), Harmonic shears (Ethicon, Somerville, NJ, USA), and linear surgical stapler (EndoGIA, Covidien, Mansfield, MA, USA; Echelon Endopath, Ethicon, Somerville, NJ, USA). Following complete parenchymal transection, an ICG clearance was performed with the inflow occluded and with outflow (hepatic vein) patent (ICG4). A final ICG clearance was performed with both inflow and outflow occlusion (ICG5). Following this step, the liver resection was completed with ligation and division of the hepatic artery, portal vein, and hepatic vein to the pertinent hemiliver.

2.6. Study Endpoints. Although this feasibility study was not designed to assess endpoints, postoperative liver failure and death due to postoperative liver insufficiency were assessed. All postoperative morbidities were recorded and graded according to the Clavien-Dindo classification [38]. Postoperative liver failure was defined according to the International Study Group of Liver Surgery (ISGLS) grading [2].

2.7. Statistics. Values for results are expressed as median with the range and mean ± standard deviation.

2.8. Results. In total, 10 patients participated in this feasibility study. Demographic and tumour information are listed in Table 1. The majority of patients underwent preoperative chemotherapy (7) and were trisegmentectomies (6) while half had preoperative portal vein embolization (5). In patients who underwent preoperative portal vein embolization, the median kinetic growth rate of the future remnant was 7.4%/week.

There were 3 cases of posthepatectomy liver failure, one of which was grade C liver failure. This patient died on the fifth postoperative day. Stratified by outcome (Table 1), the patients with posthepatectomy liver failure were older with cholangiocarcinoma.

2.8.1. CT Volumetry. The median estimated liver remnant on CT volumetry was 46% (range 26–84%). The estimated remnant in the patient who died was 38%. For the other two patients with posthepatectomy liver failure, the estimated liver remnant was 45% and 46%.

2.8.2. Standardized Volumetry. The median estimated liver remnant on standardized volumetry was 57%. This was 49% in the patient who died. In the patients with reversible liver failure, their standardized volumetry was 65% and 59%.

2.8.3. Intraoperative ICG Clearance. The intraoperative ICG clearances at the various time points are shown in Table 1. The patient who died had a lower ICG clearance at the ICG3, ICG4, and ICG5 time points (7.5, 7.2, and 7.1%/min) compared to the other patients (11.8 ± 3, 10.7 ± 2.1, and 14.4 ± 4.9%/min). The interquartile ranges stratified for outcome are displayed in Figure 2. Cardiac index was measured at each ICG time point and ranged from 1.9 to 3.6 (Table 1).

2.9. Discussion. This study describes a novel technique to assess FLR intraoperatively. In our early experience with these first ten cases, the technique was shown to be feasible and its potential for use as a safety check step was demonstrated along with alternate treatment strategies in the setting of apparent inadequacy of the FLR.

ICG clearance is a functional liver test which has been in established use for planning of surgical resection and for monitoring patients following liver resection for liver insufficiency [22–27]. Following intravenous injection, ICG is taken up by hepatocytes and excreted with bile via an ATP-dependent mechanism. As hepatic ATP is important for liver viability, regeneration, and metabolic function, ICG clearance correlates with global liver function [39].

This study assessed the use of ICG clearance intraoperatively at various time points during liver resection. Time points ICG3, ICG4, and ICG5 demonstrate increasing degrees of vascular exclusion of the FLR. Interestingly, increasing vascular exclusion led to decreased ICG clearance in some cases but, in other cases, it led to improved clearance. One explanation for this observation relates to haemodynamic variability during the different time points. Another reason is the potential for interlobar crossover flow [40] in ICG3 or retrograde hepatic vein flow [41] in both ICG3 and ICG4. This could either lead to better ICG clearance by the functional contribution of the additional parenchyma or to decreased ICG clearance due to ICG stasis in the nonexcluded but diseased parenchyma. Therefore, the ALIIVE step, which essentially replicates the hepatectomized state, should best predict the outcome.

This pilot study was not intended, nor was it powered, to determine a safety cutoff level for ICG clearance during vascular exclusion. However, an indication of a safety cutoff level can be extrapolated from the previous studies assessing ICG clearance postoperatively [22, 23, 25, 27]. In a study by Sugimoto et al., following liver resection, a PDR <7%/min on postoperative day 1 was found to be highly predictive for liver insufficiency (sensitivity 71.4%, specificity 95.5%) and death (sensitivity 100%, specificity 93.6%) [27]. In another study by Ohwada et al., patients who had liver failure following hepatectomy had a median postoperative PDR of 7.6%/min [23]. They proposed the use of an estimated remnant PDR cutoff (based on a product of CT volumetry and preoperative ICG clearance) of 9%/min to be 88% sensitive and 82% specific in the prediction of posthepatectomy liver insufficiency. In the study by de Liguori Carino et al. from Liverpool, ICG

TABLE 1: Demographic, preoperative/operative factors and ICG clearance stratified by outcome.

Demographics	Median (% or range)	Dead	Alive	Posthepatectomy liver failure	No posthepatectomy liver failure
Number	10	1	9	3	7
Sex (male : female)	8 : 2	male	7 : 2	3 male	5 : 2
Age	60.9 (19–76)	75	63.7 ± 11.8	70.8 ± 4.5	62.5 ± 13.0
BMI	23.4 (21–30)	22.8	25 ± 3.2	25.2 ± 3.1	24.8 ± 3.3
Preoperative factors					
Colorectal metastases	6	0	6	0	6
Cholangiocarcinoma	4	1	3	3	1
Preoperative chemotherapy	7	0	7	1	6
Portal vein embolisation	5	1	4	2	3
If PVE-kinetic growth rate (%/week)	7.4 (6.47–9.07)	6.6	7.38 ± 1.2	7.0 ± 0.6	7.8 ± 1.8
Trisegmentectomy	6	1	5	1	5
Right hemihepatectomy	3	0	3	2	1
Left hemihepatectomy	1	0	1	0	1
Future liver remnant volume (mL)	760 (351–1221)	710	877 ± 299	869 ± 196	859 ± 328
CT volumetry (%)	46 (26–84)	38	53 ± 18	43.0 ± 4.4	54.5 ± 19.9
Standardized volumetry (%)	57 (22–66)	49	55 ± 17	57.9 ± 8.3	53.3 ± 19.0
Bilirubin (μmol/L)	12 (5–35)	25	13 ± 10	10 ± 5.4	23 ± 13.1
Operative factors					
Blood loss (mL)	650 (200–1500)	1200	660 ± 568	700 ± 707	775 ± 585
Operating time (min)	510 (360–840)	540	518 ± 165	500 ± 69	534 ± 195
ICG clearance					
ICG 1: preoperative	21.4 (12.2–25.5)	14.2	19.2 ± 5.2	24.2 ± 1.9	17.8 ± 5.0
ICG 2: under anaesthesia ± clearance of future liver remnant	15.2 (7.0–28.3)	11.7	18.0 ± 7.7	19.7 ± 7.6	15.7 ± 7.8
ICG 3: inflow control	11.0 (7.3–16.2)	7.5	11.8 ± 3.0	8.6 ± 2.1	12.9 ± 2.7
ICG 4: inflow control following parenchymal transection	10.3 (7.8–13.8)	7.8	10.7 ± 2.1	10.4 ± 3.8	10.7 ± 2.3
ICG 5: inflow and outflow control following parenchymal transection (ALIIVE)	12.9 (7.1–24.7)	7.1	14.4 ± 4.9	10.4 ± 4.2	15.2 ± 5.1
Cardiac index (ICG2)	2.4 (2.1–3.3)	2.1	2.6 ± 0.5	2.1 ± 0.1	3.0 ± 0.4
Cardiac index (ICG3)	2.8 (1.9–3.2)	2.6	2.7 ± 0.5	2.3 ± 0.4	3.1 ± 0.2
Cardiac index (ICG4)	3.0 (2.3–3.2)	3.0	2.8 ± 0.5	2.7 ± 0.5	3.2 ± 0.5
Cardiac index (ICG5)	3.0 (2.4–3.6)	3.1	2.9 ± 0.5	2.8 ± 0.4	3.4 ± 0.5
Outcome					
Hospital stay (days)	11 days (5–48)	n/a	16 ± 14	33 ± 21	10 ± 4
Posthepatectomy liver failure	3 (30%)				
Grade A: abnormal lab parameters	1 (10%)				
Grade B: deviation from routine clinical management without invasive treatment	1 (10%)				
Grade C: deviation from routine clinical management requiring invasive treatment	1 (10%)				

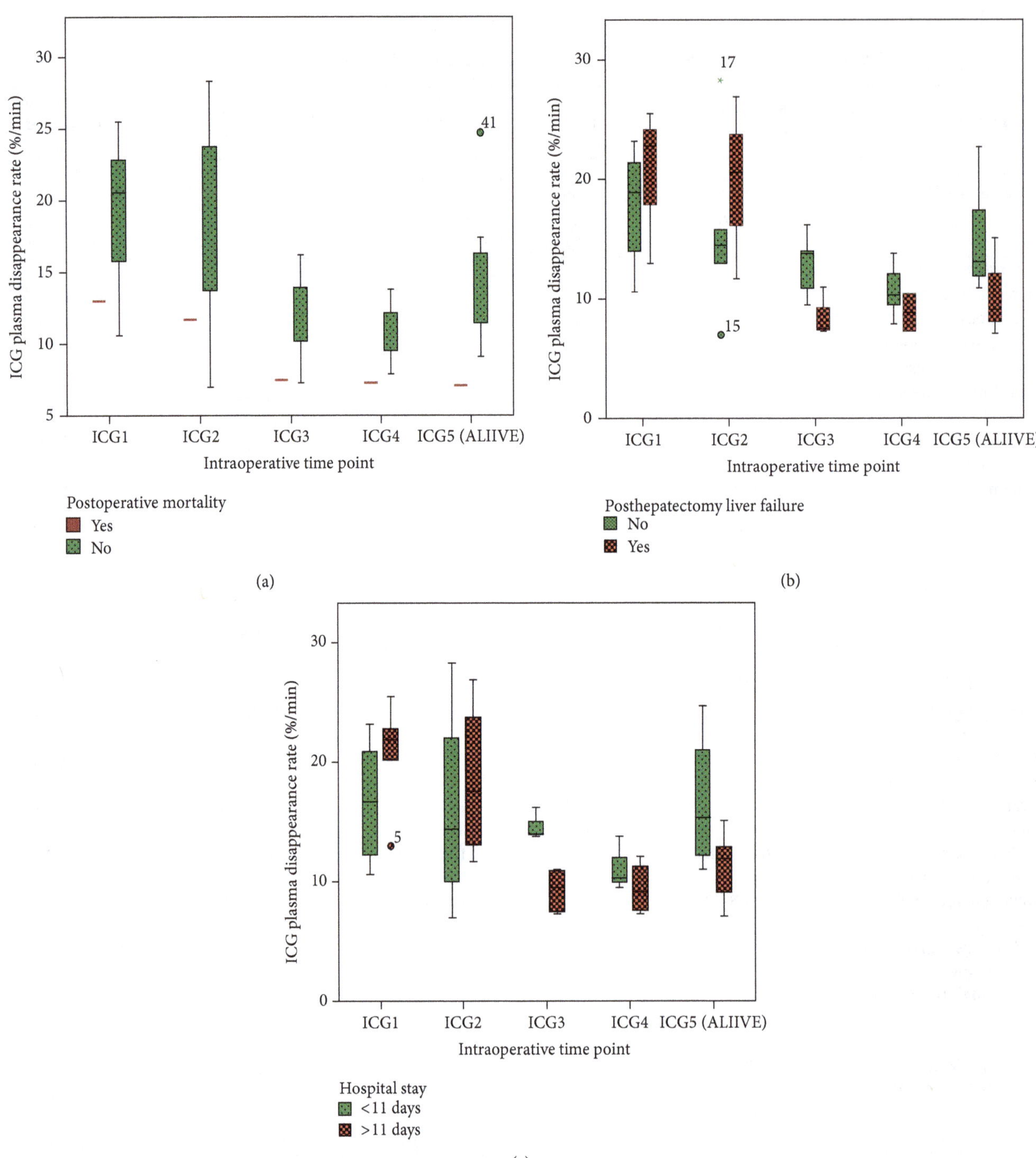

FIGURE 2: Interquartile box-plots of ICG clearance at different time points stratified by (a) postoperative mortality, (b) posthepatectomy liver failure, and (c) hospital stay.

clearance was found to be uniquely useful for the early detection of posthepatectomy liver dysfunction where those with liver dysfunction had a significantly lower postoperative day 1 PDR compared to those who did not (6.75%/min versus 13.4%/min, $P = 0.014$) [22].

As the ALIIVE technique replicates the postresection state intraoperatively, it is reasonable to assume that a PDR that can be demonstrated to be greater than 9%/min would give a margin of safety while a PDR that cannot be demonstrated to be greater than 7%/min would be at high risk of liver insufficiency and death if hepatectomy was completed.

Correspondingly, in our small series, our only postoperative mortality had an ALIIVE ICG clearance of 7.1%/min prior to completion of hepatectomy, which is significantly lower than the other ICG clearances in patients at this time point who had their hepatectomy completed. This patient had a cholangiocarcinoma who underwent preoperative portal vein embolisation before resection. FLR grew from 431 mL (24%) to 710 mL (38%) and was deemed to be sufficient based on preoperative CT and standardized volumetry. Preoperative bilirubin was slightly elevated at 25 μmol/L and histology revealed background liver parenchymal chronic cholestasis. This patient died following progressive liver failure likely due to small-for-size syndrome without sepsis or apparent surgical complications.

During this study, another patient had unexpected colorectal liver metastases on the FLR which were cleared. Following parenchymal transection, the decision was made (independent of ICG clearance) to convert the procedure to an ALPPS procedure. At this point, an ALIIVE ICG clearance was demonstrated to be 7.9%/min which, according to the studies of ICG clearance after hepatectomy, would be considered low. Two weeks later at the second stage hemihepatectomy, the ALIIVE ICG clearance had functionally increased to 11.9%/min and the liver resection was completed without complication (the ICG clearance from the first operation was not included in the overall analysis). Although management was not altered due to the ICG findings in this example, it displays the real-time intraoperative decision-making potential of the ALIIVE technique and demonstrates the functional increase of the actual future liver remnant following volume manipulation.

Following validation studies, the ALIIVE technique may potentially be used as a "check step" during major hepatectomy to avoid posthepatectomy liver failure. If there is insufficient FLR, possible alternative strategies may include conversion to a staged resection, ALPPS procedure with the addition of portal vein ligation, portal vein embolization, local ablative therapy, or palliative chemotherapy. Conversely, demonstration of sufficient FLR during a planned ALPPS procedure with the ALIIVE technique may allow confident hepatectomy and prevent unnecessary morbidity and subsequent reoperation. However, the potential benefit gained in preventing posthepatectomy liver failure will need to be balanced against the possible increase in technical difficulty with this technique as well as the potential complications in leaving the sectioned but unresected hemiliver in situ, in a prospective randomized control trial.

Although this technique would not replace preoperative volumetry, it has the potential to be a valuable adjunct to current assessment. The ALIIVE technique directly assesses FLR without making assumptions about the health of liver parenchyma, the actual resection plane, and the actual functional contribution of remnant liver parenchyma.

Liver parenchymal diseases such as nonalcoholic fatty liver disease, cirrhosis, biliary obstruction, and injury secondary to preoperative chemotherapy are associated with increased risk of liver insufficiency following liver resection. Both CT and standardized volumetry are based on the assumption of normal, homogenous liver parenchyma where a compensatory "guess" is applied with known parenchymal disease. Hepatobiliary scintigraphic functional volumetry does attempt to redress the issue of parenchymal disease but suffers the same deficiencies of being unable to predict the exact resection plane, consider the impact of impaired venous drainage, or adapt to altered intraoperative circumstances [15, 16]. The correlation of liver volume and function with more recent FLR growth techniques such as PVE and ALPPS is even less established.

A meta-analysis assessing the sensitivities of various imaging modalities following neoadjuvant chemotherapy found MRI and CT to have a pooled sensitivity of 85.7% and 69.9%, respectively, compared to intraoperative palpation with intraoperative ultrasound [42]. This means that around one out of every three to six liver tumours may be undetected on preoperative imaging requiring unplanned intraoperative resection. Additionally, the parenchymal transection plane may not follow a planned two-dimensional vertical axis as predicted by CT volumetry. Furthermore, for hemihepatectomies where the middle hepatic vein is excised the adjoining liver segments may have compromised venous drainage rendering them functionally impaired. The degree of impaired function is not taken into account with preoperative volumetric planning.

The main limitation of this technique relates to the contribution of vascular perfusion to the FLR ICG clearance. ICG clearance is a function of two processes: hepatic clearance and hepatic perfusion. The latter may be decreased by general anaesthesia, decreased cardiac output, decreased volume status, and hepatic artery vasospasm leading to impaired ICG clearance.

At each ICG clearance time point, cardiac index was measured and recorded to ensure that this was sufficient. If a low clearance was observed during the final vascular exclusion test, the vascular clamps were released and the clearance was repeated after 20 minutes with correction of any potential perfusion-limiting factors. These include increasing cardiac index with volume filling, allowing the liver to sit naturally without manipulation of the hepatic inflow, and spraying 5 mL of papaverine over the remnant liver hepatic artery to counteract potential vasospasm. Provided adequate vascular exclusion of the liver parenchyma to be resected, it is unlikely that ICG clearance assessment of the FLR can be falsely increased. The objective is to demonstrate the best possible FLR function, which, if adequate, should provide reassurance for safe resection. This technique requires the preservation of inflow and outflow until after parenchymal transection, which adds technical complexity to the operation.

This paper describes and reports the first use of the ALIIVE technique. This technique is feasible and early experience reveals it to be a compelling tool for intraoperative assessment and decision-making before irreversible vascular division to prevent posthepatectomy liver failure and death. This technique may be particularly pertinent in cases with diseased background liver parenchyma or where preoperative assessment suggests questionable future liver remnant sufficiency. The limit of safe ICG clearance during vascular exclusion remains to be confirmed by future validation studies.

References

[1] O. J. Garden, M. Rees, G. J. Poston et al., "Guidelines for resection of colorectal cancer liver metastases," *Gut*, vol. 55, supplement 3, pp. iii1–iii8, 2006.

[2] N. N. Rahbari, O. J. Garden, R. Padbury et al., "Posthepatectomy liver failure: a definition and grading by the International Study Group of Liver Surgery (ISGLS)," *Surgery*, vol. 149, no. 5, pp. 713–724, 2011.

[3] G. Garcea and G. J. Maddern, "Liver failure after major hepatic resection," *Journal of Hepato-Biliary-Pancreatic Surgery*, vol. 16, no. 2, pp. 145–155, 2009.

[4] D. Ribero, M. Amisano, F. Bertuzzo et al., "Measured versus estimated total liver volume to preoperatively assess the adequacy of the future liver remnant: which method should we use?" *Annals of Surgery*, vol. 258, no. 5, pp. 801–807, 2013.

[5] H. Bismuth, R. Adam, F. Lévi et al., "Resection of nonresectable liver metastases from colorectal cancer after neoadjuvant chemotherapy," *Annals of Surgery*, vol. 224, no. 4, pp. 509–522, 1996.

[6] K. M. Eltawil, N. Boame, R. Mimeault et al., "Patterns of recurrence following selective intraoperative radiofrequency ablation as an adjunct to hepatic resection for colorectal liver metastases," *Journal of Surgical Oncology*, vol. 110, no. 6, pp. 734–738, 2014.

[7] K. Uesaka, Y. Nimura, and M. Nagino, "Changes in hepatic lobar function after right portal vein embolization: an appraisal by biliary indocyanine green excretion," *Annals of Surgery*, vol. 223, no. 1, pp. 77–83, 1996.

[8] M. Nagino, Y. Nimura, J. Kamiya et al., "Changes in hepatic lobe volume in biliary tract cancer patients after right portal vein embolization," *Hepatology*, vol. 21, no. 2, pp. 434–439, 1995.

[9] M. E. Moussa, N. A. Habib, and A. G. Bean, "Repeated resection for malignant liver tumours," *Annals of the Royal College of Surgeons of England*, vol. 77, no. 5, pp. 364–368, 1995.

[10] A. A. Schnitzbauer, S. A. Lang, H. Goessmann et al., "Right portal vein ligation combined with in situ splitting induces rapid left lateral liver lobe hypertrophy enabling 2-staged extended right hepatic resection in small-for-size settings," *Annals of Surgery*, vol. 255, no. 3, pp. 405–414, 2012.

[11] M. Narita, E. Oussoultzoglou, P. Fuchshuber et al., "What is a safe future liver remnant size in patients undergoing major hepatectomy for colorectal liver metastases and treated by intensive preoperative chemotherapy?" *Annals of Surgical Oncology*, vol. 19, no. 8, pp. 2526–2538, 2012.

[12] J. Shindoh, C.-W. D. Tzeng, T. A. Aloia et al., "Optimal future liver remnant in patients treated with extensive preoperative chemotherapy for colorectal liver metastases," *Annals of Surgical Oncology*, vol. 20, no. 8, pp. 2493–2500, 2013.

[13] A. L. Young, D. Wilson, J. Ward et al., "Role of quantification of hepatic steatosis and future remnant volume in predicting hepatic dysfunction and complications after liver resection for colorectal metastases: a pilot study," *HPB*, vol. 14, no. 3, pp. 194–200, 2012.

[14] M. D'Onofrio, R. de Robertis, E. Demozzi, S. Crosara, S. Canestrini, and R. Pozzi Mucelli, "Liver volumetry: is imaging reliable? Personal experience and review of the literature," *World Journal of Radiology*, vol. 6, no. 4, pp. 62–71, 2014.

[15] S. Dinant, W. de Graaf, B. J. Verwer et al., "Risk assessment of posthepatectomy liver failure using hepatobiliary scintigraphy and CT volumetry," *Journal of Nuclear Medicine*, vol. 48, no. 5, pp. 685–692, 2007.

[16] W. de Graaf, K. P. van Lienden, S. Dinant et al., "Assessment of future remnant liver function using hepatobiliary scintigraphy in patients undergoing major liver resection," *Journal of Gastrointestinal Surgery*, vol. 14, no. 2, pp. 369–378, 2010.

[17] S. Sakamoto, S. Uemoto, K. Uryuhara et al., "Graft size assessment and analysis of donors for living donor liver transplantation using right lobe," *Transplantation*, vol. 71, no. 10, pp. 1407–1413, 2001.

[18] T. Schroeder, A. Radtke, H. Kuehl, J. F. Debatin, M. Malagó, and S. G. Ruehm, "Evaluation of living liver donors with an all-inclusive 3D multi-detector row CT protocol," *Radiology*, vol. 238, no. 3, pp. 900–910, 2006.

[19] A. Bégin, G. Martel, R. Lapointe et al., "Accuracy of preoperative automatic measurement of the liver volume by CT-scan combined to a 3D virtual surgical planning software (3DVSP)," *Surgical Endoscopy*, vol. 28, no. 12, pp. 3408–3412, 2014.

[20] M. Trauner, P. J. Meier, and J. L. Boyer, "Mechanisms of disease: molecular pathogenesis of cholestasis," *The New England Journal of Medicine*, vol. 339, no. 17, pp. 1217–1227, 1998.

[21] G. Cherrick, S. Stein, C. Leevy, and C. Davidson, "Indocyanine green: observations on its physical properties, plasma decay, and hepatic extraction," *The Journal of Clinical Investigation*, vol. 39, pp. 592–600, 1960.

[22] N. de Liguori Carino, D. A. O'Reilly, K. Dajani, P. Ghaneh, G. J. Poston, and A. V. Wu, "Perioperative use of the LiMON method of indocyanine green elimination measurement for the prediction and early detection of post-hepatectomy liver failure," *European Journal of Surgical Oncology*, vol. 35, no. 9, pp. 957–962, 2009.

[23] S. Ohwada, S. Kawate, K. Hamada et al., "Perioperative real-time monitoring of indocyanine green clearance by pulse spectrophotometry predicts remnant liver functional reserve in resection of hepatocellular carcinoma," *British Journal of Surgery*, vol. 93, no. 3, pp. 339–346, 2006.

[24] S. Scheingraber, S. Richter, D. Igna, S. Flesch, B. Kopp, and M. K. Schilling, "Indocyanine green disappearance rate is the most useful marker for liver resection," *Hepato-Gastroenterology*, vol. 55, no. 85, pp. 1394–1399, 2008.

[25] J. G. Tralhao, E. Hoti, B. Oliveiros, M. F. Botelho, and F. C. Sousa, "Study of perioperative liver function by dynamic monitoring of ICG-clearance," *Hepato-Gastroenterology*, vol. 59, no. 116, pp. 1179–1183, 2012.

[26] Y. Yokoyama, H. Nishio, T. Ebata, T. Igami, G. Sugawara, and M. Nagino, "Value of indocyanine green clearance of the future liver remnant in predicting outcome after resection for biliary cancer," *British Journal of Surgery*, vol. 97, no. 8, pp. 1260–1268, 2010.

[27] H. Sugimoto, O. Okochi, M. Hirota et al., "Early detection of liver failure after hepatectomy by indocyanine green elimination rate measured by pulse dye-densitometry," *Journal of Hepato-Biliary-Pancreatic Surgery*, vol. 13, no. 6, pp. 543–548, 2006.

[28] P. Faybik, C.-G. Krenn, A. Baker et al., "Comparison of invasive and noninvasive measurement of plasma disappearance rate of indocyanine green in patients undergoing liver transplantation: a prospective investigator-blinded study," *Liver Transplantation*, vol. 10, no. 8, pp. 1060–1064, 2004.

[29] L. Olmedilla, C. Ripoll, I. Garutti et al., "Early noninvasive measurement of the indocyanine green plasma disappearance rate accurately predicts early graft dysfunction and mortality after deceased donor liver transplantation," *Liver Transplantation*, vol. 15, no. 10, pp. 1247–1253, 2009.

[30] B. M. Parker, J. B. Cywinski, J. M. Alster et al., "Predicting immunosuppressant dosing in the early postoperative period with noninvasive indocyanine green elimination following orthotopic liver transplantation," *Liver Transplantation*, vol. 14, no. 1, pp. 46–52, 2008.

[31] J. J. Vos, T. W. L. Scheeren, D. J. Lukes, M. T. de Boer, H. G. D. Hendriks, and J. K. G. Wietasch, "Intraoperative ICG plasma disappearance rate helps to predict absence of early postoperative complications after orthotopic liver transplantation," *Journal of Clinical Monitoring and Computing*, vol. 27, no. 5, pp. 591–598, 2013.

[32] T. Von Spiegel, M. Scholz, G. Wietasch et al., "Perioperative monitoring of indocyanine green clearance and plasma disappearance rate in patients undergoing liver transplantation," *Anaesthesist*, vol. 51, no. 5, pp. 359–366, 2002.

[33] E. Levesque, F. Saliba, S. Benhamida et al., "Plasma disappearance rate of indocyanine green: a tool to evaluate early graft outcome after liver transplantation," *Liver Transplantation*, vol. 15, no. 10, pp. 1358–1364, 2009.

[34] L. Schneider, M. Spiegel, S. Latanowicz et al., "Noninvasive indocyanine green plasma disappearance rate predicts early complications, graft failure or death after liver transplantation," *Hepatobiliary and Pancreatic Diseases International*, vol. 10, no. 4, pp. 362–368, 2011.

[35] E. P. Misiakos, N. P. Karidis, and G. Kouraklis, "Current treatment for colorectal liver metastases," *World Journal of Gastroenterology*, vol. 17, no. 36, pp. 4067–4075, 2011.

[36] Y. Kishi, E. K. Abdalla, Y. S. Chun et al., "Three hundred and one consecutive extended right hepatectomies: evaluation of outcome based on systematic liver volumetry," *Annals of Surgery*, vol. 250, no. 4, pp. 540–547, 2009.

[37] D. Ribero, Y. S. Chun, and J.-N. Vauthey, "Standardized liver volumetry for portal vein embolization," *Seminars in Interventional Radiology*, vol. 25, no. 2, pp. 104–109, 2008.

[38] D. Dindo, N. Demartines, and P.-A. Clavien, "Classification of surgical complications: a new proposal with evaluation in a cohort of 6336 patients and results of a survey," *Annals of Surgery*, vol. 240, no. 2, pp. 205–213, 2004.

[39] K. Chijiiwa, A. Mizuta, J. Ueda et al., "Relation of biliary bile acid output to hepatic adenosine triphosphate level and biliary indocyanine green excretion in humans," *World Journal of Surgery*, vol. 26, no. 4, pp. 457–461, 2002.

[40] R. E. Koehler, M. Korobkin, and F. Lewis, "Arteriographic demonstration of collateral arterial supply to the liver after hepatic artery ligation," *Radiology*, vol. 117, no. 1, pp. 49–54, 1975.

[41] T. Sato, T. Kurokawa, T. Kusano et al., "Uptake of indocyanine green by hepatocytes under inflow occlusion of the liver," *Journal of Surgical Research*, vol. 105, no. 2, pp. 81–85, 2002.

[42] C. S. van Kessel, C. F. M. Buckens, M. A. A. J. van den Bosch, M. S. van Leeuwen, R. Van Hillegersberg, and H. M. Verkooijen, "Preoperative imaging of colorectal liver metastases after neoadjuvant chemotherapy: a meta-analysis," *Annals of Surgical Oncology*, vol. 19, no. 9, pp. 2805–2813, 2012.

10

Ischemic Preconditioning of Rat Livers from Non-Heart-Beating Donors Decreases Parenchymal Cell Killing and Increases Graft Survival after Transplantation

Robert T. Currin,[1] Xing-Xi Peng,[1] and John J. Lemasters[2]

[1] *Department of Cell & Developmental Biology, University of North Carolina, Chapel Hill, NC 27599, USA*
[2] *Center for Cell Death, Injury & Regeneration, Departments of Pharmaceutical & Biomedical Sciences and Biochemistry & Molecular Biology, Medical University of South Carolina, Charleston, SC 29425, USA*

Correspondence should be addressed to John J. Lemasters, jjlemasters@musc.edu

Academic Editor: Peter Schemmer

A critical shortage of donors exists for liver transplantation, which non-heart-beating cadaver donors could help ease. This study evaluated ischemic preconditioning to improve graft viability after non-heart-beating liver donation in rats. Ischemic preconditioning was performed by clamping the portal vein and hepatic artery for 10 min followed by unclamping for 5 min. Subsequently, the aorta was cross-clamped for up to 120 min. After 2 h of storage, livers were either transplanted or perfused with warm buffer containing trypan blue. Aortic clamping for 60 and 120 min prior to liver harvest markedly decreased 30-day graft survival from 100% without aortic clamping to 50% and 0%, respectively, which ischemic preconditioning restored to 100 and 50%. After 60 min of aortic clamping, loss of viability of parenchymal and nonparenchymal cells was 22.6 and 5.6%, respectively, which preconditioning decreased to 3.0 and 1.5%. Cold storage after aortic clamping further increased parenchymal and non-parenchymal cell killing to 40.4 and 10.1%, respectively, which ischemic preconditioning decreased to 12.4 and 1.8%. In conclusion, ischemic preconditioning markedly decreased cell killing after subsequent sustained warm ischemia. Most importantly, ischemic preconditioning restored 100% graft survival of livers harvested from non-heart-beating donors after 60 min of aortic clamping.

1. Introduction

Liver transplantation surgery is a viable alternative for patients with end-stage liver disease but the number of heart-beating cadavers suitable for liver donation remains a key limitation. In human kidney transplantation, organ donation from non-heart-beating cadavers is now employed successfully at many centers [1]. Organ donors are typically terminally ill patients who do not meet the criteria of brain death and whose life support is withdrawn at the request of the family. After cardiac arrest occurs and death is pronounced several minutes later, the organs are harvested.

The use of livers from non-heart-beating donors is also emerging as an important stratagem to expand the liver donor pool [2]. Organs from non-heart-beating cadaver donors typically experience several minutes of warm ischemia prior to cold preservation. Warm ischemic injury that occurs to livers after cardiac arrest can severely compromise graft viability. Early clinical results with livers from non-heart-beating donors were poor, and two-month graft survival was only 50% even for donors that were extubated in an operating room setting [3]. With more rapid organ harvesting, clinical outcomes have improved, but rates of primary nonfunction, initial poor function, and ischemic-type biliary strictures remain greater than with donor livers from heat-beating cadaver donors [2]. Consequently, new and different strategies are needed to block warm ischemic injury in this context and to improve the outcome of non-heart-beating cadaver donation in liver transplantation.

Ischemic conditioning is the application of brief episodes of nonlethal ischemia and reperfusion to confer protection against sustained ischemia, which is showing therapeutic

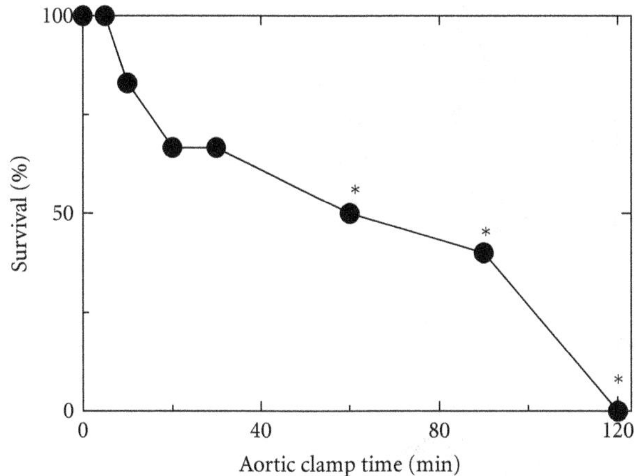

Figure 1: Loss of graft survival after aortic clamping. Aortas were clamped for 0 to 120 min. After clamping, livers were flushed with ice-cold UW solution. After 2 h of cold storage, the livers were transplanted into recipient rats, as described in section 2. Data are from 5 to 12 transplantations per time point. $^*P < 0.05$ compared to 0 min clamping by Fisher's exact test.

potential in various clinical settings [4, 5]. In rodent studies, ischemic preconditioning of the liver protects against injury after subsequent prolonged warm ischemia, particularly in fatty livers [6–8]. Decreases of transaminase release and sinusoidal endothelial cell killing also occur after cold preservation, which improve graft survival after orthotopic transplantation [9, 10]. In human liver surgery, ischemic preconditioning decreases postoperative transaminases and hepatic apoptosis, particularly in patients with mild-to-moderate steatosis, but in liver transplantation the benefit of ischemic preconditioning remains to be conclusively established [11–14]. The effect of ischemic preconditioning on graft injury and survival after transplantation of livers from non-heart-beating donors is not well studied. Here, we show that preconditioning with 10 min of warm hepatic ischemia markedly decreases hepatocellular and endothelial cell killing after subsequent sustained warm ischemia and after sustained warm ischemia followed by cold storage. Most importantly, ischemic preconditioning restores graft survival of livers harvested from non-heart-beating donors.

2. Methods

2.1. Orthotopic Rat Liver Transplantation. All animal protocols conformed to criteria of the Institutional Animal Care and Use Committee. Orthotopic rat liver transplantation was performed in male Lewis rats (220–280 g) under ether anesthesia using an arterialized two-cuff method by slight modification of the procedure of Steffen et al. [15]. For the donor operation, the liver was freed from its peritoneal attachments, and the common bile duct was cannulated with a polyethylene tube and divided. Cold University of Wisconsin (UW) solution (Viaspan, Dupont Pharma, Wilmington, DE) was infused through the portal vein. The suprahepatic inferior cava, subhepatic inferior cava, portal vein, and celiac artery were divided at the level of the diaphragm, left renal vein, splenic vein, and splenic artery, respectively. The liver was excised and placed in a bath of ice-chilled UW solution. Cuffs were then placed on the portal vein and subhepatic inferior cava before storage at 0–1°C in an ice water bath.

In recipient rats, the proper hepatic and gastroduodenal arteries were divided at their origin, leaving a stump of the common hepatic artery. The stump was clamped at the base of the dissected segment. The bifurcation of the proper hepatic and gastroduodenal arteries was cut, leaving a funnel-shaped opening to which a cuff was attached. After dividing the bile duct at the hilum, the suprahepatic inferior cava, portal vein, and subhepatic inferior cava were clamped and divided, and the recipient liver was removed. The donor liver was then rinsed with 10 mL of Ringer's solution at 37°C. Subsequently, the suprahepatic inferior cava was anastomosed with a running suture, and the portal vein, subhepatic inferior cava, and hepatic artery were connected in sequence by insertion of cuffs. The bile duct was anastomosed over an intraluminal polyethylene splint.

2.2. Ischemic Preconditioning and Aortic Clamping. To induce ischemic preconditioning, the abdomen was opened under ether anesthesia, and the hepatic artery and portal vein were occluded with a mini-bulldog vascular clamp for 10 min. The clamp was then released, and the liver was reperfused for 5 min prior to harvesting. To simulate non-heart-beating organ donation, the thorax was opened under ether anesthesia, and the ascending aorta clamped for 5 to 120 min, followed immediately by harvest of the liver.

2.3. Cell Killing. To assess cell viability after storage, livers were reperfused for 15 min with Krebs-Henseleit bicarbonate buffer (KHB) containing 500 μM trypan blue at an initial flow rate of 5 mL/min increasing to 30 mL/min over the first 5 min. In some experiments, stored livers were reperfused for 5 min with ice-cold UW solution containing 500 μM trypan blue at an initial flow rate of 5 mL/min increasing to 15 mL/min after 5 min [16, 17]. After trypan blue infusion, livers were fixed by perfusion for 2 min with 2% paraformaldehyde in 0.1 M NaPi buffer, pH 7.4. The temperature of the fixation was the same as the preceding perfusion. After this initial fixation, the left lateral lobe was cut into 1 cm slices and placed in ice-cold fixative. The tissue was then embedded in paraffin, sectioned, and stained with eosin or hematoxylin/eosin. For each liver, nuclear trypan blue uptake in parenchymal and nonparenchymal cells was determined in 5 random periportal and pericentral regions in eosin-stained sections using a 60X objective and expressed as the percentage of total nuclei counted in hematoxylin/eosin stained sections.

2.4. Statistics. Differences in survival were analyzed using Fisher's exact test, and differences between means were analyzed by analysis of variance (ANOVA). One-tailed tests were used to test unidirectional hypotheses, for example, that ischemic preconditioning decreases storage/reperfusion

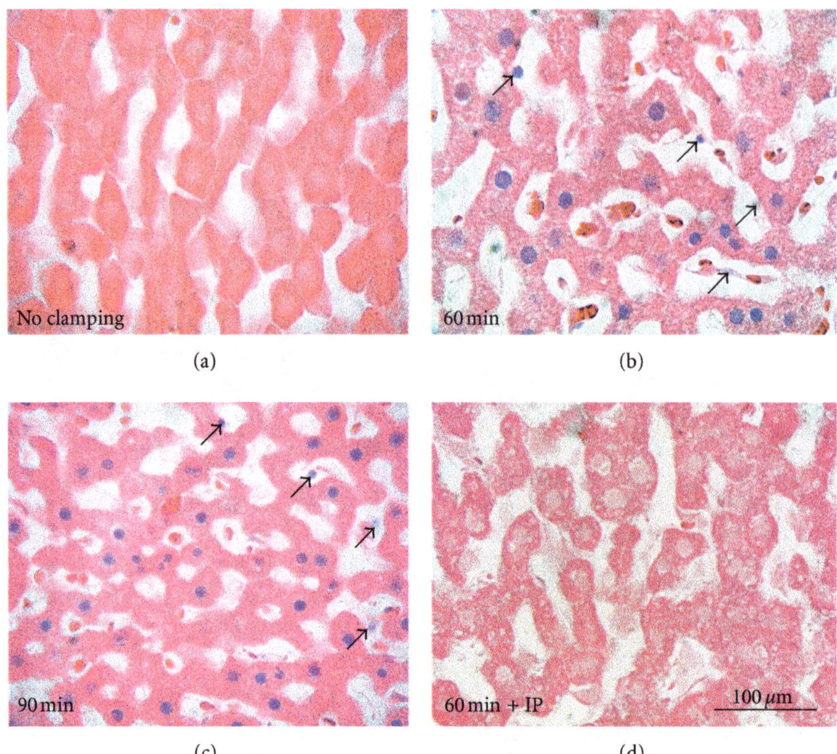

Figure 2: Light microscopy of livers after aortic clamping. In (a, b, c), the aortas of anesthetized rats were clamped for 0, 60, and 90 min, respectively, and their livers were then infused with cold UW solution containing trypan blue to label nonviable cells, as described in section 2. In d, a liver was first subjected to 10 min of ischemia followed by 5 min of reperfusion before 60 min aortic clamping. Trypan blue was then infused, as described for (a–c). Blue nuclei in eosin-counterstained sections represent mostly nonviable parenchymal cells. Arrows identify examples of nonviable nonparenchymal cells.

injury and improves graft survival. Group sizes are given in the legends to the figures. Errors represent the standard error of the mean. *P* values of less than 0.05 were considered to be significant.

3. Results

3.1. Decreased Graft Survival after Warm Ischemia Prior to Liver Harvest. Harvesting livers from non-heart-beating cadaver donors represents a potential means to expand the donor pool for human clinical liver transplantation. Accordingly, we harvested rat livers after various periods of aortic clamping and transplanted them into syngeneic recipient Lewis rats. When the aorta was not cross-clamped prior to liver harvest, 30-day graft survival was 100% after 2 h of cold storage (Figure 1). Graft survival was also 100% after 5 min of aortic clamping. After 10 min and longer, graft survival decreased progressively from 83% after 10 min to 50% after 60 min and 0% after 120 min. Thus, the livers tolerated only a very short period of warm ischemia before graft survival after transplantation began to decline. Necropsies revealed that none of the deaths was due to an obvious surgical error, such as a leaky arterial or venous anastomosis.

3.2. Loss of Parenchymal and Nonparenchymal Cell Viability after Warm Ischemia and Warm Ischemia Followed by Cold Storage. In another set of experiments, we assessed what cell types were losing viability as a consequence of various periods of warm ischemia. Aortas were cross-clamped, and after various periods of time, cold UW solution containing trypan blue was infused for 5 min followed by perfusion fixation with cold phosphate-buffered paraformaldehyde. Viable cells exclude trypan blue, whereas nonviable cells take up trypan blue into their nuclei. Thus, by counting trypan blue positive nuclei in eosin-counterstained histological sections, loss of viability of both parenchymal and nonparenchymal cells was determined.

Without aortic cross-clamping, trypan blue-stained nuclei were extremely rare in histological sections (Figure 2(a)). By contrast, with aortic cross-clamping, trypan blue labeling progressively increased (Figures 2(b) and 2(c) and Figure 3). Most trypan blue labeling occurred in hepatic parenchymal cells (hepatocytes), but some nonparenchymal cells also began to label after longer periods of clamping (Figures 2(b) and 2(c), arrowheads). The percentage of trypan blue-labeled parenchymal and nonparenchymal nuclei was averaged for several livers subjected to various times of aortic cross-clamping. After 0 and 5 min of aortic cross-clamping, trypan blue labeling of parenchymal or nonparenchymal cells was less than 0.5% (Figure 3). After longer times of cross-clamping, parenchymal cell killing (loss of viability) steadily increased from 12% after 30 min to 40% after 90 min. Nonparenchymal cell killing increased to a lesser extent to a maximum of 6% after 60 min. Nonparenchymal

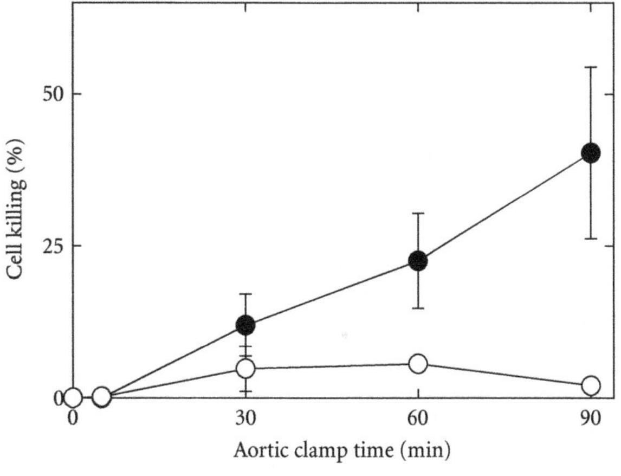

FIGURE 3: Increased parenchymal and nonparenchymal cell killing after aortic clamping. Aortas were clamped for 0 to 90 min. After clamping, livers were immediately infused with cold UW solution containing trypan blue and fixed, as described in Figure 2. Data represent means ± S.E.M. from 3 to 5 rats per group per time point.

killing appeared to decrease after 90 min, but this finding may be artifactual due to masking of nonparenchymal labeling by parenchymal nuclear labeling or to washout of nuclei of nonviable nonparenchymal cells as the livers were infused with trypan blue-containing UW solution.

To assess the additional effect of cold storage and reperfusion, aortas were cross-clamped for 0 to 90 min, and the livers were then infused with cold UW solution and stored for 2 h. After storage, livers were reperfused at 37°C for 15 min with KHB containing trypan blue and fixed for histology. Cold storage and reperfusion in the absence of aortic clamping led to virtually no trypan blue staining of either parenchymal or nonparenchymal cells (Figure 4(a)). With increasing times of aortic clamping followed by cold storage and reperfusion, parenchymal cell killing increased markedly (Figures 4(b), 4(c), and 5). After 30 and 60 min of cross-clamping and cold storage, parenchymal cell killing was 3.8 and 1.8 times that observed after clamping but no cold storage (Figure 5 compared to Figure 3, $P < 0.05$). After 90 min of cross-clamping, cold storage caused 28% more parenchymal cell killing than in the absence of cold storage, but this difference was not statistically significant (Figure 4(d) and Figure 5). None of the differences between nonparenchymal cell killing after clamping alone and nonparenchymal cell killing after clamping plus storage were statistically significant.

3.3. Improved Survival after Ischemic Preconditioning of Liver Grafts Subjected to Warm Ischemia and Cold Storage. In an effort to make donor livers resistant to the deleterious effects of aortic clamping prior to organ harvest and cold storage, we performed an ischemic preconditioning protocol whereby the hepatic artery and portal vein were occluded for 10 min. Subsequently, the vascular clamp was removed to allow the reflow of blood to the liver. After 5 more min, the aorta was cross-clamped for 60 to 120 min, and the livers were harvested, stored 2 h in UW solution, and transplanted. In comparison to non-preconditioned liver grafts, 30-day survival of liver grafts subjected to ischemic preconditioning increased from 50 to 100% after 60 min of aortic clamping ($P < 0.05$), 40 to 67% after 90 min of clamping ($P = 0.39$), and 0 to 50% after 120 minute of clamping ($P < 0.05$) (Figure 6). When it occurred, graft failure developed relatively rapidly. After clamp times of 60, 90 and 120 min, survival of animals that did not live to 30 days averaged 2.4, 2.5, and 4.8 days, respectively, without preconditioning. With preconditioning, average time to death of animals not surviving 30 days was 3.0 and 4.8 days after 90, and 120 min of aortic clamping.

3.4. Decreased Parenchymal and Nonparenchymal Cell Killing by Ischemic Preconditioning in Livers Subjected to Warm Ischemia. Since ischemic preconditioning improved survival of liver grafts subjected to warm ischemia before storage, we investigated how ischemic preconditioning influenced cell killing during these treatments. Livers were subjected to ischemic preconditioning or a sham operation. Subsequently, aortic clamping was imposed for 60 min, and the livers were infused with cold trypan blue-containing UW solution followed by fixation for histology. Our goal was to determine how ischemic preconditioning affected parenchymal and nonparenchymal cell killing prior to cold storage. As shown in Figure 7, ischemic preconditioning (IP) decreased parenchymal (a) and nonparenchymal (b) cell killing determined by trypan blue labeling to 3.0 to 1.5%, respectively, from 22.5% and 5.6 % after sham treatment (control) ($P < 0.05$).

Similarly, we subjected livers to ischemic preconditioning (IP) or sham treatment followed by 1 h of aortic clamping and 2 h of cold storage in UW solution. At the end of storage, the livers were either flushed with cold trypan blue-containing UW solution to assess cell killing at the end of storage (unreperfused) or reperfused with warm trypan blue-containing KHB for 15 min to assess cell killing after reperfusion (reperfused). As shown in Figure 8, parenchymal (left panel) and nonparenchymal (right panel) cell killing without preconditioning was about the same in stored livers that were not reperfused as in those that were reperfused. By contrast, ischemic preconditioning prior to aortic clamping and cold storage caused large and statistically significant decreases of both parenchymal and nonparenchymal cell killing measured at the end of cold storage with and without reperfusion.

4. Discussion

The success of liver transplantation surgery for patients with end-stage liver disease has caused growth worldwide of waiting lists for liver transplantation surgery, which greatly outnumber the available donor livers. The use of livers from non-heart-beating donors is one potential source for increasing the organ donation pool. Non-heart-beating donors have become an important source of kidney

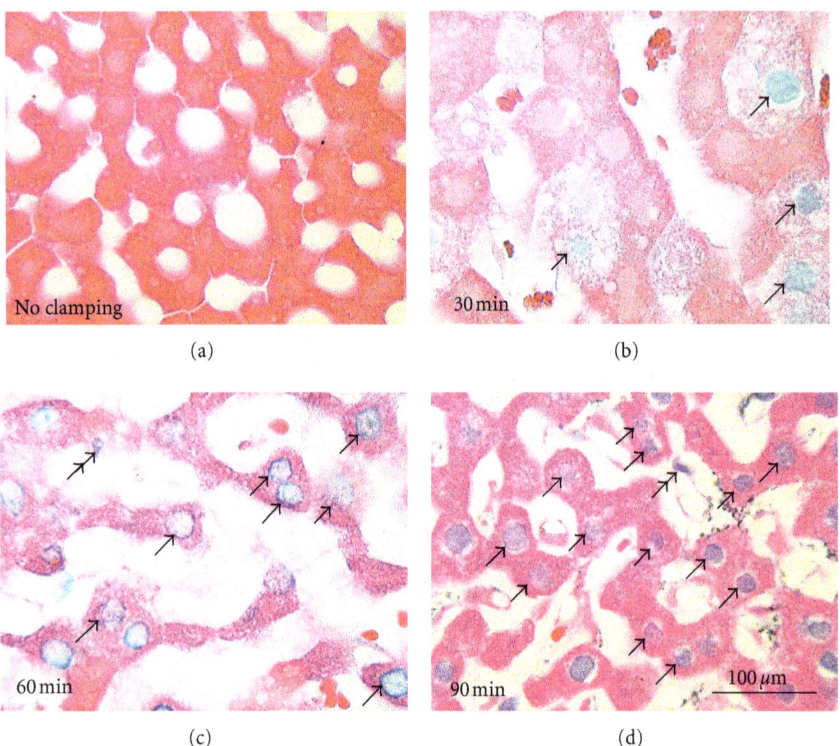

FIGURE 4: Light microscopy of livers after aortic clamping and cold storage/reperfusion. Aortas were clamped for 0 to 90 min. After clamping, livers were stored for 2 h in cold UW solution, followed by 15 min of warm reperfusion with KHB containing trypan blue to label nonviable cells, as described in section 2. Blue nuclei in eosin-counterstained sections represent nonviable parenchymal and nonparenchymal cells, as illustrated by arrows and double arrows respectively.

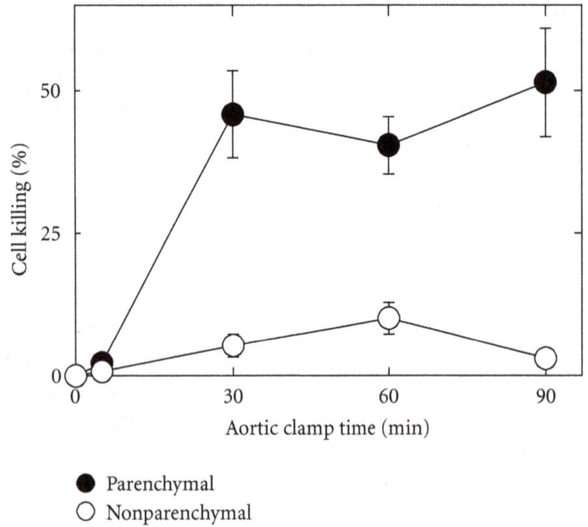

FIGURE 5: Parenchymal and nonparenchymal cell killing after aortic clamping and cold storage/reperfusion. Aortas were clamped for 0 to 90 min, and livers were cold stored and reperfused, as described in Figure 4. Data represent means ± S.E.M. from 5 rats per group per time point.

donations and are becoming an increasing source for liver donation [1, 2]. However unlike kidney grafts, liver grafts must recover function much more quickly and appear to be more susceptible to harvest, preservation, and reperfusion injury.

In our non-heart-beating model, the aortas of Lewis rats were cross-clamped for a specified period of time, stored for 2 h in UW solution, and transplanted. After as little as 10 min of aortic clamping, graft survival decreased after orthotopic rat liver transplantation (Figure 1). With increasing aortic clamp time, there was a continued decline in graft survival to 50% after 60 min of aortic clamping and 0% after 120 min of warm ischemia.

To better understand the injury caused by aortic clamping, we infused trypan blue at the end of aortic clamping to label nonviable cells. To minimize the effects of reperfusion we infused cold UW solution containing trypan blue for 5 min. Trypan blue labeling indicated that cellular killing was predominately to parenchymal cells (Figure 2). Trypan blue nuclear labeling signifies onset of necrotic cell death. Although not analyzed in detail, apoptosis was largely absent as shown by the lack of nuclear condensation, lobulation, and chromatin aggregation, which is consistent with earlier studies of both warm and cold ischemia (reviewed in [18]). Parenchymal cell killing started after as little as 10 min of aortic clamping and steadily increased over time (Figure 3). Parenchymal cell killing increased further after subsequent cold storage in UW solution and reperfusion, but no significant differences in nonparenchymal cell killing were

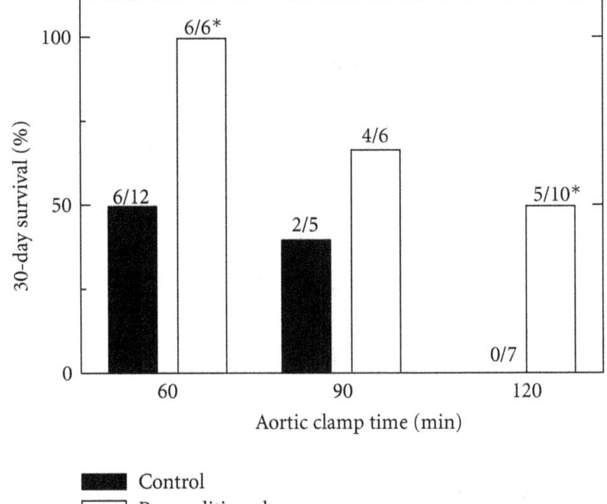

FIGURE 6: Improved graft survival by ischemic preconditioning before aortic clamping. Anesthetized rats were given a sham operation (control) or ischemic preconditioning by clamping of the hepatic artery and portal vein for 10 min followed by 5 min of blood reperfusion (preconditioned). The aortas of the rats were then clamped for 60, 90, or 120 min. After clamping, livers were infused with cold UW solution, and stored for 2 h. After storage, livers were transplanted into recipient rats, and recipient survival after 30 days was determined. Numbers above the bars indicate survivors/total transplants. $*P < 0.05$ versus control by Fisher's exact test.

observed between aortic clamping and aortic clamping plus cold storage and reperfusion (Figures 4 and 5). Unlike cold ischemia [19, 20], warm ischemia involved principally parenchymal cells. Injury to parenchymal cells began to increase after 10 min of aortic clamping and continued to increase over time, which correlated with transplantation studies where graft failure also began to occur and progressively increased after 10 min or more of aortic clamping.

In heart and other organs including liver, preconditioning by short periods of ischemia followed by reperfusion protects against longer periods of ischemia [4]. Our model of ischemic preconditioning entailed clamping the hepatic artery and portal vein for 10 min, followed by 5 min of blood reperfusion. Such ischemic preconditioning markedly increased graft survival after 60 and 120 min of aortic cross-clamping (Figure 6). Substantial survival after as much as 120 min of aortic cross-clamping illustrates the robustness of protection by ischemic preconditioning. Likewise, ischemic preconditioning decreased parenchymal and nonparenchymal cell killing after aortic clamping and after aortic clamping followed by cold storage plus reperfusion (Figures 7 and 8). In some models, repetitive (up to 3) intervals of short ischemia/reperfusion further improve protection by ischemic preconditioning [4, 5]. Future studies will be needed to optimize preconditioning in terms of ischemia time and number of repetitions for non-heart-beating liver donation, although use of repetitions of ischemia/reperfusion may be impractical in a clinical donor situation. Ischemic-type biliary strictures can develop 1 to 4 months after liver transplantation whose incidence increases with non-heart-beating donation [2, 21, 22]. Future studies will also be needed to determine if ischemic preconditioning can also decrease the incidence of such strictures.

The mechanisms of action for ischemic preconditioning of the liver involve a variety of factors and pathways, including adenosine, nitric oxide, and activation of protein kinases (e.g., phosphatidylinositol 3-kinase, protein kinase C, p38 MAP kinase) and transcription factors (e.g., signal transducer and activator of transcription 3, nuclear factor-kB and hypoxia-inducible factor 1) [5]. In the context of cold storage/reperfusion injury to liver, we and others showed in a rat model of orthotopic liver transplantation that ischemic preconditioning improves survival of liver grafts harvested from heart-beating rat donors [10, 23, 24]. Improved graft survival is associated with decreased sinusoidal endothelial cell killing and Kupffer activation mediated at least in part by an adenosine A_2 receptor pathway coupled to increased cAMP [9]. Ischemic preconditioning also decreases hepatic injury, attenuates mitochondrial dysfunction, reduces free radical formation, and improves regeneration of small-for-size liver grafts, possibly by increasing mitochondrial superoxide dismutase expression [25]. Increasingly, ischemic preconditioning is being employed clinically to decrease hepatic injury after liver transplantation and other surgeries [12].

By contrast to the predominantly nonparenchymal cell injury that occurs after cold storage/reperfusion, the findings of the present study show that warm ischemia induced by aortic clamping caused loss of viability predominantly to parenchymal cells, namely, the hepatocytes. This lethal parenchymal cell injury then led to graft failure after orthotopic rat liver transplantation. Reperfusion was not a key factor contributing to cell killing after aortic clamping, since cell death could be shown in the absence of warm reperfusion by direct infusion of cold UW solution containing trypan blue. Nonetheless, subsequent brief cold storage and warm reperfusion did increase cell killing moderately. The change in cell type and role of reperfusion in hepatic cell killing after warm versus cold ischemia suggests different mechanisms of injury. Since parenchymal cell injury after aortic clamping occurred before cold storage, assessment of the suitability of donor livers from non-heart-beating cadavers might be possible before cold storage by examining trypan blue labeling in biopsies.

In conclusion, ischemic preconditioning protected strongly against parenchymal cell killing after aortic clamping and markedly improved survival of grafts from non-heart-beating donors. In a clinical setting, uncontrolled episodes of hypoxia and hypoperfusion may contribute to protective preconditioning, but organ manipulations such as ischemic preconditioning are currently prohibited prior to declaration of donor death. However, future changes in living wills and accepted ethical practices may permit use of ischemic preconditioning in terminally ill donors just prior to withdrawal of life support. Moreover, better understanding of the mechanisms underlying protection by ischemic preconditioning in the specific context of non-heart-beating liver donation may permit

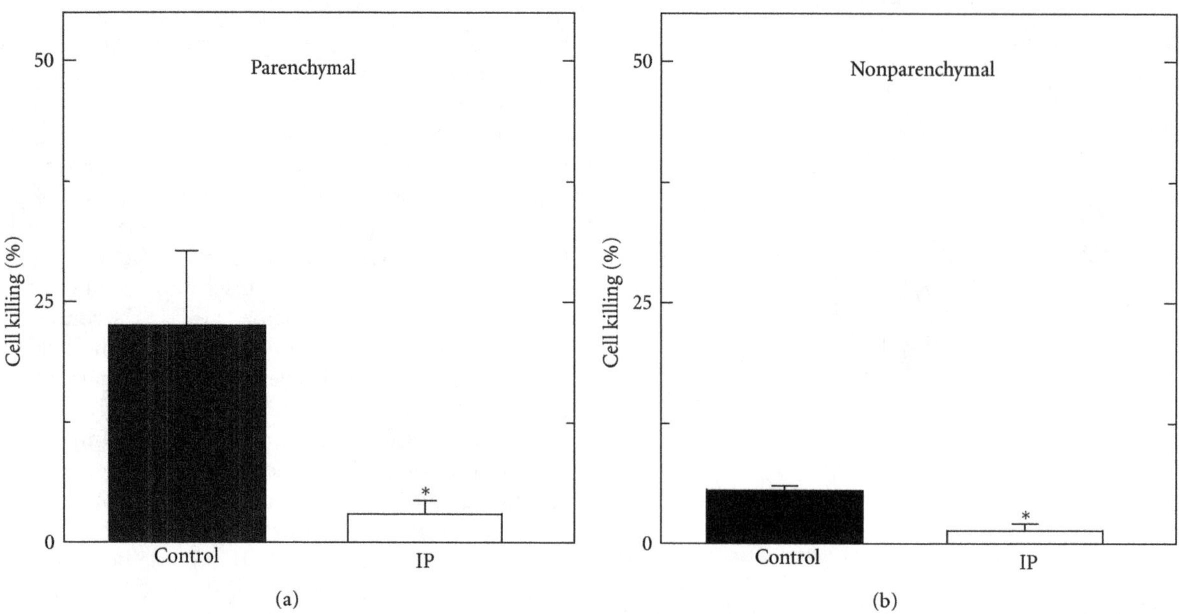

FIGURE 7: Decreased parenchymal and nonparenchymal cell killing by ischemic preconditioning after aortic clamping. Anesthesized rats were given a sham operation (control) or ischemic preconditioning by clamping of the hepatic artery and portal vein for 10 min followed by 5 min of blood reperfusion (IP). The aortas of the rats were then clamped for 60 min. After clamping, the livers were infused with cold UW solution containing trypan blue to label nonviable parenchymal (a) and nonparenchymal (b) cells. Data represent means ± S.E.M. from 5 rats per group per time point. $^*P < 0.05$ versus control by ANOVA.

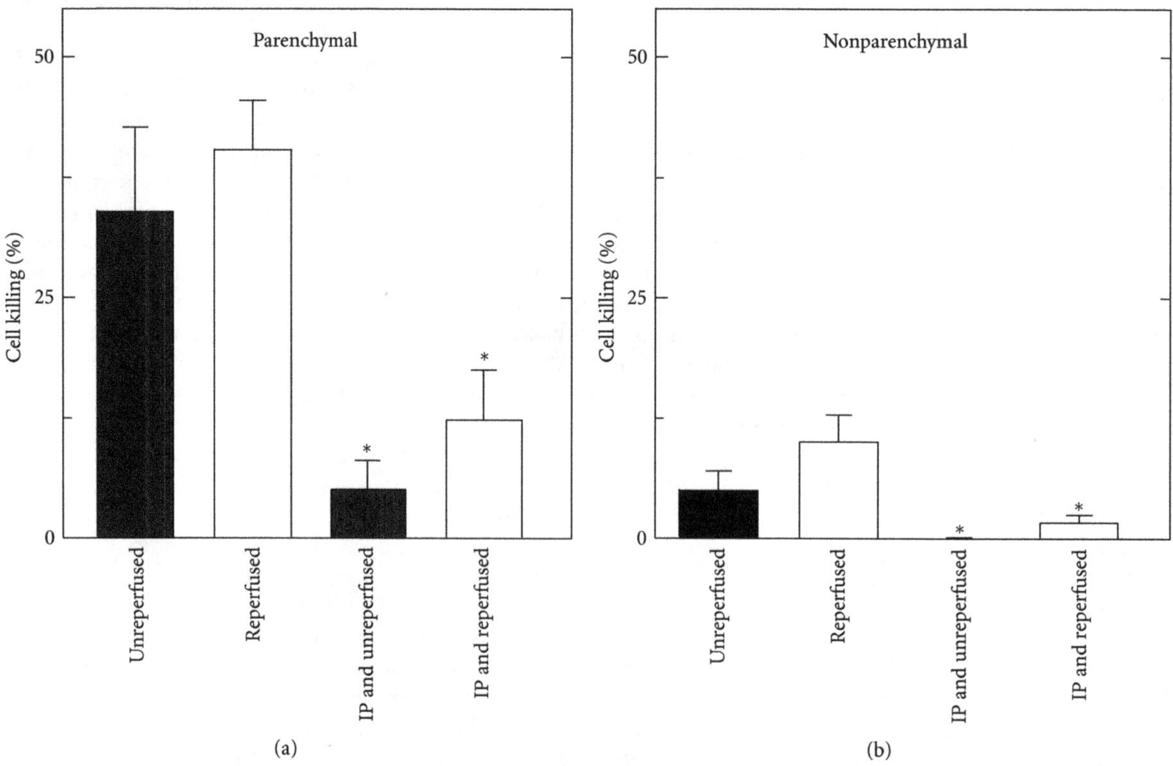

FIGURE 8: Decreased parenchymal and nonparenchymal cell killing by ischemic preconditioning after aortic clamping and cold storage with and without reperfusion. Anesthesized rats were given a sham operation or ischemic preconditioning (IP) by clamping of the hepatic artery and portal vein for 10 min followed by 5 min of blood reperfusion. The aortas of the rats were then clamped for 60 min. After clamping, the livers were stored for 2 h in cold UW solution. Subsequently, the livers were infused for 5 min with cold UW solution containing trypan blue to label nonviable cells in the absence of warm reperfusion (unreperfused) or infused for 15 min with warm KHB containing trypan blue to label nonviable cells after warm reperfusion (reperfused), as described in section 2. Nonviable parenchymal cells (a) and nonparenchymal cells (b) were counted from 5 livers per group. $^*P < 0.05$ compared to the corresponding non-IP group by ANOVA.

use of pharmacological strategies to simulate ischemic preconditioning. In this way, ischemic preconditioning or its pharmacological surrogate might one day be applied clinically in advance of liver donation after planned removal of life-sustaining treatment such as mechanical ventilation.

Acknowledgments

This work was supported, in part, by Grants DK37034 and DK073336 from the National Institutes of Health. Imaging facilities for this research were supported, in part, by Cancer Center Support Grant P30 CA138313 to the Hollings Cancer Center, Medical University of South Carolina.

References

[1] A. R. Evenson, "Utilization of kidneys from donation after circulatory determination of death," *Current Opinion in Organ Transplantation*, vol. 16, no. 4, pp. 385–389, 2011.

[2] D. Monbaliu, J. Pirenne, and D. Talbot, "Liver transplantation using Donation after Cardiac Death donors," *Journal of Hepatology*, vol. 56, pp. 474–485, 2012.

[3] A. Casavilla, C. Ramirez, R. Shapiro et al., "Experience with liver and kidney allografts from non-heart-beating donors," *Transplantation*, vol. 59, no. 2, pp. 197–203, 1995.

[4] D. J. Hausenloy and D. M. Yellon, "The therapeutic potential of ischemic conditioning: an update," *Nature Reviews Cardiology*, vol. 8, pp. 619–629, 2011.

[5] E. Alchera, C. Dal Ponte, C. Imarisio, E. Albano, and R. Carini, "Molecular mechanisms of liver preconditioning," *World Journal of Gastroenterology*, vol. 16, no. 48, pp. 6058–6067, 2010.

[6] C. Peralta, G. Hotter, D. Closa, E. Gelpí, O. Bulbena, and J. Roselló-Catafau, "Protective effect of preconditioning on the injury associated to hepatic ischemia-reperfusion in the rat: role of nitric oxide and adenosine," *Hepatology*, vol. 25, no. 4, pp. 934–937, 1997.

[7] T. Yoshizumi, K. Yanaga, Y. Soejima, T. Maeda, H. Uchiyama, and K. Sugimachi, "Amelioration of liver injury by ischaemic preconditioning," *British Journal of Surgery*, vol. 85, no. 12, pp. 1636–1640, 1998.

[8] A. Serafín, J. Roselló-Catafau, N. Prats, C. Xaus, E. Gelpí, and C. Peralta, "Ischemic preconditioning increases the tolerance of fatty liver to hepatic ischemia-reperfusion injury in the rat," *American Journal of Pathology*, vol. 161, no. 2, pp. 587–601, 2002.

[9] M. Arai, R. G. Thurman, and J. J. Lemasters, "Contribution of adenosine A2 receptors and cyclic adenosine monophosphate to protective ischemic preconditioning of sinusoidal endothelial cells against storage/reperfusion injury in rat livers," *Hepatology*, vol. 32, no. 2, pp. 297–302, 2000.

[10] D. P. Yin, H. N. Sankary, A. S. F. Chong et al., "Protective effect of ischemic preconditioning on liver preservation-reperfusion injury in rats," *Transplantation*, vol. 66, no. 2, pp. 152–157, 1998.

[11] P. A. Clavien, M. Selzner, H. A. Rüdiger et al., "A prospective randomized study in 100 consecutive patients undergoing major liver resection with versus without ischemic preconditioning," *Annals of Surgery*, vol. 238, no. 6, pp. 843–852, 2003.

[12] O. de Rougemont, K. Lehmann, and P. A. Clavien, "Preconditioning, organ preservation, and postconditioning to prevent ischemia-reperfusion injury to the liver," *Liver Transplantation*, vol. 15, no. 10, pp. 1172–1182, 2009.

[13] M. L. DeOliveira, R. Graf, and P. A. Clavien, "Ischemic preconditioning: promises from the laboratory to patients—sustained or disillusioned?" *American Journal of Transplantation*, vol. 8, no. 3, pp. 489–491, 2008.

[14] B. Koneru, A. Fisher, Y. He et al., "Ischemic preconditioning in deceased donor liver transplantation: a prospective randomized clinical trial of safety and efficacy," *Liver Transplantation*, vol. 11, no. 2, pp. 196–202, 2005.

[15] R. Steffen, D. M. Ferguson, and R. A. F. Krom, "A new method for orthotopic rat liver transplantation with arterial cuff anastomosis to the recipient common hepatic artery," *Transplantation*, vol. 48, no. 1, pp. 166–168, 1989.

[16] B. U. Bradford, M. Marotto, J. J. Lemasters, and R. G. Thurman, "New, simple models to evaluate zone-specific damage due to hypoxia in the perfused rat liver: time course and effect of nutritional state," *Journal of Pharmacology and Experimental Therapeutics*, vol. 236, no. 1, pp. 263–268, 1986.

[17] J. C. Caldwell-Kenkel, R. T. Currin, Y. Tanaka, R. G. Thurman, and J. J. Lemasters, "Reperfusion injury to endothelial cells following cold ischemic storage of rat livers," *Hepatology*, vol. 10, no. 3, pp. 292–299, 1989.

[18] H. Jaeschke and J. J. Lemasters, "Apoptosis versus oncotic necrosis in hepatic ischemia/reperfusion injury," *Gastroenterology*, vol. 125, no. 4, pp. 1246–1257, 2003.

[19] J. C. Caldwell-Kenkel, R. G. Thurman, and J. J. Lemasters, "Selective loss of nonparenchymal cell viability after cold ischemic storage of rat livers," *Transplantation*, vol. 45, no. 4, pp. 834–837, 1988.

[20] J. C. Caldwell-Kenkel, R. T. Currin, Y. Tanaka, R. G. Thurman, and J. J. Lemasters, "Kupffer cell activation and endothelial cell damage after storage of rat livers: effects of reperfusion," *Hepatology*, vol. 13, no. 1, pp. 83–95, 1991.

[21] P. M. Porrett, J. Hsu, and A. Shaked, "Late surgical complications following liver transplantation," *Liver Transplantation*, vol. 15, no. 2, pp. S12–S18, 2009.

[22] C. L. Jay, V. Lyuksemburg, D. P. Ladner et al., "Ischemic cholangiopathy after controlled donation after cardiac death liver transplantation: a meta-analysis," *Annals of Surgery*, vol. 253, no. 2, pp. 259–264, 2011.

[23] M. Arai, R. G. Thurman, and J. J. Lemasters, "Involvement of Kupffer cells and sinusoidal endothelial cells in ischemic preconditioning to rat livers stored for transplantation," *Transplantation Proceedings*, vol. 31, no. 1-2, pp. 425–427, 1999.

[24] M. Arai, R. G. Thurman, and J. J. Lemasters, "Ischemic preconditioning of rat livers against cold storage-reperfusion injury: role of nonparenchymal cells and the phenomenon of heterologous preconditioning," *Liver Transplantation*, vol. 7, no. 4, pp. 292–299, 2001.

[25] H. Rehman, H. D. Connor, V. K. Ramshesh et al., "Ischemic preconditioning prevents free radical production and mitochondrial depolarization in small-for-size rat liver grafts," *Transplantation*, vol. 85, no. 9, pp. 1322–1331, 2008.

11

Klatskin-Like Lesions

M. P. Senthil Kumar[1, 2] and R. Marudanayagam[1]

[1] *The Liver Unit, Queen Elizabeth Hospital Birmingham, Edgbaston, Birmingham B15 2TH, UK*
[2] *Department of HPB Surgery and Liver Transplantation, Queen Elizabeth Hospital Birmingham, 3rd Floor Nuffield House, Edgbaston, Birmingham B15 2TH, UK*

Correspondence should be addressed to M. P. SenthilKumar, sanskrity@hotmail.com

Academic Editor: Olivier Farges

Hilar cholangiocarcinoma, also known as Klatskin tumour, is the commonest type of cholangiocarcinoma. It poses unique problems in the diagnosis and management because of its anatomical location. Curative surgery in the form of major hepatic resection entails significant morbidity. About 5–15% of specimens resected for presumed Klatskin tumour prove not to be cholangiocarcinomas. There are a number of inflammatory, infective, vascular, and other pathologies, which have overlapping clinical and radiological features with a Klatskin tumour, leading to misinterpretation. This paper aims to summarise the features of such Klatskin-like lesions that have been reported in surgical literature.

1. Introduction

Hilar cholangiocarcinoma, also known as Altemeier-Klatskin tumour is a primary malignancy of the liver occurring at the confluence of the bile ducts, first reported by Altemeier et al. in 1957 and characterised by Klatskin in 1965 [1, 2]. Occurring within 2 cm of the hilar confluence, it accounts for about 50–70% of all cholangiocarcinomas [3].

Resection and in selected patients, transplantation offers the best chance of cure in Klatskin tumours. Hence, early diagnosis is vital for a radical surgical approach to be feasible and effective. Equally, it is ideal, though not always possible, to have an established diagnosis of cancer or a strong probability of malignancy before embarking on a radical liver resection in view of the potential morbidity and mortality. Klatskin tumours have to be differentiated from a number of benign pathologies and some malignant lesions that mimic the clinical presentation and the radiological appearances (Table 1). These have been variously called "Klatskin-mimicking lesions," "the malignant masquerade," and "pseudo-Klatskin tumours" [4, 5]. In most large series of hilar strictures, operated on, with a preoperative diagnosis of cholangiocarcinoma (CCA), the rate of benign lesions on final histopathology ranges from 5 to 15%, reaching up to a third in some reports (Table 1) [6–10].

Hilar cholangiocarcinoma has three morphological types: periductal infiltrative, polypoid, and exophytic (mass forming), depending on the predominant pattern of spread in relation to the duct wall. Infiltrating CCA is the commonest type of hilar CCA (70%) and typically appears as a focal thickening of bile duct with hyperattenuation on imaging. Polypoid CCA appears as an intraluminal hypoattenuating lesion. Exophytic hilar CCA is typically seen as a hypodense mass lesion with rim enhancement. Tumour markers such as CA19-9, IL-6, and neutrophil gelatinase-associated lipocalin (NGAL), although are typically raised in CCA, do not have sufficient discriminatory power to be clinically useful in Klatskin mimicking lesions [8–11]. ERCP and PTC are also useful to clarify the anatomy. Brush cytology, though it has a high specificity, suffers from a low sensitivity. Cholangioscopy with cytology and confocal laser endomicroscopy are promising evolving technologies in the evaluation of indeterminate biliary strictures [12, 13].

Multimodal imaging to include multidetector CT, MRI, and MRCP is the key. In general, vascular involvement, involvement of secondary biliary radicles, duct wall thickness >4 mm, lobar atrophy are all pointers to a cholangiocarcinoma but are not diagnostic [14, 15]. There are a few confounding issues which need attention while interpreting

Table 1: Incidence of Klatskin-like lesions.

Author (year)	Incidence (%)	Region
Myburgh (1995) [5]	3	South Africa
Verbeek (1992) [7]	13	Netherlands
Gerhards (2001) [8]	15	Netherlands
Knoefel (2003) [9]	18	Germany
Koea (2004) [10]	24	New Zealand
Wetter (1991) [6]	31	California

the clinical and imaging features in Klatskin tumours. Some of the Klatskin mimicking lesions such as tuberculosis, sarcoidosis, lymphoma, metastasis may have prominent hilar lymphadenopathy leading to a misdiagnosis of an advanced cholangiocarcinoma. Some diseases such as primary sclerosing cholangitis, intrahepatic stones, and oriental cholangiohepatitis which by themselves may mimic a Klatskin lesion also are high risk factors for the development of cholangiocarcinoma and may be harbouring them at presentation.

Hilar lesions should be interpreted in the clinical context that they present. In addition to a detailed history of current symptoms past medical and surgical history is important. Biochemical, hematological, serological, and radiological evidence of involvement of other organ systems should be sought, especially in young patients, as there may be specific clues in certain disorders such as sarcoidosis, connective tissue disorders, IgG4-related disease, eosinophilic cholangiopathy, HIV, and tuberculosis. It is important to recognize them as there are alternative treatments available. In some disorders such as portal biliopathy surgery may be dangerous and may be avoided with the correct preoperative diagnosis.

The aim of this paper is to highlight the presentation and features of various Klatskin-like lesions that have been and may be interpreted as hilar CCA. A systematic medline search was performed for relevant publications between 1966 and 2012, using the terms hilar cholangiocarcinoma, Klatskin tumour, Klatskin-mimicking lesions, and pseudo-Klatskin tumour. Retrieved publications and their references were then scrutinized for reports of lesions that mimicked Klatskin tumours. A summary of the key lesions is presented (Table 2).

Table 2: Klatskin-like lesions.

(A) Dominant stricture in PSC
(B) Hepatolithiasis and recurrent pyogenic cholangitis
(C) Mirizzi syndrome
(D) Inflammatory-infiltrative
  (a) Inflammatory pseudotumour
  (b) IgG4 related Cholangiopathy
  (c) Eosinophilic cholangiopathy
  (d) Follicular cholangiopathy
  (e) Xanthogranulomatous cholangitis
  (f) Mast cell cholangiopathy
  (g) Sarcoidosis
(E) Infective
  (a) Cholangiopathy in the immunocompromised
    (i) AIDS cholangiopathy
    (ii) Primary immunodeficiency
  (b) Bacterial
  (c) Biliary tuberculosis
  (d) Fungal
  (e) Parasitic
(F) Vascular
  (a) Portal hypertensive biliopathy
  (b) Ischaemic cholangiopathy
(G) Toxic
  (a) Postchemotherapy
  (b) Thorotrast-induced granuloma
(H) Trauma
  (a) Biliary
  (b) Systemic
(I) Tumours
  (a) Malignant
    (i) Gall bladder carcinoma
    (ii) Hepatocellular carcinoma
    (iii) Lymphoepithelioma-like carcinoma
    (iv) Neuroendocrine tumours
    (v) Granular cell tumour
    (vi) Lymphoma
    (vii) Leukemia
    (viii) Myeloma
    (ix) Other metastasis
  (b) Benign
    (i) Neurilemmoma
(J) Miscellaneous
  (a) Proliferative cholangitis
  (b) Nonparasitic cysts
  (c) Erdheim-Chester disease
  (d) Ormond's disease
  (e) Heterotopic pancreas/stomach
  (f) Cholecystohepatic duct with absent common hepatic duct
(K) Idiopathic

2. Dominant Stricture of Primary Sclerosing Cholangitis (PSC)

PSC is a chronic cholestatic disorder of possible autoimmune etiology in which a localized high grade stricture in the intra- or extrahepatic bile ducts may be the presenting feature in up to 20% of patients [16]. Though PSC classically manifests as multifocal strictures and dilatations, which are often discontinuous, leading to a beaded appearance on imaging, a dominant stricture at the hilum may be mistaken for a CCA. Central to the interpretation of strictures in PSC is the fact that the lifetime risk of cholangiocarcinoma in PSC is up to 25%. Nearly two-thirds of patients who develop a cholangiocarcinoma in the context of PSC have a dominant stricture, and hilar lesions in PSC have a higher risk of being malignant [16, 17].

Clinically, the association of inflammatory bowel disease (in up to 80% of patients) is a useful clue. Serum tumour markers and noninvasive imaging modalities have a low sensitivity and specificity in differentiating benign from malignant stricture. Bile CEA levels >30 ng/ml may be a useful discriminator [18]. While conventional brush cytology at ERCP or PTC suffers from a high false negative rate, transpapillary cholangioscopy with brush cytology is a sensitive test and also retains a high specificity [19, 20].

3. Intrahepatic Stones and Recurrent Pyogenic Cholangitis

Though hepatolithiasis may complicate any longstanding stricture or ductal dilatation, it is a classical feature of the syndrome of recurrent pyogenic cholangitis (RPC). Endemic in Southeast Asia and first described by Digby in 1930, RPC is a syndrome of recurrent infections of the biliary tree associated with intrahepatic strictures and hepatolithiasis [21]. It presents between the 3rd and 5th decades with no gender preponderance, with stones typically occurring in the left lateral segment and the right posterior segments. Classical features are Charcot's triad (recurrent fever, right upper quadrant pain and jaundice) and Reynold's pentad (+ hypotension and altered sensorium).

The etiology of intrahepatic stones is complex with an interplay of metabolic abnormalities, poor bile flow and stasis, infections or infestations, ductal mucin secretion, proliferative cholangitis, all playing a role. Ascaris and liver flukes such as Clonorchis, Opisthorchis, and Fasciola are thought to initiate the biliary injury, which is propagated by the stones, inflammatory strictures, and the invariable occurrence of multiple cycles of cholangitis. However, an alternative view is that E coli infection coupled with a low protein diet favours deconjugation of bilirubin in the bile ducts leading to sludge and later stones [22].

There are two common types of intrahepatic stones—brown pigment and cholesterol which elicit three types of inflammation—suppurative cholangitis, chronic proliferative cholangitis and chronic granulomatous cholangitis. Pigment stones with calcium bilirubinate as the chief component are the commonest type of stones, and about 90% of these are hyperintense on plain CT. The other classical features of RPC on imaging are central duct dilatation with rapid tapering (arrow head sign), poor arborisation of bile ducts in the periphery, and segmental nonfilling of ducts (absent duct sign) [22]. Hilar stricture due to hepatolithiasis has been misinterpreted as cholangiocarcinoma [23, 24]. Stones may be imaging occult especially with contrast CT, as they may be isodense. Noncontrast CT is more sensitive. MRI is the best modality to delineate the stones, the extent of the stricture and lobar atrophy.

4. Mirizzi Syndrome

Named after Pablo Luis Mirizzi, who described it in 1948, it is the obstruction of the common hepatic or bile duct by a gallstone impacted in the cystic duct or Hartmann's pouch of the gall bladder. Inflammation around the hilum may result in a stricture. Presence of a large impacted stone is an important pointer to the diagnosis, but gallstones are not always seen on a CT, and the imaging findings may mimic a periductal infiltrating type of cholangiocarcinoma [14]. MR cholangiography is the investigation of choice as it often identifies the gallstone, the extrinsic compression, the dilated proximal ducts and normal distal ducts which are the defining features of Mirizzi syndrome.

5. Inflammatory-Infiltrative

5.1. Inflammatory Pseudotumour (IPT). First recognized in 1939 in the lungs, hepatic IPT was first described by Pack and Baker in 1953 [25]. IPT is a relatively rare cause of a hilar mass lesion, which closely mimics a cholangiocarcinoma, with only about 200 reports in literature. IPT occurs in young adults and children and is commoner in the lungs, stomach, omentum, and mesentery among other sites. It is a benign nonneoplastic proliferative lesion characterized histologically by a heterogenous inflammatory infiltrate of plasma cells, lymphocytes, macrophages, eosinophils, and dendritic cells amidst a myofibroblastic background [26]. Macroscopically it forms a nonencapsulated mass lesion in the liver, which ranges from grey-white to brown-tan in appearance. Though an inflammatory response to efflux of toxic bile acids is thought to contribute to the pathogenesis, the exact etiology is unknown [27]. There are associations with Crohn's disease, phlebitis, Epstein-Barr virus infection, autoimmune pancreatitis, PSC, and recurrent pyogenic cholangitis [27, 28]. Rare instances of multiple IPTs and invasion of hepatic veins have been reported in literature [29].

On CT and MRI, there is typically no arterial phase enhancement, but there is delayed peripheral enhancement in the portal venous phase [30, 31]. Imaging modalities including CT scan, liver-specific MRI, and PET scan are not reliable in differentiating IPT from hilar cholangiocarcinoma [28, 31]. CEA and AFP are usually normal in IPT, while CA19-9 may be mildly elevated in some patients. The prognosis is good, and spontaneous resolution has been reported. Corticosteroids, antibiotics, and nonsteroidal anti-inflammatory drugs have been used with inconsistent effect.

5.2. IgG4-Related Sclerosing Cholangiopathy (ISC). IgG4-related autoimmune disease is an inflammatory multisystem disorder of which cholangiopathy may be one of the manifestations. The tissues affected range from pancreas (autoimmune pancreatitis), liver and bile ducts (autoimmune hepatitis; cholangiopathy), salivary glands (chronic sclerosing sialadenitis), lacrimal glands (Mikulicz's disease) retroperitoneum (retroperitoneal fibrosis), mediastinum (sclerosing mediastinitis) and kidneys [32]. It is characterized by infiltration of tissues by IgG4-positive plasma cells and associated with elevated levels of serum IgG4.

ISC is of two distinct types: a diffuse sclerosing cholangitis pattern and a hilar pseudotumour pattern [32]. Typically it is a disease of the large bile ducts. The distinguishing features of ISC are concentric bile duct thickening, smooth strictures, multifocal involvement, minimal proximal dilatation and the absence of ectasia, diverticula and pruning [33].

More than 90% of the patients with ISC have autoimmune pancreatitis, and it has been called IgG4-related sclerosing pancreatocholangitis [34–36]. The pancreatitis often precedes the presentation of cholangitis although it may follow it. An Ig-G4 level of >140 mg/l is considered significant for the diagnosis of Ig-G4 related disease, while a level >300 mg/l confers high specificity [32]. Other serological markers include hypergammaglobulinemia, antinuclear antibody and peripheral eosinophilia [32].

Imaging modalities including CT, MRI, and PET scans are not useful in differentiating a hilar cholangiocarcinoma from Ig-G4 cholangiopathy with certainty [32]. However, they may provide indirect evidence by detecting the associated autoimmune pancreatitis, which has distinct and diagnostic imaging features. Brush cytology is an unreliable discriminator due to the frequency of false negative and false positive results [37]. Histology, however, is reliable. The histological hallmarks of IgG4- related disease are lymphoplasmacytic infiltration especially IgG4-positive plasma cells, storiform fibrosis, obliterative phlebitis, and eosinophilia. In patients presenting with biliary strictures options to achieve histological diagnosis include a percutaneous or endoscopic biopsy of the stricture or mass lesion or a biopsy of the ampulla of vater [32].

Ig-G4 cholangiopathy runs a benign course, and the associated pancreatitis may resolve spontaneously. Ig-G4 cholangiopathy responds well to oral corticosteroids. The recommended dose based on extrapolation from the studies on autoimmune pancreatitis is prednisolone 0.6 mg/kg/d which may be tapered over 3–6 months [35, 36, 38]. Rituximab is an option for steroid refractory disease [39].

5.3. Eosinophilic Cholangiopathy (EC). Eosinophilic cholangiopathy or cholangitis is characterized by a dense transmural inflammatory infiltration of the biliary tract by eosinophils, leading to strictures and obstructive jaundice. Mass lesions are uncommon.

Although Albot et al. described eosinophilic cholecystitis in 1949, Butler et al. in 1985 were the first to characterize eosinophilic cholangiopathy [40, 41]. EC is rare with only about 10 cases reported in literature. Though EC may occur as an isolated phenomenon, it often manifests as a part of a systemic syndrome involving other organs and tissues (bone marrow, kidney, ureters, stomach, bowel pancreas, and lymph nodes). In the biliary tree, gall bladder involvement (eosinophilic cholecystitis) is slightly more common than ductal involvement.

Peripheral eosinophilia is an important clue to the possibility but is not universal feature. In patients with eosinophilic gastroenteritis and biliary stricture, the presentation may mimic primary sclerosing cholangitis with ulcerative colitis [42]. Patients with eosinophilic gastroenteritis who have serosal involvement may develop ascites, which may clinically mimic advanced cholangiocarcinoma. Ascitic fluid cytology is eosinophil rich and is a useful diagnostic test [42].

Pathologically, the differential diagnosis in view of the portal eosinophilic infiltrates includes parasitic, fungal and drug-induced liver disease, as well as primary sclerosing cholangitis, allograft rejection, autoimmune cholangitis, and primary biliary cirrhosis, depending on the context.

The etiology and pathogenesis of EC are poorly understood. There are no specific or characteristic radiological or serological tests. However, the prognosis is good with a quick and, often, a sustained response to steroids. For example, Vauthey et al. report a patient who received prednisolone at the dose of 40 mg/day for 8 weeks and had a complete resolution of the biliary lesion and was well at 18-months followup [43].

5.4. Follicular Cholangitis (FC). FC is another lymphoplasmacytic infiltrative process of unknown etiology, which is similar to ISC but in contrast to which, the characteristic feature is the presence of periductal lymphoid follicles. It was first described by Aoki et al., in 2003, and there have been a few case reports since, mostly in the eastern literature [44–47]. Patients are usually more than 40 years of age, and there is no gender preponderance. The hilar bile ducts are typically involved. It may affect the pancreas concurrently (follicular pancreatocholangitis). Plasma IgG4 levels are not raised nor is there a prominence of IgG4-positive plasma cells on histology. There are no disease associations, no specific serum markers, or diagnostic imaging features. Patients usually undergo resection for suspected cancer. There are no reported recurrences. The natural history and the response to steroids are unknown.

5.5. Mast Cell Cholangiopathy. Mast cells are fibrogenic and contribute to the pathogenesis of certain hepatic diseases where fibrosis plays a key role such as alcoholic liver disease and PSC. Though diffuse mast cell infiltration of the liver in systemic mastocytosis resulting in intrahepatic cholestasis is not uncommon, it is an extremely rare cause of secondary sclerosing cholangitis manifesting as ductal lesions, with only 2 case reports in literature [48, 49]. The patients were both women over 70 years, had systemic mastocytosis, and presented with jaundice. One patient had ascites while the other had lytic bone lesions. Bile duct thickening on CT and multiple ductal lesions on cholangiography were present. Urinary histamine and tryptase levels are raised in mastocytosis and are useful in diagnosis, as is a bone marrow biopsy.

5.6. Xanthogranulomatous Cholangitis (XGC). Xanthogranulomatous cholecystitis is an uncommon, but well-characterized chronic invasive inflammatory process of the gall bladder which may mimic gall bladder carcinoma. In a particularly aggressive form of xanthogranulomatous cholecystitis, the inflammatory fibrosis spreads to contiguous tissues and organs [50]. When this involves the hilar bile ducts, it may simulate a Klatskin tumour. Xanthogranulomatous cholecystitis almost always occurs in the presence of gall stones and is associated with a significant thickening of gall bladder wall, which is unusual in cholangiocarcinoma.

In XGC, an even rarer condition, a similar inflammation typified by infiltration of the bile duct wall by foamy macrophages with inflammatory infiltrate and fibrosis occurs, leading to thickening and smooth strictures involving the large bile ducts. XGC may occur alone or in association with xanthogranulomatous cholecystitis and may occur in children as well as adults [51–54]. There is no gender predilection. Hilar lesions are clinically indistinguishable to Klatskin tumours and have been diagnosed with certainty only after hepatic resection [54].

5.7. Sarcoidosis. Sarcoidosis is a steroid responsive multisystem granulomatous disorder of uncertain etiology which is characterized by noncaseating epitheloid granulomas, commonly affecting the lungs, lymph nodes, eyes, and the skin. Hepatic manifestations were first described by Klatskin and Yesner in 1950 and include granulomatous hepatitis, cholestasis, cirrhosis, portal fibrosis leading to presinusoidal portal hypertension, Budd-Chiari syndrome, adult ductopenia-like syndrome, and rarely chronic granulomatous sclerosing cholangitis with ductal strictures [55–57]. Nodal involvement with hilar stricture may closely resemble a hilar cholangiocarcinoma [57]. Moreover sarcoid-like nodal changes may be seen in other malignancies further confounding the issue [58]. Hepatic sarcoidosis detectable on liver biopsies may also be associated with PSC and PBC [59].

Sarcoidosis commonly occurs in women in their 3rd or 4th decades, and hepatic sarcoidosis almost always has concurrent pulmonary involvement. PET CT has been shown to be useful in targeting nodes for biopsy. Spyglass cholangioscopy with directed biopsy may clinch the diagnosis with a high degree of accuracy [57]. Hypercalcemia and elevated serum angiotensin-converting enzyme are useful corroborative tests but are neither sensitive nor specific in hepatic sarcoidosis. The mainstay of treatment of symptomatic strictures in sarcoidosis is drainage. Ursodeoxycholic acid and corticosteroids (prednisolone 40–60 mg/day for 6 months) may benefit cholestasis but may not resolve associated fibrosis or ductopenia [57, 59].

6. Infective

6.1. Cholangiopathy of Immunosuppression. HIV infection, especially when it has progressed to full-blown AIDS, is associated with characteristic biliary abnormalities, which collectively are known as AIDS cholangiopathy, first recognized in 1986 [60]. It is more common in advanced disease, poorly treated disease, and in patients with low CD4 counts (<135/mm3) and hence is a marker of poor prognosis [61, 62]. Sclerosing cholangitis is seen in more than 70% of patients with AIDS cholangiopathy, most commonly involving the large intrahepatic ducts, either alone or in association with papillary stenosis or extrahepatic duct strictures [62, 63]. There is often an elevated alkaline phosphatase, and most patients are symptomatic. Treatment is by papillotomy where necessary, and imaging directed dilatation and stenting of strictures. Specific therapy targeted against a host of opportunistic pathogens implicated such as cytomegalovirus, cryptosporidium, mycobacteria does not seem to affect the long-term outcome [64].

Sclerosing cholangitis is the commonest hepatobiliary complication in children with primary immunodeficiency. Cholangiographic abnormalities were found in 60% of patients with clinical evidence of liver disease. Cryptosporidium parvum infection was the major pathogen implicated. These patients are also prone for biliary malignancies. Hematopoietic stem cell transplant in the early stages and combined liver transplant in late stages have a therapeutic role [65, 66].

6.2. Bacterial Infections. Rarely multiple pyogenic liver abscesses may cause ductal abnormalities [67]. This has also been reported in relation to systemic gram-positive sepsis and infection with *E. coli* [68, 69]. Although the clinical context makes the diagnosis self-evident, if the underlying primary cause such as diverticulitis is clinically subtle, and the presentation is with jaundice or deranged liver function tests, then ductal dilatation and strictures on imaging may be misconstrued as possible cholangiocarcinoma.

6.3. Tuberculosis. Four types of hepatobiliary tuberculosis caused by Mycobacterium tuberculosis are recognized—military tuberculosis of the liver, granulomatous hepatitis, local parenchymal disease, and the rarer focal sclerosing type due to direct involvement of bile ducts resulting in strictures [70, 71]. In addition periportal tuberculous lymphadenitis is a well-documented cause of hilar biliary obstruction, which may mimic a cholangiocarcinoma [72].

Though hepatic involvement in TB is common as a part of disseminated disease, isolated biliary TB affecting the ducts is rare. Hilar strictures in biliary TB are difficult to distinguish from cholangiocarcinoma, but the younger age (<40 years in two-thirds), history of low-grade fever before the onset of jaundice, presence of extra hepatic TB and calcifications in the liver are suggestive [72]. Brush cytology demonstrating acid-fast bacilli (AFB), biopsies showing caseating granulomas, and bile PCR for AFB are useful tests [71, 73, 74]. Hilar nodal disease and compression from granulomas may also cause ductal abnormalities on imaging. Fibrotic strictures may need specific intervention in addition to the standard antituberculous chemotherapy.

There has been a case report of systemic Mycobacterium genavense causing sclerosing cholangitis [75].

6.4. Fungal. Invasive fungal infections involving the liver are often seen in immunocompromised patients and often are a marker of a disseminated infection. The microabscesses of candidiasis and the granulomas of histoplasmosis, aspergillosis, blastomycosis are well studied, but, in general, these do not mimic a cholangiocarcinoma.

However, in mucormycosis insidious progression of focal liver lesions may present with mass lesions and hilar ductal strictures [76]. There have also been a few case reports of disseminated cryptococcosis manifesting as cholangitis [77–83]. This may even occur in the immunocompetent host. Some patients have ductal lesions with or without lymphadenopathy mimicking hilar cholangiocarcinoma [83]. Bile culture, nodal FNA, and culture, serum cryptococcal antigen screen are useful diagnostic tools. The lesions respond to antifungal treatment.

6.5. Parasitic. Parasites such as ascaris and liver flukes are known to be associated with the syndrome of oriental cholangiohepatitis. Rarely, focal duct strictures of the major hepatic ducts resembling a cholangiocarcinoma may be caused by Clonorchis infestation [84].

7. Vascular

7.1. Portal Hypertensive Biliopathy (PHB). There are recognizable changes that occur in the biliary tree as a consequence of portal hypertension and cavernomatous transformation of the portal vein, which have been collectively and variously labeled as portal hypertensive biliopathy, cholangiopathy associated with portal hypertension and portal cavernoma-associated cholangiopathy [85].

PHB in essence is due to the pressure and ischemia on the biliary tree from the engorged collateral veins that evolve in portal hypertension. The epicholedochal venous plexus of Saint (a fine reticular web that hugs the bile ducts) and the paracholedochal venous plexus of Petren (a longitudinally oriented network of larger caliber veins) are central to the pathophysiology. The epicholedochal plexus is thought to cause fine irregularities in the bile ducts, while the paracholedochal plexus causes the mass effect. With chronicity, a solid connective tissue scaffold forms around the leash of collaterals encasing the bile duct [85–87].

PHB is more common in extrahepatic portal venous obstruction, occurring in more than 80% of patients than in cirrhosis, where the frequency is up to 30%. There is a male predominance and being a slowly progressive disease, they often present in the fourth decade of life. Smooth strictures and segmental dilatations are typical and may be intrahepatic or extrahepatic. Other abnormalities include angulation, indentation, pruning, and clustering of intrahepatic ducts [85]. In cirrhotics the strictures are predominantly intrahepatic, while in extrahepatic portal venous obstruction, they are both extra- and intrahepatic [88]. The left duct is involved nearly twice as commonly as the right duct [85].

A stricture at the hilum with the mass effect caused by the cavernoma mimics a cholangiocarcinoma and has been termed "pseudocholangiocarcinoma sign" [89]. Intrahepatic strictures in PHB may resemble primary sclerosing cholangitis at cholangiography, and the term "pseudosclerosing cholangitis" has been used to describe this [90]. The key distinguishing characteristic of the strictures in PBH is that they are smooth as opposed to the typically irregular contour seen in cholangiocarcinoma.

There is an increased incidence of biliary lithiasis (about 20%), and this in fact may bring the problem to light. Most patients, however, are asymptomatic and are often discovered incidentally on imaging for other clinical problems. About a fifth to a third of patients become symptomatic with pain, jaundice, recurrent cholangitis or present with significantly deranged liver function tests [85]. Though ultrasound, either transabdominal or endoscopic, is useful to assess the varices, MR portography and MR cholangiography are the investigations of choice in suspected PHB.

Portosystemic shunt is known to cause resolution of the varices and the biliary strictures, and hence this should be considered as an important therapeutic option [87, 91–93]. Symptomatic patients will require percutaneous or endoscopic biliary dilatation and repeated stent changes every 4–6 months.

A special challenge in these patients is the risk of hemobilia after biliary interventions. Periampullary varices increase the risk of postsphincterotomy bleed, and intracholedochal varices may mimic stones on a cholangiogram and may result in significant bleeding if traumatised by a Dormia basket. Open surgery may equally be difficult due to a wall of varices around the bile duct and at the hilum making safe access a challenge. For distal lesions, it has been suggested that these patients undergo a portosystemic shunt (mesocaval; lienorenal; TIPPS), if there is a shuntable vein, as the first stage and then considered for a second stage biliary enteric anastomosis after stone clearance [85]. Selected patients may benefit from liver transplantation [94].

7.2. Ischaemic Cholangiopathy. Ischemic injury results in tissue death resulting ultimately in fibrosis. The biliary tree is solely dependent on the hepatic arterial flow unlike the parenchyma and hence is very susceptible to ischaemic insults. The commonest region to be affected by ischemic cholangiopathy is the midcommon bile duct followed by the hepatic ductal confluence [95].

Multifocal nonanastomotic ischaemic biliary stricture following liver transplant is the prototype ischemic cholangiopathy. This is most evident in donation after cardiac death (DCD) grafts with long warm or cold ischaemic time and after hepatic artery thrombosis. But because of the context there is hardly any uncertainty about the diagnosis.

Similarly strictures following iatrogenic bile duct injury at cholecystectomy are evident from the clinical context. Inadvertent right hepatic arterial injury at laparoscopic cholecystectomy is estimated to occur in 7% of cholecystectomies and in about 25% of patients who have a bile duct injury [96]. The contribution of ischemia to strictures following bile duct reconstruction after repair of iatrogenic bile duct injuries is difficult to estimate. However, it is known that a certain proportion of patients develop hilar and intrahepatic strictures and consequent recurrent cholangitis ultimately needing liver resection [97].

A secondary sclerosing cholangitis of the critically ill, of presumed ischaemic origin has been recognized [98, 99]. This typically occurs in patients who have had septic shock of a diverse etiology and consequently had to spend a prolonged time in the intensive care unit with respiratory and cardiovascular support. Enterococcus faecium was consistently isolated from many patients in one study [99].

Ischemic biliary strictures have been described in hepatic artery atherosclerosis [100]; sickle cell disease [101], polyarteritis nodosa [102]; paroxysmal nocturnal hemoglobinuria [103]; hereditary haemorrhagic telangiectasia [104]; henoch-schonlein purpura [105]; systemic lupus erythematosus and scleroderma [95]. On occasion, when they occur close to the hilum, they may potentially raise the suspicion of a malignant stricture. External beam radiotherapy-induced strictures have been described in the extrahepatic bile duct, and intrahepatic strictures may occur after selective internal radiation therapy (SIRT) or after transcatheter hepatic arterial embolization, but often the clinical context makes the diagnosis apparent [106–108].

8. Trauma

Blunt trauma is a rare cause of biliary strictures, and the commonest site is the supraduodenal CBD [109, 110]. However, hilar stricture resembling a Klatskin tumour has been reported [111]. Presentation often is delayed for many weeks to years. Interestingly, remote severe trauma or severe sepsis, not directly involving the biliary tree, may also result in a posttraumatic sclerosing cholangitis [98, 112]. The pathogenesis is presumed to have an ischemic origin as most patients at least in one series had hemodynamic instability following trauma [113].

9. Toxic

Chemotherapy-induced biliary sclerosis (CIBS) is well documented after intra-arterial infusional chemotherapy with 5-FU and may occur in up to half the patients receiving the treatment [114]. The hilar bifurcation and the proximal common hepatic duct are the commonest sites [115, 116]. Intrahepatic infiltration of cisplatin, mitomycin C, and formaldehyde are also known to lead to biliary sclerosing lesions [28]. Direct toxicity and vasculitis are thought to be the mechanisms.

10. Tumours

A number of malignancies involving the hilum may mimic a CCA. The key among them is gall bladder carcinoma, hepatocellular carcinoma, neuroendocrine tumours, colorectal metastasis, lymphoma, leukemia, and myeloma.

Gall bladder cancers usually have a dominant lesion in the gall bladder, but a primary arising from region of the neck and infiltrating the hilum is difficult to differentiate from a Klatskin tumour. Infiltrating HCC typically has early arterial phase enhancement with a washout. Neuroendocrine tumours are typically hyperattenuating. Periportal lymphangitic metastasis occurring at the hilum may mimic a cholangiocarcinoma, but they do not show ductal dilatation and involve both sides of the liver [117]. Lymphoepithelioma-like carcinomas are rare malignancies which are associated with Epstein-Barr virus infection. They have an intense lymphocytic infiltrate and may even occur alongside cholangiocarcinomas [118]. Parenchymal hepatic metastasis, that may involve the hilum, is characterized by a central necrosis and hence a hypoattenuating centre. This is rare in CCA. Benign tumours of the bile duct such as neurilemmoma occurring at the hilum may be difficult to differentiate from hilar CCA [119].

11. Miscellaneous

Proliferative cholangitis (Cholangitis glandularis proliferans) is a benign intraductal proliferative disorder described by Krukowski et al. in 1983 [120]. It typically involves the extrahepatic biliary tree but may involve the hilum. Proliferative cholangitis has been implicated in hepatolithiasis; whether this is a cause or a consequence is debated. Erdheim-Chester disease is a rare multisystem infiltrative disorder characterized by non-Langhans cell histiocytosis. Biliary hilar infiltration may produce Klatskin-like lesions [121]. Ormond's disease characterized by retroperitoneal fibrosis may present with hilar inflammatory stricture [122]. Heterotopic pancreatic tissue is commonly found in the stomach and duodenum but may occur in the hilar confluence [123] as can heterotopic gastric mucosa [124]. Cholecystohepatic duct with absence of common hepatic duct where the right and left ducts drain into the gall bladder has been mistaken for a malignant hilar stricture on preoperative imaging [125]. Idiopathic nonspecific fibrosis of hilar ducts has also been reported in many series [10, 126, 127].

12. Conclusion

In many instances of hilar strictures, resection would probably continue to be the only definitive means of achieving a diagnosis with certainty. This is perhaps justified in comparison to missing a therapeutic window in a potentially operable Klatskin tumour. However, awareness of the varied pathological entities that may mimic a Klatskin tumour and the interpretation of the radiological and pathological data in the clinical context may help identify at least a small proportion of patients who may be deferred the morbidity of surgery. Most such identified patients could be successfully managed by interventional or medical means.

References

[1] W. A. Altemeier, E. A. Gall, M. M. Zinninger, and P. I. Hoxworth, "Sclerosing carcinoma of the major intra hepatic bile ducts," *Archives of Surgery*, vol. 75, no. 3, pp. 450–461, 1957.

[2] G. Klatskin, "Adenocarcinoma of the hepatic duct at its bifurcation within the porta hepatis. An unusual tumor with distinctive clinical and pathological features," *The American Journal of Medicine*, vol. 38, no. 2, pp. 241–256, 1965.

[3] S. A. Khan, H. C. Thomas, B. R. Davidson, and S. D. Taylor-Robinson, "Cholangiocarcinoma," *The Lancet*, vol. 366, no. 9493, pp. 1303–1314, 2005.

[4] N. S. Hadjis, N. A. Collier, and L. H. Blumgart, "Malignant masquerade at the hilum of the liver," *British Journal of Surgery*, vol. 72, no. 8, pp. 659–661, 1985.

[5] J. A. Myburgh, "Resection and bypass for malignant obstruction of the bile duct," *World Journal of Surgery*, vol. 19, no. 1, pp. 108–112, 1995.

[6] L. A. Wetter, E. J. Ring, C. A. Pellegrini, and L. W. Way, "Differential diagnosis of sclerosing cholangiocarcinomas of the common hepatic duct (Klatskin tumors)," *American Journal of Surgery*, vol. 161, no. 1, pp. 57–63, 1991.

[7] P. C. Verbeek, D. J. van Leeuwen, L. T. de Wit et al., "Benign fibrosing disease at the hepatic confluence mimicking Klatskin tumors," *Surgery*, vol. 112, no. 5, pp. 866–871, 1992.

[8] M. F. Gerhards, P. Vos, T. M. van Gulik, E. A. Rauws, A. Bosma, and D. J. Gouma, "Incidence of benign lesions in patients resected for suspicious hilar obstruction," *British Journal of Surgery*, vol. 88, no. 1, pp. 48–51, 2001.

[9] W. T. Knoefel, K. L. Prenzel, M. Peiper et al., "Klatskin tumors and Klatskin mimicking lesions of the biliary tree," *European Journal of Surgical Oncology*, vol. 29, no. 8, pp. 658–661, 2003.

[10] J. Koea, A. Holden, K. Chau, and J. McCall, "Differential diagnosis of stenosing lesions at the hepatic hilus," *World Journal of Surgery*, vol. 28, no. 5, pp. 466–470, 2004.

[11] K. Leelawat, S. Narong, J. Wannaprasert, and S. Leelawat, "Serum NGAL to clinically distinguish cholangiocarcinoma from benign biliary tract diseases," *International Journal of Hepatology*, vol. 2011, Article ID 873548, 6 pages, 2011.

[12] Y. K. Chen, R. J. Shah, D. K. Pleskow et al., "Miami classification (MC) of probe-based confocal laser endomicroscopy (pCLE) findings in the pancreaticobiliary (PB) system for evaluation of indeterminate strictures: interim results from an international multicenter registry," *Gastrointestinal Endoscopy*, vol. 71, no. 5, p. AB134, 2010.

[13] A. Meining, Y. K. Chen, D. Pleskow et al., "Direct visualization of indeterminate pancreaticobiliary strictures with probe-based confocal laser endomicroscopy: a multicenter experience," *Gastrointestinal Endoscopy*, vol. 74, pp. 961–968, 2011.

[14] C. O. Menias, V. R. Surabhi, S. R. Prasad, H. L. Wang, V. R. Narra, and K. N. Chintapalli, "Mimics of cholangiocarcinoma: spectrum of disease," *RadioGraphics*, vol. 28, no. 4, pp. 1115–1129, 2008.

[15] W. J. Lee, H. Lim, K. M. Jang et al., "Radiologic spectrum of cholangiocarcinoma: emphasis on unusual manifestations and differential diagnoses," *RadioGraphics*, vol. 21, pp. S97–S116, 2001.

[16] M. Aljiffry, P. D. Renfrew, M. J. Walsh, M. Laryea, and M. Molinari, "Analytical review of diagnosis and treatment strategies for dominant bile duct strictures in patients with primary sclerosing cholangitis," *International Hepato-Pancreato-Biliary Association*, vol. 13, no. 2, pp. 79–90, 2011.

[17] U. Beuers, U. Spengler, W. Kruis et al., "Ursodeoxycholic acid for treatment of primary sclerosing cholangitis: a placebo-controlled trial," *Hepatology*, vol. 16, no. 3, pp. 707–714, 1992.

[18] A. Nakeeb, P. A. Lipsett, K. D. Lillemoe et al., "Biliary carcinoembryonic antigen levels are a marker for cholangiocarcinoma," *American Journal of Surgery*, vol. 171, no. 1, pp. 147–153, 1996.

[19] A. E. Berstad, L. Aabakken, H. J. Smith, S. Aasen, K. M. Boberg, and E. Schrumpf, "Diagnostic accuracy of magnetic resonance and endoscopic retrograde cholangiography in primary sclerosing cholangitis," *Clinical Gastroenterology and Hepatology*, vol. 4, no. 4, pp. 514–520, 2006.

[20] J. J. Tischendorf, M. Krüger, C. Trautwein et al., "Cholangioscopic characterization of dominant bile duct stenoses in patients with primary sclerosing cholangitis," *Endoscopy*, vol. 38, no. 7, pp. 665–669, 2006.

[21] K. H. Digby, "Common-duct stones of liver origin," *British Journal of Surgery*, vol. 17, no. 68, pp. 578–591, 1930.

[22] W. M. Tsui, Y. Chan, C. Wong, Y. Lo, Y. Yeung, and Y. Lee, "Hepatolithiasis and the syndrome of recurrent pyogenic cholangitis: clinical, radiologic, and pathologic features," *Seminars in Liver Disease*, vol. 31, no. 1, pp. 33–48, 2011.

[23] B. Javaid and R. M. Faizallah, "Intrahepatic stones might mimic cholangiocarcinoma on ERCP," *Gastrointestinal Endoscopy*, vol. 53, no. 4, pp. 535–538, 2001.

[24] Y. Senda, H. Nishio, T. Ebata et al., "Hepatolithiasis in the hepatic hilum mimicking hilar cholangiocarcinoma: report of a case," *Surgery Today*, vol. 41, no. 9, pp. 1243–1246, 2011.

[25] G. T. Pack and H. W. Baker, "Total right hepatic lobectomy. Report of a case," *Annals of surgery*, vol. 138, no. 2, pp. 253–258, 1953.

[26] L. P. Dehner, "Inflammatory myofibroblastic tumor: the continued definition of one type of so-called inflammatory pseudotumor," *American Journal of Surgical Pathology*, vol. 28, no. 12, pp. 1652–1654, 2004.

[27] W. Faraj, H. Ajouz, D. Mukherji, G. Kealy, A. Shamseddine, and M. Khalife, "Inflammatory pseudo-tumor of the liver: a rare pathological entity," *World Journal of Surgical Oncology*, vol. 9, article 5, 2011.

[28] R. Abdalian and E. J. Heathcote, "Sclerosing cholangitis: a focus on secondary causes," *Hepatology*, vol. 44, no. 5, pp. 1063–1074, 2006.

[29] K. Kai, S. Matsuyama, T. Ohtsuka, K. Kitahara, D. Mori, and K. Miyazaki, "Multiple inflammatory pseudotumor of the liver, mimicking cholangiocarcinoma with tumor embolus in the hepatic vein: report of a case," *Surgery Today*, vol. 37, no. 6, pp. 530–533, 2007.

[30] F. H. Yan, K. R. Zhou, Y. P. Jiang, and W. B. Shi, "Inflammatory pseudotumor of the liver: 13 cases of MRI findings," *World Journal of Gastroenterology*, vol. 7, no. 3, pp. 422–424, 2001.

[31] M. E. Tublin, A. J. Moser, J. W. Marsh, and T. C. Gamblin, "Biliary inflammatory pseudotumor: imaging features in seven patients," *American Journal of Roentgenology*, vol. 188, no. 1, pp. W44–W48, 2007.

[32] Y. Zen and Y. Nakanuma, "Ig G4 cholangiopathy," *International Journal of Hepatology*, vol. 2012, Article ID 472376, 6 pages, 2012.

[33] H. C. Oh, M. H. Kim, K. T. Lee et al., "Clinical clues to suspicion of IgG4-associated sclerosing cholangitis disguised as primary sclerosing cholangitis or hilar cholangiocarcinoma," *Journal of Gastroenterology and Hepatology*, vol. 25, no. 12, pp. 1831–1837, 2010.

[34] A. Ghazale, S. T. Chari, L. Zhang et al., "Immunoglobulin G4-associated cholangitis: clinical profile and response to therapy," *Gastroenterology*, vol. 134, no. 3, pp. 706–715, 2008.

[35] G. W. Erkelens, F. P. Vleggaar, W. Lesterhuis, H. R. van Buuren, and S. D. van der Werf, "Sclerosing pancreato-cholangitis responsive to steroid therapy," *The Lancet*, vol. 354, no. 9172, pp. 43–44, 1999.

[36] A. Horiuchi, S. Kawa, H. Hamano, Y. Ochi, and K. Kiyosawa, "Sclerosing pancreato-cholangitis responsive to corticosteroid therapy: report of 2 case reports and review," *Gastrointestinal Endoscopy*, vol. 53, no. 4, pp. 518–522, 2001.

[37] V. Trent, K. K. Khurana, and L. R. Pisharodi, "Diagnostic accuracy and clinical utility of endoscopic bile duct brushing in the evaluation of biliary strictures," *Archives of Pathology and Laboratory Medicine*, vol. 123, no. 8, pp. 712–715, 1999.

[38] T. Kamisawa, T. Shimosegawa, K. Okazaki et al., "Standard steroid treatment for autoimmune pancreatitis," *Gut*, vol. 58, no. 11, pp. 1504–1507, 2009.

[39] M. Topazian, T. E. Witzig, T. C. Smyrk et al., "Rituximab therapy for refractory biliary strictures in immunoglobulin G4-associated cholangitis," *Clinical Gastroenterology and Hepatology*, vol. 6, no. 3, pp. 364–366, 2008.

[40] G. Albot, F. Poilleux, and C. Oliver, "Les cholécystitis a éosinophiles," *La Presse Médicale*, vol. 57, pp. 558–559, 1949.

[41] T. W. Butler, T. A. Feintuch, and W. P. Caine Jr., "Eosinophilic cholangitis, lymphadenopathy, and peripheral eosinophilia: a case report," *American Journal of Gastroenterology*, vol. 80, no. 7, pp. 572–574, 1985.

[42] C. Nashed, S. V. Sakpal, V. Shusharina, and R. S. Chamberlain, "Eosinophilic cholangitis and cholangiopathy: a sheep in wolves clothing," *HPB Surgery*, vol. 2010, Article ID 906496, 7 pages, 2010.

[43] J. N. Vauthey, E. Loyer, P. Chokshi, and S. Lahoti, "Case 57: eosinophilic cholangiopathy," *Radiology*, vol. 227, no. 1, pp. 107–112, 2003.

[44] T. Aoki, K. Kubota, T. Oka, K. Hasegawa, I. Hirai, and M. Makuuchi, "Follicular cholangitis: another cause of benign biliary stricture," *Hepato-Gastroenterology*, vol. 50, no. 51, pp. 639–642, 2003.

[45] J. Y. Lee, J. H. Lim, and H. K. Lim, "Follicular cholangitis mimicking hilar cholangiocarcinoma," *Abdominal Imaging*, vol. 30, no. 6, pp. 744–747, 2005.

[46] T. Fujita, M. Kojima, N. Gotohda et al., "Incidence, clinical presentation and pathological features of benign sclerosing cholangitis of unknown origin masquerading as biliary carcinoma," *Journal of Hepato-Biliary-Pancreatic Sciences*, vol. 17, no. 2, pp. 139–146, 2010.

[47] Y. Zen, A. Ishikawa, S. Ogiso, N. Heaton, and B. Portmann, "Follicular cholangitis and pancreatitis—clinicopathological features and differential diagnosis of an under-recognized entity," *Histopathology*, vol. 60, pp. 261–269, 2012.

[48] G. I. Papachristou, A. J. Demetris, F. Craig, K. K. W. Lee, and M. Rabinovitz, "Cholestatic jaundice and bone lesions in an elderly woman," *Nature Clinical Practice Gastroenterology and Hepatology*, vol. 1, no. 1, pp. 53–57, 2004.

[49] T. H. Baron, R. E. Koehler, W. H. Rodgers, M. B. Fallon, and S. M. Ferguson, "Mast cell cholangiopathy: another cause of sclerosing cholangitis," *Gastroenterology*, vol. 109, no. 5, pp. 1677–1681, 1995.

[50] A. H. Kwon, Y. Matsui, and Y. Uemura, "Surgical procedures and histopathologic findings for patients with xanthogranulomatous cholecystitis," *Journal of the American College of Surgeons*, vol. 199, no. 2, pp. 204–210, 2004.

[51] S. Kawate, S. Ohwada, H. Ikota, K. Hamada, K. Kashiwabara, and Y. Morishita, "Xanthogranulomatous cholangitis causing obstructive jaundice: a case report," *World Journal of Gastroenterology*, vol. 12, no. 27, pp. 4428–4430, 2006.

[52] T. Kawana, S. Suita, T. Arima et al., "Xanthogranulomatous cholecystitis in an infant with obstructive jaundice," *European Journal of Pediatrics*, vol. 149, no. 11, pp. 765–767, 1990.

[53] P. Prasil, S. Cayer, M. Lemay, L. Pelletier, R. Cloutier, and S. Leclerc, "Juvenile xanthogranuloma presenting as obstructive jaundice," *Journal of Pediatric Surgery*, vol. 34, no. 7, pp. 1072–1073, 1999.

[54] R. P. Krishna, A. Kumar, R. K. Singh, S. Sikora, R. Saxena, and V. K. Kapoor, "Xanthogranulomatous inflammatory strictures of extrahepatic biliary tract: presentation and surgical management," *Journal of Gastrointestinal Surgery*, vol. 12, no. 5, pp. 836–841, 2008.

[55] G. Klatskin and R. Yesner, "Hepatic manifestations of sarcoidosis and other granulomatous diseases; a study based on histological examination of tissue obtained by needle biopsy of the liver," *The Yale Journal of Biology and Medicine*, vol. 23, no. 3, pp. 207–248, 1950.

[56] K. G. Ishak, "Sarcoidosis of the liver and bile ducts," *Mayo Clinic Proceedings*, vol. 73, no. 5, pp. 467–472, 1998.

[57] J. M. Petersen, "Klatskin-like biliary sarcoidosis: a cholangioscopic diagnosis," *Gastroenterology and Hepatology*, vol. 5, no. 2, pp. 137–140, 2009.

[58] A. Onitsuka, Y. Katagiri, S. Kiyama et al., "Hilar cholangiocarcinoma associated with sarcoid reaction in the regional lymph nodes," *Journal of Hepato-Biliary-Pancreatic Surgery*, vol. 10, no. 4, pp. 316–320, 2003.

[59] A. Karagiannidis, M. Karavalaki, and A. Koulaouzidis, "Hepatic sarcoidosis," *Annals of Hepatology*, vol. 5, no. 4, pp. 251–256, 2006.

[60] S. J. Margulis, C. L. Honig, R. Soave, A. F. Govoni, J. A. Mouradian, and I. M. Jacobson, "Biliary tract obstruction in the acquired immunodeficiency syndrome," *Annals of Internal Medicine*, vol. 105, no. 2, pp. 207–210, 1986.

[61] S. Pol, C. A. Romana, S. Richard et al., "Microsporidia infection in patients with the human immunodeficiency virus and unexplained cholangitis," *The New England Journal of Medicine*, vol. 328, no. 2, pp. 95–99, 1993.

[62] J. P. Cello and M. F. Chan, "Long-term follow-up of endoscopie retrograde cholangiopancreatography sphincterotomy for patients with acquired immune deficiency syndrome papillary stenosis," *American Journal of Medicine*, vol. 99, no. 6, pp. 600–603, 1995.

[63] Y. Benhamou, E. Caumes, Y. Gerosa et al., "AIDS-related cholangiopathy. Critical analysis of a prospective series of 26 patients," *Digestive Diseases and Sciences*, vol. 38, no. 6, pp. 1113–1118, 1993.

[64] A. Forbes, C. Blanshard, and B. Gazzard, "Natural history of AIDS related sclerosing cholangitis: a study of 20 cases," *Gut*, vol. 34, no. 1, pp. 116–121, 1993.

[65] A. R. Hayward, J. Levy, F. Facchetti et al., "Cholangiopathy and tumors of the pancreas, liver, and biliary tree in boys with X-linked immunodeficiency with hyper-IgM," *Journal of Immunology*, vol. 158, no. 2, pp. 977–983, 1997.

[66] F. Rodrigues, E. G. Davies, P. Harrison et al., "Liver disease in children with primary immunodeficiencies," *Journal of Pediatrics*, vol. 145, no. 3, pp. 333–339, 2004.

[67] A. H. Steinhart, M. Simons, R. Stone, and J. Heathcote, "Multiple hepatic abscesses: cholangiographic changes simulating sclerosing cholangitis and resolution after percutaneous drainage," *American Journal of Gastroenterology*, vol. 85, no. 3, pp. 306–308, 1990.

[68] W. Scheppach, G. Druge, G. Wittenberg et al., "Sclerosing cholangitis and liver cirrhosis after extrabiliary infections: report on three cases," *Critical Care Medicine*, vol. 29, no. 2, pp. 438–441, 2001.

[69] N. Urushihara, N. Ariki, T. Oyama et al., "Secondary sclerosing cholangitis and portal hypertension after O157

enterocolitis: extremely rare complications of hemolytic uremic syndrome," *Journal of Pediatric Surgery*, vol. 36, no. 12, pp. 1838–1840, 2001.

[70] S. Z. Alvarez, "Hepatobiliary tuberculosis," *Journal of Gastroenterology and Hepatology*, vol. 13, no. 8, pp. 833–839, 1998.

[71] V. H. Chong, P. U. Telisinghe, S. K. S. Yapp, and A. Jalihal, "Biliary strictures secondary to tuberculosis and early ampullary carcinoma," *Singapore Medical Journal*, vol. 50, no. 3, pp. e94–e96, 2009.

[72] S. S. Saluja, S. Ray, S. Pal et al., "Hepatobiliary and pancreatic tuberculosis: a two decade experience," *BMC Surgery*, vol. 7, article 10, 2007.

[73] Y. Özin, E. Parlak, Z. M. Kiliç, T. Temuçin, and N. Şaşmaz, "Sclerosing cholangitis-like changes in hepatobiliary tuberculosis," *Turkish Journal of Gastroenterology*, vol. 21, no. 1, pp. 50–53, 2010.

[74] M. Inal, E. Aksungur, E. Akgül, Ö. Demirbaş, M. Oguz, and E. Erkoçak, "Biliary tuberculosis mimicking cholangiocarcinoma: treatment with metallic biliary endoprothesis," *American Journal of Gastroenterology*, vol. 95, no. 4, pp. 1069–1071, 2000.

[75] H. Albrecht, S. Rüsch-Gerdes, H. J. Stellbrink, H. Greten, and S. Jäckle, "Disseminated Mycobacterium genavense infection as a cause of pseudo-whipple's disease and sclerosing cholangitis," *Clinical Infectious Diseases*, vol. 25, no. 3, pp. 742–743, 1997.

[76] K. W. Li, T. F. Wen, and G. D. Li, "Hepatic mucormycosis mimicking hilar cholangiocarcinoma: a case report and literature review," *World Journal of Gastroenterology*, vol. 16, no. 8, pp. 1039–1042, 2010.

[77] J. I. Lin, M. A. Kabir, H. C. Tseng, N. Hillman, J. Moezzi, and N. Gopalswamy, "Hepatobiliary dysfunction as the initial manifestation of disseminated cryptococcosis," *Journal of Clinical Gastroenterology*, vol. 28, no. 3, pp. 273–275, 1999.

[78] J. S. Kim, B. I. Choi, and M. C. Han, "Cryptococcal cholangiohepatitis with intraductal cryptococcoma," *American Journal of Roentgenology*, vol. 163, no. 4, pp. 995–996, 1994.

[79] H. B. Lefton, R. G. Farmer, R. Buchwald, and R. Haselby, "Cryptococcal hepatitis mimicking primary sclerosing cholangitis. A case report," *Gastroenterology*, vol. 67, no. 3, pp. 511–515, 1974.

[80] J. L. Gollan, G. P. Davidson, K. Anderson, T. A. White, and C. L. Kimber, "Visceral cryptococcosis without central nervous system or pulmonary involvement: presentation as hepatitis," *Medical Journal of Australia*, vol. 1, no. 10, pp. 469–471, 1972.

[81] M. K. Goenka, S. Mehta, S. K. Yachha, B. Nagi, A. Chakraborty, and A. K. Malik, "Hepatic involvement culminating in cirrhosis in a child with disseminated cryptococcosis," *Journal of Clinical Gastroenterology*, vol. 20, no. 1, pp. 57–60, 1995.

[82] J. C. Bucuvalas, K. E. Bove, R. A. Kaufman et al., "Cholangitis associated with cryptococcus neoformans," *Gastroenterology*, vol. 88, no. 4, pp. 1055–1059, 1985.

[83] H. Hameed, F. Sultan, Y. I. Khan, M. Hussain, and R. Azhar, "An unusual cause of obstructive jaundice," *Journal of the Royal College of Physicians of Edinburgh*, vol. 39, no. 3, pp. 221–223, 2009.

[84] B. G. Kim, D. H. Kang, C. W. Choi et al., "A case of clonorchiasis with focal intrahepatic duct dilatation mimicking an intrahepatic cholangiocarcinoma," *Clinical Endoscopy*, vol. 44, no. 1, pp. 55–58, 2011.

[85] R. K. Dhiman, A. Behera, Y. K. Chawla, J. B. Dilawari, and S. Suri, "Portal hypertensive biliopathy," *Gut*, vol. 56, no. 7, pp. 1001–1008, 2007.

[86] B. Condat, V. Vilgrain, T. Asselah et al., "Portal cavernoma-associated cholangiopathy: a clinical and MR cholangiography coupled with MR portography imaging study," *Hepatology*, vol. 37, no. 6, pp. 1302–1308, 2003.

[87] A. Chaudhary, P. Dhar, A. Sachdev et al., "Bile duct obstruction due to portal biliopathy in extrahepatic portal hypertension: surgical management," *British Journal of Surgery*, vol. 85, no. 3, pp. 326–329, 1998.

[88] G. H. Malkan, S. J. Bhatia, K. Bashir et al., "Cholangiopathy associated with portal hypertension: diagnostic evaluation and clinical implications," *Gastrointestinal Endoscopy*, vol. 49, no. 3, pp. 344–348, 1999.

[89] Y. Bayraktar, F. Balkanci, A. Ozenc et al., "The "pseudo-cholangiocarcinoma sign" in patients with cavernous transformation of the portal vein and its effect on the serum alkaline phosphatase and bilirubin levels," *American Journal of Gastroenterology*, vol. 90, no. 11, pp. 2015–2019, 1995.

[90] J. B. Dilawari and Y. K. Chawla, "Pseudosclerosing cholangitis in extrahepatic portal venous obstruction," *Gut*, vol. 33, no. 2, pp. 272–276, 1992.

[91] A. Gorgul, B. Kayhan, I. Dogan, and S. Ünal, "Disappearance of the pseudo-cholangiocarcinoma sign after TIPSS," *American Journal of Gastroenterology*, vol. 91, no. 1, pp. 150–154, 1996.

[92] Y. Bayraktar, M. A. Ozturk, T. Egesel, S. Çekirge, and F. Balkanci, "Disappearance of "pseudocholangiocarcinoma sign" in a patient with portal hypertension due to complete thrombosis of left portal vein and main portal vein web after web dilatation and transjugular intrahepatic portosystemic shunt," *Journal of Clinical Gastroenterology*, vol. 31, no. 4, pp. 328–332, 2000.

[93] R. Khare, S. S. Sikora, G. Srikanth et al., "Extrahepatic portal venous obstruction and obstructive jaundice: approach to management," *Journal of Gastroenterology and Hepatology*, vol. 20, no. 1, pp. 56–61, 2005.

[94] F. Filipponi, L. Urbani, G. Catalano et al., "Portal biliopathy treated by liver transplantation," *Transplantation*, vol. 77, no. 2, pp. 326–327, 2004.

[95] P. Deltenre and D. C. Valla, "Ischemic cholangiopathy," *Seminars in Liver Disease*, vol. 28, no. 3, pp. 235–246, 2008.

[96] S. M. Strasberg and W. S. Helton, "An analytical review of vasculobiliary injury in laparoscopic and open cholecystectomy," *International Hepato-Pancreato-Biliary Association*, vol. 13, no. 1, pp. 1–14, 2011.

[97] T. Ota, R. Hirai, K. Tsukuda, M. Murakam, M. Naitou, and N. Shimizu, "Biliary reconstruction with right hepatic lobectomy due to delayed management of laparoscopic bile duct injuries: a case report," *Acta Medica Okayama*, vol. 58, no. 3, pp. 163–167, 2004.

[98] S. Engler, C. Elsing, C. Flechtenmacher, L. Theilmann, W. Stremmel, and A. Stiehl, "Progressive sclerosing cholangitis after septic shock: a new variant of vanishing bile duct disorders," *Gut*, vol. 52, no. 5, pp. 688–693, 2003.

[99] C. M. Gelbmann, P. Rümmele, M. Wimmer et al., "Ischemic like cholangiopathy with secondary sclerosing cholangitis in critically ill patients," *American Journal of Gastroenterology*, vol. 102, no. 6, pp. 1221–1229, 2007.

[100] A. Saiura, N. Umekita, S. Inoue et al., "Benign biliary stricture associated with atherosclerosis," *Hepato-Gastroenterology*, vol. 48, no. 37, pp. 81–82, 2001.

[101] M. Ahmed, M. Dick, G. Mieli-Vergani, P. Harrison, J. Karani, and A. Dhawan, "Ischaemic cholangiopathy and sickle cell disease," *European Journal of Pediatrics*, vol. 165, no. 2, pp. 112–113, 2006.

[102] E. S. Barquist, N. Goldstein, and M. J. Zinner, "Polyarteritis nodosa presenting as a biliary stricture," *Surgery*, vol. 109, no. 1, pp. 16–19, 1991.

[103] D. L. T. Huong, D. Valla, D. Franco et al., "Cholangitis associated with paroxysmal nocturnal hemoglobinuria: another instance of ischemic cholangiopathy?" *Gastroenterology*, vol. 109, no. 4, pp. 1338–1343, 1995.

[104] G. Garcia-Tsao, J. R. Korzenik, L. Young et al., "Liver disease in patients with hereditary hemorrhagic telangiectasia," *The New England Journal of Medicine*, vol. 343, no. 13, pp. 931–936, 2000.

[105] S. Viola, M. Meyer, M. Fabre et al., "Ischemic necrosis of bile ducts complicating Schonlein-Henoch purpura," *Gastroenterology*, vol. 117, no. 1, pp. 211–214, 1999.

[106] K. L. Chandrasekhara and S. K. Iyer, "Obstructive jaundice due to radiation-induced hepatic duct stricture," *American Journal of Medicine*, vol. 77, no. 4, pp. 723–724, 1984.

[107] S. S. M. Ng, S. C. H. Yu, P. B. S. Lai, and W. Y. Lau, "Biliary complications associated with selective internal radiation (SIR) therapy for unresectable liver malignancies," *Digestive Diseases and Sciences*, vol. 53, no. 10, pp. 2813–2817, 2008.

[108] M. Makuuchi, M. Sukigara, T. Mori et al., "Bile duct necrosis: complication of transcatheter hepatic arterial embolization," *Radiology*, vol. 156, no. 2, pp. 331–334, 1985.

[109] D. H. Park, M. Kim, T. N. Kim et al., "Endoscopic treatment for suprapancreatic biliary stricture following blunt abdominal trauma," *American Journal of Gastroenterology*, vol. 102, no. 3, pp. 544–549, 2007.

[110] K. H. Yoon, H. K. Ha, M. H. Kim et al., "Biliary stricture caused by blunt abdominal trauma: clinical and radiologic features in five patients," *Radiology*, vol. 207, no. 3, pp. 737–741, 1998.

[111] K. Osei-Boateng, N. Ravendhran, O. Haluszka, and P. E. Darwin, "Endoscopic treatment of a post-traumatic biliary stricture mimicking a Klatskin tumor," *Gastrointestinal Endoscopy*, vol. 55, no. 2, pp. 274–276, 2002.

[112] M. Schmitt, C. B. Kölbel, M. K. Müller, C. S. Verbeke, and M. V. Singer, "Sclerosing cholangitis after burn injury," *Zeitschrift fur Gastroenterologie*, vol. 35, no. 10, pp. 929–934, 1997.

[113] J. Benninger, R. Grobholz, Y. Oeztuerk et al., "Sclerosing cholangitis following severe trauma: description of a remarkable disease entity with emphasis on possible pathophysiologic mechanisms," *World Journal of Gastroenterology*, vol. 11, no. 27, pp. 4199–4205, 2005.

[114] D. Hohn, J. Melnick, R. Stagg et al., "Biliary sclerosis in patients receiving hepatic arterial infusions of floxuridine," *Journal of Clinical Oncology*, vol. 3, no. 1, pp. 98–102, 1985.

[115] J. F. Botet, R. C. Watson, N. Kemeny, J. M. Daly, and S. Yeh, "Cholangitis complicating intraarterial chemotherapy in liver metastasis," *Radiology*, vol. 156, no. 2, pp. 335–337, 1985.

[116] S. Phongkitkarun, S. Kobayashi, V. Varavithya, X. Huang, S. A. Curley, and C. Charnsangavej, "Bile duct complications of hepatic arterial infusion chemotherapy evaluated by helical CT," *Clinical Radiology*, vol. 60, no. 6, pp. 700–709, 2005.

[117] H. Tada, M. Morimoto, T. Shima et al., "Progressive jaundice due to lymphangiosis carcinomatosa of the liver: CT appearance," *Journal of Computer Assisted Tomography*, vol. 20, no. 4, pp. 650–652, 1996.

[118] E. Henderson-Jackson, N. A. Nasir, A. Hakam, A. Nasir, and D. Coppola, "Primary mixed lymphoepithelioma-like carcinoma and intra-hepatic cholangiocarcinoma: a case report and review of literature," *International Journal of Clinical and Experimental Pathology*, vol. 3, no. 7, pp. 736–741, 2010.

[119] F. Kamani, A. Dorudinia, F. Goravanchi, and F. Rahimi, "Extrahepatic bile duct neurilemmoma mimicking Klatskin tumor," *Archives of Iranian Medicine*, vol. 10, no. 2, pp. 264–267, 2007.

[120] Z. H. Krukowski, J. L. McPhie, A. G. H. Farquharson, and N. A. Matheson, "Proliferative cholangitis (cholangitis glandularis proliferans)," *British Journal of Surgery*, vol. 70, no. 3, pp. 166–171, 1983.

[121] F. Gundling, A. Nerlich, W. U. Heitland, and W. Schepp, "Biliary manifestation of Erdheim-Chester disease mimicking Klatskin's carcinoma," *American Journal of Gastroenterology*, vol. 102, no. 2, pp. 452–454, 2007.

[122] M. Quante, B. Appenrodt, S. Randerath, M. Wolff, H. P. Fischer, and T. Sauerbruch, "Atypical Ormond's disease associated with bile duct stricture mimicking cholangiocarcinoma," *Scandinavian Journal of Gastroenterology*, vol. 44, no. 1, pp. 116–120, 2009.

[123] C. Heer, M. Pförtner, U. Hamberger, U. Raute-Kreinsen, M. Hanraths, and D. K. Bartsch, "Heterotopic pancreatic tissue in the bifurcation of the bile duct: rare diagnosis mimicking a Klatskin tumour ," *Chirurg*, vol. 81, no. 2, pp. 151–154, 2010.

[124] P. G. Kalman, R. M. Stone, and M. J. Phillips, "Heterotopic gastric tissue of the bile duct," *Surgery*, vol. 89, no. 3, pp. 384–386, 1981.

[125] N. Dubale, N. K. Anupama, M. Tandon, R. Pradeep, D. N. Reddy, and G. V . Rao, "Anomalous biliary duct mistaken as hilar stricture. A case report," *Journal of Gastroenterology and Hepatology*, vol. 1, no. 1, pp. 34–36, 2011.

[126] R. Santoro, E. Santoro, G. M. Ettorre, C. Nicolas, and E. Santoro, "Benign hilar stenosis mimicking Klatskin tumor," *Annales de Chirurgie*, vol. 129, no. 5, pp. 297–300, 2004.

[127] D. Uhlmann, M. Wiedmann, F. Schmidt et al., "Management and outcome in patients with Klatskin-mimicking lesions of the biliary tree," *Journal of Gastrointestinal Surgery*, vol. 10, no. 8, pp. 1144–1150, 2006.

12

The Changing Spectrum of Surgically Treated Cystic Neoplasms of the Pancreas

Jennifer K. Plichta, Jacqueline A. Brosius, Sam G. Pappas, Gerard J. Abood, and Gerard V. Aranha

Department of Surgery, Loyola University Health System, Maywood, IL 60153, USA

Correspondence should be addressed to Gerard V. Aranha; garanha@lumc.edu

Academic Editor: Richard Charnley

Introduction. While the incidence of pancreatic cystic lesions has steadily increased, we sought to evaluate the changes in their surgical management. *Methods.* Patients with pancreatic cystic lesions who underwent surgical resection from 2003 to 2013 were identified. Clinicopathologic factors were analyzed and compared to a similar cohort from 1992 to 2002. *Results.* There were 134 patients with pancreatic cystic lesions who underwent surgical resection from 2003 to 2013, compared to 73 from 1992 to 2002. The most common preoperative imaging was a CT scan, although 66% underwent EUS and 63% underwent biopsy. Pathology included 18 serous, 47 mucinous, 11 pseudopapillary, and 58 intraductal papillary mucinous neoplasms (IPMN). In comparing cohorts, there were significantly fewer serous lesions and more IPMN. Postoperative complication rates were similar, and perioperative mortality rates were comparable. *Conclusion.* There has been a dramatic change in surgically treated pancreatic cystic tumors over the past two decades. Our data suggests that the incorporation of new imaging and diagnostic tests has led to greater detection of cystic tumors and a decreased rate of potentially unnecessary resections. Therefore, all patients with cystic pancreatic lesions should undergo a focused CT-pancreas, and an EUS biopsy should be considered, in order to best select those that would benefit from surgical resection.

1. Introduction

Neoplasms comprise 50% of cystic lesions of the pancreas [1]. They are divided into four main subtypes: serous cystic neoplasms (SCN), mucinous cystic neoplasms (MCN), solid pseudopapillary neoplasms (SPN), and intraductal papillary mucinous neoplasms (IPMN). Most frequently, these neoplasms are found incidentally, and the number of patients diagnosed with a neoplasm by imaging done for an unrelated reason is >2% [2]. The rise in routine use of computed tomography (CT) scans and magnetic resonance imaging (MRI) has led to an increase in the diagnosis of asymptomatic cystic neoplasms [3].

In general, IPMN, mucinous cysts, and SPN are removed surgically, given their significant potential for malignant transformation. Serous cystadenomas, in contrast, have a negligible rate of malignant transformation, although these lesions are more likely to be larger and cause symptoms due to mass effect [4]. It is considered standard of care to resect symptomatic serous cystadenomas that cause significant morbidity. However, the decision to resect asymptomatic masses has been more controversial, and management varies greatly by institution [4]. In the past, a more aggressive approach has been utilized for serous cystadenomas, due to concern for misdiagnosis based on standard, older imaging [4].

Pancreas-specific CT, developed in the mid-1990s, is a multidetector CT (MDCT) that allows for visualization of arterial, pancreatic, and portal venous phases and drastically enhances the diagnostic accuracy of pancreatic tumors [5]. The introduction of this technology along with endoscopic ultrasound- (EUS-) guided biopsies (fine needle aspiration FNA) has provided us with new ways to confirm pathology before operative intervention is undertaken. These advancements in imaging and technology have subsequently influenced the management of these neoplasms.

The objective of this study was to review our institution's experience with pancreatic cystic lesions and to characterize their presentation, diagnosis, and perioperative management. In order to determine how the spectrum of surgically treated cystic neoplasms of the pancreas may have changed over the years, we compared these patients to a previous study conducted by our institution from 1992 to 2002 [6].

2. Methods

Through a retrospective chart review, patients with pancreatic cystic lesions who underwent surgical resection from 2003 to 2013 at Loyola University Medical Center were identified (modern cohort). Patients with a prior history of pancreatic cancer were excluded. Clinicopathologic factors were assessed from the medical record, including clinical presentation, preoperative evaluation/imaging, surgeries performed, pathologic results, postoperative complications, and mortalities. The Social Security Death Index was utilized to determine current living status of patients in the modern cohort.

In the preoperative setting, a CT scan was typically the initial imaging performed. For patients with a contrast allergy or nonspecific findings on CT, an MRI was obtained. The main criterion for doing an EUS in the modern cohort was to get an accurate diagnosis of serous and mucinous tumors. If CT clearly showed a SPN or main duct IPMN, then EUS was not performed. However, EUS was done for asymptomatic branch duct IPMN to evaluate it for possible malignant features. In general, when an EUS was performed at our institution in the modern cohort, cyst fluid was sent for mucin, CEA (carcinoembryonic antigen), amylase, and cytology. Cysts that were high in amylase with no mucin or CEA and negative cytology were considered to be pseudocysts and were excluded. Fluids that had no mucin, low amylase, and low CEA were considered serous and were operated upon only if symptomatic. Cysts high in mucin with high CEA and atypical or malignant cytology went to surgery.

Select results were compared to a similar cohort of patients from 1992 to 2002 (data previously collected [6]). Statistical analyses were conducted using Stata 10.0 (StataCorp, College Station, TX). Categorical variables were analyzed using Chi-squared (χ^2) tests, and continuous variables were analyzed using Mann-Whitney U tests or Student's t-tests. Statistical significance was defined as $P \leq 0.05$ (2-sided). This study was approved by the Loyola University Health Systems Institutional Review Board.

3. Results

From 2003 to 2013, there were 134 patients with pancreatic cystic lesions who underwent surgical resection (modern cohort). The median age of the modern cohort was 66 years (range 18–88 years old). The historic cohort was comprised of patients who underwent surgical resection from 1992 to 2002 and included 73 patients. Patients were predominately females in both populations (67% versus 67%). The most common presenting symptom was abdominal pain (48%, $n = 62$), which was less common than observed in the historic cohort (64%, $P = 0.013$). However, the same number of lesions in the modern cohort was found incidentally on imaging (48%, $n = 62$). Other common clinical presentations for the modern cohort included 34 with weight loss, 11 with pancreatitis, and 7 with jaundice (Figure 1).

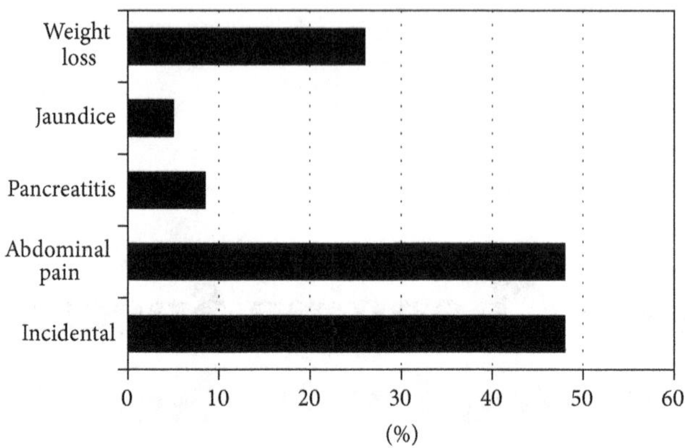

FIGURE 1: The most common clinical presentations in patients with pancreatic cystic lesions who underwent surgical resection from 2003 to 2013.

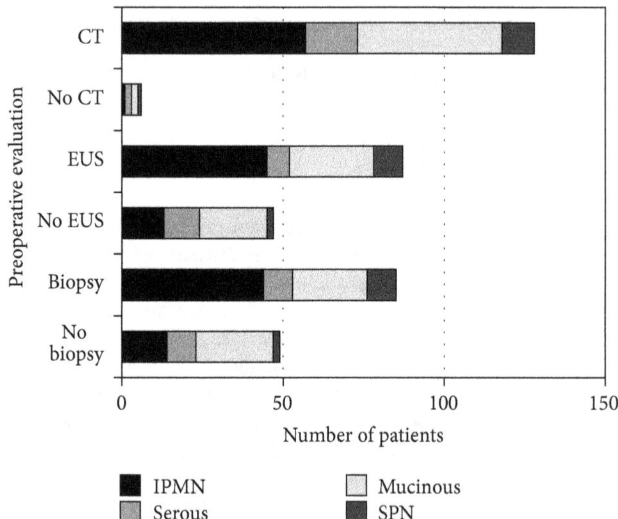

FIGURE 2: Preoperative evaluation of the modern cohort, including CT scans, endoscopic ultrasounds, and biopsy in select patients, stratified by the type of pancreatic cystic neoplasm. CT: computed tomography scan; EUS: endoscopic ultrasound.

Prior to surgery, the majority of recent patients had a CT scan (98%, $n = 128$), while only 66% underwent EUS ($n = 87$) and 63% underwent biopsy ($n = 85$); the data is summarized in Figure 2 and is stratified by the type of cystic neoplasm. This data (preoperative imaging and biopsy) is not available in our records for the historic cohort, and we were unable to collect this data retrospectively. For the patients who underwent a biopsy (or fine needle aspiration), the indications for surgery included 14 patients with malignant lesions, 25 patients with atypical cells, 13 patients with mucin ±, an elevated CEA, and 4 patients with specific indications including (1) main duct IPMN; (2) an elevated CA19-9; (3)

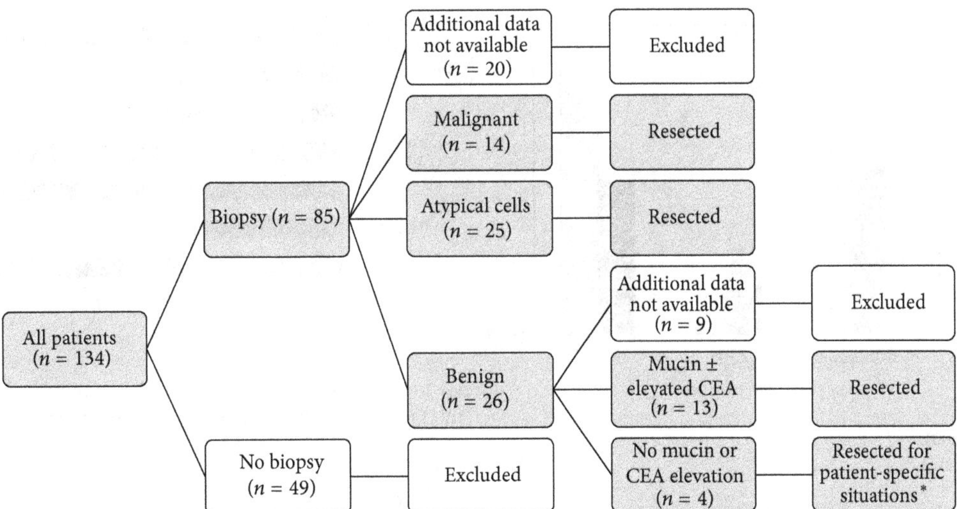

FIGURE 3: Results of preoperative biopsies and the algorithm for deciding when to operate. *The four patients resected who did not meet standard biopsy criteria were for (1) main duct IPMN; (2) elevated serum CA19-9; (3) two separate pancreatic tumors in a patient with Von Hippel-Lindau disease (one serous and one pancreatic neuroendocrine tumor); and (4) patient symptoms. IPMN: intraductal papillary mucinous neoplasms; CA: cancer antigen; CEA: carcinoembryonic antigen.

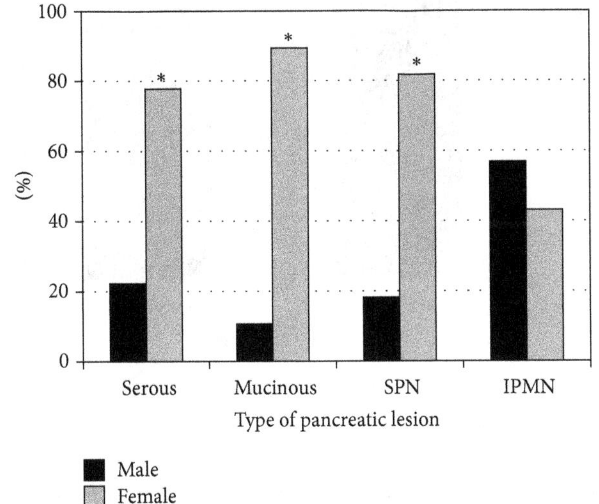

FIGURE 4: Comparison of pancreatic cystic lesions by gender in the modern cohort; $^*P < 0.05$. SPN: solid pseudopapillary neoplasms; IPMN: intraductal papillary mucinous neoplasms.

TABLE 1: Types of surgeries performed based upon the pathology of the pancreatic cystic lesions.

Type of tumor	PD	DP	CP	TP	Other
SCN	9	8	0	0	1
Mucinous (MCN)	17	26	1	1	2
Cystadenoma	12	23	1	1	2
Cystadenocarcinoma	5	3	0	0	0
SPN	3	8	0	0	0
IPMN	33	22	3	0	0
Total	62	64	4	1	3

SCN: serous cystic neoplasms; MCN: mucinous cystic neoplasms; SPN: solid pseudopapillary neoplasms; IPMN: intraductal papillary mucinous neoplasms; PD: pancreaticoduodenectomy; DP: distal pancreatectomy; CP: central pancreatectomy; TP: total pancreatectomy.

two separate pancreatic tumors in a patient with Von Hippel-Lindau disease (one serous, one pancreatic neuroendocrine tumor); and (4) patient symptoms. These results are outlined in Figure 3. The results of the biopsy were not available in 29 patients, as some patients were referred to our institution from an outside hospital and the records available were limited.

The main pathologic subtypes in the modern cohort included 18 serous lesions, 47 mucinous lesions, 11 SPN, and 58 IPMN. Most of the lesions were more common in females (serous $P = 0.018$, mucinous $P = 0.000$, and SPN $P = 0.035$), while IPMN lesions were similarly distributed (Figure 4). Malignancy was noted in 17% of the mucinous lesions and 38% of the IPMN. Compared to the historic cohort, there were significantly fewer serous lesions (13% versus 36%, $P = 0.0002$) and more IPMN (43% versus 25%, $P = 0.008$). There was no difference in the incidence of mucinous lesions or SPN (Figure 5).

The majority of patients in the modern cohort underwent pancreaticoduodenectomy ($n = 62$) or distal pancreatectomy ($n = 64$). In addition, there were 4 central pancreatectomies, 1 total pancreatectomy, and 3 other procedures (Table 1). In the historic cohort, the most common surgical resection was also the distal pancreatectomy (59%, $n = 43$); however, pancreaticoduodenectomies were significantly more common in the modern cohort (27% versus 46%, $P = 0.008$; Figure 6). Postoperatively, the most common complications in the modern cohort were wound infections ($n = 7$), intra-abdominal abscesses ($n = 7$), and urinary tract infections ($n = 6$). Other complications included 5 pancreatic fistulas, 5 with delayed gastric emptying, 3 gastrointestinal bleeds, and

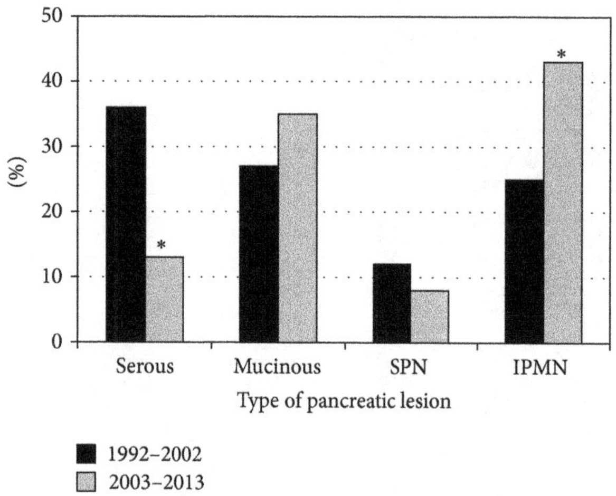

FIGURE 5: Comparison of pancreatic cystic lesions by patient cohort; $^*P < 0.01$. SPN: solid pseudopapillary neoplasms; IPMN: intraductal papillary mucinous neoplasms.

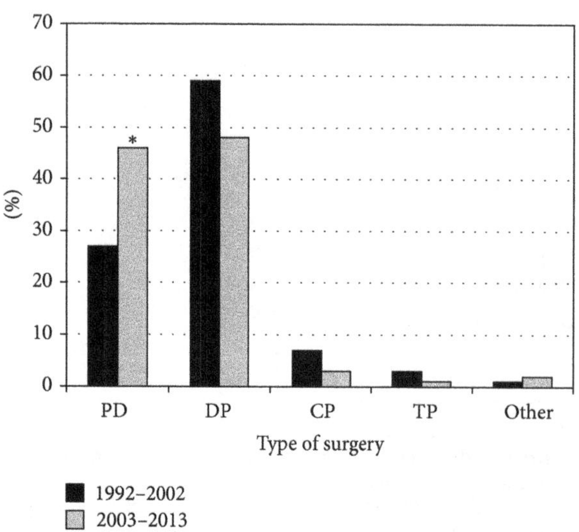

FIGURE 6: Comparison of surgeries performed by patient cohort; $^*P < 0.01$. PD: pancreaticoduodenectomy; DP: distal pancreatectomy; CP: central pancreatectomy; TP: total pancreatectomy.

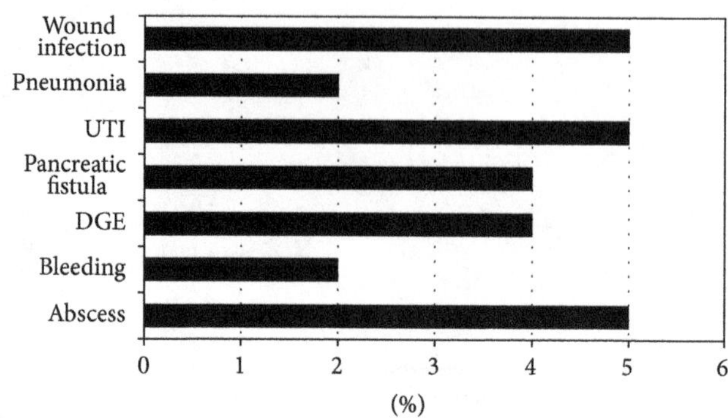

FIGURE 7: Most common postoperative complications. UTI: urinary tract infection; DGE: delayed gastric emptying.

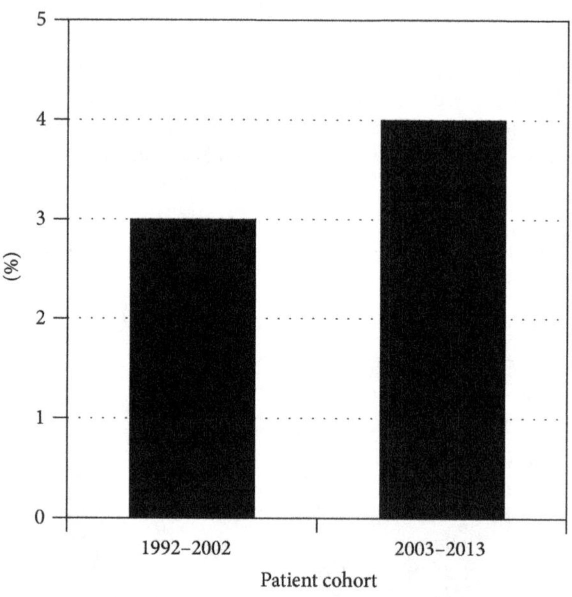

FIGURE 8: Comparison of mortalities by patient cohort.

2 pneumonias (Figure 7). Overall complication rates between the modern and historic cohorts were similar (32% versus 27%, $P = 0.42$), while pancreatic fistula rates were slightly less common in the modern cohort (4% versus 10%, $P = 0.085$). Perioperative mortality rates were comparable between both cohorts (3% versus 4%, $P = 0.67$; Figure 8).

4. Discussion

The increasing use of multidetector computed tomography (MDCT), magnetic resonance imaging (MRI), and endoscopic ultrasound (EUS) has specifically resulted in the increased recognition of pancreatic cystic lesions [7]. While some of these lesions are associated with malignancy, many of the lesions are asymptomatic at the time of diagnosis and benign in pathology. This has led to controversy in the surgical management of cystic pancreatic lesions [8]. Cystic lesions of the pancreas may be classified into neoplasms and pseudocysts [7]. The most common cystic neoplasms of the pancreas are serous cystic neoplasms (SCN), mucinous cystic neoplasms (MCN), solid pseudopapillary neoplasms (SPN), and intraductal papillary mucinous neoplasms (IPMN) [6].

We previously published our experience with the surgical management of cystic neoplasms between January 1992 and September 2002 [6]. In that decade, the most common cystic tumors surgically treated were SCN followed by MCN and both cystadenomas and cystadenocarcinomas, followed by IPMN, with SPN being the least common. Since that time, we and others [6, 9] have noted a change in the indications for surgery in pancreatic cystic neoplasms. At present, the most common indication for resection of a pancreatic cystic lesion is suspicion of malignancy, typically in IPMN and MCN. The prevalence of SCN has remained stable, while surgery for SCN has decreased dramatically. Why have all of these shifts occurred? The reasons are threefold: (1) SCN are often asymptomatic; (2) the incidence of malignancy in these tumors is quite low [10–13]; (3) the incidence of invasive carcinoma in IPMN is 15% at initial diagnosis and is cumulative over time [14]. Furthermore, improvements in MDCT, MRI, and EUS with cyst fluid analysis have helped differentiate the subtypes of cystic tumors prior to surgical treatment [15–17]. In a study by Lee et al., three radiologists were asked to interpret MDCTs and MRIs of 63 patients with cystic tumors of the pancreas, and the ability of each to predict malignancy was 77.8%, 73%, and 73%. These predictions were the same whether it was MDCT or MRI. The combination of MRI and MDCT was not significantly better but may merit future investigation [15].

The use of EUS in addition to CT (or MRI) has been recently evaluated by Khashab et al. [18]. This study evaluated 154 patients who underwent EUS and subsequent surgical resection and compared the diagnostic yield of the various imaging modalities. After CT or MRI, EUS increased the rate of correctly identifying neoplastic cysts by 36% and 54%, respectively, and thus appears to be a useful adjunct in the preoperative evaluation of patients with cystic neoplasms. In the modern cohort of our patients, there were slightly more patients with serous lesions that did not undergo preoperative evaluation with EUS, which may suggest that the addition of this study may have yielded a more accurate diagnosis preoperatively and possibly avoided surgical resection in select cases. Overall, the decreased rate of surgical resection for serous lesions is likely related to the increased use of CT scans and confirmation by EUS when necessary.

Cyst fluid analysis from EUS has also demonstrated utility in diagnosing SCN [13, 19, 20]. In one study at Indiana University Medical Center, analysis of the cyst fluid using VEGF-A correlated with pathologic diagnosis [13]. For SCN specifically, a high level of VEGF-A (8500 pg/mL) had a sensitivity of 100% and specificity of 97%. With a cutoff of 200 pg/mL, VEGF-C identified SCN with 100% sensitivity and 90% specificity. Another study from Massachusetts General Hospital demonstrated a low CEA level and a low amylase level in SCN lesions [19]. Therefore, the surgical intervention in SCN today is limited to those patients who are symptomatic, those who have large tumors, and those who have enlarging lesions. Our policy on asymptomatic SCN is to get a MDCT at six-month intervals for two years and then yearly for a period of five years.

Currently, the major controversy surrounding cystic tumors of the pancreas is related to IPMN. IPMN lesions can be classified into 3 subtypes: (1) main duct IPMN (MD-IPMN); (2) mixed duct IPMN; and (3) branch duct IPMN (BD-IPMN). In a review of a published series of 50 or more cases, the frequency of malignancy was 61.6% and the frequency of invasive IPMN was 43.1%. Considering these incidences, it was felt that surgical resections were strongly recommended in all fit patients in whom the main duct was dilated greater than 5 mm in diameter and in those who presented with symptoms of jaundice, pancreatitis, diabetes, and/or steatorrhea [21]. However, much of the controversy surrounds the decision to resect or observe BD-IPMN lesions. Tanaka et al. [21] published international consensus guidelines in 2012 for the management of IPMN of the pancreas. The frequency of malignancy in resected BD-IPMN was 25.5% (range 6.3–46.5%); the frequency of invasive cancer was 17.7% (range 1.4–36.7%). This may warrant consideration of resection in many patients; however, BD-IPMN are often discovered incidentally [8] and occur in elderly patients who may have comorbid conditions. Therefore, in these patients, surgery may be indicated when the cyst is greater than 3 cm, imaging follow-up reveals growth, a mural nodule is present, and/or positive cytology is obtained [21]. In the absence of these clinical indications, the consensus group concluded that BD-IPMN lesions less than 3 cm could be observed, particularly in elderly patients. In comparison, other authors have recommended consideration of enucleation for BD-IPMN [22]. However, the incidence of pancreatic fistula was 43%, and, as such, we have not undertaken enucleation for BD-IPMN. In reviewing our own data (reported previously [23]), preoperative testing did not reliably differentiate main versus branch duct lesions, and thus the decision to observe should be undertaken cautiously. Nevertheless, there does appear to be a role for observation in patients with lesions that are asymptomatic and not showing growth with no mural nodules.

Tanaka et al. also published guidelines for MCN. MCN is defined by the presence of ovarian stroma and has a low prevalence of invasive carcinoma [21]. These tumors often occur in young women, and the risk of progression to invasion, though not accurately known, is possible [24, 25]. Based on this, the consensus in MCN is to resect, which can often be achieved laparoscopically when involving the body of the pancreas [21]. In the frail elderly patient, ablation may be considered [21]. Because of the potential for surgical management, it is important to distinguish mucinous from nonmucinous cystic neoplasms in the preoperative evaluation. The utility of EUS cytology and cyst fluid analysis (CEA and amylase) has previously been assessed and proven to be highly specific for differentiating these tumors, while EUS morphology alone did not distinguish between the two groups [20].

SPN of the pancreas is an entity that occurs mainly in young women in the third decade of life; however, as in our series, others have seen a few cases which occur in men [26, 27]. These tumors have both solid and cystic elements and can present with solitary lesions in the head, body, and tail of the pancreas, and a certain percentage of patients will present with metastases at the time of diagnoses [26, 27]. Because these lesions occur mainly in young women and have a malignant potential, the general consensus is to resect, depending on the location of the tumor, either by pancreaticoduodenectomy or distal pancreatectomy ± splenectomy. Cure rates are high, and patients often do well after removal of metastases when they occur in the liver [26, 27].

Although our work represents an update on the management of pancreatic cystic neoplasms, it has several limitations. It is a retrospective review of data from one institution and thus has an inevitable selection bias. The ideal study would include data on those patients with pancreatic cystic lesions who do not undergo surgery, which could then serve as a population for comparison. Patients managed nonoperatively, however, are followed up by several types of physicians, often including nonsurgeons, which makes identification of such patients difficult. In addition, some are only followed up for a few years and are then released from follow-up. Because of these pitfalls, the overall incidence of pancreatic cystic neoplasms could not be calculated in our study. However, there were approximately 75 patients followed up by surgeons during the second era, based on CT and EUS criteria; in the first era, we operated on all cystic lesions that were proven not to be pseudocysts and were evaluated by a surgeon. The majority of these were serous cystic adenomas, and they are followed up with CT scans every six months for two years and yearly scans for three years. Only one branch duct IPMN became symptomatic during this time period and required surgical intervention.

5. Conclusions

In summary, our experience with cystic tumors of the pancreas in the modern era reveals a dramatic change in the indication for surgery, which is mainly related to SCN and IPMN. In the first decade reviewed, SCN was the most commonly resected cystic tumor, and, in the second decade, IPMN was the most commonly resected tumor and SCN was the second least. This is likely related to the advancements in imaging and fluid analysis using EUS. Our present approach to SCN is to surgically resect those that are symptomatic, those that are large, and those that are growing on sequential follow-up imaging. Because of the possibility of a benign MCN undergoing malignant transformation, we recommend resection of these tumors. SPN lesions often occur in young women, can harbor malignancy, and sometimes present with metastases. Therefore, we suggest that resection is indicated in relation to the site of the tumor in the pancreas. These patients may also benefit from metastasectomy. MD-IPMN patients who present with jaundice, pancreatitis, steatorrhea, diabetes, and/or main duct diameter greater than 5 mm should undergo surgical resection. This may include pancreaticoduodenectomy or a total pancreatectomy. In BD-IPMN, surgery is reserved for those who are symptomatic, those with enlarging lesions on follow-up imaging, those whose cytology reveals atypia, and those with a mural nodule on imaging. For those with mixed type IPMN, surveillance is performed for high risk patients with comorbidities and those who have a borderline dilated duct that is less than 5 mm. However, in those patients who have major pancreatic duct dilatation and have cytology that is atypical, we recommend resection. It is our contention that the proper use of imaging and cyst fluid analysis has led to less surgery in asymptomatic SCN and increased recognition of IPMN where the prevalence of malignancy is a reality.

Acknowledgment

The authors would like to acknowledge the funding provided by the Department of Surgery, Loyola University Health System.

References

[1] T. A. Laffan, K. M. Horton, A. P. Klein et al., "Prevalence of unsuspected pancreatic cysts on MDCT," *The American Journal of Roentgenology*, vol. 191, no. 3, pp. 802–807, 2008.

[2] K. S. Spinelli, T. E. Fromwiller, R. A. Daniel et al., "Cystic pancreatic neoplasms: observe or operate," *Annals of Surgery*, vol. 239, no. 5, pp. 651–659, 2004.

[3] C. Fernández-Del Castillo, J. Targarona, S. P. Thayer et al., "Incidental pancreatic cysts: clinicopathologic characteristics and comparison with symptomatic patients," *Archives of Surgery*, vol. 138, no. 4, pp. 427–434, 2003.

[4] C. M. Pyke, J. A. van Heerden, T. V. Colby, M. G. Sarr, and A. L. Weaver, "The spectrum of serous cystadenoma of the pancreas: clinical, pathologic, and surgical aspects," *Annals of Surgery*, vol. 215, no. 2, pp. 132–139, 1992.

[5] V. Chaudhary and S. Bano, "Imaging of the pancreas: recent advances," *Indian Journal of Endocrinology and Metabolism*, vol. 15, no. 5, pp. S25–S32, 2011.

[6] M. K. Sheehan, K. Beck, J. Pickleman et al., "Spectrum of cystic neoplasms of the pancreas and their surgical management," *Archives of Surgery*, vol. 138, no. 6, pp. 657–662, 2003.

[7] B. G. Turner and W. R. Brugge, "Pancreatic cystic lesions: when to watch, when to operate, and when to ignore," *Current Gastroenterology Reports*, vol. 12, no. 2, pp. 98–105, 2010.

[8] J. J. Farrell and C. Fernández-Del Castillo, "Pancreatic cystic neoplasms: management and unanswered questions," *Gastroenterology*, vol. 144, no. 6, pp. 1303–1315, 2013.

[9] N. P. Valsangkar, V. Morales-Oyarvide, S. P. Thayer et al., "851 resected cystic tumors of the pancreas: a 33-year experience at the Massachusetts General Hospital," *Surgery*, vol. 152, no. 3, pp. S4–S12, 2012.

[10] M. Fukasawa, H. Maguchi, K. Takahashi et al., "Clinical features and natural history of serous cystic neoplasm of the pancreas," *Pancreatology*, vol. 10, no. 6, pp. 695–701, 2011.

[11] J. C. King, T. T. Ng, S. C. White, G. Cortina, H. A. Reber, and O. J. Hines, "Pancreatic serous cystadenocarcinoma: a case report and review of the literature," *Journal of Gastrointestinal Surgery*, vol. 13, no. 10, pp. 1864–1868, 2009.

[12] J. F. Tseng, A. L. Warshaw, D. V. Sahani et al., "Serous cystadenoma of the pancreas: tumor growth rates and recommendations for treatment," *Annals of Surgery*, vol. 242, no. 3, pp. 413–421, 2005.

[13] M. T. Yip-Schneider, H. Wu, R. P. Dumas et al., "Vascular endothelial growth factor, a novel and highly accurate pancreatic fluid biomarker for serous pancreatic cysts," *Journal of the American College of Surgeons*, vol. 218, no. 4, pp. 608–617, 2014.

[14] C. M. Schmidt, "Is surgical intervention for cystic neoplasms of the pancreas being underutilized?" *Journal of Gastrointestinal Surgery*, vol. 18, no. 1, pp. 184–186, 2014.

[15] H.-J. Lee, M.-J. Kim, J.-Y. Choi, H.-S. Hong, and K. A. Kim, "Relative accuracy of CT and MRI in the differentiation of benign from malignant pancreatic cystic lesions," *Clinical Radiology*, vol. 66, no. 4, pp. 315–321, 2011.

[16] Y. Nakai, H. Isayama, T. Itoi et al., "Role of endoscopic ultrasonography in pancreatic cystic neoplasms: where do we stand and where will we go?" *Digestive Endoscopy*, vol. 26, no. 2, pp. 135–143, 2014.

[17] T. Tirkes, K. Sandrasegaran, R. Sanyal et al., "Secretin-enhanced MR cholangiopancreatography: spectrum of findings," *Radiographics*, vol. 33, no. 7, pp. 1889–1906, 2013.

[18] M. A. Khashab, K. Kim, A. M. Lennon et al., "Should we do EUS/FNA on patients with pancreatic cysts? the incremental diagnostic yield of EUS over CT/MRI for prediction of cystic neoplasms," *Pancreas*, vol. 42, no. 4, pp. 717–721, 2013.

[19] K. B. Lewandrowski, J. F. Southern, M. R. Pins, C. C. Compton, and A. L. Warshaw, "Cyst fluid analysis in the differential diagnosis of pancreatic cysts: a comparison of pseudocysts, serous cystadenomas, mucinous cystic neoplasms, and mucinous cystadenocarcinoma," *Annals of Surgery*, vol. 217, no. 1, pp. 41–47, 1993.

[20] S. Attasaranya, S. Pais, J. LeBlanc, L. McHenry, S. Sherman, and J. M. DeWitt, "Endoscopic ultrasound-guided fine needle aspiration and cyst fluid analysis for pancreatic cysts," *Journal of the Pancreas*, vol. 8, no. 5, pp. 553–563, 2007.

[21] M. Tanaka, C. Fernández-Del Castillo, V. Adsay et al., "International consensus guidelines 2012 for the management of IPMN and MCN of the pancreas," *Pancreatology*, vol. 12, no. 3, pp. 183–197, 2012.

[22] O. Turrini, C. M. Schmidt, H. A. Pitt et al., "Side-branch intraductal papillary mucinous neoplasms of the pancreatic head/uncinate: resection or enucleation?" *HPB*, vol. 13, no. 2, pp. 126–131, 2011.

[23] J. K. Plichta, K. Ban, Z. Fridirici et al., "Should all branch-duct intraductal papillary mucinous neoplasms be resected?" *The American Journal of Surgery*, vol. 209, no. 3, pp. 478–482, 2015.

[24] M. G. Sarr, H. A. Carpenter, L. P. Prabhakar et al., "Clinical and pathologic correlation of 84 mucinous cystic neoplasms of the pancreas. Can one reliably differentiate benign from malignant (or premalignant) neoplasms?" *Annals of Surgery*, vol. 231, no. 2, pp. 205–212, 2000.

[25] R. E. Jimenez, A. L. Warshaw, K. Z'graggen et al., "Sequential accumulation of K-ras mutations and p53 overexpression in the progression of pancreatic mucinous cystic neoplasms to malignancy," *Annals of Surgery*, vol. 230, no. 4, pp. 501–511, 1999.

[26] S. Reddy, J. L. Cameron, J. Scudiere et al., "Surgical management of solid-pseudopapillary neoplasms of the pancreas (Franz or Hamoudi tumors): a large single-institutional series," *Journal of the American College of Surgeons*, vol. 208, no. 5, pp. 950–957, 2009.

[27] J. M. Butte, M. F. Brennan, M. Gönen et al., "Solid pseudopapillary tumors of the pancreas. Clinical features, surgical outcomes, and long-term survival in 45 consecutive patients from a single center," *Journal of Gastrointestinal Surgery*, vol. 15, no. 2, pp. 350–357, 2011.

13

An Evaluation of Neoadjuvant Chemoradiotherapy for Patients with Resectable Pancreatic Ductal Adenocarcinoma

Hui Jiang,[1] Chi Du,[2] Mingwei Cai,[2] Hai He,[2] Cheng Chen,[1] Jianguo Qiu,[3] and Hong Wu[3]

[1] *Department of Hepatobiliary Pancreatic Surgery, The Second People's Hospital of Neijiang, Luzhou Medical College, Neijiang, Sichuan 641003, China*

[2] *Department of Cancer, The Second People's Hospital of Neijiang, Luzhou Medical College, Neijiang, Sichuan 641003, China*

[3] *Department of Hepatobiliary Pancreatic Surgery, West China Hospital, Sichuan University, Chengdu, Sichuan 610041, China*

Correspondence should be addressed to Hui Jiang; jwangyang@sina.com

Academic Editor: Attila Olah

Aims. The aim of this study is to compare our results of preoperative chemotherapy followed by pancreaticoduodenectomy (PD) with those of surgery alone in patients with localized resectable pancreatic ductal adenocarcinoma (PDAC). *Methods.* Outcome data for 112 patients of resectable PDAC who received preoperative chemoradiotherapy followed by PD (group I) between January 2004 and April 2010 were retrospectively analyzed and were compared with selected 120 patients who underwent PD alone (group II) in the same period. *Results.* Patients in group I had an incidence of locoregional recurrence of 17.1% compared to 30.8% in group II ($P = 0.03$). There were no statistically significant differences in postoperative morbidity (27.7% versus 30.8%) and mortality (2.67% versus 3.33%). The 1-, 2-, and 3-year survival rates were estimated at 82.1%, 54%, and 28%, respectively, with NCRT and 65.8%, 29.1%, and 10% without ($P = 0.006$). Nevertheless, preoperative chemotherapy did not reduce the 1-, 3-, and 5-year disease-free survival rates, which were estimated at 58%, 36.6%, and 12.5% with NCRT and 51.7%, 18.3%, and 7.5% without ($P = 0.058$). *Conclusions.* The treatment of NCRT followed by PD in patients with PDAC has a significantly lower rate of locoregional recurrence and a longer overall survival than those with surgery alone.

1. Introduction

Pancreatic ductal adenocarcinoma (PDAC) is a kind of remarkably highly lethal malignancy, foremost the 5th root cause of loss of life throughout the world [1]. Surgical resection has always been really the only most likely healing alternative. Even so, because of its ambitious tumor expansion as well as recurrence rate [2–4], in addition to the fact that a small section of patients are surgery candidates [5, 6], the actual survival rate of affected individuals is inadequate and simply ranges from 10% to 25.4% [7–10] at 5 years. The unsatisfying benefits of surgical treatment are only able to be enhanced by employing multidisciplinary treatments with adjuvant and neoadjuvant chemoradiotherapy (NCRT).

The additional current publications revealed survival advantages for PDAC patients with the use of adjuvant therapy postoperatively. A meta-analysis has been carried out by Stocken et al. [11] in 2005 from 5 randomized controlled trails, which revealed a 25% diminishment in risk of death in those who obtained chemotherapy and substantial 2 years of survival rates for those who received chemoradiotherapy, in contrast to those who did not (38% versus 25%). Alternatively, up to 30% of individuals had been incapable to complete the course of adjuvant treatment or to receive the designed amount of radiation or chemotherapy typically mainly because of the morbidity and continuous recuperation intervals following surgical treatment [12, 13].

In the contrast, the full course of prescribed chemotherapy is easily completed in NCRT without any delay, and it will presumably enhance effectiveness of chemoradiotherapy.

Even though an extreme variety of phase I/II studies [14, 15] have been published on the potential benefits for

NCRT for patients with both resectable and unresectable PDAC, in addition to minimizing the possibilities of local tumor recurrence [16, 17], achieving better local tumor control [17, 18], or tumor downstaging with a subsequent potentially resectable tumor [19–21], unfortunately, no randomized controlled phase III trials comparing NCRT plus surgery versus surgical treatment only have been reported up till now, and as a consequence there are certainly no evidence-based medicine proofs that NCRT can offer any benefits for patients with PDAC. Within the distinction, the entire duration of prescribed chemoradiotherapy is definitely carried out with virtually no holdoff, and it can presumptively improve usefulness for PDAC patients.

Here we reported the principal experience with our large single institution by comparing 5-FU-based NCRT accompanied by PD with surgery alone. It is needed to be realized that NCRT is characterized as any preoperative chemoradiotherapy planning to increase the rate of microscopic tumor clearance and also to reduce the rate of tumor recurrence in this study.

2. Materials and Methods

2.1. Patients. Between January 2004 and April 2010, 232 consecutive patients with PDAC (limited to TI/T2 TNM staging) who were admitted to the Department of Hepatobiliary Pancreatic Surgery in our institution underwent PD, among whom 112 (48.7%) patients were treated with NCRT preoperatively, whereas the remaining 120 (51.3%) patients underwent PD alone. Patients were included in the study if they were pathologically proven to be PDAC cases postoperatively, and they were excluded if they were not amenable to operation, or if they were other cancer cases or with no cancers.

The approach to NCRT was determined and carried out by individual surgeons. The unique situation in our department was that 1 team of surgeons favored the use of NCRT and 1 team did not. Their choice of treatment was consistent over the period of the study, and this allowed for comparison of treatment between the 2 groups.

Preoperative evaluation of the staging of tumor consisted of physical examination, chest-radiography, abdomen contrast-enhanced computed tomography (CT), magnetic resonance imaging (MRI), and endoscopic retrograde cholangiopancreatography (ERCP). All patients were required to meet the following eligible criteria for tumor resectability: tumors which do not involve major vascular structures including the celiac axis (CA), superior mesenteric artery (SMA), and superior mesenteric/portal vein complex and without extensive peripancreatic lymphadenopathy and/or the absence of distant metastases which were diagnosed radiologically before surgery.

After the completion of chemoradiotherapy, all patients were treated with pancreatic resection for curative intents and underwent no adjuvant chemoradiotherapy postoperatively. The median follow-up time for Group I was 28.6 months (range: 4–70 months) and 24.3 months (range: 9–67 months) for Group II.

2.2. Chemoradiotherapy. Chemotherapy was performed as neoadjuvant treatment in 81 of the 112 patients (96.4%). The main agents were 5-FU (600 mg/m^2, d 1, 8, and 15 for 1 cycle) and gemcitabine (1000 mg/m^2, d 1, 8, and 15 for 1 cycle). In the study that used only one regimen (n = 60), 38 (46.9%) patients were treated using 5-FU, and 35 (43.2%) patients used a gemcitabine-based regimen. Furthermore, gemcitabine and oxaliplatin combinations were used in 8 (9.8%) patients.

Thirty-one of the 112 patients (27.6%) received neoadjuvant radiotherapy (extrabody radiotherapy, EBRT). Doses applied ranged from 46 Gy/23 F to 50 Gy/23 F. No patients received both chemotherapy and radiotherapy.

2.3. Operative Finding. After four weeks of chemoradiotherapy, the planned pancreaticoduodenectomy (PD) or partial/total pancreatectomy were performed in all patients for curative intents. In our study, 124 patients (53.5%) underwent a classic PD (Whipple) and 76 (32.7%) underwent a pylorus-preserving PD (PPPD). Partial or total pancreatectomy was performed in 32 (14.8%) patients. R0 resection was achieved in 189 (81.4%) patients, of whom 92 patients were in the NCRT group and 97 patients were in the surgery-alone group. Pathologic specimens were reviewed and staged according to the American Joint Committee on Cancer (AJCC) Guidelines. Pathologic data regarding TNM staging, tumor size, histological differentiation grade, lymph node involvement, lymphovascular invasion, perineural invasion, and surgical margins were recorded.

2.4. Followup and Endpoints. All of the included patients were enrolled in our strict follow-up system. After discharge, serum CA-199 and an abdominal ultrasonography (US) and/or contrast-enhanced computed tomography scan was performed approximately 1 month for the initial three months after operation. Thereafter, we screened patients by tumor marker measurement and US every 3 months, and by helical CT every 6 months, and by ERCP or MRI when recurrence was suspected.

The endpoint of this study was time-to-recurrence which was defined as the period between initial pancreatectomy and the diagnosis of recurrence and time-to-death which calculated the duration from the date of transplantation to the date of death for any reasons. All followup data were summarized as of the end of August 2010.

2.5. Statistical Analysis. The Chi-square test or the Fisher exact test was used to evaluate the significant differences between the two groups. A proportion of patients with perioperative morbidity and mortality as well as tumor recurrence were compared between the two groups. The Kaplan-Meier curves were constructed for overall survival and disease-free survival, and the log-rank test was applied to compare the survival between the 2 groups of patients. A value of $P < 0.05$ was considered statistically significant.

3. Results

3.1. Comparison between the Two Groups. Patient demographics, including age, sex, body weight, height, and concurrent illness, were well matched in the two groups (Table 1). The size of the lesion, the histological differentiation, and the depth of tumor invasion in the two groups were also comparable (Table 2). Of the 232 patients, there were 144 (62.1%) males with a median age of 46.2 years (range: 17–67 years) and 88 (37.9%) females with a median age of 38.5 years (range: 24–54 years).

3.2. Postoperative Morbidity and Mortality. Data regarding morbidity following neoadjuvant treatment and pancreatic resection were presented for 68 of 232 patients (Table 3). Morbidity included pancreatic fistula, which was defined as all suspect drainage with more than 300 IU/mL amylase-counting for more than 3 days; postoperative intraperitoneal hemorrhage (from arterial or venous vessel, operative field, and gastrointestinal track); lymphorrhea (colorless drainage of more than 300 mL for more than 10 postoperative days); diarrhea (more than three liquid exonerations per day for more than 10 days); delayed gastric emptying, which was calculated by the nasogastric tube (NGT) left in place for 3 days or reinsered because of repeated emesis after removal of the NGT being unable to tolerate a solid diet after the 7th postoperative day; abdominal infection (after the 3rd postoperative day, fever, abdominal distension, and intestinal paralysis appear and last for 24–48 hours, with leukocytosis, hypoproteinemia, and anemia; fluid accumulation is found radiologically); small bowel infraction; pulmonary embolization; atelectasis; and wound infections (Table 4).

The postoperative mortality was calculated as death from any causes within 45 days postoperatively. Postoperative mortality was 2.67% for patients in Group I and 3.33% in Group II. Mortality was not statistically different in the two groups.

3.3. Overall Survivals (OS). The analysis of the OS curves between the two groups was revealed in Figure 1, which demonstrated that there was a statistically significant difference between the two groups ($P = 0.006$). The overall survival rates for the 112 patients in NCRT group at 1, 3, and 5 years were 76%, 55%, and 22%, respectively, whereas they were 44%, 25%, and 9% in the surgery-alone group, respectively.

3.4. Disease-Free Survivals (DFS). The Kaplan-Meier DFS curves of patients between the two groups were compared in Figure 2, which revealed that the DFS was longer in the NCRT group, with the disease-free survival rate of 58% at 1 year, 36.6% at 3 years, and 12.5% at 5 years, and it was 51.7% at 1 year, 22% at 3 years, and 7.5% at 5 years in the surgery-alone group. However, the DFS was not significantly different when the two groups were compared ($P = 0.058$).

3.5. Tumor Recurrences. Tumor recurrences were observed in 176 patients. The recurrence rates were 35.3% for the NCRT group and 40.5% for the surgery-alone group, respectively. Focusing on the clinical pathological features of all patients, there were no significant differences between the two groups ($P < 0.05$). Intrahepatic and locoregional lymph nodes metastases were the main first or primary locations of cancer recurrence in both groups (Table 5). Although the overall tumor recurrence rates were not statistically different between the two groups, patients receiving NCRT were more likely to have lower frequency of local lymph node metastasis than patients receiving surgery alone. The frequencies of other locations of postoperative tumor recurrence were similar between the two groups (4.9% versus 5.3%; $P = 0.02$).

4. Discussion

Preoperative chemoradiotherapy is usually a neoadjuvant treatment method. Even though the effective use of adjuvant chemotherapy and radiotherapy in addition to intraoperative radiotherapy (IORT) or EBRT (extrabody radiotherapy) can partially control the local tumor growth and reduce tumor recurrence, there seemed to be tiny impact on the increase of the rate of survival of patients who underwent such procedure, so neoadjuvant therapies are actually suggested by some surgeons, aiming to enhance the resection rate and the 5-year survivals. Theoretically, preoperative chemoradiotherapy has the following advantages when compared with the adjuvant therapy in patients with pancreatic cancer. (1) It can complete the path of adjuvant treatment or obtain the organized quantity of chemotherapy or radiation with no delay virtually [22]; (2) it can downstage tumor classification enabling an improved tumor oncological clearance along with a higher negative surgical margin (R0 resection) [23, 24]; (3) it limits the possible likelihood of cancerous growth seeding due to intraoperative manipulation [25]; (4) it is much more prone to endure it (chemoradiotherapy) prior to surgery; (5) it blocks the oxygen supply to the tumor cells and kills them effectively; and (6) it minimizes the potential risk of pancreatic anastomotic leakage.

NCRT may additionally improve survival after resection for patients with PDAC. Nonetheless, there is actually constrained information concerning the role of NCRT for pancreatic cancer in clinical practice. Preoperative chemotherapy and radiotherapy are nevertheless a place of disputes. Pendurthi et al. [26] retrospectively abbreviated the information of 70 patients who received preoperative and postoperative chemoradiotherapy and found that 27 patients who underwent preoperative chemoradiotherapy were more unlikely to possess lymph node involvement (28% versus 87%, $P < 0.0006$) and a lower rate of positive surgery margins (28% versus 56%, P = ns) compared with the 43 patients who obtained chemoradiotherapy after surgery, but there were no significant differences between the two groups in overall survival rates and local tumor control. Similarly, Evans and Pisters [27] from the Department of Anderson Cancer Center confirmed that preoperative chemoradiotherapy did not increase postoperative morbidity, the 3-year survival rate reached 23%, and a less probability of local tumor recurrence was witnessed as a result of a long-term follow-up. In addition, in the Stanford Cancer Center, Joseph Cetal [28] found that preoperative chemoradiotherapy was tolerated in

TABLE 1: Clinical characteristics of the patients.

Demographics	Group I	Group II	*P* values
Sex (male/female)	75/37	69/51	0.773
Age (year)	45.9 ± 9.8	45.5 ± 9.3	0.672
Heights (cm)	166.5 ± 6.1	165.2 ± 5.8	0.914
Body weight (kg/m^2)	57.6 ± 10.3	59.9 ± 7.6	0.254
Concurrent illness			
Hypertension	21	24	.ns*
Pulmonary tuberculosis	4	3	.ns
Diabetes mellitus	13	10	.ns
COPD*	11	14	.ns
Cholelithiasis	16	22	.ns
GERD*	5	7	.ns
Endometriosis	4	4	.ns
Others	13	16	.ns

*COPD: chronic obstructive pulmonary diseases; *GERD: Gastroesophageal reflux disease; ns: not significant.

TABLE 2: Operative and pathological characteristics of both groups.

Characteristics	Group I	Group II	*P* values
Tumor location (head/body/tail)	98/14	96/24	.ns
Tumor size (mm)	3.2 ± 1.3	3.5 ± 0.8	.ns
Serum CA199 (U/mL)	210.7 ± 45.6	284.3 ± 55.7	.ns
Types of surgery			
Whipple*	65	59	.ns
PPPD*	35	41	.ns
Partial or total pancreatectomy	12	20	.ns
Pathological differentiation (well/moderate/poor/others)	12/74/23/3	14/76/25/5	.ns
TNM* staging (I/II/III-IV)	58/49/5	49/64/7	.ns
Surgery margins (R0/R1/R2)	95/17/0	96/24/0	.ns
Operative time (min)	615 ± 180	635 ± 210	.ns
Blood loss (mL)	1120 ± 350	1240 ± 430	.ns
Hospital stay (day)	11.5 ± 4.3	12.3 ± 3.5	.ns

*Whipple: standard pancreatoduodenectomy. PPPD: pylorus-preserving pancreatic resection. T: tumor. N: lymph nodes. M: metastasis.

TABLE 3: Postoperative mortality and morbidity between the two groups.

Objects	All patients	Group I	Group II	*P* values
Morbidity	29.3%	27.7%	30.8%	0.123
Mortality	3.02%	2.67%	3.33%	0.123

TABLE 4: Number of complications between the two groups.

Complications	Group I	Group II
Pancreatic fistula	7	9
Intraperitoneal hemorrhage	3	4
Lymphorrhea	5	6
Small bowel infarction	2	2
Diarrhea	4	5
Pulmonary embolization	2	1
Atelectasis	3	2
Delayed gastric emptying	5	8
Total	31	37

TABLE 5: Comparison between the two groups regarding the first location of tumor recurrences.

Metastasis site	Group I (no. and %)	Group II (no. and %)	P values
Intrahepatic	35 (42.7%)	31 (33.1%)	.ns
Locoregional	14 (17.1%)	29 (30.8%)	0.032
Peritoneal	12 (14.8%)	11 (11.7%)	.ns
Pulmonary	10 (12.2%)	12 (12.9%)	.ns
Retroperitoneal	7 (8.5%)	6 (6.4%)	.ns
Others	4 (4.9%)	5 (5.3%)	.ns

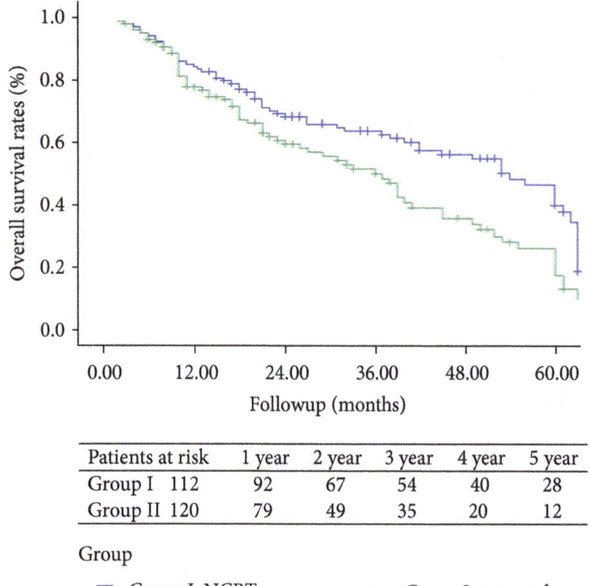

FIGURE 1: Showing the Kaplan-Meier overall survival curve for the 112 patients receiving NCRT and the 120 patients receiving surgery resection alone. There was no significant difference in overall survival between the two groups ($P = 0.006$).

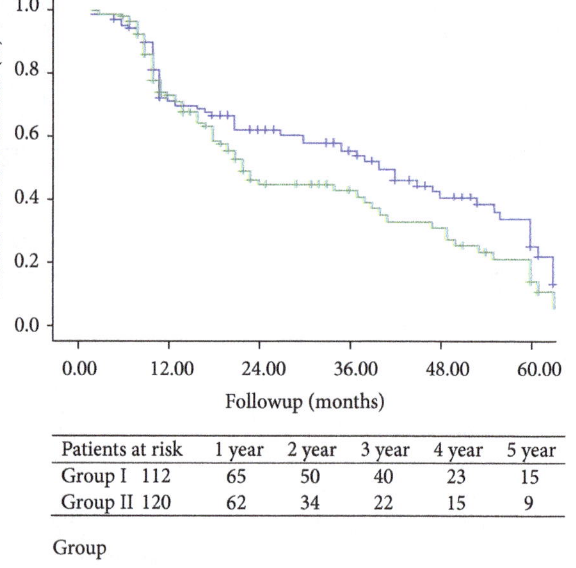

FIGURE 2: Showing the Kaplan-Meier disease-free survival curve for patients undergoing NCRT ($n = 112$) compared with those patients undergoing surgery resection alone ($n = 120$). There was no statistical difference between the two groups ($P = 0.058$).

locally advanced tumors without having to incorporate the operation risk and downstage the tumor TNM stage, as well as to increase the oncological clearance rate.

The role of preoperative chemoradiotherapy in extended survival for patients with pancreatic cancer remains not noticeable currently, but NCRT has been considered as one of the most reliable treatment methods within the treatments for individuals with locally advanced pancreatic cancer.

The parameters used to classify the pancreatic cancer into resectable category are typically depending on primary tumor TNM stage, lymph nodes status, and adjacent major organs conditions. The surgical resection margin status and the existence of lymph nodes metastases were found to be the most significant determinants of survival after surgery [29, 30]. In our study, patients who received pancreatectomy alone were more prone to have local lymph node metastasis ($P < 0.001$). Overall survival was statistically different for those who received neoadjuvant therapy when compared with those who received surgery alone ($P = 0.969$), even though there was no statistical difference in disease-free survivals among the two groups.

Our study can be criticized for its patient selection and lack of pathological diagnosis preoperatively, as well as the retrospective nature of assessment of outcome. Nonetheless, considering the existing debate in the application of NCRT for PDAC, it highlights several significant things for surgeons. First, it is very important to determine which patients are more or less likely to benefit from the use of NCRT. Second, the preoperative criteria and definitions for resectability and unresectability are clearly keys and have to be standardized, and the necessity for a histological diagnosis is additionally an essential point for the patients who are initially unresectable. Third, it is also considerable to distinguish between the prognostically favorable groups of patients with intrapancreatic bile duct cancer from individuals with PADC due to the effects of the neoadjuvant treatment on histology of the primary tumor. Additionally, the survival rates reported in our research also compare and contrast positively towards the survival data of other retrospective neoadjuvant treatment series.

5. Conclusion

The frequently acknowledged conventional strategy to affected individuals with resectable pancreatic tumors is pancreaticoduodenectomy accompanied by 5-FU-based chemotherapy or radiotherapy. In the absence of randomized controlled trails, the application of neoadjuvant therapy for resectable pancreatic cancer remains disputable. For marginally unresectable tumors, neoadjuvant chemoradiotherapy may turn out to be a highly effective strategy for determining which patients might possibly benefit from surgical exploration and experimented with resection.

Authors' Contribution

Hui Jiang and Chi Du contributed equally to the study.

References

[1] S. L. Parker, T. Tong, S. Bolden, and P. A. Wingo, "Cancer statistics, 1996," *Ca-A Cancer Journal for Clinicians*, vol. 46, no. 1, pp. 5–27, 1996.

[2] T. Manabe, G. Ohshio, N. Baba et al., "Radical pancreatectomy for ductal cell carcinoma of the head of the pancreas," *Cancer*, vol. 64, no. 5, pp. 1132–1137, 1989.

[3] H. Baumel, M. Huguier, J. C. Manderscheid, J. M. Fabre, S. Houry, and H. Fagot, "Results of resection for cancer of the exocrine pancreas: a study from the French Association of Surgery," *British Journal of Surgery*, vol. 81, no. 1, pp. 102–107, 1994.

[4] J. F. Griffin, S. R. Smalley, W. Jewell et al., "Patterns of failure after curative resection of pancreaticcarcinoma," *Cancer*, vol. 66, pp. 56–61, 1990.

[5] V. K. Mehta, G. Fisher, J. A. Ford et al., "Preoperative chemoradiation for marginally resectable adenocarcinoma of the pancreas," *Journal of Gastrointestinal Surgery*, vol. 5, no. 1, pp. 27–35, 2001.

[6] P. Ghaneh, A. Sultana, S. Shore, D. Stocken, and J. Neoptolemos, "The case for adjuvant chemotherapy in pancreatic cancer," *Best Practice and Research*, vol. 20, no. 2, pp. 383–401, 2006.

[7] J. L. Cameron, T. S. Riall, J. Coleman, and K. A. Belcher, "One thousand consecutive pancreaticoduodenectomies," *Annals of Surgery*, vol. 244, no. 1, pp. 10–15, 2006.

[8] A. Richter, M. Niedergethmann, J. W. Sturm, D. Lorenz, S. Post, and M. Trede, "Long-term results of partial pancreaticoduodenectomy for ductal adenocarcinoma of the pancreatic head: 25-Year experience," *World Journal of Surgery*, vol. 27, no. 3, pp. 324–329, 2003.

[9] M. Wagner, C. Redaelli, M. Lietz, C. A. Seiler, H. Friess, and M. W. Büchler, "Curative resection is the single most important factor determining outcome in patients with pancreatic adenocarcinoma," *British Journal of Surgery*, vol. 91, no. 5, pp. 586–594, 2004.

[10] K. C. Conlon, D. S. Klimstra, and M. F. Brennan, "Long-term survival after curative resection for pancreatic ductal adenocarcinoma: clinicopathologic analysis of 5-year survivors," *Annals of Surgery*, vol. 223, no. 3, pp. 273–279, 1996.

[11] D. D. Stocken, M. W. Büchler, C. Dervenis et al., "Meta-analysis of randomised adjuvant therapy trials for pancreatic cancer," *British Journal of Cancer*, vol. 92, no. 8, pp. 1372–1381, 2005.

[12] F. R. Spitz, J. L. Abbruzzese, J. E. Lee et al., "Preoperative and postoperative chemoradiation strategies in patients treated with pancreaticoduodenectomy for adenocarcinoma of the pancreas," *Journal of Clinical Oncology*, vol. 15, no. 3, pp. 928–937, 1997.

[13] J. H. Klinkenbijl, J. Jeekel, T. Sahmoud et al., "Adjuvant radiotherapy and 5-fluorouracil after curative resection of cancer of the pancreas and periampullary region: phase III trial of the EORTC Gastrointestinal Tract Cancer Cooperative Group," *Annals of Surgery*, vol. 230, no. 6, pp. 776–784, 1999.

[14] O. Turrini, F. Viret, L. Moureau-Zabotto et al., "Neoadjuvant chemoradiation and pancreaticoduodenectomy for initially locally advanced head pancreatic adenocarcinoma," *European Journal of Surgical Oncology*, vol. 35, no. 12, pp. 1306–1311, 2009.

[15] O. Turrini, M. Ychou, L. Moureau-Zabotto et al., "Neoadjuvant docetaxel-based chemoradiation for resectable adenocarcinoma of the pancreas: new neoadjuvant regimen was safe and provided an interesting pathologic response," *European Journal of Surgical Oncology*, vol. 36, no. 10, pp. 987–992, 2010.

[16] A. M. Stessin, J. E. Meyer, and D. L. Sherr, "Neoadjuvant radiation is associated with improved survival in patients with resectable pancreatic cancer: an analysis of data from the surveillance, epidemiology, and end results (SEER) registry," *International Journal of Radiation Oncology Biology Physics*, vol. 72, no. 4, pp. 1128–1133, 2008.

[17] C. P. Raut, D. B. Evans, C. H. Crane, P. W. T. Pisters, and R. A. Wolff, "Neoadjuvant therapy for resectable pancreatic cancer," *Surgical Oncology Clinics of North America*, vol. 13, no. 4, pp. 639–661, 2004.

[18] R. R. White and D. S. Tyler, "Neoadjuvant therapy for pancreatic cancer: the Duke experience," *Surgical Oncology Clinics of North America*, vol. 13, no. 4, pp. 675–684, 2004.

[19] H. J. Kim, K. Czischke, M. F. Brennan, and K. C. Conlon, "Does neoadjuvant chemoradiation downstage locally advanced pancreatic cancer?" *Journal of Gastrointestinal Surgery*, vol. 6, no. 5, pp. 763–769, 2002.

[20] V. Moutardier, O. Turrini, L. Huiart et al., "A reappraisal of preoperative chemoradiation for localized pancreatic head ductal adenocarcinoma in a 5-year single-institution experience," *Journal of Gastrointestinal Surgery*, vol. 8, no. 4, pp. 502–510, 2004.

[21] K. M. Brown, V. Siripurapu, M. Davidson et al., "Chemoradiation followed by chemotherapy before resection for borderline pancreatic adenocarcinoma," *American Journal of Surgery*, vol. 195, no. 3, pp. 318–321, 2008.

[22] R. V. Tse, L. A. Dawson, A. Wei, and M. Moore, "Neoadjuvant treatment for pancreatic cancer-A review," *Critical Reviews in Oncology/Hematology*, vol. 65, no. 3, pp. 263–274, 2008.

[23] S. P. Cleary, R. Gryfe, M. Guindi et al., "Prognostic factors in resected pancreatic adenocarcinoma: analysis of actual 5-year survivors," *Journal of the American College of Surgeons*, vol. 198, no. 5, pp. 722–731, 2004.

[24] J. F. Pingpank, J. P. Hoffman, E. A. Ross et al., "Effect of preoperative chemoradiotherapy on surgical margin status of resected adenocarcinoma of the head of the pancreas," *Journal of Gastrointestinal Surgery*, vol. 5, no. 2, pp. 121–130, 2001.

[25] O. Ishikawa, H. Ohigashi, S. Imaoka et al., "Is the long-term survival rate improved by preoperative irradiation prior to

Whipple's procedure for adenocarcinoma of the pancreatic head?" *Archives of Surgery*, vol. 129, no. 10, pp. 1075–1080, 1994.

[26] T. K. Pendurthi, J. P. Hoffman, E. Ross, D. E. Johnson, and B. L. Eisenberg, "Preoperative versus postoperative chemoradiation for patients with resected pancreatic adenocarcinoma," *American Surgeon*, vol. 64, no. 7, pp. 686–692, 1998.

[27] D. B. Evans and P. W. T. Pisters, "Commentary: preoperative chemoradiation therapy for pancreatic cancer," *Surgical Clinics of North America*, vol. 81, no. 3, pp. 709–713, 2001.

[28] J. C. Poen, J. M. Ford, and J. E. Niederhuber, "Chemoradiotherapy in the management of localized tumors of the pancreas," *Annals of Surgical Oncology*, vol. 6, no. 1, pp. 117–122, 1999.

[29] J. Hein Allema, M. E. Reinders, T. M. van Gulik, M. J. W. Koelemay, D. J. van Leeuwen, L. Th. de Wit et al., "Prognostic factors for survival after pancreaticoduodenectomy for patients with carcinoma of the pancreatic head region," *Cancer*, vol. 75, pp. 2069–2076, 1995.

[30] J. E. Lim, M. W. Chien, and C. C. Earle, "Prognostic factors following curative resection for pancreatic adenocarcinoma: a population-based, linked database analysis of 396 patients," *Annals of Surgery*, vol. 237, no. 1, pp. 74–85, 2003.

14

Laparoscopy in Liver Transplantation: The Future Has Arrived

Quirino Lai,[1] Rafael S. Pinheiro,[2] Giovanni B. Levi Sandri,[1] Gabriele Spoletini,[1] Fabio Melandro,[1] Nicola Guglielmo,[1] Marco Di Laudo,[1] Fabrizio M. Frattaroli,[1] Pasquale B. Berloco,[1] and Massimo Rossi[1]

[1] *Department of General Surgery and Organ Transplantation, Sapienza University of Rome, Umberto I Policlinic of Rome, Viale del Policlinico 155, 00161 Rome, Italy*
[2] *Department of Liver Transplantation, University of São Paulo, 01005 010 São Paulo, SP, Brazil*

Correspondence should be addressed to Quirino Lai, lai.quirino@libero.it

Academic Editor: Andrea Lauterio

In the last two decades, laparoscopy has revolutionized the field of surgery. Many procedures previously performed with an open access are now routinely carried out with the laparoscopic approach. Several advantages are associated with laparoscopic surgery compared to open procedures: reduced pain due to smaller incisions and hemorrhaging, shorter hospital length of stay, and a lower incidence of wound infections. Liver transplantation (LT) brought a radical change in life expectancy of patients with hepatic end-stage disease. Today, LT represents the standard of care for more than fifty hepatic pathologies, with excellent results in terms of survival. Surely, with laparoscopy and LT being one of the most continuously evolving challenges in medicine, their recent combination has represented an astonishing scientific progress. The intent of the present paper is to underline the current role of diagnostic and therapeutic laparoscopy in patients waiting for LT, in the living donor LT and in LT recipients.

1. Introduction

In the last decades, laparoscopy has revolutionized the field of surgery. Video laparoscopy was officially born in 1987, when Professor Phillipe Mouret performed the first cholecystectomy in Lyons, France [1]. Many procedures previously performed with the open technique are now carried out with the laparoscopic approach. Several advantages are associated with laparoscopic surgery compared to open procedures: reduced pain due to smaller incisions and haemorrhaging, shorter hospital length of stay, and a lower incidence of wound infections are all arguments that gave strength to the widespread of laparoscopy.

Similarly, liver transplantation (LT) has radically changed the care for many patients with hepatic end-stage diseases. The first human LT was performed in 1963 by Professor Thomas Starzl [2] in Denver, United States; however, due to its initial poor results, LT remained an experimental therapy for several years. Only introduction of cyclosporine [3] markedly improved patient outcomes, turning LT to a standard clinical treatment for more than fifty adult and paediatric liver pathologies and, at the same time, allowing to achieve excellent results in terms of survival.

The intent of the present paper is to underline the current role of diagnostic and therapeutic laparoscopy in patients waiting for LT, in the living donor LT and in LT recipients.

2. Pretransplant Surgery

2.1. Laparoscopic Liver Resection. The first nonanatomical laparoscopic hepatectomy was performed by Gagner in 1992 [4] and the first anatomical one by Azagra in 1996 [5]. Since these first experiences, laparoscopic approach for hepatic resection has been adopted in different centres, showing its feasibility and safety in well-selected patients [6–10] and also confirming its prerogatives (shorter operative times, less bleeding) even in this very complex type of surgery [7, 11].

However, malignant tumors were initially considered a contraindication for mini-invasive approach. Only in the last years, this risk has been reconsidered, showing no difference in margin-free resection, port-site recurrence, or tumour seeding rates between open and laparoscopic techniques [12–15]. Consequently, malignant tumors do not represent anymore a contraindication for an expert surgeon in choosing a laparoscopic approach [16]. Until now, more than 3,000 minimally invasive hepatic resections have been reported in the literature [17], and-small-to medium sized procedures have become commonplace in many centres [18].

Recently, a consensus conference [19] has underlined that acceptable indications for laparoscopic liver resection are (a) solitary lesions with a diameter ≤5 cm, located in segments II–VI; (b) laparoscopic approach to left lateral sectionectomy (LLS) should be considered as a standard practice; (c) although all types of liver resection can be run laparoscopically, major liver resections (e.g., right or left hepatectomies) should be reserved for experienced surgeons facile with more advanced laparoscopic hepatic resections.

The main indication for resection in patients waiting for LT is represented by hepatocellular carcinoma (HCC). Transplant surgeons are well aware that a LT after previous surgery could represent a real challenge, increasing technical difficulty caused by adhesions [20–22]. Basing on these considerations, laparoscopy as bridge to LT may reduce such problems [23].

Despite no prospective randomized controlled trials have been performed yet, some studies based on matched comparisons showed similar mortality and even lower morbidity rates after laparoscopy with respect to open liver resection. After laparoscopy, 3-year patient survival rates of 60–93% and 3-year disease-free survivals of 52–64% have been reported [8, 24–29].

Advent of robotic surgery has further improved the opportunity of mini-invasive treatment of HCC. The robotic approach may enable liver resection in patients with cirrhosis, allowing for technical refinements of laparoscopic liver resection due to 3-dimensional visualization of the operative field and instruments with wrist-type end-effectors [30–32].

2.2. Laparoscopic Radiofrequency Ablation. Radiofrequency (RF) ablation represents a nonsurgical locoregional treatment, used in very well-selected patients with nonresectable HCC waiting for LT. In the last years, laparoscopic or hand-assisted RF has shown promising necrosis and survival rates [33, 34], providing a substrate for their safe adoption [35]. The main advantage of laparoscopic RF with respect to percutaneous approach is the opportunity to detect pre-operatively undetectable lesions using an intraoperative ultrasound (IOUS) [36, 37]. IOUS remains the most sensitive imaging modality for HCC, being able to detect new lesions in 13.1% to 30% of cases [38–42]. In a study comparing laparoscopic liver resection and RF, Santambrogio et al. [43] identified 15 (20%) of 74 cases with previously undetected lesions in the RF group. Laparoscopic RF also consents to treat lesions considered inappropriate for percutaneous RF due to the high risk of injury in the diaphragm, stomach, or bowel [44–46]. Similarly, laparoscopic RF minimizes the risk of complications in patients previously operated in the upper abdominal quadrants [47].

2.3. Laparoscopic Kasai Procedure in Children with Biliary Atresia. Laparoscopic portoenterostomy, also named Kasai procedure, for biliary atresia was first reported by Esteves et al. in 2002 [48]. Besides its safety and feasibility, laparoscopic Kasai can provide the advantage of a lower hepatic adhesions rate, which ease the potential "salvage" LT. Martinez-Ferro et al. reported 41 cases of laparoscopic Kasai, with only one conversion [49], and encouraging results in terms of postoperative bile flow rates. However, the only prospective study comparing open and laparoscopic procedure was stopped after observing that laparoscopic patients showed a significantly shorter time between Kasai procedure and LT [50]. Therefore, the role of laparoscopic Kasai remains unclear [51], being reserved to paediatric centres with high specialization in minimally invasive surgery.

3. Laparoscopic Living Donor-Hepatectomy

The early idea of solid organ transplantation using living donors began with kidney transplants; similarly, laparoscopy for living donation was initially developed for kidney transplantation, with the intent to offer a less aggressive procedure to the donor. In fact, laparoscopic nephrectomy is associated with less postoperative pain, decreased length of hospital stay, faster return to normal activity, smaller scars, and less morbidity [52]. As a consequence, an increased number of kidney transplants using living donors have been recently observed in many centres [53, 54].

Living-donor liver transplantation is a complex procedure, with major risks of morbidity and mortality with respect to kidney donation: the reported mortality of this procedure has varied from 0.2% to 0.5% [55]. Clearly, donor risk increases according to the type of hepatectomy (LLS < left hepatectomy < right hepatectomy (RH)).

Typically, a LLS or a left hepatectomy is sufficient in a paediatric living liver donation, while a RH is necessary for an adult-to-adult donation.

However, despite different surgical approaches could be adopted, open living donation always requires a large abdominal incision. This aspect, combined with postoperative pain, long hospital stay, and long periods of recovery, represents a barrier to donation, especially in young women [56].

Recently, experimental model has demonstrated the feasibility of laparoscopic living donation using the available technology [57].

Concurrent improvement in laparoscopic surgery for hepatic tumours enhanced feasibility and safety of more complex procedures [18], leading to the establishment of laparoscopic surgery for liver living donors. Soubrane et al. [58] reflected on the quality of the graft and the morbidity rates in the donor: they reported comparable results in both conventional and laparoscopic techniques apart from longer operative times and lower blood losses in the laparoscopy group.

3.1. Paediatric Donation. Paediatric living donation provides similar or better short-term graft function and long-term survival rates with respect to postmortem donor LT: the first case of laparoscopic donation was reported by Cherqui et al. [56]. In 2006, Soubrane et al. [58] reported the safety of laparoscopic LLS in 16 consecutive live donors compared with the conventional LLS. According to the first series experienced, the liver graft typically includes the LLS (i.e., segments II and III according to Couinaud's classification), left branch of hepatic artery, left portal branch, left bile duct, and left hepatic vein. After these initial experiences, several other new series have been reported worldwide [59, 60].

Recently, Kim et al. compared 11 laparoscopic LLS for living donation with 11 open ones, showing that the laparoscopic group had significantly shorter hospital stay, whilst duration of operation, blood loss, warm ischemia time, and out-of-pocket medical costs were comparable between groups [61].

A similar study from Washington DC compared 15 laparoscopic or laparoscopic-assisted left or right hepatectomies for liver donation with 15 hepatectomies with open access: no substantial differences were observed in terms of early graft function, allograft biliary, and vascular complications and survivals (1-year graft and patient survival: 100% versus 93% in laparoscopic and open group, resp.) [62].

3.2. Adult Donation. In 2006, Koffron et al. [63] described the first hand-assisted laparoscopic RH for live donation. Kurosaki et al. [64] reported in the same period 13 consecutive video-assisted adult-to-adult laparoscopic hepatectomies (3 RH and 10 left ± segment I hepatectomies): surgical manipulation was obtained via ports or via a 12 cm incision whilst view resulted by a combination of direct and laparoscopic vision. Reported median operation time was 363 ± 33 minutes and a median blood loss of 302 ± 191 mL. No complications were reported, restoration of liver function was smooth, and analgesics use was inferior with respect to the historical control (median: 1.2 versus 3.8 times).

In 2008, the transplant group from Seoul [65, 66] commented on the first series of hand-assisted laparoscopic modified RH preserving the middle hepatic vein; the authors reported 2 cases of laparoscopic RH and 7 cases of laparoscopy-assisted RH with a hand-port device. Hilar dissection and parenchymal transection were performed under pneumoperitoneum ($n = 2$) or through a minilaparotomy incision ($n = 7$). The graft was extracted through the site of the hand-port device or the minilaparotomy. Operative time was 765 and 898 min in the laparoscopic RH patients, and it ranged from 310 to 575 min for the laparoscopy-assisted surgery. In one case, a fluid collection along the liver resection margin was reported, but it was resolved after percutaneous drainage.

At the Northwestern University, Baker et al. [67] retrospectively compared 33 open versus 33 laparoscopic living donor RHs, suggesting that laparoscopy could present equivalent safety, resource utilization, and effectiveness, with several adjunctive physical and psychological benefits. Donor operative times were shorter for the laparoscopic group (265 min versus 316 min). Blood loss and length of stay were comparable. Additionally, total hospitalization costs were equivalent. Finally, the group from Seoul compared single-port laparoscopy-assisted donor right hepatectomy ($n = 40$) with laparoscopy-assisted donor right hepatectomy ($n = 20$) and open donor right hepatectomy ($n = 90$); postoperative complication and reoperation rates revealed no significant differences, the single-port group showing the lowest level of postoperative pain [68].

Although very limited experiences have been reported worldwide until now, no mortalities have been encountered in laparoscopic living donor hepatectomy, whether adult or paediatric. Larger experience is needed in this field, but only centres with a coincident expertise in hepatic mini-invasive surgery and living donor LT should approach this type of surgery.

4. Laparoscopic-Assisted Liver Transplantation

The first nine cases of living donor LT through a short-midline incision combined with hand-assisted laparoscopic surgery have been reported in Japan [69]. All the patients were cirrhotic (median MELD score 14). Total hepatectomy was carried out through a hand-assisted laparoscopic approach with an 8 cm upper midline incision. Explantation of the diseased liver was obtained through the upper midline incision which was extended to 12 to 15 cm. Partial liver grafts were implanted through the upper midline incision. Median surgical time was 741 min, and the median blood loss was 3,940 g.

This preliminary report of application of laparoscopy during LT procedure represents an extraordinary innovation, opening new porspectives in this fascinating surgical field. Further evolutions in the use of mini-invasive surgery in LT are expected in the next years.

5. Laparoscopic Posttransplant Surgery

Postoperative laparoscopic management of LT patients is less common with respect to renal transplant recipients: in fact, laparoscopy is easily applied after kidney transplantation, given the fact that in this type of transplant the dissection is completely extraperitoneal.

In postLT patients, laparoscopy is a useful tool to solve a number of surgical complications; however, its use is strictly connected to surgeon's experience and versatility.

5.1. Laparoscopic Incisional Hernia Repair. Incisional hernia is caused by several aetiologies, many of whose could be concomitantly observed in LT recipients: advanced age, wound infection, ascites, steroids, diabetes, surgical techniques, suture material, retransplantation, bilateral subcostal incision with midline extension, and, not less important, surgeon's experience. The most common site for incisional hernia in LT patients is located at the junction of the transverse and upper midline incisions [70]. In literature, the incidence of incisional hernia varies from 5% to 17% [71]. Large incisional and ventral hernias in nontransplant patients are now routinely repaired using laparoscopic technique. Laparoscopic ventral hernia repair seems to have a reduced risk of recurrence and infection compared to standard repair [72]. In LT patients, laparoscopic hernia repair is safe and with similar results when compared with open repair [70, 73].

Andreoni et al. [74] successfully completed 12 out of 13 attempted incisional hernia repairs by the laparoscopic technique in LT patients. Gore-Tex mesh was used. At the time of publication, they report no recurrence. They concluded that laparoscopic mesh repair of incisional hernias is practical and safe in patients with a surgical history of LT transplantation, with a low incidence of infections and no recurrence. However, in a monocentre study [74], a higher rate of postoperative seroma was observed in LT with respect to nontransplanted patients [75]. A study from Germany analyzed a population of 29 solid organs recipients: 15 cases were treated with intraperitoneal onlay mesh repair and 14 with conventional hernia repair [76]. Recurrence rate was 6% versus 50%, and complication rate was 33% versus 21% in laparoscopy and conventional groups, respectively.

A study from Spain described 20 cases of laparoscopic incisional hernia repair in patients after LT, using a Bard Composix mesh, showing excellent results and few complications [77]. Observing the excellent results obtained using laparoscopy for the treatment of incisional hernia in LT patients, we can conclude that it could be safely performed also in this particular type of patients, and it could be considered a standard practice, mainly in an expert surgeon's hands.

5.2. Other Indications. In the last years, different uses of laparoscopy have been attempted in LT recipients. Merenda et al. [78] reported two cases of intestinal occlusion caused by adhesions and three cases of lymphocele, all approached with laparoscopic surgery. In all cases but one, the authors were able to complete the surgery by laparoscopic means; in one of the two occlusions, the procedure was switched to laparotomy because of a choledochojejunal anastomosis lesion.

Gill et al. [79] reported a single case of a right adrenalectomy after LT in a 63-year-old female patient with a right adrenal mass and a previous story of left radical nephrectomy for a renal cell carcinoma and LT for primary biliary cirrhosis. A laparoscopic right adrenalectomy via the retroperitoneoscopic approach was successfully performed, and the patient was discharged home on the first postoperative day.

DeRoover and Sudan [80] documented the case of a 46-year-old female transplanted for primary sclerosing cholangitis who presented multiple splenic aneurysms and abdominal pain: after a laparoscopic splenectomy, the patient was discharged on postoperative day 3 free of symptoms. A Japanese experience [81] reported 5 cases of hand-assisted laparoscopic splenectomy for hypersplenism in living donor LT recipients. On the basis of the excellent results, the authors consider it as a possible standard procedure after LT.

Robles et al. [82] commented on 2 cases of biliary peritonitis after T-tube removal who failed conservative treatment and subsequently underwent laparoscopy: lysis of adhesions was carried out in the right upper quadrant, a Penrose drain was placed, and both patients were discharged home on postoperative day 4. In 2010, Zhu et al. [83] reported the first total laparoscopic hysterectomy after LT. Authors confirmed that no viscera adhesions were observed to the undersurface of the umbilicus.

In 2011, Lee et al. [84] were the first to successfully complete a laparoscopic total gastrectomy in a previously transplanted 72-year-old patient, showing that laparoscopy is a feasible method for gastric cancer treatment in LT patients.

Finally, the Hannover group reflected on the applicability of laparoscopy in the management of posttransplantation lymphoproliferative disorder in a pediatric population: 6 out of 34 (18%) solid organs recipients underwent laparoscopic biopsies because of the lack of superficial lesions, with a 83% success rate. In one patient, a trocar metastasis was identified and treated successfully with chemotherapy [85].

Despite few cases have been reported until now, we can affirm that several "conceptual" barriers in the field of laparoscopy have been overcome: previous LT no longer represents an absolute contraindication for laparoscopy; not only in case of small procedures (biopsies) or submesocolic and pelvic surgery, but also when supramesocolic organs are involved. Further experience is needed in this field and only surgeons with a high expertise in mini-invasive procedures must approach this type of surgery. However, the authors are confident that in the future laparoscopic or robotic surgery will substitute open surgery in many cases even in previously transplanted patients.

6. Conclusion

Use of laparoscopy in the field of LT is safe and feasible. Mini-invasive approach is commonly adopted in the bridge treatment of HCC in patients waiting for LT: in case of LLS, laparoscopic procedure is recognized as the gold standard therapy. In living donor hepatectomy, and, recently, in LT, pure mini-invasive approaches or hybrid forms of laparoscopic and open surgery have been attempted. However, a limited number of reports are currently available on this subject, and great ability and confidence are recommended for starting these laparoscopy-assisted programs. Laparoscopy for abdominal surgery after LT has been demonstrated to be feasible and safe, not only in patients candidates for pelvic surgery, but also in case of surgery in the upper abdominal quadrants. In the next future, welcome improvement in technologies will give impulse to further expansion of this surgical area.

Authors' Contribution

Q. Lai designed the study; Q. Lai, R. S. Pinheiro, G. B. L. Sandri and G. Spoltini wrote the paper; F. Melandro, N. Gugliemo, M. D. Laudo, F. M. Frattaroli, P. B. Berloco and M. Rossi participated in the critical evaluation of the paper.

References

[1] A. Cuschieri, F. Dubois, J. Mouiel et al., "The European experience with laparoscopic cholecystectomy," *American Journal of Surgery*, vol. 161, no. 3, pp. 385–387, 1991.

[2] T. E. Starzl, T. L. Marchioro, K. N. Vonkaulla, G. Hermann, R. S. Brittain, and W. R. Waddell, "Homotransplantation of the liver in humans," *Surgery, Gynecology & Obstetrics*, vol. 117, pp. 659–676, 1963.

[3] R. Y. Calne, S. Thiru, and D. J. G. White, "Cyclosporin A in patients receiving renal allografts from cadaver donors," *The Lancet*, vol. 2, no. 8104, pp. 1323–1327, 1978.

[4] M. Gagner, M. Rheault, and J. Dubuc, "Laparoscopic partial hepatectomy for liver tumor," *Surgical Endoscopy*, vol. 6, article 99, 1992.

[5] J. S. Azagra, M. Goergen, E. Gilbart, and D. Jacobs, "Laparoscopic anatomical (hepatic) left lateral segmentectomy—technical aspects," *Surgical Endoscopy*, vol. 10, no. 7, pp. 758–761, 1996.

[6] T. Mala, B. Edwin, A. R. Rosseland, I. Gladhaug, E. Fosse, and Ø. Mathisen, "Laparoscopic liver resection: experience of 53 procedures at a single center," *Journal of Hepato-Biliary-Pancreatic Surgery*, vol. 12, no. 4, pp. 298–303, 2005.

[7] B. Descottes, F. Lachachi, M. Sodji et al., "Early experience with laparoscopic approach for solid liver tumors: initial 16 cases," *Annals of Surgery*, vol. 232, no. 5, pp. 641–645, 2000.

[8] D. Cherqui, A. Laurent, C. Tayar et al., "Laparoscopic liver resection for peripheral hepatocellular carcinoma in patients with chronic liver disease: midterm results and perspectives," *Annals of Surgery*, vol. 243, no. 4, pp. 499–506, 2006.

[9] L. Biertho, A. Waage, and M. Gagner, "Laparoscopic hepatectomies," *Annales de Chirurgie*, vol. 127, no. 3, pp. 164–170, 2002.

[10] I. Dagher, J. M. Proske, A. Carloni, H. Richa, H. Tranchart, and D. Franco, "Laparoscopic liver resection: results for 70 patients," *Surgical Endoscopy and Other Interventional Techniques*, vol. 21, no. 4, pp. 619–624, 2007.

[11] C. Simillis, V. A. Constantinides, P. P. Tekkis et al., "Laparoscopic versus open hepatic resections for benign and malignant neoplasms-a meta-analysis," *Surgery*, vol. 141, no. 2, pp. 203–211, 2007.

[12] K. Ito, H. Ito, C. Are et al., "Laparoscopic versus open liver resection: a matched-pair case control study," *Journal of Gastrointestinal Surgery*, vol. 13, no. 12, pp. 2276–2283, 2009.

[13] X. J. Cai, J. Yang, H. Yu et al., "Clinical study of laparoscopic versus open hepatectomy for malignant liver tumors," *Surgical Endoscopy and Other Interventional Techniques*, vol. 22, no. 11, pp. 2350–2356, 2008.

[14] Y. Endo, M. Ohta, A. Sasaki et al., "A comparative study of the long-term outcomes after laparoscopy-assisted and open left lateral hepatectomy for hepatocellular carcinoma," *Surgical Laparoscopy, Endoscopy and Percutaneous Techniques*, vol. 19, no. 5, pp. e171–e174, 2009.

[15] B. Topal, S. Fieuws, R. Aerts, H. Vandeweyer, and F. Penninckx, "Laparoscopic versus open liver resection of hepatic neoplasms: comparative analysis of short term results," *Surgical Endoscopy and Other Interventional Techniques*, vol. 22, no. 10, pp. 2208–2213, 2008.

[16] I. Dagher, G. Di Giuro, J. Dubrez, P. Lainas, C. Smadja, and D. Franco, "Laparoscopic versus open right hepatectomy: a comparative study," *American Journal of Surgery*, vol. 198, no. 2, pp. 173–177, 2009.

[17] H. H. Kim, E. K. Park, J. S. Seoung et al., "Liver resection for hepatocellular carcinoma: case-matched analysis of laparoscopic versus open resection," *Journal of the Korean Surgical Society*, vol. 80, no. 6, pp. 412–419, 2011.

[18] R. I. Troisi, J. Van Huysse, F. Berrevoet et al., "Evolution of laparoscopic left lateral sectionectomy without the Pringle maneuver: through resection of benign and malignant tumors to living liver donation," *Surgical Endoscopy and Other Interventional Techniques*, vol. 25, no. 1, pp. 79–87, 2011.

[19] J. F. Buell, D. Cherqui, D. A. Geller et al., "The international position on laparoscopic liver surgery: the Louisville Statement, 2008," *Annals of Surgery*, vol. 250, pp. 825–830, 2009.

[20] R. Adam and D. Azoulay, "Is primary resection and salvage transplantation for hepatocellular carcinoma a reasonable strategy?" *Annals of Surgery*, vol. 241, no. 4, pp. 671–672, 2005.

[21] V. Mazzaferro, S. Todo, A. G. Tzakis, A. C. Stieber, L. Makowka, and T. E. Starzl, "Liver transplantation in patients with previous portasystemic shunt," *American Journal of Surgery*, vol. 160, no. 1, pp. 111–116, 1990.

[22] A. Steib, G. Freys, C. Lehmann, C. Meyer, and G. Mahoudeau, "Intraoperative blood losses and transfusion requirements during adult liver transplantation remain difficult to predict," *Canadian Journal of Anesthesia*, vol. 48, no. 11, pp. 1075–1079, 2001.

[23] A. Laurent, C. Tayar, M. Andréoletti, J. Y. Lauzet, J. C. Merle, and D. Cherqui, "Laparoscopic liver resection facilitates salvage liver transplantation for hepatocellular carcinoma," *Journal of Hepato-Biliary-Pancreatic Surgery*, vol. 16, no. 3, pp. 310–314, 2009.

[24] E. C. H. Lai, C. N. Tang, J. P. Y. Ha, and M. K. W. Li, "Laparoscopic liver resection for hepatocellular carcinoma ten-year experience in a single center," *Archives of Surgery*, vol. 144, no. 2, pp. 143–148, 2009.

[25] I. Dagher, P. Lainas, A. Carloni et al., "Laparoscopic liver resection for hepatocellular carcinoma," *Surgical Endoscopy and Other Interventional Techniques*, vol. 22, no. 2, pp. 372–378, 2008.

[26] L. Aldrighetti, E. Guzzetti, C. Pulitanò et al., "Case-matched analysis of totally laparoscopic versus open liver resection for HCC: short and middle term results," *Journal of Surgical Oncology*, vol. 102, no. 1, pp. 82–86, 2010.

[27] H. Tranchart, G. Di Giuro, P. Lainas et al., "Laparoscopic resection for hepatocellular carcinoma: a matched-pair comparative study," *Surgical Endoscopy and Other Interventional Techniques*, vol. 24, no. 5, pp. 1170–1176, 2010.

[28] G. Belli, P. Limongelli, C. Fantini et al., "Laparoscopic and open treatment of hepatocellular carcinoma in patients with cirrhosis," *British Journal of Surgery*, vol. 96, no. 9, pp. 1041–1048, 2009.

[29] B. S. Hu, K. Chen, H. M. Tan et al., "Comparison of laparoscopic vs open liver lobectomy (segmentectomy) for hepatocellular carcinoma," *World Journal of Gastroenterology*, vol. 17, pp. 4725–4728, 2011.

[30] F. Panaro, T. Piardi, M. Cag et al., "Robotic liver resection as a bridge to liver transplantation," *Journal of the Society of Laparoendoscopic Surgeons*, vol. 15, pp. 86–89, 2011.

[31] E. C. H. Lai, C. N. Tang, G. P. C. Yang, and M. K. W. Li, "Multimodality laparoscopic liver resection for hepatic malignancy—from conventional total laparoscopic approach to robot-assisted laparoscopic approach," *International Journal of Surgery*, vol. 9, no. 4, pp. 324–328, 2011.

[32] S. B. Choi, J. S. Park, J. K. Kim et al., "Early experiences of robotic-assisted laparoscopic liver resection," *Yonsei Medical Journal*, vol. 49, no. 4, pp. 632–638, 2008.

[33] Y. Asahina, H. Nakanishi, and N. Izumi, "Laparoscopic radiofrequency ablation for hepatocellular carcinoma: review," *Digestive Endoscopy*, vol. 21, no. 2, pp. 67–72, 2009.

[34] A. Siperstein, A. Garland, K. Engle et al., "Laparoscopic radiofrequency ablation of primary and metastatic liver tumors: technical considerations," *Surgical Endoscopy*, vol. 14, no. 4, pp. 400–405, 2000.

[35] F. Panaro, T. Piardi, M. Audet et al., "Laparoscopic ultrasound-guided radiofrequency ablation as a bridge to liver transplantation for hepatocellular carcinoma: preliminary results," *Transplantation Proceedings*, vol. 42, no. 4, pp. 1179–1181, 2010.

[36] V. R. Tandan, M. Asch, M. Margolis, A. Page, and S. Gallinger, "Laparoscopic vs. open intraoperative ultrasound examination of the liver: a controlled study," *Journal of Gastrointestinal Surgery*, vol. 1, no. 2, pp. 146–151, 1997.

[37] M. Montorsi, R. Santambrogio, P. Bianchi et al., "Laparoscopy with laparoscopic ultrasound for pretreatment staging of hepatocellular carcinoma: a prospective study," *Journal of Gastrointestinal Surgery*, vol. 5, no. 3, pp. 312–315, 2001.

[38] N. Kokudo, Y. Bandai, H. Imanishi et al., "Management of new hepatic nodules detected by intraoperative ultrasonography during hepatic resection for hepatocellular carcinoma," *Surgery*, vol. 119, no. 6, pp. 634–640, 1996.

[39] Y. Takigawa, Y. Sugawara, J. Yamamoto et al., "New lesions detected by intraoperative ultrasound during liver resection for hepatocellular carcinoma," *Ultrasound in Medicine and Biology*, vol. 27, no. 2, pp. 151–156, 2001.

[40] G. Torzilli and M. Makuuchi, "Intraoperative ultrasonography in liver cancer," *Surgical Oncology Clinics of North America*, vol. 12, no. 1, pp. 91–103, 2003.

[41] H. Cerwenka, J. Raith, H. Bacher et al., "Is intraoperative ultrasonography during partial hepatectomy still necessary in the age of magnetic resonance imaging?" *Hepato-Gastroenterology*, vol. 50, no. 53, pp. 1539–1541, 2003.

[42] K. Zhang, N. Kokudo, K. Hasegawa et al., "Detection of new tumors by intraoperative ultrasonography during repeated hepatic resections for hepatocellular carcinoma," *Archives of Surgery*, vol. 142, no. 12, pp. 1170–1176, 2007.

[43] R. Santambrogio, E. Opocher, M. Zuin et al., "Surgical resection versus laparoscopic radiofrequency ablation in patients with hepatocellular carcinoma and child-pugh class a liver cirrhosis," *Annals of Surgical Oncology*, vol. 16, no. 12, pp. 3289–3298, 2009.

[44] K. K. Tanabe, S. A. Curley, G. D. Dodd, A. E. Siperstein, and S. N. Goldberg, "Radiofrequency ablation: the experts weigh in," *Cancer*, vol. 100, no. 3, pp. 641–650, 2004.

[45] T. Livraghi, L. Solbiati, M. F. Meloni, G. S. Gazelle, E. F. Halpern, and S. N. Goldberg, "Treatment of focal liver tumors with percutaneous radio-frequency ablation: complications encountered in a multicenter study," *Radiology*, vol. 226, no. 2, pp. 441–451, 2003.

[46] A. Casaril, M. Abu Hilal, A. Harb, T. Campagnaro, G. Mansueto, and N. Nicoli, "The safety of radiofrequency thermal ablation in the treatment of liver malignancies," *European Journal of Surgical Oncology*, vol. 34, no. 6, pp. 668–672, 2008.

[47] K. C. Yun, H. Rhim, S. A. Yong, Y. K. Mi, and K. L. Hyo, "Percutaneous radiofrequency ablation therapy of hepatocellular carcinoma using multitined expandable electrodes: comparison of subcapsular and nonsubcapsular tumors," *American Journal of Roentgenology*, vol. 186, supplement 5, pp. S269–S274, 2006.

[48] E. Esteves, E. C. Neto, M. O. Neto, J. Devanir, and R. E. Pereira, "Laparoscopic Kasai portoenterostomy for biliary atresia," *Pediatric Surgery International*, vol. 18, no. 8, pp. 737–740, 2002.

[49] M. Martinez-Ferro, E. Esteves, and P. Laje, "Laparoscopic treatment of biliary atresia and choledochal cyst," *Seminars in Pediatric Surgery*, vol. 14, no. 4, pp. 206–215, 2005.

[50] B. M. Ure, J. F. Kuebler, N. Schukfeh, C. Engelmann, J. Dingemann, and C. Petersen, "Survival with the native liver after laparoscopic versus conventional kasai portoenterostomy in infants with biliary atresia: a prospective trial," *Annals of Surgery*, vol. 253, no. 4, pp. 826–830, 2011.

[51] K. W. E. Chan, K. H. Lee, J. W. C. Mou, S. T. G. Cheung, and Y. H. P. Tam, "The outcome of laparoscopic portoenterostomy for biliary atresia in children," *Pediatric Surgery International*, vol. 27, no. 7, pp. 671–674, 2011.

[52] J. L. Flowers, S. Jacobs, E. Cho et al., "Comparison of open and laparoscopic live donor nephrectomy," *Annals of Surgery*, vol. 226, no. 4, pp. 483–490, 1997.

[53] L. E. Ratner, L. R. Kavoussi, M. Sroka et al., "Laparoscopic assisted live donor nephrectomy—a comparison with the open approach," *Transplantation*, vol. 63, no. 2, pp. 229–233, 1997.

[54] L. E. Ratner, J. Hiller, M. Sroka et al., "Laparoscopic live donor nephrectomy removes disincentives to live donation," *Transplantation Proceedings*, vol. 29, no. 8, pp. 3402–3403, 1997.

[55] P. Intaraprasong, A. Sobhonslidsuk, and S. Tongprasert, "Donor outcomes after Living Donor Liver Transplantation (LDLT)," *Journal of the Medical Association of Thailand*, vol. 93, no. 11, pp. 1340–1343, 2010.

[56] D. Cherqui, O. Soubrane, E. Husson et al., "Laparoscopic living donor hepatectomy for liver transplantation in children," *The Lancet*, vol. 359, no. 9304, pp. 392–396, 2002.

[57] E. Lin, R. Gonzalez, K. R. Venkatesh et al., "Can current technology be integrated to facilitate laparoscopic living donor hepatectomy?" *Surgical Endoscopy and Other Interventional Techniques*, vol. 17, no. 5, pp. 750–753, 2003.

[58] O. Soubrane, D. Cherqui, O. Scatton et al., "Laparoscopic left lateral sectionectomy in living donors: safety and reproducibility of the technique in a single center," *Annals of Surgery*, vol. 244, no. 5, pp. 815–820, 2006.

[59] R. Troisi, R. Debruyne, and X. Rogiers, "Laparoscopic living donor hepatectomy for pediatric liver transplantation," *Acta Chirurgica Belgica*, vol. 109, no. 4, pp. 559–562, 2009.

[60] J. C. U. Coelho, A. C. T. de Freitas, and J. E. F. Mathias, "Laparoscopic resection of the left lateral segment of the liver in living donor liver transplantation," *Revista do Colegio Brasileiro de Cirurgioes*, vol. 36, no. 6, pp. 537–538, 2009.

[61] K. H. Kim, D. H. Jung, K. M. Park et al., "Comparison of open and laparoscopic live donor left lateral sectionectomy," *British Journal of Surgery*, vol. 98, pp. 1302–1308, 2011.

[62] A. Thenappan, R. C. Jha, T. Fishbein et al., "Liver allograft outcomes after laparoscopic-assisted and minimal access live donor hepatectomy for transplantation," *American Journal of Surgery*, vol. 201, no. 4, pp. 450–455, 2011.

[63] A. J. Koffron, R. Kung, T. Baker, J. Fryer, L. Clark, and M. Abecassis, "Laparoscopic-assisted right lobe donor hepatectomy," *American Journal of Transplantation*, vol. 6, no. 10, pp. 2522–2525, 2006.

[64] I. Kurosaki, S. Yamamoto, C. Kitami et al., "Video-assisted living donor hemihepatectomy through a 12-cm incision for adult-to-adult liver transplantation," *Surgery*, vol. 139, no. 5, pp. 695–703, 2006.

[65] K. S. Suh, N. J. Yi, J. Kim et al., "Laparoscopic hepatectomy for a modified right graft in adult-to-adult living donor liver transplantation," *Transplantation Proceedings*, vol. 40, no. 10, pp. 3529–3531, 2008.

[66] K. S. Suh, N. J. Yi, T. Kim et al., "Laparoscopy-assisted donor right hepatectomy using a hand port system preserving the middle hepatic vein branches," *World Journal of Surgery*, vol. 33, no. 3, pp. 526–533, 2009.

[67] T. B. Baker, C. L. Jay, D. P. Ladner et al., "Laparoscopy-assisted and open living donor right hepatectomy: a comparative study of outcomes," *Surgery*, vol. 146, no. 4, pp. 817–825, 2009.

[68] H. J. Choi, Y. K. You, G. H. Na et al., "Single-port laparoscopy-assisted donor right hepatectomy in living donor liver transplantation: sensible approach or unnecessary hindrance?" *Transplantation Proceedings*, vol. 44, pp. 347–352, 2012.

[69] S. Eguchi, M. Takatsuki, A. Soyama et al., "Elective living donor liver transplantation by hybrid hand-assisted laparoscopic surgery and short upper midline laparotomy," *Surgery*, vol. 150, pp. 1002–1005, 2011.

[70] A. Kurmann, G. Beldi, S. A. Vorburger, C. A. Seiler, and D. Candinas, "Laparoscopic incisional hernia repair is feasible and safe after liver transplantation," *Surgical Endoscopy and Other Interventional Techniques*, vol. 24, no. 6, pp. 1451–1455, 2010.

[71] T. Piardi, M. Audet, F. Panaro et al., "Incisional hernia repair after liver transplantation: role of the mesh," *Transplantation Proceedings*, vol. 42, no. 4, pp. 1244–1247, 2010.

[72] B. T. Heniford, A. Park, B. J. Ramshaw, G. Voeller, J. G. Hunter, and R. J. Fitzgibbons, "Laparoscopic repair of ventral hernias: nine years' experience with 850 consecutive hernias," *Annals of Surgery*, vol. 238, no. 3, pp. 391–400, 2003.

[73] K. Mekeel, D. Mulligan, K. S. Reddy, A. Moss, and K. Harold, "Laparoscopic incisional hernia repair after liver transplantation," *Liver Transplantation*, vol. 13, no. 11, pp. 1576–1581, 2007.

[74] K. A. Andreoni, H. Lightfoot, D. A. Gerber, M. W. Johnson, and J. H. Fair, "Laparoscopic incisional hernia repair in liver transplant and other immunosuppressed patients," *American Journal of Transplantation*, vol. 2, no. 4, pp. 349–354, 2002.

[75] K. Harold, K. Mekeel, J. Spitler et al., "Outcomes analysis of laparoscopic ventral hernia repair in transplant patients," *Surgical Endoscopy and Other Interventional Techniques*, vol. 23, no. 8, pp. 1835–1838, 2009.

[76] H. Scheuerlein, F. Rauchfuss, A. Gharbi, M. Heise, and U. Settmacher, "Laparoscopic incisional hernia repair after solid-organ transplantation," *Transplantation Proceedings*, vol. 43, no. 5, pp. 1783–1789, 2011.

[77] R. Gianchandani, E. Moneva, P. Marrero et al., "Feasibility and effectiveness of laparoscopic incisional hernia repair after liver transplantation," *Transplantation Proceedings*, vol. 43, no. 3, pp. 742–744, 2011.

[78] R. Merenda, G. E. Gerunda, D. Neri et al., "Laparoscopic surgery after orthotopic liver transplantation," *Liver Transplantation*, vol. 6, no. 1, pp. 104–107, 2000.

[79] I. S. Gill, A. M. Meraney, J. T. Mayes, and E. L. Bravo, "Laparoscopic right adrenalectomy after liver transplantation," *Transplantation*, vol. 71, no. 9, pp. 1350–1351, 2001.

[80] A. DeRoover and D. Sudan, "Treatment of multiple aneurysms of the splenic artery after liver transplantation by percutaneous embolization and laparoscopic splenectomy," *Transplantation*, vol. 72, no. 5, pp. 956–958, 2001.

[81] H. Uehara, H. Kawanaka, T. Akahoshi et al., "The feasibility and effectiveness of a hand-assisted laparoscopic splenectomy for hypersplenism in patients after living-donor liver transplantation," *Surgical Laparoscopy, Endoscopy and Percutaneous Techniques*, vol. 19, no. 6, pp. 484–487, 2009.

[82] R. Robles, P. Parrilla, J. A. Lujan, J. A. Torralba, P. Ramirez, and F. S. Bueno, "Laparoscopic treatment of biliary peritonitis after T tube removal in patients undergoing orthotopic liver transplantation," *British Journal of Surgery*, vol. 84, no. 9, p. 1244, 1997.

[83] H. B. Zhu, Y. Jin, S. T. Xu, Y. X. Xia, and L. P. Xie, "Total laparoscopic hysterectomy after liver transplantation," *Hepatobiliary and Pancreatic Diseases International*, vol. 9, no. 4, pp. 438–440, 2010.

[84] M. S. Lee, E. Y. Kim, J. H. Lee et al., "Laparoscopy-assisted distal gastrectomy for gastric cancer after liver transplantation," *Journal of the Korean Surgical Society*, vol. 80, supplement 1, pp. S1–S5, 2011.

[85] M. L. Metzelder, T. Schober, L. Grigull et al., "The role of laparoscopic techniques in children with suspected post-transplantation lymphoproliferative disorders.," *Journal of Laparoendoscopic & Advanced Surgical Techniques*, vol. 21, pp. 767–770, 2011.

15

The Interaction between Diabetes, Body Mass Index, Hepatic Steatosis, and Risk of Liver Resection: Insulin Dependent Diabetes Is the Greatest Risk for Major Complications

M. G. Wiggans,[1,2] J. T. Lordan,[1] G. Shahtahmassebi,[3] S. Aroori,[1] M. J. Bowles,[1] and D. A. Stell[1,2]

[1] *Hepatopancreatobiliary Surgery, Plymouth Hospitals NHS Trust, Derriford Hospital, Derriford Road, Plymouth, Devon PL6 8DH, UK*
[2] *Peninsula College of Medicine and Dentistry, University of Exeter and Plymouth University, John Bull Building, Plymouth, Devon PL6 8BU, UK*
[3] *School of Science and Technology, Nottingham Trent University, Nottingham NG1 4BU, UK*

Correspondence should be addressed to M. G. Wiggans; matthew.wiggans@doctors.org.uk

Academic Editor: Georgios Glantzounis

Background. This study aimed to assess the relationship between diabetes, obesity, and hepatic steatosis in patients undergoing liver resection and to determine if these factors are independent predictors of major complications. *Materials and Methods.* Analysis of a prospectively maintained database of patients undergoing liver resection between 2005 and 2012 was undertaken. Background liver was assessed for steatosis and classified as <33% and ≥33%. Major complications were defined as Grade III–V complications using the Dindo-Clavien classification. *Results.* 504 patients underwent liver resection, of whom 56 had diabetes and 61 had steatosis ≥33%. Median BMI was 26 kg/m^2 (16–54 kg/m^2). 94 patients developed a major complication (18.7%). BMI ≥ 25 kg/m^2 ($P = 0.001$) and diabetes ($P = 0.018$) were associated with steatosis ≥33%. Only insulin dependent diabetes was a risk factor for major complications ($P = 0.028$). Age, male gender, hypoalbuminaemia, synchronous bowel procedures, extent of resection, and blood transfusion were also independent risk factors. *Conclusions.* Liver surgery in the presence of steatosis, elevated BMI, and non-insulin dependent diabetes is not associated with major complications. Although diabetes requiring insulin therapy was a significant risk factor, the major risk factors relate to technical aspects of surgery, particularly synchronous bowel procedures.

1. Introduction

Liver failure occurs in up to 32% of patients following liver resection [1–5] and is a major contributor to both morbidity [6] and mortality [7]. Liver resection is technically more difficult in patients with parenchymal liver disease [8] and the risks of liver resection are increased due to impaired hepatic regeneration [9].

Nonalcoholic fatty liver disease (NAFLD) is the commonest cause of liver disease in the West [10] and is also the commonest cause of a sustained rise in serum transaminases in patients with no history of chronic liver disease [11]. NAFLD encompasses steatosis (excess accumulation of triglycerides), steatohepatitis (hepatocyte damage, inflammatory infiltrate, and fibrosis), and cirrhosis [12] and can be demonstrated with routine histological staining. NAFLD is associated with diabetes mellitus and obesity [13, 14] which are also undergoing a global epidemic [15, 16]. However, not all patients with obesity and diabetes develop NAFLD and similarly not all patients with NAFLD suffer either diabetes or obesity [17].

Liver-directed chemotherapy is also associated with hepatotoxicity. Steatohepatitis has been shown to occur in 20% of patients who receive irinotecan and 5% of those who receive fluorouracil (5FU) [18], with a resulting increase in complications after surgery. Oxaliplatin is associated with sinusoidal obstruction syndrome [18, 19]. Recreational alcohol use is also a major cause of hepatic steatosis [20].

A meta-analysis has shown that hepatic steatosis is associated with increased risk of postoperative complications and that moderate and severe steatosis are associated with increased mortality compared to patients with normal liver parenchyma or mild steatosis [21]. However, this analysis is based on four studies, only two of which included both BMI and diabetes in multivariate analyses [8, 22–24]. Obesity, diabetes, and hepatic steatosis often coexist in the metabolic syndrome [25], and the increased risk of operating in the presence of steatosis may be due to associated comorbidity. Diabetes mellitus and obesity are independent risk factors for postoperative complications following other types of major surgery, including infectious [26–28], cardiovascular [28, 29], and renal complications [26, 28, 29]. Furthermore in the four studies included in the meta-analysis heterogeneous definitions of postoperative complications were used, and often relatively minor complications were included. Recently complications after liver surgery have been classified by the Dindo-Clavien system [30], which stratifies severity of complications and allows comparison of outcomes between centres.

The aim of this study was to assess the relationship between the incidence of diabetes, obesity, and hepatic steatosis in patients undergoing liver resection after a period of abstention from alcohol consumption and to determine if these factors are independent predictors of major complications following liver resection, using the Dindo-Clavien system.

2. Materials and Methods

A retrospective analysis of a prospectively maintained database of all patients undergoing liver resection between July 2005 and September 2012 was undertaken. Patient characteristics, laboratory data, and intraoperative details were retrieved. BMI was recorded preoperatively and the cohort was divided into three categories: 18.5–24.99 kg/m^2 (normal), 25–29.99 kg/m^2 (overweight), and ≥30 kg/m^2 (obese). Diabetes was categorised according to the requirement for insulin. The presence of preexisting chronic liver disease was confirmed by histology. American Association of Anesthesiologists (ASA) grade was determined by the responsible anaesthetist and the physiologic score calculated according to the POSSUM system [31]. Selected patients were treated with neoadjuvant chemotherapy. All patients underwent preoperative counselling by a nurse specialist where abstention from alcohol was mandated. This instruction was also contained in a patient information sheet. The normal interval from preoperative counselling to surgery in this series is approximately 30 days.

Liver resections were defined according to the Brisbane classification [32] and undertaken using standard techniques, using hepatic inflow occlusion selectively. Major resections were defined as resections of three or more segments. Synchronous liver and bile-duct resections were performed in the presence of hilar cholangiocarcinoma. Radiofrequency ablation was used where small lesions were not accessible for surgical resection.

Major complications were defined as Grade III–V complications using the Dindo-Clavien classification where Grade III complications are those requiring surgical, endoscopic, or radiological intervention, Grade IV includes life threatening complications including organ failure, and Grade V is death [30]. Posthepatectomy liver failure (PHLF) was defined in accordance with the International Study Group of Liver Surgery (ISGLS) [33] as an increased prothrombin time (PT) and serum bilirubin concentration on or after postoperative day five. In patients with preoperatively increased PT or serum bilirubin concentration PHLF was defined as an increasing serum bilirubin concentration and PT on or after postoperative day 5, compared with the values of the previous day. Renal dysfunction was defined as an increase in serum creatinine of ≥1.5-fold from the preoperative baseline, according to RIFLE criteria [34].

Serum biochemistry tests and coagulation assays were performed preoperatively, in the first 24 postoperative hours, and then repeated according to clinical course. The peak measurement of bilirubin, prothrombin time (PT), and creatinine was recorded. Clotting factors were not administered between postoperative days (POD) 1–5. At histological examination the background liver parenchyma at least 1 cm from the tumour edge was assessed for degree of steatosis using the Brunt classification (the proportion of hepatocytes containing fat droplets; 1: <33%, 2: 33–66%, and 3: >66%) [35]. For analysis the data was divided into <33% (mild or none) and ≥33% (moderate or severe).

The minimum postoperative followup was 90 days and mortality was recorded along with details of postoperative intervention and complications.

To determine potential associations between patient characteristics and steatosis and between patient, operative, and histological characteristics and major complications univariate logistic regression or chi-square test at the level of $P < 0.25$ [36] was performed, as appropriate. Significant variables in the univariate analysis were included in the multivariate logistic regression model and were considered to be significant if $P < 0.05$. All analyses were carried out using the statistical package R 2.1.14 [37].

3. Results

Of 504 patients treated in the study period, surgery was undertaken for metastatic disease in 358 (71.0%), of whom 308 (61.1%) had colorectal liver metastases. Resections were performed for primary hepatic malignancy in 106 patients (21.0%) including hepatocellular carcinoma in 39 (7.7%) and cholangiocarcinoma in 31 (6.2%) patients. In 40 patients (7.9%) resection was performed for benign tumours. Major resection was undertaken in 299 patients (59.3%). In twenty-three patients a synchronous bowel procedure was performed including 10 colonic resections, 11 small bowel procedures, one gastric resection, and one Whipple's procedure. Fifty-six patients were diabetic (11.1%), of whom 15 were insulin dependent (26.8%). The median BMI of patients undergoing resection was 26 kg/m^2 (range 16–54 kg/m^2). Elevated BMI

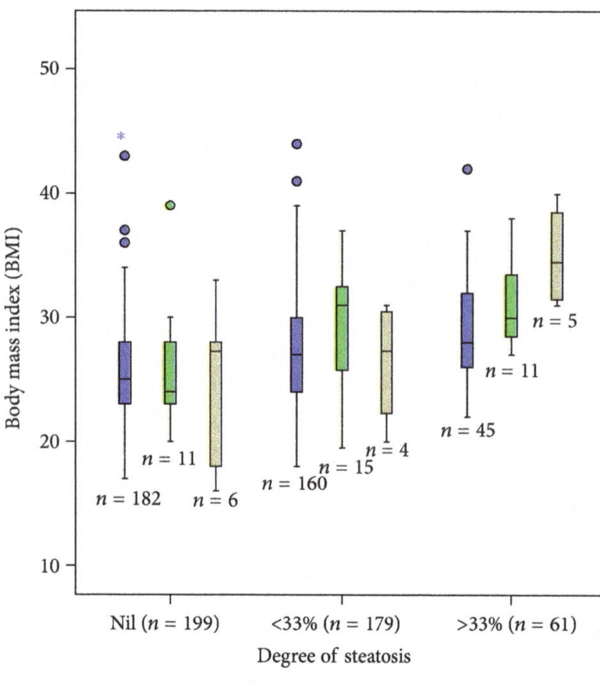

FIGURE 1: Box plot of body mass index (BMI), diabetic status, and degree of hepatic steatosis in 439 patients undergoing liver resection. Nil versus <33% ($P < 0.001$), <33 versus ≥33% ($P = 0.001$).

(≥25 kg/m^2) was noted in 332 patients (65.9%) and 123 patients (24.4%) were obese (≥30 kg/m^2). Five patients had no BMI recorded and were excluded from analysis. Preoperative liver-directed chemotherapy was used in 168 patients (33.3%). The most commonly used regime was oxaliplatin and capecitabine which was used in 118 patients (70.2%). Irinotecan was used in six patients (3.6%).

Histopathological examination revealed zero, mild, moderate, and severe steatosis in 199 (39.5%), 179 (35.5%), 54 (10.7%), and seven (1.4%) patients, respectively. Degree of steatosis was not recorded in 65 patients (12.9%). The distribution of BMI, diabetes, and steatosis is shown in Figure 1. The median BMI of patients with no steatosis (25 kg/m^2, range 16–45) was lower than those with mild steatosis (27 kg/m^2, range 18–44) ($P < 0.001$), which was lower than patients with moderate/severe steatosis (29 kg/m^2, range 22–42) ($P = 0.001$). The median BMI of diabetic patients was 29 kg/m^2 (16–40) compared to 26 kg/m^2 (17–54) in nondiabetic patients ($P = 0.002$). There was no difference in the median BMI of patients with insulin dependent diabetes (IDDM) (29 kg/m^2, range 16–40) and those with non-insulin dependent diabetes (NIDDM) (29 kg/m^2, range 20–39) ($P = 0.816$). The rate of mild steatosis among diabetics was 16/52 (30.8%) compared to 45/387 (11.6%) in nondiabetics ($P = 0.001$), but there was no significant difference in the rates of mild steatosis in patients with NIDDM (11/37) and those with IDDM (5/15). The rate of moderate/severe steatosis was 6/135 (4.4%) in normal weight, nondiabetic patients, 39/249 (15.6%) in overweight nondiabetics ($P = 0.001$), 0/12 in normal weight diabetics, and 15/39 (38.5%) in overweight diabetics ($P < 0.001$).

Elevated preoperative transaminase levels were noted in 18 of 60 patients (30%) with moderate/severe steatosis and 61 of 369 patients (16.5%) with steatosis <33% ($P = 0.019$). The sensitivity and specificity of elevated transaminases for predicting the presence of moderate or severe steatosis were 30% and 83%, respectively.

Multivariate analysis revealed that elevated BMI ≥ 25 kg/m^2 ($P = 0.001$) and the presence of diabetes ($P = 0.018$) were significantly associated with moderate/severe hepatic steatosis (Table 1). BMI ≥ 25 kg/m^2 increased the risk by a factor of 2.97 and diabetes increased the risk by a factor of 2.69. Among diabetic patients insulin dependence increased the risk of moderate/severe steatosis by a factor of 4.31 ($P = 0.037$). However, BMI ≥ 30 kg/m did not increase the risk of moderate/severe steatosis compared to BMI of 25–29.9 ($P = 0.144$). Raised preoperative transaminase levels also increased the risk of moderate/severe steatosis by a factor of 3.82 ($P < 0.001$), and raised preoperative alkaline phosphatase concentrations decreased the risk by a factor of 0.15 ($P = 0.001$). Hepatic steatosis was not associated with liver-directed chemotherapy or other biochemical markers of liver dysfunction (preoperative hypoalbuminemia and hyperbilirubinemia).

During the study period 94 patients developed a major postoperative complication. Twenty-three patients died within 90 days of surgery (4.6%) and 71 patients who survived beyond 90 days suffered a major complication (14.1%). The most common cause of mortality was liver failure (nine patients).

Of patients who developed Grade IV complications 34/64 (53.1%) developed PHLF and 31/64 developed renal failure (48.4%). Of the 34 patients who developed PHLF 29 had undergone major liver resection. Twenty-three patients developed bile leaks, and seven required relaparotomy/relaparoscopy. Multivariate analysis revealed that older age, male gender, hypoalbuminaemia, synchronous bowel procedures, number of segments resected, and blood transfusion were independent risk factors for major postoperative complications (Table 2). There was no association between NIDDM, BMI, or degree of hepatic steatosis and major postoperative complications. IDDM more than trebled the risk of major complication compared to nondiabetics and those with NIDDM. The complications in these groups are shown in Table 3. The greatest risk however occurred when liver resection was undertaken in conjunction with a synchronous bowel procedure, which increased the risk of major complication almost six times that of a liver-only resection. Ten of 23 patients developed major postoperative complications, six of whom had colonic resections (three right sided and three left sided), three had small bowel procedures, and one had a gastric resection.

In the 299 patients who underwent major resection, there was no significant difference in the proportion of patients with steatosis ≥33% between patients who did (10/64, 15.6%) or did not (23/201, 11.4%) develop major complications

TABLE 1: Analysis of factors associated with hepatic steatosis (≥33%) in 439 patients undergoing liver resection.

N = 439	Steatosis < 33% (n = 378) Median (range)	Count (%)	Steatosis ≥ 33% (n = 61) Median (range)	Count (%)	Univariate P value	Comparison	Multivariate Odds ratio (95% CI)	P value
Age	65 (21–90)		65 (41–87)		0.622			
Gender								
Female		168 (44.4)		24 (39.3)	0.544			
Male		210 (55.6)		37 (60.7)				
Liver-directed chemotherapy								
Yes		132 (34.9)		20 (32.8)	1.000			
No		246 (65.1)		41 (67.2)				
Preexisting chronic liver disease								
Yes		6 (1.6)		3 (4.9)	0.228*			0.869
No		372 (98.4)		58 (95.1)				
Preoperative jaundice (≥50 micromoles/L)								
Yes		5 (1.3)		0	0.800			
No		373 (98.7)		61 (100)				
Hypoalbuminaemia (<35 g/L)								
Yes		15 (4.0)		1 (1.6)				
No		360 (95.2)		59 (96.7)	0.602			
Not recorded		3 (0.8)		1 (1.6)				
Raised preoperative alkaline phosphatase								
Yes		92 (24.3)		5 (8.2)				
No		283 (74.9)		55 (90.2)	0.008*		0.15 (0.05–0.46)	0.001**
Not recorded		3 (0.8)		1 (1.6)				
Raised preoperative transaminase								
Yes		61 (16.1)		18 (29.5)				
No		308 (81.5)		42 (68.9)	0.021*		3.82 (1.85–7.89)	<0.001**
Not recorded		9 (2.4)		1 (1.6)				
Diabetic status								
Nondiabetic		342 (90.5)		45 (73.8)		Diabetic versus nondiabetic	2.69 (1.18–6.13)	0.018**
Non-insulin dependent		26 (6.9)		11 (18.0)	0.001*			
Insulin dependent		10 (2.6)		5 (8.2)		Insulin dependent versus non-insulin dependent	4.31 (1.09–16.98)	0.037**
Body mass index (kg/m^2)								
<25		141 (37.3)		6 (10)		<25 versus ≥25	2.97 (1.59–5.57)	0.001**
25–29.9		153 (40.5)		27 (45.0)	<0.001*			
≥30		81 (21.4)		27 (45.0)		25–29.9 versus ≥30		0.144
Not recorded		3 (0.8)		1 (1.6)				

*Significant at the level of 0.25 for univariate analysis and included in multivariate analysis.
**Significant at the level of 0.05 for multivariate analysis.

TABLE 2: Analysis of factors associated with major complications following liver resection in 504 patients.

$N = 504$	No complication ($n = 410$)	Major complication ($n = 94$)	Univariate	Multivariate	
			P value	Odds ratio (95% CI)	P value
Median age (range)	64 (21–90)	67 (32–88)	0.015*	1.03 (0.99–1.07)	0.004**
Gender (%)					
Male	211 (51.5)	67 (71.3)	0.001*	2.36 (1.34–4.17)	0.028**
Female	199 (48.5)	27 (28.7)			
Pathology (%)					
Benign	34 (8.3)	6 (6.4)			
Primary	83 (20.2)	23 (24.5)	0.622		
Secondary	293 (71.5)	65 (69.1)	0.308		
Liver-directed chemotherapy (%)	130 (31.7)	33 (35.1)	0.608		
Preexisting chronic liver disease (%)	10 (2.4)	1 (1.1)	0.666		
Preoperative jaundice (≥50 micromoles/L) (%)	6 (1.5)	3 (3.2)	0.266		
Hypoalbuminaemia (<35 g/L) (%)	9 (2.2)	8 (8.5)	0.004*	2.97 (1.01–8.74)	0.047**
Raised preoperative alkaline phosphatase (%)	95 (23.2)	24 (25.5)	0.721		
Raised preoperative transaminase (%)	74 (18.0)	21 (22.3)	0.320		
Preoperative glomerular filtration rate (%)					
≤90 mL/min	274 (66.8)	63 (67.0)	0.892		
Median preoperative haemoglobin (g/dL) (range)	13 (9–17)	13 (9–16)	0.025*		0.439
Median preoperative white cell count (/L) (range)	7 (3–17)	7 (3–25)	0.422		
Diabetic status (%)					
Nondiabetic	370 (90.2)	78 (83.0)			0.912
Non-insulin dependent (versus nondiabetic)	32 (7.8)	9 (9.6)	0.014*		
Insulin dependent diabetes (versus non-insulin dependent and nondiabetics)	8 (2.0)	7 (7.4)		3.86 (1.17–12.75)	0.028**
Body mass index (kg/m^2) (%)					
<25	139 (33.9)	28 (29.8)			
25–30	167 (40.7)	42 (44.7)	0.697		
>30	99 (24.1)	24 (25.5)			
American Association of Anesthesiologists (ASA) grade (%)			0.198*		
1 versus 2					
1	46 (11.2)	6 (6.4)			0.611
2	266 (64.9)	58 (61.7)			
2 versus 3 and 4					
3	95 (23.2)	30 (31.9)			0.783
4	2 (0.5)	0			
Median P-POSSUM physiologic score (range)	16 (12–32)	18 (12–30)	0.003*		0.764

Table 2: Continued.

N = 504	No complication (n = 410)	Major complication (n = 94)	Univariate	Multivariate	
			P value	Odds ratio (95% CI)	P value
Operative approach (%)					
Laparoscopic	46 (11.2)	4 (4.3)	0.065*		0.812
Open	364 (88.8)	90 (95.7)			
Radiofrequency ablation included (%)	18 (4.4)	5 (5.3)	0.698		
Wedge resection included (%)	181 (44.1)	22 (23.4)	<0.001*		0.353
Bile-duct reconstruction (%)	34 (8.3)	12 (12.8)	0.246*		0.585
Synchronous bowel procedure (%)	13 (3.2)	10 (10.6)	0.003*	5.99 (2.25–15.96)	<0.001**
Median number of segments resected (range)	3 (1–6)	4 (1–6)	<0.001	1.51 (1.26–1.80)	<0.001**
Repeat operation (%)	31 (7.6)	6 (6.4)	0.861		
Intraoperative blood loss (%)					
<500 mL	218 (53.2)	29 (30.9)	<0.001		0.463
≥500 mL	188 (45.9)	65 (69.1)			
Blood transfusion required (%)	65 (15.9)	41 (43.6)	<0.001	2.48 (1.44–4.30)	0.001**
Steatosis (%)					
<33%	308 (75.1)	70 (74.5)	1.000		
≥33%	50 (12.2)	11 (11.7)			

*Significant at the level of 0.25 for univariate analysis and included in multivariate analysis.
**Significant at the level of 0.05 for multivariate analysis.

TABLE 3: Postoperative complications, 90-day mortality, and diabetic status in 504 patients undergoing liver resection (patients may have had more than one complication).

$N = 504$	All patients ($n = 504$) Count (%)	Nondiabetic ($n = 448$) Count (%)	Non-insulin dependent diabetes ($n = 41$) Count (%)	Insulin dependent diabetes ($n = 15$) Count (%)	P value Nondiabetic versus non-insulin dependent diabetic	P value Nondiabetic versus insulin dependent diabetic
Any major complication	94 (18.7)	78 (17.4)	9 (21.9)	7 (46.6)	0.521	0.010
90-day mortality (Grade V)						
Liver failure	9 (1.8)	5 (1.1)	3	1	0.023*	0.180
Sepsis	4 (0.8)	3 (0.7)	1	0	0.296	1.000
Malignancy	4 (0.8)	3 (0.7)	0	1	1.000	0.124
Pulmonary embolus	1 (0.2)	1 (0.2)	0	0	1.000	1.000
Anastomotic leak	1 (0.2)	1 (0.2)	0	0	1.000	1.000
Peptic ulcer	1 (0.2)	1 (0.2)	0	0	1.000	1.000
Strangulated hernia	1 (0.2)	1 (0.2)	0	0	1.000	1.000
Peritonitis	1 (0.2)	1 (0.2)	0	0	1.000	1.000
Heart failure	1 (0.2)	1 (0.2)	0	0	1.000	1.000
Total	**23 (4.6)**	**17 (3.8)**	**4**	**2**	**0.089**	**0.122**
Grade IV complications						
Posthepatectomy liver failure (PHLF)	34 (6.7)	30 (6.7)	4	0	0.515	0.613
Renal dysfunction	31 (6.2)	24 (5.4)	4	3	0.280	0.050
Respiratory failure requiring intensive care	2 (0.4)	2 (0.4)	0	0	1.000	1.000
Total	**67 (13.3)**	**56 (12.5)**	**8**	**3**	**0.224**	**0.421**
Grade III complications						
Bile leak						
Drain	12 (2.4)	11 (2.5)	0	1	0.611	0.330
ERCP	11 (2.2)	10 (2.2)	1	0	1.000	1.000
Relaparotomy/relaparoscopy						
Washout	3 (0.6)	1 (0.2)	1	1	0.161	0.064
Adhesiolysis	2 (0.4)	2 (0.4)	0	0	1.000	1.000
Defunction for anastomotic leak	1 (0.2)	0	1	0	0.084	1.000
Small bowel leak	1 (0.2)	1 (0.2)	0	0	1.000	1.000
Drainage						
Liver abscess	1 (0.2)	1 (0.2)	0	0	1.000	1.000
Pleural effusion	1 (0.2)	0	0	1	1.000	0.032
Pneumothorax	1 (0.2)	1 (0.2)	0	0	1.000	1.000
Subphrenic collection	2 (0.4)	2 (0.4)	0	0	1.000	1.000
Total	**35 (6.9)**	**29 (6.5)**	**3**	**3**	**0.743**	**0.077**

(P = 0.388). Similarly there was no significant difference in the proportion of patients with steatosis ≥33% between patients who did (4/22, 15.6%) or did not (29/243, 11.9%) develop PHLF (P = 0.495).

4. Discussion

The principal finding of this study is that although diabetes mellitus and higher BMI are risk factors for steatosis in patients undergoing liver resection, the majority of cases of steatosis occur in nondiabetic patients with mildly elevated BMI (25–30). Secondly, steatosis and elevated BMI are not associated with major complications after liver resection, and diabetes is a risk factor for these complications only if patients are insulin dependent. Other predictors of major complications are older age, male gender, preoperative hypoalbuminaemia, synchronous bowel procedures, number of segments resected, and requirement for blood transfusion.

The 90-day mortality (4.6%) and morbidity (14.7%) rate are similar to published series [4, 18, 38], although other series have included minor (Grade I and II) complications [39–41]. Composite outcomes similar to the one used in this study have been used previously in studies evaluating outcomes following gastrointestinal surgery [42, 43]. The present study confirms the association between hepatic steatosis and BMI [44]. Whilst the rate of moderate/severe steatosis was greatest in overweight diabetic patients (38.5%), it also occurred in patients of normal weight without diabetes (4.4%). This suggests that other risk factors may be involved in the aetiology of the disease. Undernutrition [17], impaired glucose tolerance [45], and genetic factors [46] have also been implicated in the development of NAFLD. Alcohol consumption is an unlikely cause of steatosis in this series as all patients are asked to abstain from alcohol consumption prior to surgery, although compliance with this instruction has not been assessed.

Elevated transaminase levels are associated with hepatic steatosis, but the sensitivity of abnormal transaminases in detecting moderate or severe NAFLD is poor, as 70% of these patients had normal transaminase levels. This is in keeping with other studies [47]. Interestingly, raised preoperative alkaline phosphatase concentration was associated with decreased incidence of steatosis. Elevated alkaline phosphatase may be found in cases of biliary obstruction, and of the 119 patients with this finding 16.8% had cholangiocarcinomas compared to only 2.9% of the 380 patients with normal alkaline phosphatase. This group is more likely to be systemically unwell as a consequence of biliary obstruction and to have suffered a period of anorexia and weight loss, which may affect the degree of hepatic steatosis.

Preoperative chemotherapy was not shown to be associated with steatosis. Studies have shown an association between steatohepatitis and irinotecan therapy [18], which was rarely used in this series. In addition the policy in this unit is to use only four cycles of chemotherapy and to allow a period of recovery before undertaking liver resection, to allow resolution of hepatotoxicity.

Previous studies have shown that steatosis increases the risk of PHLF [8, 21]. The rate of PHLF in this series was low (6.7%) and occurred in 6.6% patients with moderate/severe steatosis and 6.1% of the patients with none/mild steatosis. The majority of cases of PHLF followed major liver resection (29/34). It is possible that there is an independent association between steatosis and PHLF, which is not revealed in this study which uses a composite outcome including other complications in the multivariate analysis. Steatosis may be a risk factor for liver failure in patients undergoing extended hepatectomy, although not in major hepatectomy in this series, where the risk of this complication is greatest. Previous studies have recommended liver biopsy to investigate the presence of steatosis prior to resection [48, 49]. The current study suggests that the risk of this investigation is not justified due to the lack of effect of steatosis on outcome.

The rate of bile leak requiring intervention (4.6%) was not affected by the degree of hepatic steatosis suggesting that hepatic steatosis does not make parenchymal division more difficult to perform.

Elevated BMI was not associated with major complications in this series, although it may be associated with more minor complications such as wound infection which has not been explored in this study.

Diabetes was an independent risk factor for complications after liver surgery which confirms the findings of previous studies [5, 50–52], although identification of insulin dependence as the major risk factor is a novel finding. Whilst there was no significant difference in the risk of major complications between nondiabetic patients and those with non-insulin dependent diabetes, the risk of complications was more than trebled in those with insulin dependent diabetes. This finding reflects the multisystem nature of diabetic end-organ damage. Diabetic nephropathy is a major cause of renal dysfunction [53] and was the most common complication in patients with IDDM. Renal dysfunction was also twice as common amongst patients with IDDM compared to those with NIDDM.

Older age, male gender, preoperative hypoalbuminaemia, number of liver segments resected, and requirement for blood transfusion have all been previously identified as risk factors for postoperative complications [38]. The finding that performing synchronous bowel procedures is associated with worse outcome is similar to that of a previous study which found that the risk of a major complication was 20.4% after a synchronous colonic resection compared to 14.9% after a liver-only resection [54]. Although a recent systematic review suggested no difference in terms of overall morbidity or mortality between synchronous and staged resections [55] the results of the present study reveal the risk of developing a major complication after a synchronous bowel procedure was almost six times that of a liver-only resection. It should also be noted that the synchronous procedures included a gastric resection and Whipple's procedure which may pose different risks to colonic resections. Most of the increased risk in this context relates to leaks from enteric anastomoses.

5. Conclusions

The results of this study allow clinicians to advise patients regarding the risks of liver resection and to place them in context. In particular, liver surgery in the presence of steatosis, elevated BMI, and NIDDM does not lead to greatly increased operative risk. While insulin dependence is a significant risk factor for complications after liver surgery, the major risk factors in this series related to technical details of the operation, particularly the performance of simultaneous bowel procedures.

References

[1] O. Farges, B. Malassagne, J. F. Flejou, S. Balzan, A. Sauvanet, and J. Belghiti, "Risk of major liver resection in patients with underlying chronic liver disease: a reappraisal," *Annals of Surgery*, vol. 229, no. 2, pp. 210–215, 1999.

[2] J. Belghiti, K. Hiramatsu, S. Benoist, P. P. Massault, A. Sauvanet, and O. Farges, "Seven hundred forty-seven hepatectomies in the 1990s: an update to evaluate the actual risk of liver resection," *Journal of the American College of Surgeons*, vol. 191, no. 1, pp. 38–46, 2000.

[3] A. Cucchetti, G. Ercolani, M. Vivarelli et al., "Impact of model for end-stage liver disease (MELD) score on prognosis after hepatectomy for hepatocellular carcinoma on cirrhosis," *Liver Transplantation*, vol. 12, no. 6, pp. 966–971, 2006.

[4] J. T. Mullen, D. Ribero, S. K. Reddy et al., "Hepatic insufficiency and mortality in 1,059 noncirrhotic patients undergoing major hepatectomy," *Journal of the American College of Surgeons*, vol. 204, no. 5, pp. 854–862, 2007.

[5] M. G. Wiggans, G. Shahtahmassebi, M. J. Bowles, S. Aroori, and D. A. Stell, "Renal dysfunction is an independent risk factor for mortality after liver resection and the main determinant of outcome in posthepatectomy liver failure," *HPB Surgery*, vol. 2013, Article ID 875367, 7 pages, 2013.

[6] R. T. Poon, S. T. Fan, C. M. Lo et al., "Improving perioperative outcome expands the role of hepatectomy in management of benign and malignant hepatobiliary diseases," *Annals of Surgery*, vol. 240, no. 4, pp. 698–708, 2004.

[7] W. R. Jarnagin, M. Gonen, Y. Fong et al., "Improvement in perioperative outcome after hepatic resection: analysis of 1,803 consecutive cases over the past decade," *Annals of Surgery*, vol. 236, no. 4, pp. 397–407, 2002.

[8] K. E. Behrns, G. G. Tsiotos, N. F. DeSouza, M. K. Krishna, J. Ludwig, and D. M. Nagorney, "Hepatic steatosis as a potential risk factor for major hepatic resection," *Journal of Gastrointestinal Surgery*, vol. 2, no. 3, pp. 292–298, 1998.

[9] R. Veteläinen, A. van Vliet, D. J. Gouma, and T. M. van Gulik, "Steatosis as a risk factor in liver surgery," *Annals of Surgery*, vol. 245, no. 1, pp. 20–30, 2007.

[10] Y. Takahashi, T. Fukusato, A. Inui, and T. Fujisawa, "Nonalcoholic fatty liver disease and nonalcoholic steatohepatitis," *World Journal of Gastroenterology*, vol. 70, no. 10, pp. 1–29, 2012.

[11] J. M. Clark, F. L. Brancati, and A. M. Diehl, "The prevalence and etiology of elevated aminotransferase levels in the United States," *American Journal of Gastroenterology*, vol. 98, no. 5, pp. 960–967, 2003.

[12] S. Chitturi, G. C. Farrell, E. Hashimoto, T. Saibara, G. K. K. Lau, and J. D. Sollano, "Non-alcoholic fatty liver disease in the Asia-Pacific region: definitions and overview of proposed guidelines," *Journal of Gastroenterology and Hepatology*, vol. 22, no. 6, pp. 778–787, 2007.

[13] G. Bedogni, L. Miglioli, F. Masutti, C. Tiribelli, G. Marchesini, and S. Bellentani, "Prevalence of and risk factors for nonalcoholic fatty liver disease: the dionysos nutrition and liver study," *Hepatology*, vol. 42, no. 1, pp. 44–52, 2005.

[14] Y. Falck-Ytter, Z. M. Younossi, G. Marchesini, and A. J. McCullough, "Clinical features and natural history of nonalcoholic steatosis syndromes," *Seminars in Liver Disease*, vol. 21, no. 1, pp. 17–26, 2001.

[15] World Health Organization, *Obesity: Preventing and Managing the Global Epidemic*, World Health Organization, Geneva, Switzerland, 2000.

[16] G. Danaei, M. M. Finucane, Y. Lu et al., "National, regional, and global trends in fasting plasma glucose and diabetes prevalence since 1980: systematic analysis of health examination surveys and epidemiological studies with 370 country-years and 2·7 million participants," *The Lancet*, vol. 378, no. 9785, pp. 31–40, 2011.

[17] K. Das, K. Das, P. S. Mukherjee et al., "Nonobese population in a developing country has a high prevalence of nonalcoholic fatty liver and significant liver disease," *Hepatology*, vol. 51, no. 5, pp. 1593–1602, 2010.

[18] J. Vauthey, T. M. Pawlik, D. Ribero et al., "Chemotherapy regimen predicts steatohepatitis and an increase in 90-day mortality after surgery for hepatic colorectal metastases," *Journal of Clinical Oncology*, vol. 24, no. 13, pp. 2065–2072, 2006.

[19] L. Rubbia-Brandt, V. Audard, P. Sartoretti et al., "Severe hepatic sinusoidal obstruction associated with oxaliplatin-based chemotherapy in patients with metastatic colorectal cancer," *Annals of Oncology*, vol. 15, no. 3, pp. 460–466, 2004.

[20] L. M. DeCarli and C. S. Lieber, "Fatty liver in the rat after prolonged intake of ethanol with a nutritionally adequate new liquid diet.," *Journal of Nutrition*, vol. 91, no. 3, pp. 331–336, 1967.

[21] V. E. de Meijer, B. T. Kalish, M. Puder, and J. N. M. IJzermans, "Systematic review and meta-analysis of steatosis as a risk factor in major hepatic resection," *British Journal of Surgery*, vol. 97, no. 9, pp. 1331–1339, 2010.

[22] D. A. Kooby, Y. Fong, A. Suriawinata et al., "Impact of steatosis on perioperative outcome following hepatic resection," *Journal of Gastrointestinal Surgery*, vol. 7, no. 8, pp. 1034–1044, 2003.

[23] D. Gomez, H. Z. Malik, G. K. Bonney et al., "Steatosis predicts postoperative morbidity following hepatic resection for colorectal metastasis," *The British Journal of Surgery*, vol. 94, no. 11, pp. 1395–1402, 2007.

[24] L. McCormack, H. Petrowsky, W. Jochum, K. Furrer, and P. Clavien, "Hepatic steatosis is a risk factor for postoperative complications after major hepatectomy: a matched case-control study," *Annals of Surgery*, vol. 245, no. 6, pp. 923–930, 2007.

[25] International Diabetes Federation, "The IDF concensus worldwide definition of the metabolic syndrome," 2006.

[26] A. K. Mathur, A. A. Ghaferi, N. H. Osborne et al., "Body mass index and adverse perioperative outcomes following hepatic resection," *Journal of Gastrointestinal Surgery*, vol. 14, no. 8, pp. 1285–1291, 2010.

[27] K. Dhatariya, N. Levy, A. Kilvert et al., "NHS Diabetes guideline for the perioperative management of the adult patient with diabetes," *Diabetic Medicine*, vol. 29, no. 4, pp. 420–433, 2012.

[28] A. Frisch, P. Chandra, D. Smiley et al., "Prevalence and clinical outcome of hyperglycemia in the perioperative period in noncardiac surgery," *Diabetes Care*, vol. 33, no. 8, pp. 1783–1788, 2010.

[29] K. Dhatariya, D. Flanagan, L. Hilton et al., "Management of adults with diabetes undergoing surgery and elective procedures: improving standards," 2011.

[30] D. Dindo, N. Demartines, and P.-A. Clavien, "Classification of surgical complications: a new proposal with evaluation in a cohort of 6336 patients and results of a survey," *Annals of Surgery*, vol. 240, no. 2, pp. 205–213, 2004.

[31] G. P. Copeland, D. Jones, and M. Walters, "POSSUM: a scoring system for surgical audit," *The British Journal of Surgery*, vol. 78, no. 3, pp. 355–360, 1991.

[32] J. Belghiti, P.-A. Clavien, E. Gadzijev et al., "The Brisbane 2000 terminology of hepatic anatomy and resections," *The Holiday Property Bond*, vol. 2, no. 3, pp. 333–339, 2000.

[33] N. N. Rahbari, O. J. Garden, R. Padbury et al., "Posthepatectomy liver failure: a definition and grading by the International Study Group of Liver Surgery (ISGLS)," *Surgery*, vol. 149, no. 5, pp. 713–724, 2011.

[34] R. Bellomo, C. Ronco, J. A. Kellum, R. L. Mehta, and P. Palevsky, "Acute renal failure—definition, outcome measures, animal models, fluid therapy and information technology needs: the Second International Consensus Conference of the Acute Dialysis Quality Initiative (ADQI) Group," *Critical Care*, vol. 8, no. 4, pp. R204–R212, 2004.

[35] E. M. Brunt, C. G. Janney, A. M. Di Bisceglie, B. A. Neuschwander-Tetri, and B. R. Bacon, "Nonalcoholic steatohepatitis: a proposal for grading and staging the histological lesions," *American Journal of Gastroenterology*, vol. 94, no. 9, pp. 2467–2474, 1999.

[36] A. Agresti, *An Introduction to Categorical Data Analysis*, John Wiley & Sons, Hoboken, NJ, USA, 2nd edition, 2002.

[37] "R Project for Statistical Computing," 2011, http://www.r-project.org/.

[38] C. D. Mann, T. Palser, C. D. Briggs et al., "A review of factors predicting perioperative death and early outcome in hepatopancreaticobiliary cancer surgery," *HPB*, vol. 12, no. 6, pp. 380–388, 2010.

[39] S. Virani, J. S. Michaelson, M. M. Hutter et al., "Morbidity and mortality after liver resection: results of the patient safety in surgery study," *Journal of the American College of Surgeons*, vol. 204, no. 6, pp. 1284–1292, 2007.

[40] A. Andres, C. Toso, B. Moldovan et al., "Complications of elective liver resections in a center with low mortality: a simple score to predict morbidity," *Archives of Surgery*, vol. 146, no. 11, pp. 1246–1252, 2011.

[41] C. Reissfelder, N. N. Rahbari, M. Koch et al., "Postoperative course and clinical significance of biochemical blood tests following hepatic resection," *British Journal of Surgery*, vol. 98, no. 6, pp. 836–844, 2011.

[42] R. M. Pearse, D. A. Harrison, N. MacDonald et al., "Effect of a perioperative, cardiac output-guided hemodynamic therapy algorithm on outcomes following major gastrointestinal surgery: a randomized clinical trial and systematic review," *The Journal of the American Medical Association*, vol. 311, no. 21, pp. 2181–2190, 2014.

[43] H. Abu Daya, M. Eloubeidi, H. Tamim et al., "Opposing effects of aspirin and anticoagulants on morbidity and mortality in patients with upper gastrointestinal bleeding," *Journal of Digestive Diseases*, vol. 15, no. 6, pp. 283–292, 2014.

[44] J. E. Everhart and K. M. Bambha, "Fatty liver: think globally," *Hepatology*, vol. 51, no. 5, pp. 1491–1493, 2010.

[45] C. Ortiz-Lopez, R. Lomonaco, B. Orsak et al., "Prevalence of prediabetes and diabetes and metabolic profile of patients with Nonalcoholic Fatty Liver Disease (NAFLD)," *Diabetes Care*, vol. 35, no. 4, pp. 873–878, 2012.

[46] S. Romeo, J. Kozlitina, C. Xing et al., "Genetic variation in PNPLA3 confers susceptibility to nonalcoholic fatty liver disease," *Nature Genetics*, vol. 40, no. 12, pp. 1461–1465, 2008.

[47] J. D. Browning, L. S. Szczepaniak, R. Dobbins et al., "Prevalence of hepatic steatosis in an urban population in the United States: impact of ethnicity," *Hepatology*, vol. 40, no. 6, pp. 1387–1395, 2004.

[48] F. G. Fernandez, J. Ritter, J. W. Goodwin, D. C. Linehan, W. G. Hawkins, and S. M. Strasberg, "Effect of steatohepatitis associated with irinotecan or oxaliplatin pretreatment on resectability of hepatic colorectal metastases," *Journal of the American College of Surgeons*, vol. 200, no. 6, pp. 845–853, 2005.

[49] D. Zorzi, A. Laurent, T. M. Pawlik, G. Y. Lauwers, J. Vauthey, and E. K. Abdalla, "Chemotherapy-associated hepatotoxicity and surgery for colorectal liver metastases," *The British Journal of Surgery*, vol. 94, no. 3, pp. 274–286, 2007.

[50] M. Shimada, T. Matsumata, K. Akazawa et al., "Estimation of risk of major complications after hepatic resection," *American Journal of Surgery*, vol. 167, no. 4, pp. 399–403, 1994.

[51] A. Taketomi, D. Kitagawa, S. Itoh et al., "Trends in Morbidity and Mortality after Hepatic Resection for Hepatocellular Carcinoma: an Institute's Experience with 625 Patients," *Journal of the American College of Surgeons*, vol. 204, no. 4, pp. 580–587, 2007.

[52] M. Shimada, K. Takenaka, Y. Fujiwara et al., "Risk factors linked to postoperative morbidity in patients with hepatocellular carcinoma," *British Journal of Surgery*, vol. 85, no. 2, pp. 195–198, 1998.

[53] Y.-M. Sun, Y. Su, J. Li, and L.-F. Wang, "Recent advances in understanding the biochemical and molecular mechanism of diabetic nephropathy," *Biochemical and Biophysical Research Communications*, vol. 433, no. 4, pp. 359–361, 2013.

[54] O. H. Hamed, N. H. Bhayani, G. Ortenzi et al., "Simultaneous colorectal and hepatic procedures for colorectal cancer result in increased morbidity but equivalent mortality compared with colorectal or hepatic procedures alone: Outcomes from the National Surgical Quality Improvement Program," *HPB*, vol. 15, no. 9, pp. 695–702, 2013.

[55] P. M. Lykoudis, D. O'Reilly, K. Nastos, and G. Fusai, "Systematic review of surgical management of synchronous colorectal liver metastases," *British Journal of Surgery*, vol. 101, no. 6, pp. 605–612, 2014.

16

Contemporary Strategies in the Management of Hepatocellular Carcinoma

Shirin Elizabeth Khorsandi and Nigel Heaton

Institute of Liver Studies, King's College Hospital, Denmark Hill, London SE5 9RS, UK

Correspondence should be addressed to Shirin Elizabeth Khorsandi, s.khorsandi@imperial.ac.uk

Academic Editor: Andrea Lauterio

Liver transplantation is the treatment of choice for selected patients with hepatocellular carcinoma (HCC) on a background of chronic liver disease. Liver resection or locoregional ablative therapies may be indicated for patients with preserved synthetic function without significant portal hypertension. Milan criteria were introduced to select suitable patients for liver transplant with low risk of tumor recurrence and 5-year survival in excess of 70%. Currently the incidence of HCC is climbing rapidly and in a current climate of organ shortage has led to the re-evaluation of locoregional therapies and resectional surgery to manage the case load. The introduction of biological therapies has had a new dimension to care, adding to the complexities of multidisciplinary team working in the management of HCC. The aim of this paper is to give a brief overview of present day management strategies and decision making.

1. Introduction

Hepatocellular carcinoma (HCC) is the fifth most common cancer in the world. Ninety percent of primary liver cancers are HCC, the majority of which develop on the background of cirrhosis. Over the past decade, medical management of the patient with chronic liver disease has improved. In parallel, the prevalence of hepatitis B (HBV), hepatitis C virus (HCV), alcohol related liver disease, and NASH has increased and combined with an ageing population has led to a surge in the number of cases worldwide [1–3]. As a consequence, HCC is an important complication of cirrhosis and a leading indication for liver transplantation (LT), accounting for approximately a third of patients on transplant waiting lists [4]. The introduction of surveillance using alphafetoprotein and ultrasound has led to the earlier recognition of HCC and increases the therapeutic options available [5]. In the absence of treatment the overall 5-year survival is <10% [6]. These include LT, resection, locoregional, and systemic therapies. For a solitary HCC with preserved liver function and low hepatic vein pressure gradient, liver resection still remains the first choice.

Historically, survival rates were 35–62% at 3 years and 17–50% at 5 years for patients with cirrhosis undergoing resection for HCC [6, 7]. However, tumor recurrence rates were high, up to 70%, and progression to liver failure was common [6, 8–10]. LT is an attractive treatment option as it treats both the cancer and underlying liver disease. In the 1980s, patients presenting with large HCC were considered good candidates for LT as they were in better condition than patients with chronic liver disease and were more likely to survive the perioperative period but they had large or multifocal tumors. This resulted in a high recurrence rate of up to 65%, a 5 year survival of 10–35%, and a median survival of those with recurrence of 6 months, coupled with increasing demand for donor livers led to a more restrictive selection process [11–13]. Recognition that small tumors appeared to fare better after LT led Mazzaferro to introduce the Milan criteria to select patients leading to improved survival with low rates of tumor recurrence [14]. By adhering to the Milan criteria of undertaking LT for HCC with a solitary tumor ≤ 5 cm or 3 tumors ≤ 3 cm each, a 5 year survival greater than 70% and recurrence rates of <10% were produced.

2. Staging

A staging system for HCC poses problems because the presence of liver disease and tumor varies due to the different epidemiological backgrounds and risk factors. The ideal staging system needs to include prognostic information regarding both the cancer and liver functional status and take account of clinical factors that influence response to treatment. The TNM classification is an oncology standard useful in conjunction with the presence of microvascular invasion of examined resection or explanted tumors/liver and provides information regarding the risk of tumor recurrence but does not take account of the liver functional status. As TNM requires pathological data (microvascular invasion) and only 20% HCC are resected for which it is good at discriminating stages for, its usability is limited. The Okuda staging system has been widely used since 1985. It uses four criteria of ascites, albumin, bilirubin, and tumor size to assess liver functional status and tumor stage. It is a good system for stratifying advanced/symptomatic disease but less useful in early stage to guide treatment choices. Other available systems are the French classification, the Cancer of the Liver Italian Program (CLIP) classification, and the Barcelona-Clínic Liver Cancer (BCLC) staging system; the Chinese University Prognostic Index (CUPI score) and the Japan Integrated Staging (JIS) or bm-JIS if biomarkers are included [15]. The CUPI and CLIP scores mainly stratify patients at advanced stages; only two include prognostic variables (BCLC, CUPI) and only one allocates treatment according to specific prognostic subclasses (BCLC). The BCLC is emerging as the standard staging system for HCC in the West and has been externally validated and incorporates prognostic variables related to tumor (size, number, vascular invasion, N1, M1), liver function (Child-Pugh), and health status (ECOG-Eastern Cooperative Oncology Group Performance Status). As well as incorporating variables that influence therapy such as bilirubin, portal hypertension, and presence of symptoms to assist in treatment decision making (see Figure 1).

3. Liver Transplant

LT is the treatment of choice for small multifocal HCC ≤ 3 tumors and ≤ 3 cm or a single tumor ≤ 5 cm with significant liver functional impairment. Better selection of patients has improved 5 year survival to >70% and recurrence <10%. The major limitation to LT as treatment for HCC is the scarcity of cadaveric donors and the associated waiting time that results in a 20% drop-out rate and potentially increases the risk of recurrence from extension of vascular invasion. The use of tumor size and number to try to reflect tumor biology has been successful. However, it is clear that some patients with favourable "biology" are excluded. A number of groups have tried to expand indications beyond the Milan criteria and claim to achieve similar survival rates [16, 17]. The University of California San Francisco (UCSF) criteria are probably the best known and include one tumor ≤ 6.5 cm or multiple tumors of which the largest is 4.5 cm and the sum of all diameters is ≤ 8 cm [16]. More recently the up-to-7 criteria, where the HCC scores 7 based on the sum of the largest tumor (diameter cm) and the total number of tumors, have been introduced [17]. The majority of the studies supporting extension of the Milan Criteria are based on retrospective histological analysis of the tumor burden in the explant liver and have not been validated prospectively [16–19].

Another area where the principles of the Milan Criteria have been challenged is in salvage LT. Salvage LT has been advocated by some to manage HCC within Milan Criteria after resection [20]. In selected cases, similar overall 5 year survival for salvage LT as primary LT for HCC has been achieved (provided the comparison is from time listed for LT rather than date of LT, that is, intention to treat bias). There is continuing debate regarding whether previous resection compromises the subsequent LT [21]. Other groups have found salvage LT to have a high operative mortality, 23.5% versus 2.1% for primary LT, higher recurrence rates, and poorer overall 5 year survival of 41% [22]. Salvage LT remains controversial at a time of a limited resource with tumor characteristics, background liver (cirrhotic or noncirrhotic), and centre experience appearing to be the main determinants of recurrence and survival.

An alternative strategy to expanding the criteria for LT is to downstage to within Milan Criteria aiming to achieve patient survival and recurrence free survival rates similar to those treated at an earlier stage. This is distinct from bridging therapy. Bridging therapy is utilised to maintain the tumor within listing criteria while a suitable graft is awaited for on the waiting list. Bridging therapy is a widely accepted practice whereas downstaging for LT is not [23, 24]. To be eligible for downstaging locoregional therapy, there should be no radiological evidence of vascular invasion. There is no consensus limit to tumor number or size [25]. Predictors of downstaging failure are tumors with an infiltrative pattern [26] and an AFP > 1000 ng/mL [27]. There is evidence to suggest that downstaging of HCC to within Milan Criteria can produce reasonable results [25, 27]. But the data is difficult to interpret as the studies utilise different inclusion criteria (tumor size and number), locoregional therapies either individually or in combination, and endpoints. Current published data reveal that after downstaging, surgical resection rates vary widely between 7% and 18% producing 5 year survival rates of between 25% and 57% [28] and LT rates range between 24% and 90%, with an intention to treat post HCC treatment survival of between 60% and 70% at 3 years [27, 29, 30].

Living donor LT (LDLT) is a good graft option for HCC as it allows neoadjuvant treatment to be organized around a LT. It provides a high-quality graft and removes a competing HCC recipient from the waiting list. But higher recurrence rates and reduced survival have been reported when compared to cadaveric LT [31–33]. Explanations for this observation include growth factors released from the regenerating liver may stimulate cancer cell growth. The shorter waiting time for LDLT may remove the observation period that occurs on the waiting list to assess tumor biology and a 3 month cooling off period has been advocated before undertaking LDLT. Surgical oncological clearance may also be compromised as the IVC has to be preserved for LDLT

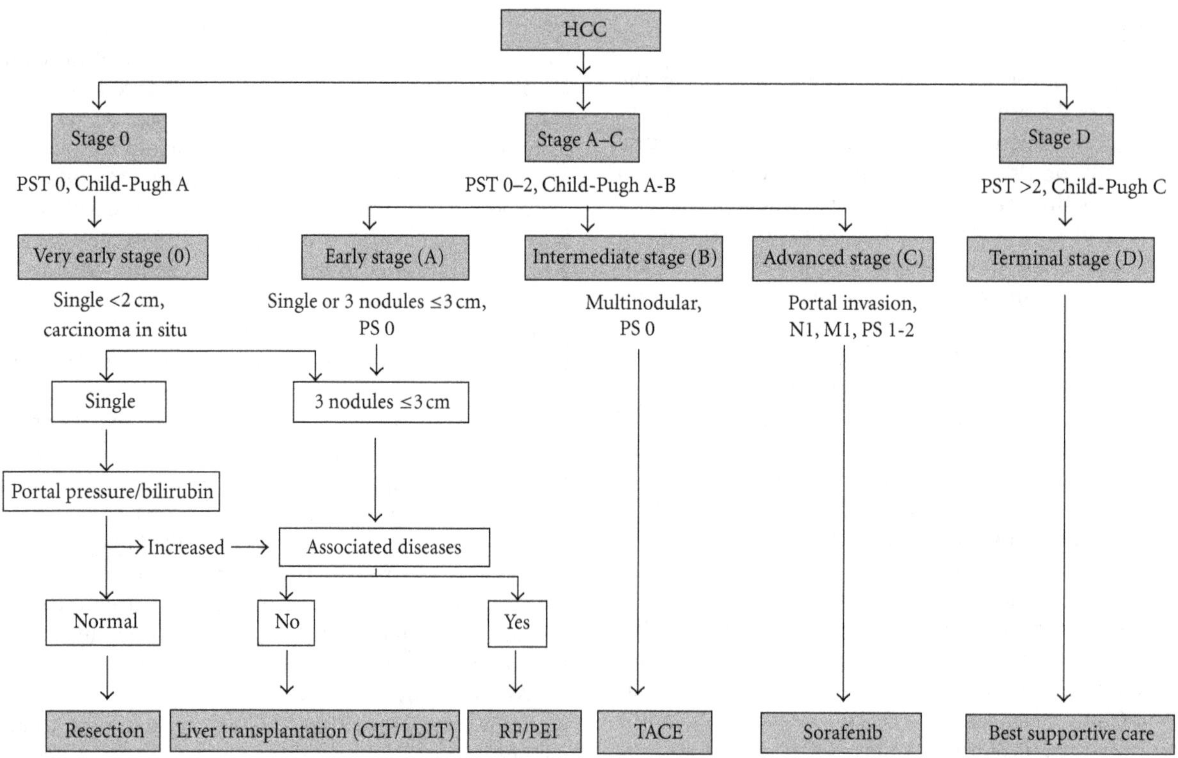

Figure 1: The Barcelona-Clínic Liver Cancer (BCLC) staging system for HCC. M: metastasis classification; N: node classification; PST: performance status; RFA: radiofrequency ablation; TACE: transarterial chemoembolization.

[34]. In addition, an element of institutional bias may lead to LDLT in HCC with a higher risk of recurrence. On multivariate analysis of published studies on LDLT versus cadaveric LT, graft type, and waiting time have not been found to be significant risk factors for recurrence post LT. If LDLT is undertaken for HCC outside regional criteria and the graft fails retransplantation with cadaveric LT is ethically contentious [35]. The donor risk and the degree of benefit to the recipient needed to justify LDLT for advanced HCC are still undetermined and for now many centres have adopted the same criteria/therapeutic goals for LDLT as cadaveric LT [36].

4. Liver Resection

Resection is the treatment of choice in noncirrhotics. Noncirrhotic HCC accounts for 5% of cases in the West and 40% of cases in Asia. Patients with cirrhosis suitable for resection need preserved liver function and a hepatic venous pressure gradient ≤10 mmHg. Anatomic resection is advocated by some as being more preferable to nonanatomic, as it is thought to produce better outcome by eliminating intrahepatic metastases in the related portal vein tributary [37]. In patients with cirrhosis selected on liver functional status, the main predictors for survival are tumor size, multiplicity, and vascular invasion. Five-year survival for tumors ≤2 cm, 2–5 cm, and >5 cm are 66%, 52%, and 37%, respectively. For single tumors the 5 year survival is 57% and for multiple 26% but some centres are achieving >50% in multiple HCC within the Milan Criteria but otherwise are not suitable for LT [38]. Recurrence remains problematic occurring in 70% at 5 years; true recurrence/intrahepatic metastases generally occur within 2 years of resection; if greater than 2 years it is generally regarded as a de novo tumor or late recurrence [39]. At present there is no evidence that neoadjuvant/adjuvant therapy has any efficacy in reducing recurrence after resection [40]. Downstaging locoregional therapy can be employed to facilitate resection in disease which is initially regarded as unresectable and can achieve reasonable outcome, with 5 year survivals of 25–67%, with the possibility of cure [28]. Preoperative portal vein embolisation can be employed to increase future remnant liver volume to allow more extensive resections to be undertaken but the complication rate in cirrhotics is 10–20% and its effectiveness in this patient group is not fully established [41]. A laparoscopic approach to resection in cirrhotics has been proposed by some to reduce the operative insult and the risk of decompensation [42].

5. Locoregional Therapy: Ablation, TACE, and Radiation

There are a number of different locoregional strategies available or being developed but the largest experience is with transarterial chemoembolization (TACE) and radiofrequency ablation (RFA). Percutaneous ethanol injection (PEI) was the first chemical ablative technique utilised. When applied to small tumors <2 cm PEI produces 90% necroses and a 5-year survival of 47–53% but is limited by high recurrence rates of approximately 40%. Chemical ablation has now been superseded by thermal techniques such as radiofrequency ablation (RFA). RFA is the most well-studied alternative to PEI producing better local tumor control with a 2 year recurrence of 2–18% and a 5 year survival of 40–70% or better when the treatment groups have been selected [43]. Meta-analyses of randomised control trials have confirmed that RFA is a more effective way to obtain local tumor control and survival benefit compared to PEI, establishing it as a standard locoregional treatment [44, 45].

RFA can be performed percutaneously, laparoscopically, or at open surgery depending on tumor location [46, 47]. RFA is effective for early small HCC <3 cm when resection or LT are not feasible [48–51], whereas larger tumors may be inadequately treated. Overall 10–25% of tumors will not be suitable for RFA because of location such as subcapsular, adjacent to the gall bladder or major vessels which increases the risk of complication and inadequate ablation because of heat sink. The recurrence rate after RFA for selected early small HCC can be comparable to that of surgery [50, 51]. In highly selected HCC < 2 cm RFA has the potential to be curative with a rate of complete response approaching 97% and a 5 year survival of 68%. However, randomised control trials of RFA against resection for small HCC < 3 cm have failed to show that RFA is as effective as resection but the majority of studies were underpowered or had incomplete follow up [49, 52]. Increasingly, RFA is being considered as an alternative initial "curative" treatment option for small centrally placed HCC as it offers the advantages of preserving parenchyma, potentially removes competition from the transplant waiting list and based on location, effective tumor necrosis can be obtained [43, 48].

Solitary HCC > 3 cm but <5 cm RFA becomes less effective. But when TACE followed by RFA for this size tumor is applied, the therapeutic effect of RFA is significantly increased and reduces tumor progression rate to 6% compared to 39% for RFA alone [53]. In larger HCC > 5 cm outside LT criteria or not suitable for resection, ablative strategies may not work in a predictable manner. TACE also has inconsistent results and no advantage has been demonstrated by combining therapies [54]. When RFA is not suitable either because of tumor location or size, novel thermal or nonthermal ablative techniques may overcome the limits of RFA. Promising thermal ablative strategies include microwave producing large areas of ablation with less heat sink and high intensity focused US (HIFU) that can be used in patients with ascites. Alternative non thermal ablative techniques of interest include irreversible electroporation (IE). Ablative technology is improving and further experience will determine its applicability. In assessing the effectiveness of ablation radiologically, the widely used RECIST (the response evaluation criteria in solid tumours) has limitations as it includes both necrotic and viable tumor areas [55] and the modified RECIST that includes the assessment of viable tumor showing uptake in the arterial phase is more reliable.

Based on a meta-analysis TACE is emerging as the standard of care for asymptomatic HCC outside Milan criteria [56], demonstrating improved survival compared to best supportive care. A partial response of 15–55% can be observed producing a survival benefit, increasing median survival time from 16 months to 20 months with 49% survival at 2 years [56]. But individually the studies did not clearly demonstrate a benefit, mainly because of heterogenous patient study groups and varying TACE techniques. This implies that good results with TACE are achieved when it is used on a selective basis. Generally TACE is not suitable in decompensated liver disease where there is ascites or jaundice to the avoid major complications and minimize treatment related deaths to less than 2% [57]. For optimal results TACE needs to be as selective as possible, producing sustained and high localised concentrations within the tumor minimizing systemic exposure. Alternative ways to be delivering chemotherapy instead of the standard ethiodized oil (lipiodol) suspensions are drug-eluting beads [58]. In the PRECISION V trial [59], a randomized control trial, comparing drug-eluting beads with doxorubicin to conventional TACE with doxorubicin found it was better tolerated, with reduced liver toxicity and improved treatment response. Owing to the improved safety and tolerance drug-eluting beads could be applicable in higher risk patient groups. Further ways of optimising the therapeutic benefit of TACE is by combining with systemic drugs. Using agents that target the angiogenic pathways that are switched on by the local hypoxia produced by TACE is being evaluated [45]. Generally, if there is no response after two TACE sessions, alternative treatment strategies should be considered, which in the majority will be systemic therapy. In highly selected patients consideration should be given to combination of treatments such as ablation/radioembolization.

Advanced HCC that is symptomatic, exhibiting vascular invasion and/or has extrahepatic disease have a short median survival of 6 months with 25% surviving a year [60]. Systemics are often the only treatment option for palliation but there is a subset that benefit from locoregional therapy such as where vascular invasion is limited to a venous branch receiving intra-arterial therapies such as TACE [61] or radioembolization [62]. Radioembolization using yttrium-90 (90Y) labelled microspheres a beta emitter, appears promising, and may also be effective as a precursor to radical therapy with outcomes similar to TACE [30, 63] and Sorafenib [64]. There is a need to be aware of intestinal and lung shunting which may provoke serious complications. There is a minimal embolic effect so when there is main portal vein involvement and TACE is contraindicated radioembolization with yttrium may be a good option. In the absence of portal vein involvement radioembolization in Child A survival is 15.5 months, Child B is 13 months, with a portal vein involvement survival of both Child A + B being 5.6 months [65] with 25–50% response rates [64].

Cyberknife is a new stereotactic body radiation therapy (SBRT) or stereotactic ablative radiotherapy (SABR) in combination with a robotic system that tracks the tumor during respiration and is able to deliver high dose radiation accurately sparing adjacent normal tissue in a small number of fractions. A number of studies in HCC not suitable for standard locoregional treatment or resection have reported promising results. In HCC < 100 ml progression free survival rates at 6 months, 1 year, and 3 years of 83%, 72%, and 68% respectively, with overall survival at 1 year, and 3 years of 92.9% and 58.6% have been reported. It also has utility as local salvage treatment after TACE achieving local control in 95% [66]. To this date no serious SBRT related toxicities being reported [67–69] but it is not clear whether it can be applied to patients with more severe liver diseases as its threshold for tolerance is not defined.

6. Systemic Therapies: Antiviral Therapy, Immunosuppression, Biologicals, and Chemotherapy

Worldwide 78% of HCC are viral related with 53% attributed to HBV and 25% to HCV [70]. Risk of HCC recurrence after treatment is increased with progression of active hepatitis and fibrosis. Antiviral therapy is used as an adjuvant treatment with the aim to reduce viral load and fibrosis with the aim of halting progression of viral induced liver disease and reducing the risk of further HCC developing. Hepatitis B (HBV) infection increases the risk of HCC recurrence particularly for the patient who is HBeAg + and/or has a high serum HBV DNA level [71, 72]. Treatment with nucleoside analogues entecavir or tenofovir suppresses HBV DNA levels improving liver function in decompensated liver disease and may reduce the risk of HCC development over time [73]. HBV antiviral therapy reduces risk of recurrence by 41% and overall mortality by 73%, mainly because death from liver failure is reduced by 77% [74]. Use of longterm lamivudine treatment resistance can occur in 70% over 5 years has given way to alternative nucleoside analogues such as entecavir, telbivudine, and nucleotide analogues such as tenofovir but longterm data is lacking for their effect on reducing HCC recurrence.

Chronic infection with HCV appears to increase the rate of HCC development in a similar way to HBV. The risk does not change with genotype (G) but a recent meta-analysis suggests that HCV G1b maybe more at risk of HCC transformation [75]. Meta-analysis of adjuvant alpha IFN shows reduction in HCC recurrence and mortality in curatively ablated viral hepatitis related HCC. Individually these studies report no effect. Antiviral potency and the ability to produce a sustained viral response (SVR) in HCV appear to be associated with reducing the risk of HCC recurrence [76]. More longterm data is needed from the newer protease inhibitors (boceprevir, telaprevir) to determine whether the higher SVR they are able to produce translates into lower risk of HCC longterm.

Immunosuppressive agents compound malignant behaviour as immune surveillance for cancer cells is impaired. Mammalian target of rapamycin (mTOR) inhibitors, for example, Sirolimus is an exception to this rule. mTOR is overexpressed in approximately 2/3 of HCC making it an attractive therapeutic target [77]. To establish whether the immunosuppressive regime affects recurrence rates, data from the SiLVER Study is awaited. The SiLVER Study is a randomised multicenter clinical trial comparing Sirolimus containing to a mTOR inhibitor free immunosuppressive regimes. The study consists of a 3-year enrolment period and a 5-year followup. At present, there is little evidence on whether the immunosuppression regime should be completely changed to a mTOR inhibitor or whether these agents should be added to the preexisting immunosuppressive regime when recurrent HCC presents post LT [35, 78, 79]. CNI exposure should be minimised as there is evidence that this reduces the risk of tumor recurrence long term [80].

HCC is an unique chemoresistant tumor and until 2007 no systemic drug was recommended for its management. In the early 1990s, a number of randomised controlled studies assessed the role of adjuvant chemotherapy but no benefit or efficacy was demonstrated. Multiple agents have been assessed but doxorubicin, an anthracycline, has been most rigorously studied [81, 82]. The main patient groups that should be considered for adjuvant chemotherapy are those being transplanted for extended criteria or have a high risk of recurrence based on the explant pathology. As patients selected for LT should be at low risk of recurrence the majority will not gain any benefit from routine adjuvant chemotherapy.

Since 2007 Sorafenib, an oral tyrosine kinase inhibitor, has become the standard of care. Based upon the SHARP study that demonstrated Sorafenib improved median survival from 7.9 months to 10.7 months and slowed time to progression from 2.8 to 5.5 months [83]. It is well tolerated with diarrhoea in 8-9% and hand-foot skin reaction in 8–16%, with side effects leading to its discontinuation in 15%. Sorafenib is regarded as the standard therapy for metastatic disease and for HCC progressing despite optimal locoregional therapy [84]. A number of ongoing studies are establishing Sorafenib's adjuvant role in resection, local ablation (Sorafenib as Adjuvant Treatment in the Prevention of Recurrence of Hepatocellular Carcinoma (STORM)), and TACE. Additionally, a phase 1 study is being undertaken in high-risk patients post-LT that on explant are outside Milan criteria with microvascular or macrovascular invasion or histologically poorly differentiated HCC. At present there is no evidence of increased toxicity in LT recipients and Sorafenib can produce a response based on published case reports [85, 86]. Other biological agents entering phase 2 or 3 trials for HCC include EGFR (erlotinib) and VEGFR/FGFR (brivanib) tyrosine kinase inhibitors [87].

7. Conclusions

Management of HCC continues to evolve and interventional radiology in the form of TACE ± RFA increasingly dominates management either as a bridge to LT or to downstage facilitating LT or resection. As locoregional therapy technology advances patients that can be considered either for palliation or potential cure will increase. Criteria for LT listing need to become more sophisticated by incorporating tumor biology in decision making, presently inferred from clinical behaviour but in the future by the use of molecular markers. This will facilitate stratification and individualization of HCC treatment. Ultimately, the aim of LT, irrespective of disease etiology is to give the maximum benefit from a limited organ pool.

References

[1] H. B. El-Serag and A. C. Mason, "Rising incidence of hepatocellular carcinoma in the United States," *The New England Journal of Medicine*, vol. 340, no. 10, pp. 745–750, 1999.

[2] F. X. Bosch, J. Ribes, M. Díaz, and R. Cléries, "Primary liver cancer: worldwide incidence and trends," *Gastroenterology*, vol. 127, supplement 1, pp. S5–S16, 2004.

[3] H. B. El-Serag and K. L. Rudolph, "Hepatocellular carcinoma: epidemiology and molecular carcinogenesis," *Gastroenterology*, vol. 132, no. 7, pp. 2557–2576, 2007.

[4] D. Samuel, M. Colombo, H. El-Serag, R. Sobesky, and N. Heaton, "Toward optimizing the indications for orthotopic liver transplantation in hepatocellular carcinoma," *Liver Transplantation*, vol. 17, supplement 2, pp. S6–S13, 2011.

[5] V. Santi, F. Trevisani, A. Gramenzi et al., "Semiannual surveillance is superior to annual surveillance for the detection of early hepatocellular carcinoma and patient survival," *Journal of Hepatology*, vol. 53, no. 2, pp. 291–297, 2010.

[6] J. M. Llovet, J. Fuster, and J. Bruix, "Intention-to-treat analysis of surgical treatment for early hepatocellular carcinoma: resection versus transplantation," *Hepatology*, vol. 30, no. 6, pp. 1434–1440, 1999.

[7] D. Franco, L. Capussotti, C. Smadja et al., "Resection of hepatocellular carcinomas. Reults in 72 European patients with cirrhosis," *Gastroenterology*, vol. 98, no. 3, pp. 733–738, 1990.

[8] S. Okada, K. Shimada, J. Yamamoto et al., "Predictive factors for postoperative recurrence of hepatocellular carcinoma," *Gastroenterology*, vol. 106, no. 6, pp. 1618–1624, 1994.

[9] M. Minagawa, M. Makuuchi, T. Takayama, and N. Kokudo, "Selection criteria for repeat hepatectomy in patients with recurrent hepatocellular carcinoma," *Annals of Surgery*, vol. 238, no. 5, pp. 703–710, 2003.

[10] R. T. P. Poon, S. T. Fan, C. M. Lo, C. L. Liu, and J. Wong, "Intrahepatic recurrence after curative resection of hepatocellular carcinoma: long-term results of treatment and prognostic factors," *Annals of Surgery*, vol. 229, no. 2, pp. 216–222, 1999.

[11] J. G. O'Grady, R. J. Polson, K. Rolles, R. Y. Calne, and R. Williams, "Liver transplantation for malignant disease," *Annals of Surgery*, vol. 207, no. 4, pp. 373–379, 1988.

[12] B. Ringe, R. Pichlmayr, C. Wittekind, and G. Tusch, "Surgical treatment of hepatocellular carcinoma: experience with liver resection and transplantation in 198 patients," *World Journal of Surgery*, vol. 15, no. 2, pp. 270–285, 1991.

[13] P. Moreno, E. Jaurrieta, J. Figueras et al., "Orthotopic liver transplantation: treatment of choice in cirrhotic patients with hepatocellular carcinoma?" *Transplantation Proceedings*, vol. 27, no. 4, pp. 2296–2298, 1995.

[14] V. Mazzaferro, E. Regalia, R. Doci et al., "Liver transplantation for the treatment of small hepatocellular carcinomas in patients with cirrhosis," *The New England Journal of Medicine*, vol. 334, no. 11, pp. 693–699, 1996.

[15] K. M. Olthoff, A. Forner, S. Hübscher, and J. Fung, "What is the best staging system for hepatocellular carcinoma in the setting of liver transplantation?" *Liver Transplantation*, vol. 17, supplement 2, pp. S26–S33, 2011.

[16] F. Y. Yao, L. Ferrell, N. M. Bass et al., "Liver transplantation for hepatocellular carcinoma: expansion of the tumor size limits does not adversely impact survival," *Hepatology*, vol. 33, no. 6, pp. 1394–1403, 2001.

[17] V. Mazzaferro, J. M. Llovet, R. Miceli et al., "Predicting survival after liver transplantation in patients with hepatocellular carcinoma beyond the Milan criteria: a retrospective, exploratory analysis," *The Lancet Oncology*, vol. 10, no. 1, pp. 35–43, 2009.

[18] S. Roayaie, J. S. Frischer, S. H. Emre et al., "Long-term results with multimodal adjuvant therapy and liver transplantation for the treatment of hepatocellular carcinomas larger than 5 centimeters," *Annals of Surgery*, vol. 235, no. 4, pp. 533–539, 2002.

[19] N. M. Kneteman, J. Oberholzer, M. Al Saghier et al., "Sirolimus-based immunosuppression for liver transplantation in the presence of extended criteria for hepatocellular carcinoma," *Liver Transplantation*, vol. 10, no. 10, pp. 1301–1311, 2004.

[20] P. E. Majno, F. P. Sarasin, G. Mentha, and A. Hadengue, "Primary liver resection and salvage transplantation or primary liver transplantation in patients with single, small hepatocellular carcinoma and preserved liver function: an outcome-oriented decision analysis," *Hepatology*, vol. 31, no. 4, pp. 899–906, 2000.

[21] D. Fuks, S. Dokmak, V. Paradis, M. Diouf, F. Durand, and J. Belghiti, "Benefit of initial resection of hepatocellular carcinoma followed by transplantation in case of recurrence: an intention-to-treat analysis," *Hepatology*, vol. 55, no. 1, pp. 132–140, 2012.

[22] R. Adam, D. Azoulay, D. Castaing et al., "Liver resection as a bridge to transplantation for hepatocellular carcinoma on cirrhosis: a reasonable strategy?" *Annals of Surgery*, vol. 238, no. 4, pp. 508–519, 2003.

[23] P. E. Majno, R. Adam, H. Bismuth et al., "Influence of preoperative transarterial lipiodol chemoembolization on resection and transplantation for hepatocellular carcinoma in patients with cirrhosis," *Annals of Surgery*, vol. 226, no. 6, pp. 688–703, 1997.

[24] I. W. Graziadei, H. Sandmueller, P. Waldenberger et al., "Chemoembolization followed by liver transplantation for hepatocellular carcinoma impedes tumor progression while on the waiting list and leads to excellent outcome," *Liver Transplantation*, vol. 9, no. 6, pp. 557–563, 2003.

[25] F. Y. Yao, S. Breitenstein, C. E. Broelsch et al., "Does a patient qualify for liver transplantation after the down-staging of hepatocellular carcinoma?" *Liver Transplantation*, vol. 17, supplement 2, pp. S109–S116, 2011.

[26] O. Barakat, R. P. Wood, C. F. Ozaki et al., "Morphological features of advanced hepatocellular carcinoma as a predictor of downstaging and liver transplantation: an intention-to-treat analysis," *Liver Transplantation*, vol. 16, no. 3, pp. 289–299, 2010.

[27] F. Y. Yao, R. K. Kerlan Jr., R. Hirose et al., "Excellent outcome following down-staging of hepatocellular carcinoma prior to liver transplantation: an intention-to-treat analysis," *Hepatology*, vol. 48, no. 3, pp. 819–827, 2008.

[28] W. Y. Lau and E. C. H. Lai, "Salvage surgery following downstaging of unresectable hepatocellular carcinoma—a strategy to increase resectability," *Annals of Surgical Oncology*, vol. 14, no. 12, pp. 3301–3309, 2007.

[29] M. Ravaioli, G. L. Grazi, F. Piscaglia et al., "Liver transplantation for hepatocellular carcinoma: results of down-staging in patients initially outside the Milan selection criteria,"

American Journal of Transplantation, vol. 8, no. 12, pp. 2547–2557, 2008.

[30] R. J. Lewandowski, L. M. Kulik, A. Riaz et al., "A comparative analysis of transarterial downstaging for hepatocellular carcinoma: chemoembolization versus radioembolization," *American Journal of Transplantation*, vol. 9, no. 8, pp. 1920–1928, 2009.

[31] L. Kulik and M. Abecassis, "Living donor liver transplantation for hepatocellular carcinoma," *Gastroenterology*, vol. 127, supplement 1, pp. S277–S282, 2004.

[32] S. Di Sandro, A. O. Slim, A. Giacomoni et al., "Living donor liver transplantation for hepatocellular carcinoma: long-term results compared with deceased donor liver transplantation," *Transplantation Proceedings*, vol. 41, no. 4, pp. 1283–1285, 2009.

[33] K. Vakili, J. J. Pomposelli, Y. L. Cheah et al., "Living donor liver transplantation for hepatocellular carcinoma: Increased recurrence but improved survival," *Liver Transplantation*, vol. 15, no. 12, pp. 1861–1866, 2009.

[34] R. S. Mangus, J. A. Fridell, R. M. Vianna, A. B. Cooper, D. T. Jones, and A. J. Tector, "Use of the piggyback hepatectomy technique in liver transplant recipients with hepatocellular carcinoma," *Transplantation*, vol. 85, no. 10, pp. 1496–1499, 2008.

[35] P. A. Clavien, M. Lesurtel, P. M. Bossuyt et al., "Recommendations for liver transplantation for hepatocellular carcinoma: an international consensus conference report," *The Lancet Oncology*, vol. 13, pp. e11–e22, 2012.

[36] P. Bhangui, E. Vibert, P. Majno et al., "Intention-to-treat analysis of liver transplantation for hepatocellular carcinoma: living versus deceased donor transplantation," *Hepatology*, vol. 53, no. 5, pp. 1570–1579, 2011.

[37] J. Chen, K. Huang, J. Wu et al., "Survival after anatomic resection versus nonanatomic resection for hepatocellular carcinoma: a meta-analysis," *Digestive Diseases and Sciences*, vol. 56, no. 6, pp. 1626–1633, 2011.

[38] R. T. P. Poon, S. T. Fan, C. M. Lo et al., "Extended hepatic resection for hepatocellular carcinoma in patients with cirrhosis: is it justified?" *Annals of Surgery*, vol. 236, no. 5, pp. 602–611, 2002.

[39] H. Imamura, Y. Matsuyama, E. Tanaka et al., "Risk factors contributing to early and late phase intrahepatic recurrence of hepatocellular carcinoma after hepatectomy," *Journal of Hepatology*, vol. 38, no. 2, pp. 200–207, 2003.

[40] M. Samuel, P. K. Chow, E. Chan Shih-Yen, D. Machin, and K. C. Soo, "Neoadjuvant and adjuvant therapy for surgical resection of hepatocellular carcinoma," *Cochrane Database of Systematic Reviews*, no. 1, article CD001199, 2009.

[41] A. Abulkhir, P. Limongelli, A. J. Healey et al., "Preoperative portal vein embolization for major liver resection: a meta-analysis," *Annals of Surgery*, vol. 247, no. 1, pp. 49–57, 2008.

[42] K. P. Croome and M. H. Yamashita, "Laparoscopic vs open hepatic resection for benign and malignant tumors: an updated meta-analysis," *Archives of Surgery*, vol. 145, no. 11, pp. 1109–1118, 2010.

[43] T. Livraghi, F. Meloni, M. Di Stasi et al., "Sustained complete response and complications rates after radiofrequency ablation of very early hepatocellular carcinoma in cirrhosis: is resection still the treatment of choice?" *Hepatology*, vol. 47, no. 1, pp. 82–89, 2008.

[44] Y. K. Cho, J. K. Kim, M. Y. Kim, H. Rhim, and J. K. Han, "Systematic review of randomized trials for hepatocellular carcinoma treated with percutaneous ablation therapies," *Hepatology*, vol. 49, no. 2, pp. 453–459, 2009.

[45] R. Lencioni, "Loco-regional treatment of hepatocellular carcinoma," *Hepatology*, vol. 52, no. 2, pp. 762–773, 2010.

[46] S. Tanaka, M. Shimada, K. Shirabe et al., "Surgical radiofrequency ablation for treatment of hepatocellular carcinoma: an endoscopic or open approach," *Hepato-Gastroenterology*, vol. 56, no. 93, pp. 1169–1173, 2009.

[47] F. Di Benedetto, G. Tarantino, R. Montalti et al., "Laparoscopic radiofrequency ablation in the caudate lobe for hepatocellular carcinoma before liver transplantation," *Journal of Laparoendoscopic & Advanced Surgical Techniques*, vol. 22, no. 4, pp. 400–402, 2012.

[48] Y. K. Cho, J. K. Kim, W. T. Kim, and J. W. Chung, "Hepatic resection versus radiofrequency ablation for very early stage hepatocellular carcinoma: a markov model analysis," *Hepatology*, vol. 51, no. 4, pp. 1284–1290, 2010.

[49] M. S. Chen, J. Q. Li, Y. Zheng et al., "A prospective randomized trial comparing percutaneous local ablative therapy and partial hepatectomy for small hepatocellular carcinoma," *Annals of Surgery*, vol. 243, no. 3, pp. 321–328, 2006.

[50] C. Cammà, V. Di Marco, A. Orlando et al., "Treatment of hepatocellular carcinoma in compensated cirrhosis with radiofrequency thermal ablation (RFTA): a prospective study," *Journal of Hepatology*, vol. 42, no. 4, pp. 535–540, 2005.

[51] R. Tateishi, S. Shiina, T. Teratani et al., "Percutaneous radiofrequency ablation for hepatocellular carcinoma: an analysis of 1000 cases," *Cancer*, vol. 103, no. 6, pp. 1201–1209, 2005.

[52] J. Huang, L. Yan, Z. Cheng et al., "A randomized trial comparing radiofrequency ablation and surgical resection for HCC conforming to the Milan criteria," *Annals of Surgery*, vol. 252, no. 6, pp. 903–912, 2010.

[53] M. Morimoto, K. Numata, M. Kondou, A. Nozaki, S. Morita, and K. Tanaka, "Midterm outcomes in patients with intermediate-sized hepatocellular carcinoma: a randomized controlled trial for determining the efficacy of radiofrequency ablation combined with transcatheter arterial chemoembolization," *Cancer*, vol. 116, no. 23, pp. 5452–5460, 2010.

[54] A. Veltri, P. Moretto, A. Doriguzzi, E. Pagano, G. Carrara, and G. Gandini, "Radiofrequency thermal ablation (RFA) after transarterial chemoembolization (TACE) as a combined therapy for unresectable non-early hepatocellular carcinoma (HCC)," *European Radiology*, vol. 16, no. 3, pp. 661–669, 2006.

[55] A. Forner, C. Ayuso, M. Varela et al., "Evaluation of tumor response after locoregional therapies in hepatocellular carcinoma: are response evaluation criteria in solid tumors reliable?" *Cancer*, vol. 115, no. 3, pp. 616–623, 2009.

[56] J. M. Llovet and J. Bruix, "Systematic review of randomized trials for unresectable hepatocellular carcinoma: chemoembolization improves survival," *Hepatology*, vol. 37, no. 2, pp. 429–442, 2003.

[57] J. L. Raoul, B. Sangro, A. Forner et al., "Evolving strategies for the management of intermediate-stage hepatocellular carcinoma: available evidence and expert opinion on the use of transarterial chemoembolization," *Cancer Treatment Reviews*, vol. 37, no. 3, pp. 212–220, 2011.

[58] M. Varela, M. I. Real, M. Burrel et al., "Chemoembolization of hepatocellular carcinoma with drug eluting beads: efficacy and doxorubicin pharmacokinetics," *Journal of Hepatology*, vol. 46, no. 3, pp. 474–481, 2007.

[59] J. Lammer, K. Malagari, T. Vogl et al., "Prospective randomized study of doxorubicin-eluting-bead embolization in the treatment of hepatocellular carcinoma: results of the PRECISION v study," *CardioVascular and Interventional Radiology*, vol. 33, no. 1, pp. 41–52, 2010.

[60] G. Cabibbo, M. Enea, M. Attanasio, J. Bruix, A. Craxì, and C. Cammá, "A meta-analysis of survival rates of untreated patients in randomized clinical trials of hepatocellular carcinoma," *Hepatology*, vol. 51, no. 4, pp. 1274–1283, 2010.

[61] J. Luo, R. P. Guo, E. C. H. Lai et al., "Transarterial chemoembolization for unresectable hepatocellular carcinoma with portal vein tumor thrombosis: a prospective comparative study," *Annals of Surgical Oncology*, vol. 18, no. 2, pp. 413–420, 2011.

[62] L. M. Kulik, B. I. Carr, M. F. Mulcahy et al., "Safety and efficacy of 90Y radiotherapy for hepatocellular carcinoma with and without portal vein thrombosis," *Hepatology*, vol. 47, no. 1, pp. 71–81, 2008.

[63] L. M. Kulik, B. Atassi, L. van Holsbeeck et al., "Yttrium-90 microspheres (TheraSphere) treatment of unresectable hepatocellular carcinoma: downstaging to resection, RFA and bridge to transplantation," *Journal of Surgical Oncology*, vol. 94, no. 7, pp. 572–586, 2006.

[64] B. Sangro, M. Iñarrairaegui, and J. I. Bilbao, "Radioembolization for hepatocellular carcinoma," *Journal of Hepatology*, vol. 56, no. 2, pp. 464–473, 2012.

[65] R. Salem, R. J. Lewandowski, L. Kulik et al., "Radioembolization results in longer time-to-progression and reduced toxicity compared with chemoembolization in patients with hepatocellular carcinoma," *Gastroenterology*, vol. 140, no. 2, pp. 497–507, 2011.

[66] J. K. Kang, M. S. Kim, C. K. Cho et al., "Stereotactic body radiation therapy for inoperable hepatocellular carcinoma as a local salvage treatment after incomplete transarterial chemoembolization," *Cancer*, vol. 118, no. 21, pp. 5424–5431, 2012.

[67] A. Takeda, M. Takahashi, E. Kunieda et al., "Hypofractionated stereotactic radiotherapy with and without transarterial chemoembolization for small hepatocellular carcinoma not eligible for other ablation therapies: preliminary results for efficacy and toxicity," *Hepatology Research*, vol. 38, no. 1, pp. 60–69, 2008.

[68] R. V. Tse, M. Hawkins, G. Lockwood et al., "Phase I study of individualized stereotactic body radiotherapy for hepatocellular carcinoma and intrahepatic cholangiocarcinoma," *Journal of Clinical Oncology*, vol. 26, no. 4, pp. 657–664, 2008.

[69] J. H. Kwon, S. H. Bae, J. Y. Kim et al., "Long-term effect of stereotactic body radiation therapy for primary hepatocellular carcinoma ineligible for local ablation therapy or surgical resection. Stereotactic radiotherapy for liver cancer," *BMC Cancer*, vol. 10, article 475, 2010.

[70] J. F. Perz, G. L. Armstrong, L. A. Farrington, Y. J. F. Hutin, and B. P. Bell, "The contributions of hepatitis B virus and hepatitis C virus infections to cirrhosis and primary liver cancer worldwide," *Journal of Hepatology*, vol. 45, no. 4, pp. 529–538, 2006.

[71] H. I. Yang, S. N. Lu, Y. F. Liaw et al., "Hepatitis B e antigen and the risk of hepatocellular carcinoma," *The New England Journal of Medicine*, vol. 347, pp. 168–174, 2002.

[72] H. L. Y. Chan, C. H. Tse, F. Mo et al., "High viral load and hepatitis B virus subgenotype Ce are associated with increased risk of hepatocellular carcinoma," *Journal of Clinical Oncology*, vol. 26, no. 2, pp. 177–182, 2008.

[73] Y. F. Liaw, J. J. Sung, W. C. Chow et al., "Lamivudine for patients with chronic hepatitis B and advanced liver disease," *The New England Journal of Medicine*, vol. 351, pp. 1521–1531, 2004.

[74] J. S. W. Wong, G. L. H. Wong, K. K. F. Tsoi et al., "Meta-analysis: the efficacy of anti-viral therapy in prevention of recurrence after curative treatment of chronic hepatitis B-related hepatocellular carcinoma," *Alimentary Pharmacology and Therapeutics*, vol. 33, no. 10, pp. 1104–1112, 2011.

[75] S. Raimondi, S. Bruno, M. U. Mondelli, and P. Maisonneuve, "Hepatitis C virus genotype 1b as a risk factor for hepatocellular carcinoma development: a meta-analysis," *Journal of Hepatology*, vol. 50, no. 6, pp. 1142–1154, 2009.

[76] L. T. Chen, M. F. Chen, L. A. Li et al., "Long-term results of a randomized, observation-controlled, phase III trial of adjuvant interferon Alfa-2b in hepatocellular carcinoma after curative resection," *Annals of Surgery*, vol. 255, no. 1, pp. 8–17, 2012.

[77] F. Sahin, R. Kannangai, O. Adegbola, J. Wang, G. Su, and M. Torbenson, "mTOR and P70 S6 kinase expression in primary liver neoplasms," *Clinical Cancer Research*, vol. 10, no. 24, pp. 8421–8425, 2004.

[78] A. Valdivieso, J. Bustamante, M. Gastaca et al., "Management of hepatocellular carcinoma recurrence after liver transplantation," *Transplantation Proceedings*, vol. 42, no. 2, pp. 660–662, 2010.

[79] J. M. Alamo, L. Barrera, M. D. Casado et al., "Efficacy, tolerance, and safety of mammalian target of rapamycin inhibitors as rescue immunosuppressants in liver transplantation," *Transplantation Proceedings*, vol. 41, no. 6, pp. 2181–2183, 2009.

[80] M. Vivarelli, A. Dazzi, M. Zanello et al., "Effect of different immunosuppressive schedules on recurrence-free survival after liver transplantation for hepatocellular carcinoma," *Transplantation*, vol. 89, no. 2, pp. 227–231, 2010.

[81] G. Söderdahl, L. Bäckman, H. Isoniemi et al., "A prospective, randomized, multi-centre trial of systemic adjuvant chemotherapy versus no additional treatment in liver transplantation for hepatocellular carcinoma," *Transplant International*, vol. 19, no. 4, pp. 288–294, 2006.

[82] H. Pokorny, M. Gnant, S. Rasoul-Rockenschaub et al., "Does additional doxorubicin chemotherapy improve outcome in patients with hepatocellular carcinoma treated by liver transplantation?" *American Journal of Transplantation*, vol. 5, no. 4, pp. 788–794, 2005.

[83] J. M. Llovet, S. Ricci, V. Mazzaferro et al., "Sorafenib in advanced hepatocellular carcinoma," *The New England Journal of Medicine*, vol. 359, no. 4, pp. 378–390, 2008.

[84] European Association for the Study of the Liver and European Organisation for Research and Treatment of Cancer, "EASL-EORTC clinical practice guidelines: management of hepatocellular carcinoma," *Journal of Hepatology*, vol. 56, no. 4, pp. 908–943, 2012.

[85] R. Kim, G. El-Gazzaz, A. Tan et al., "Safety and feasibility of using sorafenib in recurrent hepatocellular carcinoma after orthotopic liver transplantation," *Oncology*, vol. 79, no. 1-2, pp. 62–66, 2010.

[86] M. Yeganeh, R. S. Finn, and S. Saab, "Apparent remission of a solitary metastatic pulmonary lesion in a liver transplant recipient treated with sorafenib," *American Journal of Transplantation*, vol. 9, no. 12, pp. 2851–2854, 2009.

[87] A. Villanueva and J. M. Llovet, "Targeted therapies for hepatocellular carcinoma," *Gastroenterology*, vol. 140, no. 5, pp. 1410–1426, 2011.

17

Debakey Forceps Crushing Technique for Hepatic Parenchymal Transection in Liver Surgery: A Review of 100 Cases and Ergonomic Advantages

Sundeep Jain,[1] Bharat Sharma,[2] Mitesh Kaushik,[1] and Lokendra Jain[1]

[1] *Department of Gastrointestinal Hepatopancreatobiliary Minimal Access & Bariatric Surgery, Fortis Escorts Hospital, Jawahar Lal Nehru Marg, Malviya Nagar, Jaipur, Rajasthan 302017, India*
[2] *Department of General & Minimal Access Surgery, Soni Manipal Hospital, Sikar Road, Vidhyadhar Nagar, Jaipur, Rajasthan 302013, India*

Correspondence should be addressed to Sundeep Jain; drsundeepjain@yahoo.co.in

Academic Editor: Christos G. Dervenis

Introduction and Objective. Bleeding is an important complication in liver transections. To determine the safety and efficacy of Debakey forceps for liver parenchymal transection and its ergonomic advantages over clamp crushing method we analysed our data. *Methods.* We used Debakey crushing technique in 100 liver resections and analysed data for transection time, transfusion rate, morbidity, mortality, hospital stay, influence of different types of liver conditions, and ergonomi features of Debakey forceps. *Results.* Mean age, transection time and hospital stay of 100 patients were 52.38 ± 17.44 years, 63.36 ± 33.4 minutes, and 10.27 ± 5.7 days. Transection time, and hospital stay in patients with cirrhotic liver (130.4 ± 44.4 mins, 14.6 ± 5.5 days) and cholestatic liver (75.8 ± 19.7 mins, 16.5 ± 5.1 days) were significantly greater than in patients with normal liver (48.1 ± 20.1 mins, 6.7 ± 1.8 days) ($P < 0.01$). Transection time improved significantly with experience (first fifty versus second fifty cases—70.2 ± 31.1 mins versus 56.5 ± 34.5 mins, $P < 0.04$). Qualitative evaluation revealed that Debakey forceps had ergonomic advantages over Kelly clamp. *Conclusions.* Debakey forceps crushing technique is safe and effective for liver parenchymal transection in all kinds of liver. Transection time improves with surgeon's experience. It has ergonomic advantages over Kelly clamp and is a better choice for liver transection.

1. Introduction

Prevention of blood loss is a major concern during liver resections as it is the major determinant of operative outcome. Bleeding along with bile leak and hepatic failure is one of the major postoperative complications following liver resection [1–3]. Most blood loss occurs during the parenchymal transection of liver. Many methods have been introduced to achieve safe parenchymal transection. In 1958 Lin et al. introduced the finger fracture technique which involves crushing of liver parenchyma by surgeon's finger under inflow occlusion so as to isolate vessels and bile ducts for ligation [4]. This technique was subsequently improved through the use of small Kelly clamp for blunt dissection which gives better control, namely, clamp crushing or Kellyclasia [5–7]. People have also used finer versions of clamps similar to Kelly like Pean, Halstead, Heiss, or Bengolea clamps [6, 8].

Recently, many devices have been introduced for parenchymal transection. These include ultrasonic dissector, harmonic scalpel, LigaSure, dissecting sealer using radiofrequency, and staplers [9–11]. However, the clamp crushing technique is the most widely used method [3, 9, 12–14] and has multiple advantages over other more advanced methods including safety, speed, and cost-effectiveness [9].

Thumb forceps including Debakey forceps has significant advantages in terms of its design and ergonomics over Kelly clamp which were reported previously when compared for their usage for diathermy [15]. But so far its use in liver parenchymal transection has not been tried or reported in literature.

TABLE 1: Indications of liver resection in the study.

Indications	Numbers
Gallbladder cancer	32
Secondaries liver	15 (colorectal-11, GIST-04)
Hydatid disease	11
Hilar cholangiocarcinoma	09
Hemangioma	09
Hepatocellular carcinoma	08 (Child's A status)
Hepatoblastoma	04
Neuroendocrine tumor	02
Intrahepatic cholangiocarcinoma	02
FNH	02
Hamartoma	02
Recurrent pyogenic cholangitis	01
Hemangioendothelioma	01
Cancer hepatic flexure with local invasion of liver	01
Strictured hepaticojejunostomy with atrophy of right lobe liver with recurrent cholangitis	01
Total	**100**

TABLE 2: Types of liver resections.

Type of resection	Numbers
Right hemihepatectomy	19
Right hemihepatectomy with segment I resection	08
Left hemihepatectomy	09
Left hemihepatectomy with segment I resection	01
Right trisectionectomy	11
Left lateral sectionectomy	09
Segment IVb V resection	08
Segments IV, V, and VI resection	01
Segments V, VI, and VII resection	02
Segments V and VI resection	02
Segment III resection	01
Segment V resection	01
Segment VI resection	01
Wedge resection for gallbladder cancer	13
Right posterior sectionectomy	02
Cystopericystectomy	10
Nonanatomical resection	02
Total	**100**

We have been using Debakey forceps for liver transections in all our liver resections for the past 8 years. The purpose of this study is to present our experience of 100 consecutive elective liver resections with Debakey forceps crushing technique. We compared the outcome after liver transection on different types of liver parenchyma—normal livers, cirrhotic livers, postchemotherapy livers, and cholestatic livers. We also highlight its ergonomic advantages over clamp crushing method. To the best of our knowledge this is the first such study reporting the usage of Debakey forceps for hepatic parenchymal transection.

2. Methods

This is a retrospective study of prospectively collected data of consecutive liver resections. During the period of January 2006 to October 2013 we performed a total of 146 liver resections in three hospitals under supervision of the main author (Sundeep Jain). Of these 46 were performed in emergency setting (trauma—$n = 44$; liver necrosis—$n = 2$) and excluded from the present study. Data of remaining 100 patients are presented (Table 1). Types of liver resection, according to Brisbane terminology [16], in these 100 patients are presented in Table 2.

These patients were classified in 4 groups according to the type of underlying liver parenchyma into group A—normal liver; group B—cirrhotic liver; group C—postchemotherapy liver; and group D—cholestatic liver. These four groups were compared in terms of age, gender, comorbid conditions, transection time, total operative time, postoperative length of hospital stay, blood transfusion rates, morbidity, and mortality to evaluate the effect of type of liver parenchyma with use of Debakey forceps crushing technique for liver parenchyma transection.

The first 50 (group 1) and the last 50 (group 2) were compared to evaluate the duration of transection time, total operative time, and postoperative length of hospital stay.

2.1. Qualitative Ergonomic Evaluation. The design along with mechanism of functioning of Debakey forceps and Kelly clamps was studied and compared using photographs taken during operation. This was to ascertain the advantages of one over the other in terms of ease of usage and the versatility of the instruments. Also the ergonomic differences in the wrist joint were studied, with the help of photographs while using Debakey forceps and Kelly clamps for liver parenchymal transection.

2.2. Anaesthesia Details. All the patients were induced with fentanyl 2 μgm/kg and propofol 2-3 mg/kg of body weight and intubated with atracurium 0.5 mg/kg of body weight. Maintenance of anaesthesia was achieved using sevoflurane in an air-oxygen mixture with supplemental fentanyl. After induction, central venous catheterization was done uniformly in right internal jugular vein for central venous pressure (CVP) monitoring with the aim of keeping CVP less than 5 mmHg and as close to 0 mmHg as possible, during parenchymal transection. This was achieved by fluid restriction and diuretics (frusemide) in 0.5–1 mg/kg IV dose. In 8/100 patients we had to use nitroglycerine to reduce CVP to the desired levels. During this phase urine output and mean arterial pressures were maintained at more than 0.5 mL/kg/hr and more than 70 mmHg, respectively. This was done by 100–200 mL bolus fluid challenge and norepinephrine infusion at 0.05–0.1 μgm/kg/min. During the low CVP stage patients were kept in head-low position to prevent the risk of air embolism. Euvolemia was finally achieved after transection and hemostasis were completed.

After the surgery all patients are reversed with neostigmine 40–80 μgm/kg along with glycopyrrolate 10 μgm/kg.

2.3. Surgical Details. All the patients with malignant conditions initially had staging laparoscopy. The abdomen was explored by either bilateral subcostal or triradiate incisions depending on the site and size of the lesion. The falciform ligament was then divided and the lobe to be resected was mobilized from surrounding attachments and structures like diaphragm and vena cava. Only in two patients (both with hepatocellular carcinoma) undergoing right hemihepatectomy, Pringle's manoeuvre was used to facilitate removal of associated portal vein tumour thrombus in one and due to excessive bleeding in another. In all patients during parenchymal transection low central venous pressure (0–5 mmHg) with head-low position was maintained.

The liver parenchymal transection was started with the marking of the line of resection using monopolar electrocautery followed by cutting the parenchyma for 2–4 mm deep. Then the parenchyma was crushed using fine tip (1 mm), 8 cm long straight or 9 cm long angled Debakey forceps depending on the depth of transection followed by coagulation of the small vessels of <2 mm size using monopolar electrocautery and ligation of the biliary and larger vascular pedicles using 2-0/3-0 silk sutures. Lastly, the biliary duct was isolated and divided in appropriate cases. Once the specimen was out the haemostasis was achieved using spray cautery and fine (3-0/4-0) prolene sutures. The bile leaks were looked for and suture ligated. The Roux-en-y bilioenteric anastomosis was done with the bile ducts of the remaining lobe wherever indicated. Prophylactic drains were placed in all the patients.

2.4. Statistical Analyses. Descriptive statistics are presented. All the data were computerised and analysed using STATA 11 statistical software. Intergroup comparisons were performed using Group A as control. Numerical variables have been compared using t-test and categorical variables using Chi-square test. P value <0.05 is considered statistically significant.

3. Results

During the study period of January 2006 to October 2013 a total of 100 elective liver resections were performed for various indications using Debakey thumb forceps for the liver parenchymal transection. There were 39 females and 61 males with a mean age of 52.4 ± 17 years. Indications and the type of liver resections performed are mentioned in Tables 1 and 2. Various comorbidities included hypertension ($n = 11$), diabetes ($n = 8$), and chronic obstructive pulmonary disease (COPD) ($n = 5$), while none had coronary artery disease. Group B had 8 patients, group C had 14 patients, and group D had 25 patients while normal liver parenchyma was in 53 patients.

Majority of patients underwent liver resection for malignant diseases ($n = 73$). Of these 14 (19%) had undergone preoperative chemotherapy (hepatoblastoma 3, gastrointestinal stromal tumor 4, and colorectal cancers 7). Obstructive jaundice was in 25/100 patients (12 gallbladder cancer, 9 hilar cholangiocarcinoma, and 1 each of hydatid disease, recurrent pyogenic cholangitis and strictured hepaticojejunostomy with right lobe atrophy and recurrent cholangitis). Seven of these 25 (gallbladder cancer 4, hilar cholangiocarcinoma 2, and hydatid cyst 1) had plastic stent placed in the common bile duct. Roux-en-y bilioenteric anastomosis was done in 22/25 patients. All the eight patients of hepatocellular carcinoma (HCC) had cirrhosis of liver due to alcohol in two, hepatitis B virus in four, and hepatitis C virus in two patients. All of these were in Child's A status without any history of decompensation in the past. None of them were under consideration for transplant. Pringle's manoeuvre was used in two patients, both with HCC (alcoholic & hepatitis C related cirrhosis).

The mean age, transection time, total operative time, and postoperative length of hospital stay of 100 patients were 52.4 ± 17.4 years, 63.4 ± 33.4 mins, 154.11 ± 67.6 mins, and 10.3 ± 5.7 days. The age difference of patients in all four groups (divided on the basis of type of liver parenchyma) was not statistically significant (Table 3). Patients of group A (normal liver parenchyma) had significantly less transection time in comparison to group B (cirrhotic livers) and group D (cholestatic livers), while it did not reach statistical difference when compared with group C (postchemotherapy livers) patients, though there was a trend towards lesser transection time in group A. This may be due to less number of patients in group C. The total operative time was significantly less in group A patients in comparison to group B, C, and D patients. Also group A patients had significantly less postoperative hospital stay in comparison with group B, C, and D patients. These results show that type of liver parenchyma affects the transection time, total operative time, and postoperative recovery as reflected by the postoperative hospital stay (Table 4).

Also it was found that the transection time and total operative time in Group 1 (first 50 patients) were significantly more than in Group 2 (second 50 patients), signifying the effect of surgeon's experience on it. Though, the postoperative hospital stay was similar in both these groups (Table 5).

Total 11/100 (11%) patients needed perioperative blood transfusions, with the range of 2–4 units per case. These included 1 patient of hydatid disease, 2 of secondaries liver, 1 of hilar cholangiocarcinoma, 3 of gallbladder cancer, 3 of HCC, and 1 patient of hepatoblastoma. Total 14/100 (14%) patients developed 22 postoperative complications (Table 6). Four patients had bile leak, ten had ascites, and five had wound infections.

Bile leak occurred in each patient after left hemihepatectomy for hydatid, right trisectionectomy for gallbladder cancer, right hemihepatectomy with segment I resection for hilar cholangiocarcinoma, and cystopericystectomy for hydatid cyst, with daily amount of 50 mL, 100 mL, 90 mL, and 20 mL, respectively. All but cystopericystectomy patient had preoperative biliary stent placement for obstructive jaundice.

TABLE 3: Baseline characteristics in different groups.

Characteristics	Group A (control) $N = 53$	Group B (cirrhosis) $N = 8$	Group C (CT) $N = 14$	Group D (cholestatic) $N = 25$
Sex				
Male (%)	24 (45.28)	8 (100)	9 (64.29)	20 (80)
Female (%)	29 (54.72)	0 (0.00)	5 (35.71)	5 (20)
Underlying diseases (%)				
Hypertension	7 (13.21)	3 (37.50)	1 (7.14)	0
DM	4 (7.55)	2 (25.00)	0	2 (8.00)
COPD	1 (1.89)	3 (37.50)	0	1 (4.00)
CAD	0	0	0	0

Control: normal liver parenchyma.
CT: postchemotherapy.
Cholestatic: obstructive jaundice.
DM: diabetes mellitus.
COPD: chronic obstructive pulmonary disease.
CAD: coronary artery disease.

TABLE 4: Comparison of age, transection time, total operative time, and postoperative hospital stay between four groups.

Characteristics	Group A (control) $N = 53$	Group B (cirrhosis) $N = 8$	Group C (CT) $N = 14$	Group D (cholestatic) $N = 25$	A versus B P value	A versus C P value	A versus D P value
Age (years)							
(Mean ± SD)	48.94 ± 16.27	57.25 ± 11.38	48.46 ± 22.93	47.32 ± 13.69	0.91	0.59	0.44
(Range)	23–85	40–70	4–71	25–77			
Transection time (minutes)							
(Mean ± SD)	48.09 ± 20.07	130.38 ± 44.38	60.64 ± 32.81	75.8 ± 19.72			
(Median, IQR)	48, 21	145, 69.5	52.5, 64	69, 18	0.00	0.07	0.00
(Range)	22–117	62–180	25–115	35–120			
Total operative time (minutes)							
(Mean ± SD)	110.41 ± 35.30	226.6 ± 57.8	145.21±52.91	228.52 ± 43.20			
(Median, IQR)	100, 32	218, 98.5	142.5, 94	209, 62	0.00	0.004	0.00
(Range)	68–252	150–310	75–230	152–308			
Hospital stay (days)							
(Mean ± SD)	6.72 ± 1.85	14.62 ± 5.50	10.07 ± 5.50	16.52 ± 5.11			
(Median, IQR)	7, 3	14.5, 5	9, 414	16, 6	0.00	0.0004	0.00
(Range)	4–11	8–26	4–27	9–29			

Control: normal liver parenchyma.
CT: postchemotherapy.
Cholestatic: obstructive jaundice.

In all these patients it stopped conservatively in 9, 5, 6, and 2 days, respectively.

Ascites was seen in 5 HCC patients, 4 gallbladder cancer patients (with jaundice), and 1 cholangiocarcinoma (with jaundice) patient, with the hospital stay ranging from 15 to 26 days. It was managed successfully by fluid restriction, diuretics, bed rest, and low-salt diet.

All patients with wound infections had preoperative biliary stent placement. All of these had Gram-negative organisms and were successfully managed conservatively with dressings and antibiotics based on cultures of bile taken during surgery.

There were three mortalities due to hepatic encephalopathy, liver failure, and disseminated intravascular coagulation (DIC) in patients with HCC, gallbladder cancer, and hepatoblastoma, respectively.

3.1. Qualitative Ergonomic Evaluation. Debakey forceps has some differences over Kelly clamp on the basis of its design. Kelly clamp has a hinge in the middle with two finger loops which are grasped by the thump and ring finger, while the index finger helps guide the instrument. On the other hand, Debakey forceps are held between thumb and the index finger with top end resting on the first dorsal interosseous muscle at

TABLE 5: Comparison of age, transection time, total operative time, and postoperative hospital stay in the first 50 and second 50 patients.

Characteristics	Group 1 First 50 patients	Group 2 Second 50 patients	P value
Age (years)			
(Mean ± SD)	48.08 ± 15.45	52.38 ± 17.44	0.52
(Range)	4–73	4.5–85	
Transection time (minutes)			
(Mean ± SD)	70.2 ± 31.02	56.52 ± 34.54	
(Median, IQR)	65, 33	50.5, 34	0.039
(Range)	25–160	22–180	
Total operative time (minutes)			
(Mean ± SD)	168.04 ± 66.50	140.20 ± 66.40	
(Median, IQR)	155, 117	105, 100	0.038
(Range)	68–305	74–310	
Hospital stay (days)			
(Mean ± SD)	9.66 ± 5.40	10.88 ± 5.95	
(Median, IQR)	8.5, 7	8, 7	0.28
(Range)	4–29	5–27	

TABLE 6: Postoperative complications.

Complication	Type of resection	Numbers	Disease
Bile leak	Left hemihepatectomy	01	Hydatid disease
	Cystopericystectomy	01	Hydatid disease
	Right trisectionectomy	01	Gallbladder cancer
	Right hemihepatectomy plus segment I resection	01	Hilar cholangiocarcinoma
Ascites	Right trisectionectomy	04	Gallbladder cancer
	Left hemihepatectomy plus segment I	01	Hilar cholangiocarcinoma
	Right hemihepatectomy	05	HCC
Wound infection	Left hemihepatectomy	01	Hydatid disease
	Right trisectionectomy	02	Gallbladder cancer
	Right hemihepatectomy plus segment I	01	Hilar cholangiocarcinoma
	Right hemihepatectomy	01	HCC
Hepatic encephalopathy*	Right hemihepatectomy	01	HCC
Postoperative liver failure*	Right trisectionectomy	01	Gallbladder cancer
DIC*	Right hemihepatectomy	01	Hepatoblastoma

*Signifies mortality.

the base of the thumb and index finger. Spring tension at one end holds the grasping ends apart until pressure is applied. This allows one to quickly and easily grasp small tissue and to grasp and hold tissue easily with variable pressure [17]. It is less traumatic due to its fine tip and gentle enough to fracture only the liver parenchyma without injuring the ducts or vessels. Long and angled Debakey forceps with fine tip facilitates crushing in the deeper planes of liver. There is a definite sensation of tissue being crushed while using Debakey forceps, which thus helps in releasing the pressure timely thus preventing injury to vessels.

In present study, Debakey thumb forceps is found to have similar ergonomic advantages over Kelly clamp during crushing of liver parenchyma, as was reported in one study [15] when they were compared for their usage for diathermy. These advantages are that (1) a ringed handled instrument is much more difficult to pick up from a flat surface than thumb forceps like Debakey forceps as like many surgeons we like to pick them ourselves due to the involved repetitive movements of this kind, (2) the grip between the thumb and the side of the index finger for picking up thumb forceps required less accurate placing of the hand than putting the two digits through the finger loops of Kelly clamps which can be done without having to take focus away from the area of dissection, and (3) thumb forceps are held in the classical precision grip [18] in which the ulnar digits help in supporting the instrument between thumb and the index finger in addition to the apex of the thumb thus increasing the accuracy of handling, whereas the hand is unsupported while using the Kelly clamp.

Figures 1–8 (photographs) depict wrist joint postures during liver parenchyma transection while using Kelly clamp

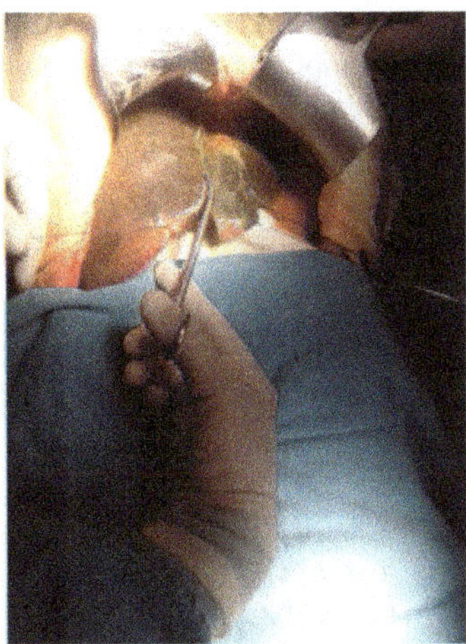

Figure 1: Abnormal posture of wrist while using Kelly clamp.

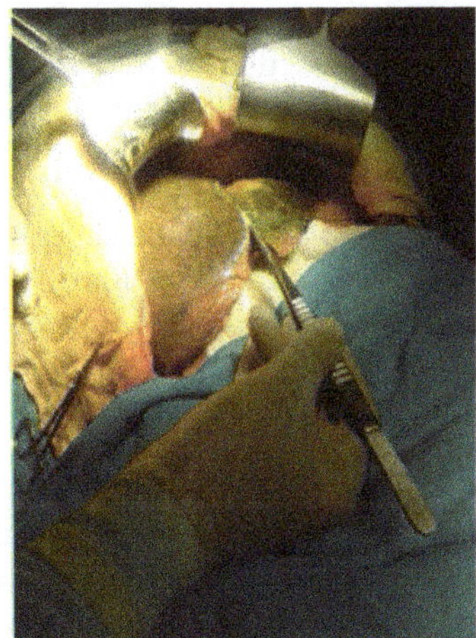

Figure 2: Neutral posture of wrist while using Debakey forceps.

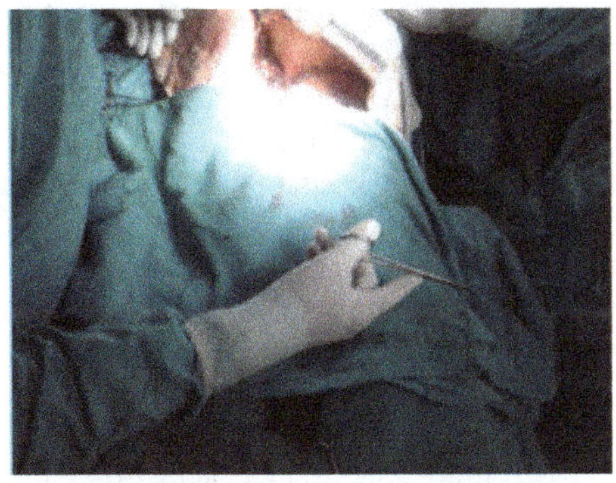

Figure 3: Position of Kelly clamp with neutral posture of wrist.

and Debakey forceps. It is clear in Figures 2, 6, 7, and 8 that the wrist joint always remains in neutral posture during liver parenchyma transection with Debakey forceps at various depths and angles. On the contrary Figures 1, 3, 4, and 5 shows that wrist joint is always in an awkward and strainful posture while using Kelly clamp for liver parenchyma transection at all the depths and angles.

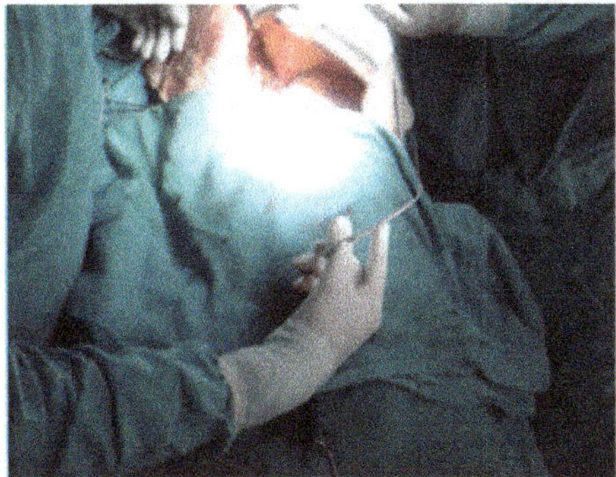

Figure 4: Position of Kelly clamp with slight flexion of wrist.

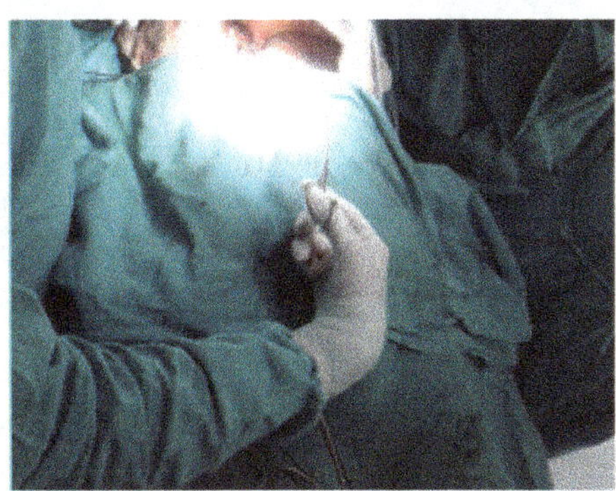

Figure 5: Functional position of Kelly clamp with awkward posture of wrist.

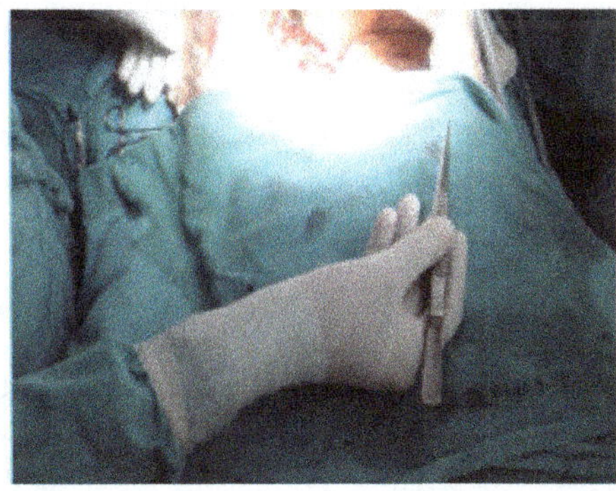

Figure 6: Position of Debakey forceps with neutral posture of wrist.

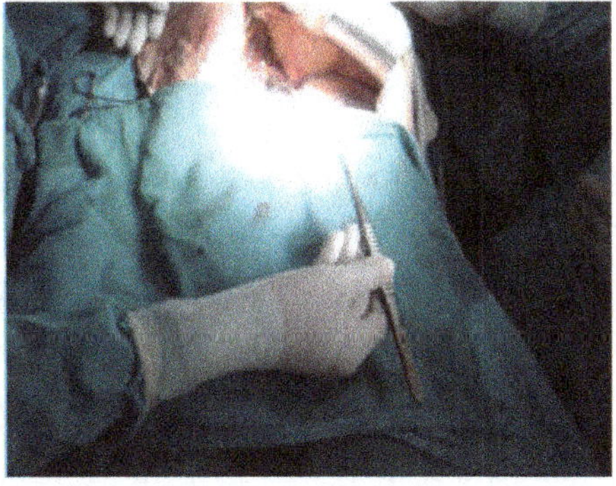

Figure 7: Inward position of Debakey forceps with neutral posture of wrist.

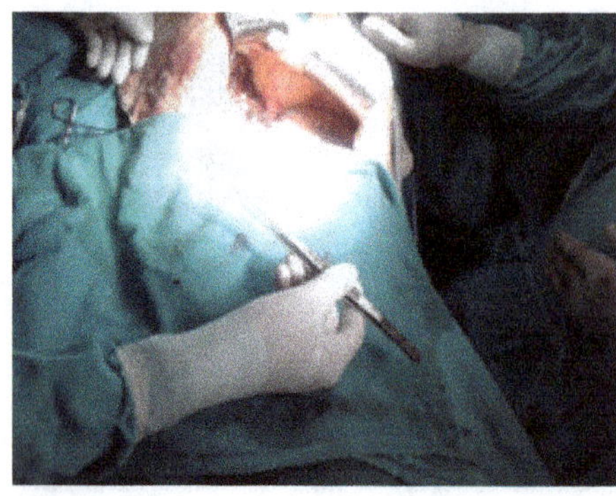

Figure 8: More inward position of Debakey forceps with neutral posture of wrist.

4. Discussion

This study shows that use of Debakey forceps crushing technique is safe and effective for liver parenchymal transection; transection time and total operative time improve with surgeon experience and it has ergonomic advantages over Kelly clamp technique.

The better understanding of liver anatomy and technical developments has helped in reducing the morbidity and mortality after liver resections [19–21]. Bleeding is the most important determinant of operative outcome after liver resection. Intraoperative blood loss with subsequent need for blood transfusion is significant risk factor for increased complication rates, poor postoperative outcomes, and shorter disease-free survival [22, 23]. Thus it is paramount to decrease the intraoperative blood loss and subsequent blood transfusions during liver resections. As most of the bleeding occurs during parenchymal transection of liver there are many methods devised from time to time to facilitate liver transection with minimal blood loss [9, 10].

Meta-analysis of 7 RCT with total 554 patients [24] has shown that there were no clinically important benefits of an alternative transection method in terms of blood loss, parenchymal injury, transection time, and hospital stay over clamp crushing method. So clamp crushing method remains the reference technique for transection of the parenchyma in elective hepatic resections. Also the 2009 Cochrane review [25] of randomized data failed to show any significant difference with regard to mortality, morbidity, and hospital stay while comparing clamp crushing technique to alternative methods. The clamp crushing avoids special equipment with similar or faster transection speed thus making it the most cost-effective technique which is 2 to 6 times cheaper than other methods depending on the number of surgeries performed each year [9, 24–28].

Our study shows that Debakey clamp is an equally effective instrument for parenchymal transection in all kinds of livers in terms of transection time and safety as is shown in previous reports using Kelly clamp technique [14]. The mean transection time in our study in normal liver was 48.1 ± 20.1 mins and it was significantly shorter than groups with patients with cirrhotic and cholestatic livers. The mean total operative time in our patients with normal liver was 110.4 ± 35.3 mins which was significantly shorter than groups with cirrhotic, postchemotherapy, and cholestatic livers.

The transfusion requirement in present study was 11% which is due to the inclusion of patients with all kinds of liver parenchyma. None of the patients with normal livers (group A) had blood transfusion which is similar to previous reports [14].

The mean postoperative length of hospital stay in subjects with normal livers was 10.3 ± 5.7 days which is similar to previous reports [9, 14, 28]. Subjects with diseased livers (groups B, C, and D) had greater hospital stay signifying the role of type of liver parenchyma on overall outcomes.

The morbidity rate in the present study is 14% (22 complications in 14 patients). Out of these 22 complications 21 have occurred in patients having cirrhotic, cholestatic, and postchemotherapy livers, while only one occurred in a patient of hydatid cyst with normal liver. The mortality in the present study is 3% with one patient each in cirrhotic, cholestatic and postchemotherapy liver groups.

All these results signify the importance of type of liver parenchyma on the transection time, total operative time, blood transfusion rates, morbidity, mortality, and postoperative hospital stay while using Debakey crush technique for liver resections.

The mean transection time and total operative time were found to be significantly more in the initial 50 cases of the total 100 cases suggesting the effect of surgeon's experience, though it did not affect the postoperative length of hospital stay (Table 5).

Technically, Debakey forceps has many advantages of Kelly clamp [14] including its efficacy and safety in all kinds of livers. It is also a cost-effective technique [25]. Ergonomically, there are two aspects which make Debakey forceps a preferred instrument compared to Kelly clamp for liver parenchymal crushing. One is the design of the instrument and the other is the posture of the wrist joint of the surgeon while operating with these instruments as described and shown above (Figures 1–8). These make Debakey forceps more useful to the operating surgeon in terms of easy handling, precise grip, ease of usage in every depth of liver resection, being less traumatic for the tissues, and giving least strain to the wrist joint by keeping it in the neutral position. This is because in neutral posture muscles are near their resting length thus making joints comfortable. For wrist joint it is neutral when forearm, wrist, and hands are all straight and in one line [29]. Awkward postures occur when wrist is in flexion or extension [30, 31]. In awkward posture muscles and ligaments of joint are either stretched or compressed. Thereby fatigue will occur more quickly, increasing the risk for injury [31].

Limitations of the present study include a nonrandomised trial design. However, this study is a single surgeon experience in consecutive cases and a large sample size with careful collection of data and is therefore important. We also performed a qualitative study of comparison of Debakey with Kelly technique and the findings are important.

In conclusion, this is the first such study showing that Debakey forceps crushing technique is as safe and effective method for liver parenchymal transection in all kinds of liver parenchyma with comparable results to Kelly clamp crushing method. It also shows that type of liver parenchyma has a significant effect on overall outcome while using Debakey crushing technique. Surgeon's experience is important. The technical and ergonomic differences between Debakey forceps and Kelly clamp, in terms of design and wrist joint posture, make Debakey forceps the preferred crushing technique for liver transection although large randomised trials are needed to confirm our findings. We therefore recommend Debakey forceps technique as the crushing method of choice for liver transection in elective liver resection operations in nontransplant setting. The ergonomic virtues of Debakey forceps should be considered while designing newer techniques and instruments for liver transection, especially in open liver resections.

Acknowledgment

The authors acknowledge inputs from Dr. Rajeev Gupta, Dr. Bhawani Mishra, and Ms. Purvi Saxena for data analyses and report writing.

References

[1] G. Gozzetti, A. Mazziotti, G. L. Grazi et al., "Liver resection without blood transfusion," *British Journal of Surgery*, vol. 82, no. 8, pp. 1105–1110, 1995.

[2] J. D. Cunningham, Y. Fong, C. Shriver, J. Melendez, W. L. Marx, and L. H. Blumgart, "One hundred consecutive hepatic resections: blood loss, transfusion, and operative technique," *Archives of Surgery*, vol. 129, no. 10, pp. 1050–1056, 1994.

[3] W. R. Jarnagin, M. Gonen, Y. Fong et al., "Improvement in perioperative outcome after hepatic resection: analysis of 1,803 consecutive cases over the past decade," *Annals of Surgery*, vol. 236, no. 4, pp. 397–407, 2002.

[4] T. Y. Lin, K. Tsu, C. Mien, and C. Chen, "Study on lobectomy of the liver," *Journal of the Formosan Medical Association*, vol. 57, pp. 742–749, 1958.

[5] H. Bismuth, "Surgical anatomy and anatomical surgery of the liver," *World Journal of Surgery*, vol. 6, no. 1, pp. 3–9, 1982.

[6] T. Y. Lin, "A simplified technique for hepatic resection: the crush method," *Annals of Surgery*, vol. 180, no. 3, pp. 285–290, 1974.

[7] T. Y. Lin, "Results in 107 hepatic lobectomies with a preliminary report on the use of a clamp to reduce blood loss," *Annals of Surgery*, vol. 177, no. 4, pp. 413–421, 1973.

[8] B. Launois, G. G. Jamieson, and T. E. Starzl, *Modern Operative Techniques in Liver Surgery*, Churchill Livingstone, Edinburgh, UK, 1st edition, 1993.

[9] M. Lesurtel, M. Selzner, H. Petrowsky, L. McCormack, and P.-A. Clavien, "How should transection of the liver be performed? A prospective randomized study in 100 consecutive patients: comparing four different transection strategies," *Annals of Surgery*, vol. 242, no. 6, pp. 814–823, 2005.

[10] R. J. Aragon and N. L. Solomon, "Techniques of hepatic resection," *Journal of Gastrointestinal Oncology*, vol. 3, pp. 28–40, 2012.

[11] P. Schemmer, H. Friess, U. Hinz et al., "Stapler hepatectomy is a safe dissection technique: analysis of 300 patients," *World Journal of Surgery*, vol. 30, no. 3, pp. 419–430, 2006.

[12] H. Imamura, Y. Seyama, N. Kokudo et al., "One thousand fifty-six hepatectomies without mortality in 8 years," *Archives of Surgery*, vol. 138, no. 11, pp. 1198–1206, 2003.

[13] H. C. Sun, L. X. Qin, L. Lu et al., "Randomized clinical trial of the effects of abdominal drainage after elective hepatectomy using the crushing clamp method," *British Journal of Surgery*, vol. 93, pp. 422–466, 2006.

[14] K. H. Kim and S. G. Lee, "Usefulness of Kelly clamp crushing technique during hepatic resection," *HPB*, vol. 10, no. 4, pp. 281–284, 2008.

[15] M. Patkin, "Ergonomics of diathermy forceps design," *Medical Journal of Australia*, vol. 2, no. 13, pp. 657–660, 1971.

[16] S. M. Strasberg, "Nomenclature of hepatic anatomy and resections: a review of the Brisbane 2000 system," *Journal of Hepato-Biliary-Pancreatic Surgery*, vol. 12, no. 5, pp. 351–355, 2005.

[17] R. P. Carlisle, *Scientific American Inventions and Discoveries: All the MilesTones in Ingenuity—From the Discovery of Fire to the Invention of the Microwave Oven*, John Wiley & Sons, New York, NY, USA, 2004.

[18] M. Patkin, "Ergonomic aspects of surgical dexterity," *Medical Journal of Australia*, vol. 2, no. 17, pp. 775–777, 1967.

[19] M. Rees, G. Plant, J. Wells, and S. Bygrave, "One hundred and fifty hepatic resections: evolution of technique towards bloodless surgery," *British Journal of Surgery*, vol. 83, no. 11, pp. 1526–1529, 1996.

[20] R. Doci, L. Gennari, P. Bignami et al., "Morbidity and mortality after hepatic resection of metastases from colorectal cancer," *British Journal of Surgery*, vol. 82, no. 3, pp. 377–381, 1995.

[21] J. Belghiti, K. Hiramatsu, S. Benoist, P. P. Massault, A. Sauvanet, and O. Farges, "Seven hundred forty-seven hepatectomies in the 1990s: an update to evaluate the actual risk of liver resection," *Journal of the American College of Surgeons*, vol. 191, no. 1, pp. 38–46, 2000.

[22] Y. Fong, J. Fortner, R. L. Sun, M. F. Brennan, and L. H. Blumgart, "Clinical score for predicting recurrence after hepatic resection for metastatic colorectal cancer: analysis of 1001 consecutive cases," *Annals of Surgery*, vol. 230, no. 3, pp. 309–321, 1999.

[23] C. B. Rosen, D. M. Nagorney, H. F. Taswell et al., "Perioperative blood transfusion and determinants of survival after liver resection for metastatic colorectal carcinoma," *Annals of Surgery*, vol. 216, no. 4, pp. 493–505, 1992.

[24] N. N. Rahbari, M. Koch, T. Schmidt et al., "Meta-analysis of the clamp-crushing technique for transection of the parenchyma in elective hepatic resection: back to where we started?" *Annals of Surgical Oncology*, vol. 16, no. 3, pp. 630–639, 2009.

[25] K. S. Gurusamy, V. Pamecha, D. Sharma, and B. R. Davidson, "Techniques for liver parenchymal transection in liver resection," *Cochrane Database of Systematic Reviews*, no. 1, Article ID CD006880, 2009.

[26] H. G. Rau, M. W. Wichmann, S. Schinkel et al., "Surgical techniques in hepatic resections: ultrasonic aspirator versus jet-cutter. A prospective randomized clinical trial," *Zentralblatt fur Chirurgie*, vol. 126, no. 8, pp. 586–590, 2001.

[27] Y. Sakamoto, J. Yamamoto, N. Kokudo et al., "Bloodless liver resection using the monopolar floating ball plus ligature

diathermy: preliminary results of 16 liver resections," *World Journal of Surgery*, vol. 28, no. 2, pp. 166–172, 2004.

[28] T. Takayama, M. Makuuchi, K. Kubota et al., "Randomized comparison of ultrasonic versus clamp transection of the liver," *Archives of Surgery*, vol. 136, no. 8, pp. 922–928, 2001.

[29] N. Warren and T. F. Morse, "Neutral posture," University of Connecticut Health Center, ErgoCenter, Farmington, Conn, USA, 2008, http://www.oehc.uchc.edu/ergo_neutralposture.asp.

[30] P. J. Keir, J. M. Bach, M. Hudes, and D. M. Rempel, "Guidelines for wrist posture based on carpal tunnel pressure thresholds," *Human Factors*, vol. 49, no. 1, pp. 88–99, 2007.

[31] D. Chaffin, G. B. J. Andersson, and B. J. Martin, *Occupational Biomechanics*, John Wiley & Sons, New York, NY, USA, 4th edition, 2006.

18

Mediastinal Pseudocyst: Varied Presentations and Management—Experience from a Tertiary Referral Care Centre in India

Durairaj Segamalai, Abdul Rehman Abdul Jameel, Naveen Kannan, Amudhan Anbalagan, Benet Duraisamy, Prabhakaran Raju, and Kannan Devy Gounder

Institute of Surgical Gastroenterology, Madras Medical College, Chennai 600003, India

Correspondence should be addressed to Kannan Devy Gounder; malarkan08@gmail.com

Academic Editor: Richard Charnley

Pseudocysts are a recognised complication following acute or chronic pancreatitis. Usually located in peripancreatic areas, they have also been reported to occur in atypical regions like liver, pelvis, spleen, and mediastinum. Mediastinal pseudocysts are a rare entity and present with myriad of symptoms due to their unique location. They are a clinical challenge to diagnose and manage. In this paper, we describe the clinical and radiological characteristics of mediastinal pseudocysts in 7 of our patients, as well as our experience in managing these patients along with their clinical outcome.

1. Introduction

Pancreatic pseudocysts are common findings in patients with acute or chronic pancreatitis, usually located in peripancreatic areas. Mediastinal pseudocyst is rare and often reported as case reports, exact incidence being unknown [1]. Pancreatic ductal disruption due to inflammatory injury leads to leakage of amylase rich pancreatic secretions along the paths of least resistance. Posterior disruptions can lead to thoracopancreatic fistulae while anterior disruptions produce pancreatic ascites. Thoracopancreatic fistulas are divided into four types based on the termination site of the fistula: pancreaticopleural, mediastinal pseudocyst, pancreaticobronchial, and pancreaticopericardial. Mediastinal pseudocyst by way of its unique location can present with myriad symptoms like dysphagia, chest pain, or palpitations and in extreme cases pericardial effusion, tamponade, and respiratory distress [2]. It can be a diagnostic and therapeutic challenge. High index of suspicion is often needed in diagnosing this entity. Pancreatic ductal morphology and its communication with the pseudocyst hold the key for successful management. We present our experience in managing mediastinal pseudocysts.

2. Materials and Methods

This study is a retrospective analysis of patients diagnosed to have mediastinal pseudocyst between Jan 2010 and March 2016 at our Institute. Our Institute is a high volume tertiary referral care centre in India, where more than 200 pancreatic surgeries are performed annually for various benign and malignant disorders. We reviewed clinical records and imaging database and were able to identify 7 patients with mediastinal pseudocyst. Thorough analysis regarding their clinical symptomatology, etiology of pancreatitis, radiological features, supplementary investigations, management strategy, and their follow-up was done. Basic laboratory investigation including serum amylase, lipase, and c-reactive protein was done. All patients underwent oesophagogastroduodenoscopy (OGD), ultrasound (USG) with portal Doppler, contrast enhanced computed tomography (CT) scan of abdomen and chest, and other investigations like echocardiogram, barium swallow, and magnetic resonance cholangiopancreatography (MRCP) as required. Patient presenting with ascites or pleural effusion underwent aspiration and biochemical fluid analysis. Patients who had dysphagia were graded as per dysphagia score of Knyrim et al. [3]; grade 0 denoted the ability to eat a normal diet; 1, the ability to eat some solid food; 2, the ability to eat semisolids only; 3, the ability to swallow liquids only; and grade 4 referred to complete dysphagia. Subsequent to the definitive intervention, the patients were advised to attend the follow-up clinic at our institution after 3 months or earlier if symptomatic. All patients underwent CT chest/abdomen to document the resolution of pseudocyst and to study the disease activity after 3 months following the primary intervention. Patients were advised to review with us after 6 months thereafter, to document any complications. Follow-up of patients was for a mean of 13 months (range 10 to 18 months). We did not encounter any dropouts in our series.

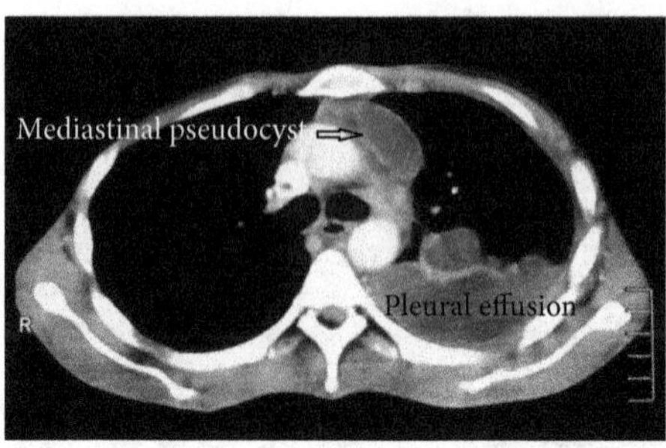

Figure 1: CT chest demonstrating mediastinal pseudocyst of size 3 cm, associated with left pleural effusion.

3. Results

The details of the patients are mentioned in Table 1. Of the 7 patients 6 were male and one was female with age ranging from 17 to 40. Our analysis reveals that chronic pancreatitis was present in 6/7 patients with mediastinal pseudocyst, with ethanol being the most common etiological factor causing chronic pancreatitis in 5/6 patients and it was idiopathic in the other patient. Acute necrotising pancreatitis was observed in one patient who had mediastinal pseudocyst.

Almost all of the patients had abdominal pain in addition to symptoms attributed to mediastinal pseudocyst like dyspnoea ($n = 3$), dysphagia ($n = 2$), chest pain ($n = 2$), and retrosternal discomfort ($n = 1$). The mean size of the mediastinal pseudocyst encountered in this series was 5.7 cm (ranging from 3 cm to 8 cm) (Figures 1 and 2). All the patients had abdominal pseudocyst. Two patients had dysphagia due to compressive effects of pseudocyst on the esophagus (Figure 3). One of the patients, who had dysphagia with considerable weight loss (>15% in 3 months), was referred to our unit as achalasia cardia on the basis of barium swallow report and he was totally relieved of his symptom following internal drainage (Figure 4). Two patients who presented with dyspnoea had severe left ventricular dysfunction, due to compressive effects on cardiac chambers (Figure 5), which improved following treatment. Pleural effusion was observed in five individuals.

We summarize our proposed treatment algorithm in Figure 6, which is based on our experience in managing such cases. We have noted in our series that mediastinal pseudocyst is invariably associated with peripancreatic pseudocyst and management directed towards the pancreatic pseudocyst leads to resolution of mediastinal component. Pancreatic ductal morphology and its communication (Figure 7) with the pseudocyst as documented by MRCP are the key parameters influencing treatment strategies. In the absence of ductal communication, ultrasound guided insertion of percutaneous catheter drains (PCDs), preferably 10–12 Fr, has been found to be helpful. From our experience, invariably multiple PCDs are required in patients with necrotic or infected collections to ensure complete resolution as they tend to block the catheters and are also not adequately drained by a single catheter. Patients with multiple ductal strictures or intraductal calculi will require a Frey's procedure to adequately drain the entire ductal system. For those with ductal communication with strictures, we advocate internal drainage in the form of cystogastrostomy or cystojejunostomy based on the anatomic proximity of the pseudocyst to the stomach wall. In our series, we performed cystogastrostomy as most of the pseudocysts were related to posterior gastric wall. We encountered pleural effusion in five patients but only two of them required insertion of intercostal drainage tube, in view of symptoms.

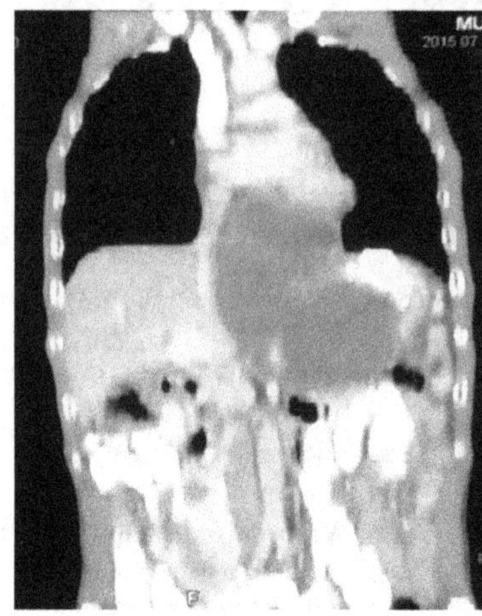

Figure 2: CT chest coronal view showing mediastinal pseudocyst of size 8 cm.

Internal drainage could also be performed by endoscopic approach, preferably with endoscopic ultrasound guidance (EUS), if expertise is available. We did not employ endoscopic approach in our series as endoscope could not be negotiated beyond oesophagogastric junction in two patients, while two patients did not require internal drainage and were managed with PCDs. One of our patients had multiple peripancreatic pseudocyst with walled-off pancreatic necrosis, for whom we felt that surgical drainage would offer better results. Endotherapy could not be considered for the patient with multiple ductal stricture associated with intraductal calculi. To summarize, internal drainage in the form of cystogastrostomy was performed in four patients, while Frey's procedure was done in one patient. Two patients were managed with multiple PCDs and intercostal drainage.

Apart from the specific management, patients were generally managed with intravenous fluids, analgesics, antiemetics, and antibiotics being initiated in those with infected

Table 1: The table shows patient demographics, presentation, clinical and radiological finding, management, and follow-up.

S. number	Age/sex	Etiology	Acute/chronic	Presenting symptoms	Size of mediastinal pseudocyst	Presence of abdominal pseudocyst	Associated complications	Management	Follow-up
1	40/M	Ethanol	Chronic	Grade 3 dysphagia[1] Weight loss Abdominal pain	5 cm	Yes Communicating with mediastinal pseudocyst	Severe OG[2] junction narrowing in barium swallow Endoscopy could not negotiate beyond oesophagogastric junction	Open cystogastrostomy	Dysphagia relieved Postop barium swallow: normal Gained weight
2	29/M	Ethanol	Acute	Dsypnoea Pain abdomen Hemoptysis, 2 weeks following intercostal drainage	8 cm	Yes 8 × 8 cm infected necrosis involving body & tail of pancreas	Pancreaticopleural fistula 40% necrosis of pancreatic body & tail Echocardiogram: severe left ventricular dysfunction EF[3] 37% Inferior phrenic & intercostal artery pseudoaneurysms	Infected necrosis was managed with 2 percutaneous drainage catheters inserted with ultrasound guidance in left subphrenic & perinephric region Intercostal drainage Angioembolisation of pseudoaneurysms	Follow-up Complete resolution of pseudocyst after 2 months Echocardiogram: EF 70%
3	31/M	Ethanol	Chronic	Abdominal pain Dsypnoea	4.5 cm	Yes Infected pseudocyst 8 × 8 cm: head and body of pancreas	Left pleural effusion Pancreatic ascites	Three PCDs inserted in left subphrenic, left perinephric region and pelvis Left intercostal drainage	2 months later, he developed splenic artery pseudoaneurysm: angioembolisation done
4	36/M	Ethanol	Chronic	Chest pain Early satiety Abdominal pain	3 cm	Yes 8 × 6 cm pseudocyst in head of pancreas	Nil	Open cystogastrostomy	Complete resolution of pseudocyst after 1 week
5	39/M	Ethanol	Chronic	Retrosternal discomfort Dsypnoea Pain abdomen	8 cm	Yes Multiple peripancreatic pseudocyst	Left pleural effusion/walled-off pancreatic necrosis Echocardiogram: severe left ventricular dysfunction EF 40%	Open cystogastrostomy, open necrosectomy, external drainage	Pseudocyst Resolved EF improved to 64%
6	33/M	Ethanol	Chronic	Chest pain Dysphagia Abdominal pain	6.5 cm	Yes. Multiple peripancreatic pseudocyst	Bilateral pleural effusion Extrinsic compression over esophagus from 34–38 cm	Open cystogastrostomy	Resolutions of symptoms
7	17/F	Idiopathic	Chronic	Abdominal pain Left sided neck pain and edema	4 cm	Yes Pseudocyst 2 × 2 cm head of pancreas Multiple parenchymal and ductal calculi	Left pleural effusion Left IJV[4]/brachiocephalic vein thrombosis	Frey's procedure	Thrombus recanalised after 6 months of anticoagulant therapy

[1]Dysphagia score cf Knyrim et al.
[2]Oesophagogastric.
[3]Ejection fraction.
[4]Internal jugular vein.

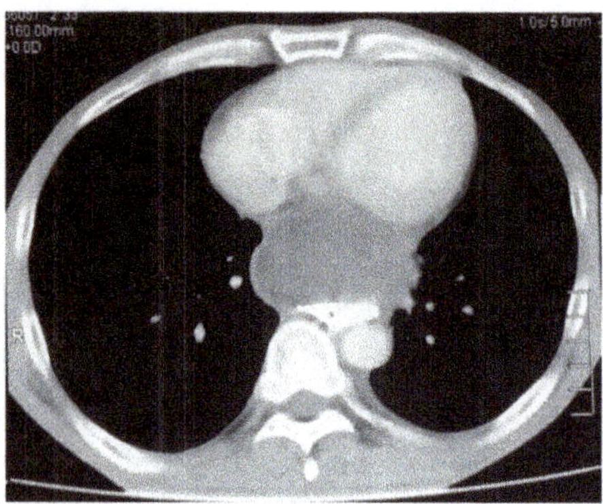

Figure 3: CT chest showing mediastinal pseudocyst compressing the esophagus.

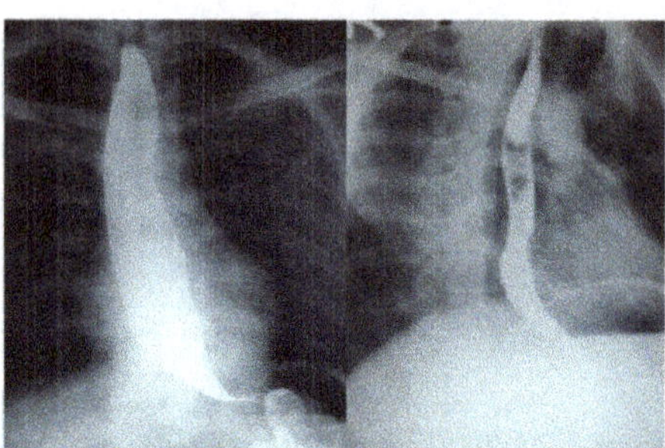

Figure 4: Barium swallow (preop and postop) demonstrating the esophageal dilatation due to mediastinal pseudocyst and resolution of compressive effects following surgery.

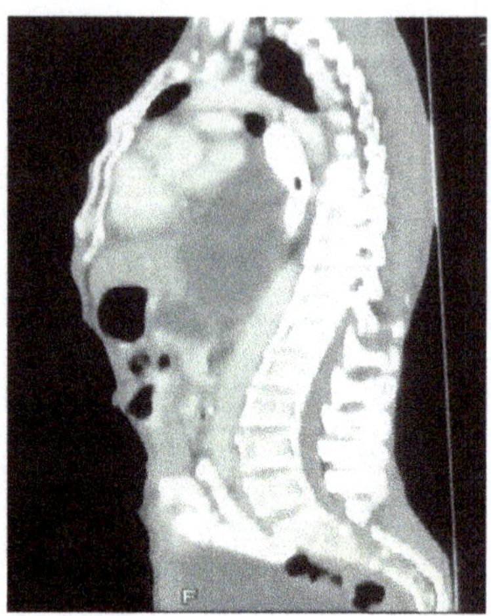

Figure 5: CT chest sagittal view demonstrating the compressive effects on cardiac chambers.

pseudocysts. Patients tolerating oral diet were encouraged to do so with low-fat diet, while those with low or no intake were put on nasojejunal feeding and total parenteral nutrition instituted when nasojejunal tube could not be placed. Our unit does not use somatostatin analogues in such patients due to lack of strong evidence in literature.

Interestingly, we noted increased incidence of vascular complications in these patients. For the patient with pancreaticopleural fistula, reported with hemoptysis 2 weeks after intercostal drainage, CT-angiogram showed multiple pseudoaneurysm involving inferior phrenic and lower intercostal arteries which was eventually managed with angioembolisation with coils (Figure 8), while another patient with infected pseudocyst developed splenic artery pseudoaneurysm in the follow-up period and required angioembolisation (Figure 9). Mediastinal pseudocyst resulted in left brachiocephalic and left internal jugular vein (IJV) thrombosis (Figure 10) in a patient who was put on anticoagulant therapy for 6 months and subsequently recanalised.

4. Discussions

Abdominal complications like pseudocyst and pancreatic necrosis are recognised complications which occur as sequelae to acute or chronic pancreatitis [4]. Mediastinal pseudocyst is a rare complication, usually detected on imaging studies performed for pancreatitis [5]. Presence of inflammation and fibrosis along the traditional peripancreatic spaces creates pathways of lesser resistance to mediastinum to form thoracopancreatic fistulas [6]. Thoracopancreatic fistulas are divided into four types based on the termination site of the fistula: pancreaticopleural, mediastinal pseudocyst, pancreaticobronchial, and pancreaticopericardial [7]. In most cases, the pseudocyst is located in the posterior mediastinum, with entry to the mediastinum via the aortic or esophageal hiatus [4].

Most patients are alcoholics with a clinical history of previous pancreatitis. The presentation is often confusing because of the paucity of clues suggestive of pancreatic disease and the preponderance of pulmonary signs and symptoms. The most common presenting symptoms are chest or abdominal pain and dyspnoea [8]. Due the mediastinal location of the pseudocyst, dysphagia occurs because of compression of the esophagus by the pseudocyst [6]. In our study, two patients had dysphagia. Since the origin of pseudocyst is a ductal disruption in the pancreas, invariably most of our patients had abdominal pain and coexistent abdominal pseudocysts.

Ultrasound is an easily available investigation to diagnose peripancreatic pseudocyst, but it is less helpful in mediastinal pseudocyst owing to its location. Computed tomography (CT) is excellent in defining pancreatic abnormalities and should be the first abdominal imaging study in suspected cases [9]. CT can also comment on the connection between the mediastinal cystic structures and the pancreas. MRI can help in delineating the communication of mediastinal pseudocysts with an abdominal pseudocyst; in addition ductal morphology like disruption, communication with pseudocyst, stricture, and dilatation are best defined by magnetic resonance cholangiopancreatography (MRCP) [5]. Endoscopic ultrasound (EUS) is an important diagnostic tool for the evaluation of mediastinal mass and cysts, and it can help in planning the optimal therapy and allow EUS guided aspiration and drainage of the cysts but is limited by availability of equipment and expertise [10].

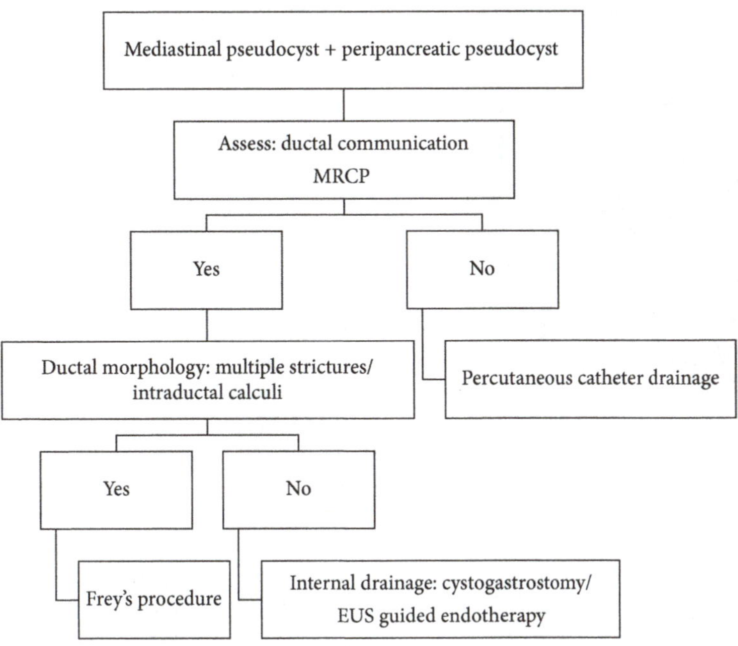

FIGURE 6: Proposed treatment algorithm for management for symptomatic mediastinal pseudocyst.

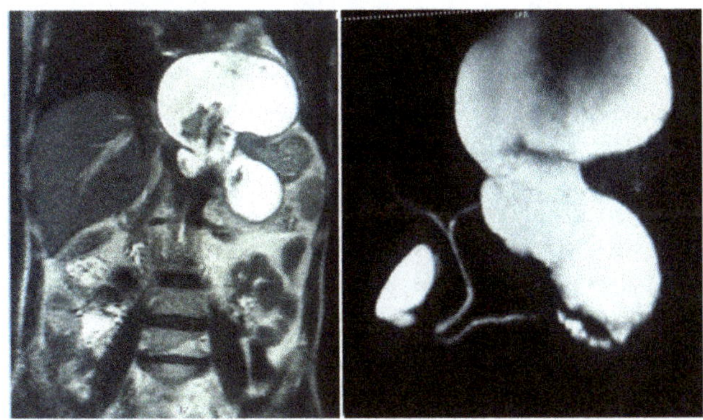

FIGURE 7: MRI abdomen showing pseudocyst involving tail of pancreas with mediastinal extension and MRCP showing ductal communication of the pseudocyst.

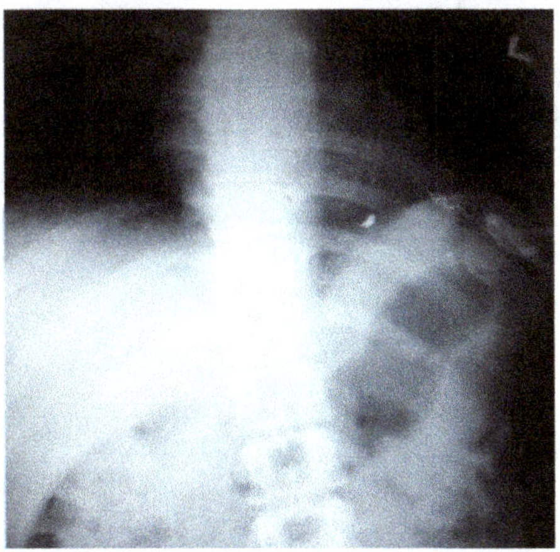

FIGURE 8: Chest X-ray demonstrating multiple coil embolization done for pseudoaneurysm of left inferior phrenic artery and multiple intercostal arteries. Note the presence of percutaneous placed catheter for drainage of peripancreatic necrosis.

The management of mediastinal pseudocysts depends on the clinical symptomatology, underlying etiology, ductal anatomy, size of the pseudocyst, and availability of expertise. Spontaneous resolution of mediastinal pseudocyst with conservative management is a rare event [11]. Endoscopic procedures have significantly influenced the management of mediastinal pseudocysts. EUS assisted endoscopic drainage through either a transoesophageal [1, 12] or transgastric approach has been described with immediate technical success in 90–95% of patients and long term success in 85–90% patients [13]. Endoscopic retrograde cholangiopancreatogram (ERCP) has been employed for transpapillary stenting of the pancreatic duct and few reports have described successful resolution of mediastinal pseudocysts with transpapillary stenting alone [12, 14]. ERCP carries with it its own set of complications, including pancreatitis, haemorrhage, duodenal perforation, and cholangitis. Complications of EUS guided cyst aspiration include perforation of the oesophagus, infection, and stricture formation [12]. The general complication rate of endoscopic management procedures for pancreatic pseudocysts is approximately 5% and pancreatic pseudocysts recur in approximately 15% of patients [15].

Surgical treatment has often been used for therapeutic management of patients with mediastinal pseudocyst and these can vary from pancreatic resections to external or internal drainage. In our study the majority of the patients were treated with surgical internal drainage like cystogastrostomy in four patients and Frey's pancreaticojejunostomy

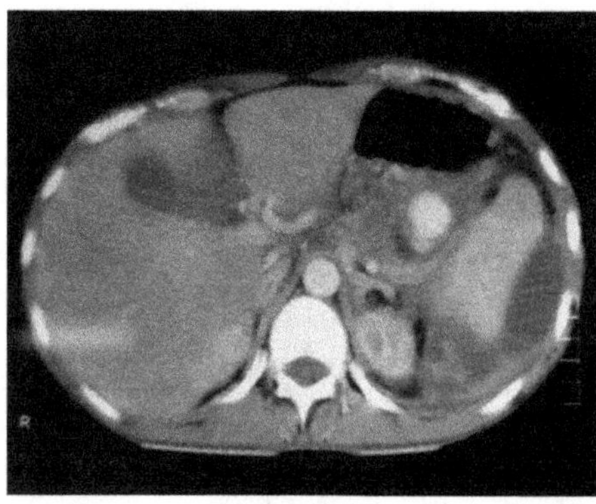

Figure 9: Contrast enhanced CT abdomen showing splenic artery pseudoaneurysm.

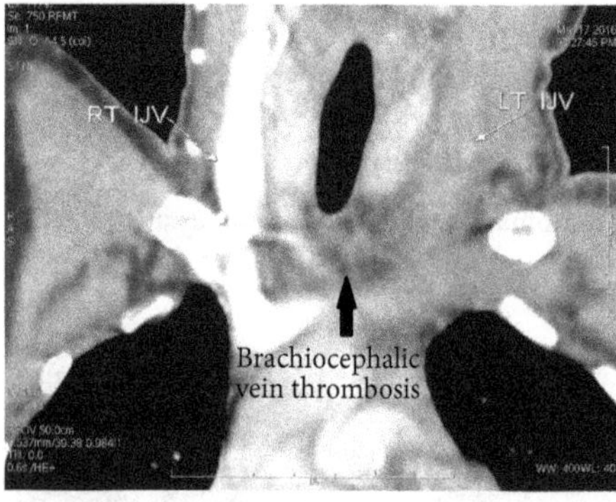

Figure 10: Contrast enhanced CT chest showing nonvisualization of left internal jugular vein and brachiocephalic vein due to thrombosis in a case of mediastinal pseudocyst.

in one patient. Successful resolution of mediastinal pseudocysts with less invasive procedures, such as combined laparoendoscopic or thoracoscopic approaches, has also been reported [16]. Interventional radiological procedures are often useful adjunct in management of complications following pancreatitis and are also useful in managing mediastinal pseudocyst. The same principle of percutaneous catheter guided drainage (step-up approach) [16] for peripancreatic collections/necrosis is applicable here as well. Drainage of the abdominal pseudocyst/necrotic collections resulted in resolution of mediastinal pseudocyst as observed in two of our patients.

Vascular complication in the background of chronic pancreatitis is a rarely observed complication but is potentially life threatening [17]. It could range from bleeding from visceral artery pseudoaneurysm to thrombosis of peripancreatic veins as encountered in our series [18, 19]. We are probably the first to report brachiocephalic vein thrombosis, due to mediastinal pseudocyst. The development of thrombosis is due to local, prothrombotic, inflammatory changes in the vascular endothelium and by extrinsic compression due to pseudocysts [20]. We would like to highlight the fact that development of a complication following pancreatitis creates an opportune environment for another complication.

There have been multiple reports of mediastinal cysts causing cardiac failure due to their compressive effects on the cardiac chambers [21]. It is interesting to note that two patients in our series had left ventricular failure with decreased ejection fraction which recovered after resolution of the cyst following treatment.

5. Conclusion

Mediastinal pseudocyst is a rare complication following acute or chronic pancreatitis, which should be kept in mind in a patient presenting with atypical symptoms. Thorough evaluation guides to the optimal treatment required. Traditional surgical drainage which treats the underlying pancreatic disease, including ductal decompression or pseudocyst decompression, is effective. Radiological interventions are a useful adjunct to surgical management. EUS guided approach, when feasible, is gaining more favour with growing expertise and advancing technology in endoscopic adjuncts. Mediastinal pseudocysts often require multiple expertise and should be managed in centers with such expertise.

Additional Points

Core Tip. Mediastinal pseudocysts are a rare entity, most of the them published as case reports; we present a series of 7 cases. The highlighting point is the varied symptomatology of the patients. The various management strategies that were employed in these were tailored to the individual patients. Interesting complications and outcomes are also recorded. This paper might serve as guide to surgeons who encounter such rare cases in their clinical practice.

Authors' Contributions

Durairaj Segamalai, Abdul Rehman Abdul Jameel, and Naveen Kannan designed the report; Amudhan Anbalagan, Benet Duraisamy, and Prabhakaran Raju collected patients clinical data; Durairaj Segamalai, Abdul Rehman Abdul Jameel, and Kannan Devy Gounder analysed the data and wrote the paper.

Disclosure

Findings of this paper have been presented to Indian Association of Surgical Gastroenterology (IASGCON 2016) conference.

References

[1] R. Gupta, J. C. Munoz, P. Garg, G. Masri, N. S. Nahman Jr., and L. R. Lambiase, "Mediastinal pancreatic pseudocyst—a case report and review of the literature," *MedGenMed Medscape General Medicine*, vol. 9, no. 2, article 8, 2007.

[2] A. V. Ajmera and T. A. Judge, "Mediastinal extension of pancreatic pseudocyst—a case with review of topic and management guidelines," *American Journal of Therapeutics*, vol. 19, no. 5, pp. e152–e156, 2012.

[3] K. Knyrim, H.-J. Wagner, N. Bethge, M. Keymling, and N. Vakil, "A controlled trial of an expansile metal stent for palliation of esophageal obstruction due to inoperable cancer," *The New England Journal of Medicine*, vol. 329, no. 18, pp. 1302–1307, 1993.

[4] N. Moorthy, A. Raveesha, and K. Prabhakar, "Pancreaticopleural fistula and mediastinal pseudocyst: an unusual presentation of acute pancreatitis," *Annals of Thoracic Medicine*, vol. 2, no. 3, pp. 122–123, 2007.

[5] D. K. Bhasin, S. S. Rana, M. Nanda et al., "Endoscopic management of pancreatic pseudocysts at atypical locations," *Surgical Endoscopy and Other Interventional Techniques*, vol. 24, no. 5, pp. 1085–1091, 2010.

[6] H. Xu, X. Zhang, A. Christe et al., "Anatomic pathways of peripancreatic fluid draining to mediastinum in recurrent acute pancreatitis: visible human project and CT study," *PLoS ONE*, vol. 8, no. 4, Article ID e62025, 2013.

[7] A. S. Fulcher, G. W. Capps, and M. A. Turner, "Thoracopancreatic fistula: clinical and imaging findings," *Journal of Computer Assisted Tomography*, vol. 23, no. 2, pp. 181–187, 1999.

[8] S. G. Kirchner, R. M. Heller, and C. W. Smith, "Pancreatic pseudocyst of the mediastinum," *Radiology*, vol. 123, no. 1, pp. 37–42, 1977.

[9] D. C. Rockey and J. P. Cello, "Pancreaticopleural fistula: report of 7 patients and review of the literature," *Medicine (Baltimore)*, vol. 69, no. 6, pp. 332–344, 1990.

[10] A. Geier, F. Lammert, C. Gartung, H. N. Nguyen, J. E. Wildberger, and S. Matern, "Magnetic resonance imaging and magnetic resonance cholangiopancreaticography for diagnosis and pre-interventional evaluation of a fluid thoracic mass," *European Journal of Gastroenterology and Hepatology*, vol. 15, no. 4, pp. 429–431, 2003.

[11] S. Santoshkumar, A. Seith, R. Rastogi, and G. C. Khilnani, "Mediastinal pseudocysts in chronic pancreatitis with spontaneous resolution," *Tropical Gastroenterology*, vol. 28, no. 1, pp. 32–34, 2007.

[12] S. S. Rana, D. K. Bhasin, C. Rao, H. Singh, V. Sharma, and K. Singh, "Esophageal stricture following successful resolution of a mediastinal pseudocyst by endoscopic transpapillary drainage," *Endoscopy*, vol. 44, no. 2, pp. E121–E122, 2012.

[13] D. Bhasin and S. Rana, "Endoscopic management of pancreatic fluid collections," *Journal of Digestive Endoscopy*, vol. 3, no. 5, pp. 40–43, 2012.

[14] D.-J. Kim, H.-W. Chung, C.-W. Gham et al., "A case of complete resolution of mediastinal pseudocyst and pleural effusion by endoscopic stenting of pancreatic duct," *Yonsei Medical Journal*, vol. 44, no. 4, pp. 727–731, 2003.

[15] D. Metaxa, A. Balakrishnan, S. Upponi, E. L. Huguet, and R. K. Praseedom, "Surgical intervention for mediastinal pancreatic pseudocysts. A case series and review of the literature," *Journal of the Pancreas*, vol. 16, no. 1, pp. 74–77, 2015.

[16] A. Bonnard, P. Lagausie, S. Malbezin, E. Sauvat, A. I. Lemaitre, and Y. Aigrain, "Mediastinal pancreatic pseudocyst in a child. A thoracoscopic approach," *Surgical Endoscopy*, vol. 15, no. 7, p. 760, 2001.

[17] J.-T. Hsu, C.-N. Yeh, C.-F. Hung et al., "Management and outcome of bleeding pseudoaneurysm associated with chronic pancreatitis," *BMC Gastroenterology*, vol. 6, article no. 3, 2006.

[18] L. Larrey Ruiz, M. Luján Sanchis, L. Peño Muñoz et al., "Pseudoaneurysm associated with complicated pancreatic pseudocysts," *Revista Española de Enfermedades Digestivas*, vol. 108, no. 9, 2016.

[19] S. Tang, "Repeated pancreatitis-induced splenic vein thrombosis leads to intractable gastric variceal bleeding: a case report and review," *World Journal of Clinical Cases*, vol. 3, no. 10, pp. 920–925, 2015.

[20] M. Kikuchi, Y. Nishizaki, K. Tsuruya et al., "Acute portal vein thrombosis due to chronic relapsing pancreatitis: a fistula between a pancreatic pseudocyst and the splenic vein," *Clinical Journal of Gastroenterology*, vol. 7, no. 1, pp. 52–57, 2014.

[21] H. Smail, J. M. Baste, J. Melki, and C. Peillon, "Mediastinal bronchogenic cyst with acute cardiac dysfunction: two-stage surgical approach," *Annals of Thoracic Surgery*, vol. 100, no. 4, pp. e79–e80, 2015.

19

Initial Experience in Single-Incision Transumbilical Laparoscopic Liver Resection: Indications, Potential Benefits, and Limitations

Giovanni Dapri,[1] Livia DiMarco,[2] Guy-Bernard Cadière,[1] and Vincent Donckier[3]

[1] *Department of Gastrointestinal Surgery, European School of Laparoscopic Surgery, Saint-Pierre University Hospital, 1000 Brussels, Belgium*
[2] *Department of Anesthesiology, Saint-Pierre University Hospital, 1000 Brussels, Belgium*
[3] *Liver Unit, Department of Abdominal Surgery, Hôpital Erasme, Université Libre de Bruxelles, 808 Route de Lennik, 1070 Brussels, Belgium*

Correspondence should be addressed to Vincent Donckier, vincent.donckier@erasme.ulb.ac.be

Academic Editor: Andrea Lauterio

Background. Single-incision transumbilical laparoscopic liver resection (SITLLR) has been recently described in limited series. We report our experience in SITLLR and discuss the future of this approach in terms of indications, potential benefits, and limitations, with a special reference to laparoscopic liver resection (LLR). *Patients and Methods.* Six patients underwent SITLLR. Indications were biliary cysts (3 cases), hydatid cysts (2), and colorectal liver metastasis (1). Procedures consisted in cysts unroofing, left lateral lobectomy, pericystectomy, and wedge resection. SITLLR was performed with 11 mm reusable trocar, 10 or 5 mm 30° scopes, 10 mm ultrasound probe, curved reusable instruments, and straight disposable bipolar shears. *Results.* Neither conversion to open surgery nor insertion of supplementary trocars was necessary. Median laparoscopic time was 105.5 minutes and median blood loss 275 mL. Median final umbilical scar length was 1.5 cm, and median length of stay was 4 days. No early or late complications occurred. *Conclusion.* SITLLR remains a challenging procedure. It is feasible in highly selected patients, requiring experience in hepatobiliary and laparoscopic surgery and skills in single-incision laparoscopy. Apart from cosmetic benefit, our experience and literature review did not show significant advantages if compared with multiport LLR, underlying that specific indications remain to be established.

1. Introduction

Since the first reports in the nineteen's [1, 2], laparoscopic liver resection (LLR) has now become a well-recognized and accepted procedure for treatment of liver tumors in selected cases. Currently, feasibility, safety, and clinical benefits of LLR have been clearly demonstrated for treatment of both benign [3] and malignant liver tumors [4]. Initially, LLR have been reserved to small lesions, located in anterior liver segments, at distance of major vascular and biliary structures, but, now, the feasibility and safety of LLR for tumors located posteriorly, centrally or requiring a major hepatic resection have been established [5]. A step forward, laparoscopic living donor hepatectomy, including left lobectomy for liver transplantation in children [6] and right hepatectomy for adult liver transplantation, has been proposed by specialized groups [7]. Single-incision transumbilical laparoscopy (SITL), firstly performed in 1992 [8], recently gained interest in general surgery. SITL represents the latest advance of the laparoscopic approach, aiming mainly to improve the cosmetic outcomes, while other potential advantages such as reduced postoperative pain, minimized operative trauma, and reduced hospital stay still need further investigations. SITL has been successfully reported for several abdominal interventions, including appendectomy, cholecystectomy, inguinal and ventral hernia, splenectomy, partial gastrectomy, and colectomy [9].

On the ground of both, the advances of multiport LLR techniques and the recent development of SITL, some surgeons reported the feasibility of single-incision transumbilical laparoscopic liver resection (SITLLR). Most reports concern clinical cases [10–20], while only few centers described series with more than 5 cases [21–28] (Table 1). Accordingly, the feasibility and beyond the potential advantages and disadvantages of this technique remain to be determined. We report herein our initial experience describing 6 patients who underwent SITLLR for benign and malignant liver lesions. We discuss the feasibility of this approach and its potential benefits and limitations, particularly compared with multiport LLR.

2. Patients and Methods

Between April 2010 and February 2012, 6 patients were submitted to SITLLR. Patients' characteristics and type of disease are represented in Table 2. The first 5 patients had no previous surgical history, whereas the patient 6 had a laparoscopic total mesorectal excision for a rectal cancer 6 months before. Surgical procedures consisted in biliary cysts unroofing (patients 1, 2, 3), left lateral lobectomy (patient 4), pericystectomy of segment 7 (patient 5), and wedge resection of segment 8 (patient 6). Preoperative work-up was performed by standard hematological and biochemical laboratory evaluations, including relevant tumor markers. All patients had preoperative liver imaging, using CT scan and/or MRI. Additionally, patient 6 had a whole body FDG-PET scan to exclude the presence of extrahepatic metastases.

2.1. Surgical Technique. The patient is placed under general anaesthesia in supine position and with the legs apart. The surgeon stands between the patient's legs and the camera-assistant to the patient's left. The original umbilical scar is incised and the fascia opened at 1 cm. A purse-string suture using 1 polydioxanone (PDS) is placed in the fascia, and an 11 mm reusable trocar is inserted inside. A 10 mm 30°, rigid and normal length scope (Karl-Storz Endoskope, Tuttlingen, Germany) is used. A curved reusable grasper (Karl-Storz Endoskope, Tuttlingen, Germany) (Figure 1(a)) is inserted at 10 o'clock position through a separate fascia opening outside the purse-string suture and without trocar. This instrument is maintained in the surgeon's nondominant hand, and it is never changed during the entire procedure.

2.1.1. Cyst Unroofing. The other instruments for the surgeon's dominant hand, like the curved reusable coagulating hook (Figure 1(b)), the curved reusable bipolar scissors (Figure 1(c)), and the curved reusable suction device, are changed during the different steps of SITLLR and inserted at 3 o'clock position inside the purse-string suture and besides the 11 mm trocar (Figure 2). The procedure starts with the exploration of the abdominal cavity and identification of the biliary cysts. The cystic domes are identified and incised enough to empty the cystic cavity. Thanks to this manoeuvre a nonconnection between the liver cysts and the biliary tree is evidenced. A meticulously complete excision of the cystic roof is performed. Thanks to the curves of the instruments, the classic working triangulation of laparoscopy is established inside the abdomen (Figure 3(a)), and surgeon is able to work in ergonomic position during the entire procedure (Figure 3(b)). The liver cyst cavities are finally checked for bleeding and left opened without omental patch.

2.1.2. Other SITLLR. A 6 mm reusable trocar is inserted at 2 o'clock position outside the purse-string suture, in order to accommodate a 5 mm 30°, rigid and longer scope. The flexible laparoscopic multifrequency linear probe is inserted in the 11 mm trocar (Figure 4), and the procedure starts with the exploration of the liver parenchyma through the intraoperative ultrasonography (IOUS), which permits to determine the transection line of the liver parenchyma. Then, the optical system is switched again into a 10 mm scope. A disposable straight bipolar shear (Ligasure V, New Haven, Covidien, CT, US) is inserted through the 6 mm trocar. The liver parenchyma is transected. An internal working triangulation is often created thanks to the curves of the grasper (Figure 5(a)), but an external conflict between the optical system and the handle of the straight bipolar shears is frequently evidenced (Figure 5(b)). If necessary, a straight 5 mm clip applier (Weck Hem-o-lock, Teleflex Medical, Sint-Stevens Woluwe, Belgium) is inserted through the 6 mm trocar.

2.1.3. End of the Procedure. A custom-made plastic bag is introduced in the abdomen through the 11 mm trocar, and the specimen is extracted transumbilically. The instruments and trocars are removed; the umbilical fascia is closed using absorbable sutures, taking care to close the separate openings for the curved grasper and for the 6 mm trocar.

3. Results

Neither conversion to open surgery nor insertion of supplementary trocars was necessary. Median total operative time (between skin incision and closure of the fascia) was 126 minutes (range: 89 to 185 min), and median laparoscopic time (between beginning of pneumoperitoneum and removal of the instruments and trocars) was 105.5 minutes (range: 71 to 160 min) (Table 3). Median total blood loss was 275 mL (range: 40 to 500 mL). No intraoperative complications occurred, excepting a major bleeding during the hydatid cyst pericystectomy (patient 5). Median final umbilical scar length was 15 mm (range: 14 to 20 mm). The patients' pain medication was kept low. No early complications were registered within the first postoperative month, and patients were discharged from the hospital between the postoperative day 3 and 5. Pathological evaluation confirmed the preoperative diagnoses of benign biliary cysts, the hydatid liver cysts, and colorectal liver metastasis; for this latter patient the margin of resection was 1 mm. After a median followup of 8 months (range: 3 to 25 months), no late complications related to recurrent disease or to the access-site were observed.

Table 1: Literature review for series of more than 5 cases.

Authors	Port	Instruments	Scope	Pathologies	Cases (n)	BMI (Kg/m^2)*	Operative time (min)*	Conversion (%)	Blood loss (mL)*	Final scar (cm)*	Hospital stay (days)*
Shetty et al. [24]	Gloveport (Sejong Medical)	Straight	5 mm Flexible	Malignant	24	NA	205$^{\#}$	8.3^{+} 16.6$^{@}$	500$^{\#}$	5	8.5$^{\#}$
Cipriani et al. [23]	Triport (ACS), Quadriport (Olympus)	Straight	5 mm Flexible	Benign and Malignant	14	24.3	187	0$^{+@}$	214	NA	5$^{\#}$
Zhao et al. [22]	Triport (ACS), 5-5-5 mm trocars	Straight and Articulating	5 mm Rigid and Flexible	Benign and Malignant	12	26.3	80.4	16.7^{+} 0$^{@}$	45	2.5	4.3
Aikawa et al. [25]	SILS port (Covidien)	Straight	5 mm Flexible	Benign and Malignant	8	NA	148	0$^{+@}$	2	3	6.2
Pan et al. [28]	10 mm and 5 mm trocars	Straight	10 mm	Benign and Malignant	8	26.2	89.7	0$^{+@}$	64.3	2.5	3.7
Tan et al. [26]	various	Straight and Articulating	5 mm Flexible	Benign and Malignant	7	NA	142$^{\#}$	NA^{+} 0$^{@}$	200$^{\#}$	NA	3$^{\#}$
Gaujoux et al. [21]	Gelport (Applied)	Straight	10 mm Flexible	Benign and Malignant	5	27.1	107	0$^{+@}$	39	5	2
Cai et al. [27]	Triport (ASC)	Straight	10 mm Rigid	Benign	5	25.8$^{\#}$	87.3$^{\#}$	0$^{+@}$	NA	NA	4.6$^{\#}$

*Mean.
#Median.
+Additional trocar.
@Open surgery.
NA: Not available.

Table 2: Patients' characteristics.

Patients	Age (years)	Sex	BMI (Kg/m^2)	Indication (liver segment)	Intervention
1	53	F	20.8	Biliary cyst (4, 7, 8)	Cyst unroofing
2	59	F	30.2	Biliary cyst (3, 4)	Cyst unroofing
3	46	F	20.5	Biliary cyst (4, 5, 6, 7)	Cyst unroofing
4	24	F	24.4	Hydatid cyst (2, 3)	Left lobectomy
5	26	F	20.6	Hydatid cyst (7)	Pericystectomy
6	65	F	23	Colorectal metastasis (8)	Wedge resection

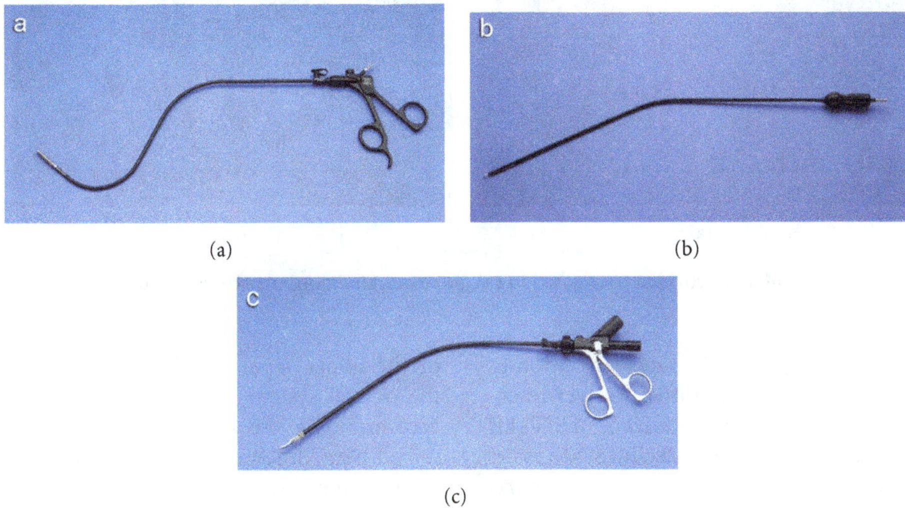

Figure 1: Curved reusable instruments according to DAPRI: grasping forceps III (a), coagulating hook (b), bipolar scissors (c) (courtesy of Karl Storz-Endoskope, Tuttlingen, Germany).

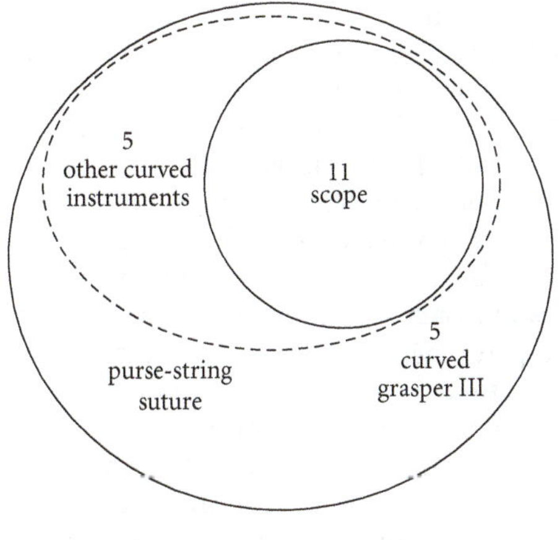

Figure 2: Umbilical access during cyst unroofing: placement of purse-string suture, 11 mm trocar for the 10 mm scope, and 5 mm curved instruments without trocars.

4. Discussion

The development of new techniques to reduce the surgical trauma and to minimize the abdominal wall damage is an obvious trend in liver surgery. Accordingly, LLR has been increasingly performed this last decade, becoming now a standardized procedure in selected cases, able to provide significant benefits as compared with classical open liver resections [29, 30]. SITLLR represents an ultimate evolution of the laparoscopic approach to the liver, being considered as very minimally invasive. The objective of SITLLR, beyond the cosmetic gain, is to further reduce the global surgical stress, potentially having a favorable impact on the postoperative evolution. At this point of the experience, several questions on SITLLR remain to be addressed, concerning the feasibility and mostly the reproducibility of this technique, the indications, selection criteria, limitations, effect on postoperative outcomes, and long-term results. It is on these bases that it would be possible to evaluate if SITLLR could become, more

TABLE 3: Operative and postoperative outcomes.

Patients	Total operative time (min)	Laparoscopic time (min)	Blood loss (mL)	Final scar length (mm)	Length of stay (days)	Followup (months)
1	90	81	50	14	3	25
2	89	71	40	14	3	13
3	138	115	400	16	4	3
4	114	96	350	20	5	9
5	185	160	500	16	5	7
6	158	140	200	15	4	6
MEDIAN	126	105.5	275	15	4	8

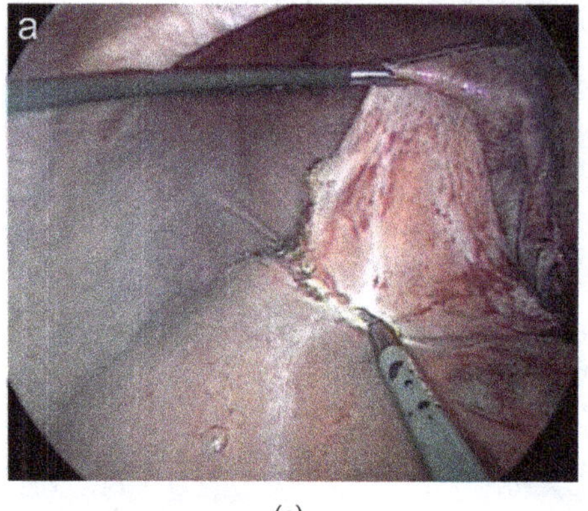

(a)

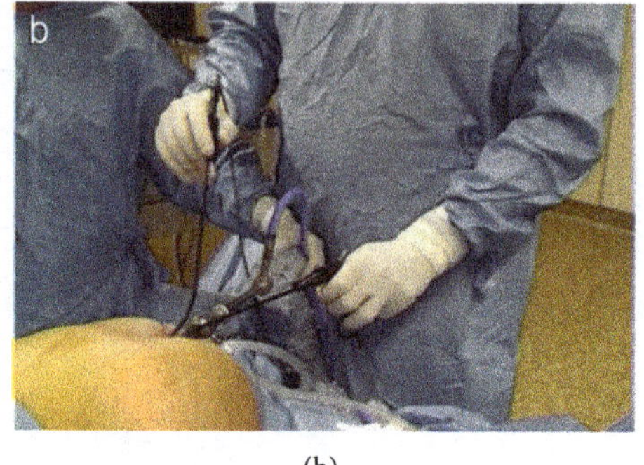

(b)

FIGURE 3: Cyst unroofing: internal working triangulation (a) and external ergonomy (b) using curved reusable instruments.

than just a technical challenge, a real therapeutic option to improve the outcomes of patients submitted to liver resections. For such evaluation, the growing experience of SITLLR should be closely confronted to the well-established results of LLR, serving as standard of comparison. Several reports have reported the feasibility of SITLLR in selected cases [21–28]. Accordingly [21, 23, 25, 26, 28], our series confirms as SITLLR can be performed without conversion to open surgery or insertion of supplementary trocars, including also the resection of the lesions located in posterior liver segments. From a technical point of view, the objective during SITLLR is to maintain the procedure as similar as possible to the principles of multiport LLR. As a matter of fact, the technique described here is basically close to multiport laparoscopy, with the main difference that it is performed through the same umbilical incision, using instruments close to each other. One of the main rules of laparoscopy, which consists in maintaining the optical system as the bisector of the working triangulation [31], is respected during SITL because the 10 mm scope is maintained in the center of the umbilical access and the instrument for the surgeon's nondominant hand (curved grasper) on the right side of the access, whereas the instruments for the surgeon's dominant hand (coagulating hook, bipolar scissors, bipolar shears, clip applier, suction device) on the left side. The curved grasper is never changed during the entire procedure, whereas the instruments for the surgeon's dominant hand are continuously changed and replaced by the 5 mm scope during the step of IOUS. This step is the only one where one of the above laparoscopic rules is not respected, because the optical system is inserted laterally to give the place to accommodate the ultrasound probe. The technique described here, differently from the common SITL [9], did not increase the cost of standard laparoscopy, because all of the material implemented is reusable, except for the straight bipolar shears used during the parenchymal transection. As during multiport LLR, SITLLR parenchymal transection can be performed using several devices like Harmonic ACE (Ethicon Endosurgery, Cincinnati, OH, US) [21, 26, 28], saline-linked sealing dissector (SH2.0, TissueLink Medical's Dover, NH, US) (12), SonoSurg (Olympus, Tokyo, Japan) [14, 23], cavitron ultrasonic surgical aspirator (CUSA Excel, Valley Lab Inc., Boulder, CO, US) [24], Surgiwand (Covidien, Mansfield, MA, US) [24], Maryland type forceps and bipolar forceps combined with suction irrigation system [25], or Ligasure (Covidien New Haven, CT, US) [26, 28]. We adopted the use of curved coagulating hook and curved bipolar scissors for cystic dome resection and straight bipolar shears for parenchyma transection. Comparing these two instruments, surgeon was immediately confronted with the problem of external conflict between the optical system and the handle of the straight bipolar shears because, differently from the curved tools, both instruments are supported by a straight shaft (Figures 4 and 5). A significant gap was observed between the total and the laparoscopic times. This interval time can be explained by the need to get access to the peritoneal cavity as well as the time to meticulously close the umbilical access and the separate fascial openings at

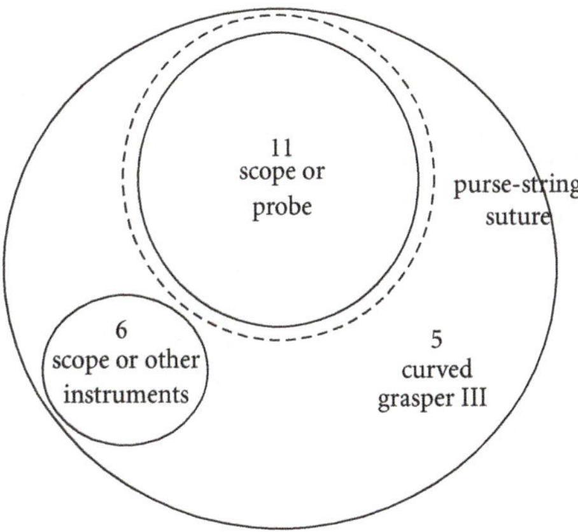

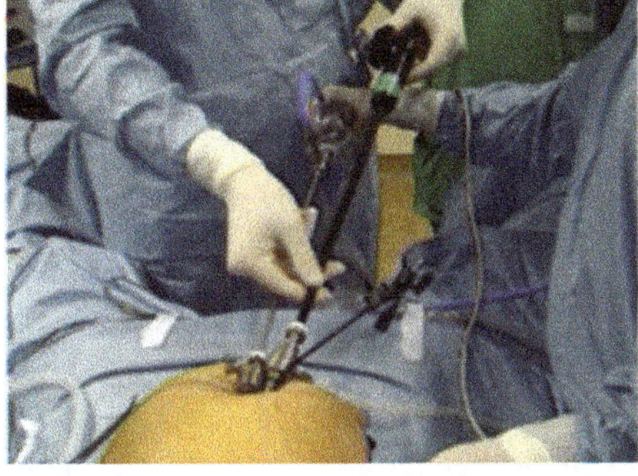

FIGURE 4: Umbilical access during other SITLLR: IOUS performed with the insertion of the ultrasound probe into the 11 mm trocar and use of long scope through the 6 mm trocar.

the end of the procedure, while laparoscopic time in this series remained similar to that previously reported [21]. This could be surely improved thanks to the surgeon's learning curve, and the time of laparoscopy could be reduced if particular devices with multiple functions like tissue division, hemostasis, irrigation, and suction are adopted [25]. Blood loss during SITLLR as well as during multiport LLR remains a factor related to the use of specific instruments for the parenchymal transection, to the extension of the parenchyma resected, to the time of transection, and, lastly, to the occurrence of intraoperative complications [21–25, 28]. In one case of this series (patient 5), a pericystectomy performed in segment 7 for a hydatid cyst, a significant bleeding was achieved, most probably in relation to the difficult access to superior and posterior liver segments and to the longer time needed for parenchymal transection. Still, no patients of the series necessitated blood transfusions, and no postoperative early complications were recorded.

After a median followup of 8 months, we did not achieve any complications related to the access site, to the remaining liver tissue, and to the general patient's conditions, but a longer followup is necessary for the evaluation of recurrent disease and for the appearance of incisional hernia at the access site. Thanks to the technique described here, the umbilical incision length is kept minimal. This result can be obtained because disposable port devices, requiring larger incision [9], are not used. Moreover, tumor's size and pathology are factors influencing the final scar length because malignant tumors superior to 30 mm of diameter need enlargement of the scar for extraction and intact specimen for pathological examination [14, 23, 26]. In our experience benign lesions, like biliary and hydatid cysts, were fragmented at the level of the umbilicus in a plastic bag, while malignant lesions were selected for SITLLR if small and with a diameter inferior to 3 cm [21, 22, 25]. In case of larger lesions, the final scar length has to be enlarged [23, 24, 26], sharing then an increased risk for development of incisional hernia [32, 33]. Such risk can also be associated to the placement of the final drain through the scar [10, 23]. As previously reported [21, 26], and similarly to our attitude during multiport LLR, we did not use a drain. In cases where a drain has to be left in the abdomen, we prefer to use a different abdominal wall punction, out of the umbilicus, in order to avoid the risk of incisional hernia. This punction can also be used during SITLLR to insert a needlescopic (3 mm) instrument [22] or a classic additional trocar [14, 23]. Hence, SITLLR becomes a technique of reduced port surgery, using two accesses, one at the umbilicus and one in another abdominal quadrant. Similarly, a supplementary instrument can also be inserted for technical problems due to tissue manipulation or compromised visualization [22] and non-controlled perioperative bleeding or limited length of instruments [24]. Other factors of selection for SITLLR are the patient's body mass index and the patient's height, because it can be a cause of conversion to multiport laparoscopy [22, 24]. According to other authors [23, 26], we did not consider previous abdominal surgery, like in our patient 6, as a contraindication to SITLLR. Potential indications for LLR have now been clearly identified, showing essentially no predefined contraindications as compared with open liver resection in terms of disease pathology, including both benign and malignant tumors, either primary hepatocellular carcinoma or liver metastases. Importantly, with the reserves due to the absence of randomized trial and many selection biases, no oncological disadvantages have been shown for laparoscopic approach as compared with standard open procedure, neither in terms of radicality of resection nor for the risk of tumor cell seeding and long-term outcomes [34–38]. At this point of the experience, there are no reasons to consider that the same would be true for SITLLR. From surgeon's side, several statements clearly underlined that LLR should be performed by surgeons experienced in liver resections, meaning knowledge of hepatic anatomy, experience in open liver surgery, and skills in the use of IOUS [30]. Additionally, extensive experience in laparoscopic surgery and ability to identify and control major vascular and biliary structures laparoscopically are mandatory before embarking on multiport LLR [34]. Regarding the application of SITL to the liver, it is most probably reasonable to go back to the initial development of LLR, both in terms of indications and surgeon's experience. Accordingly, small anterior tumors, including malignant lesions, could be selected for SITL if the transection plane is well defined and at distance of the major biliary and vascular structures. Shetty et al. [24] described

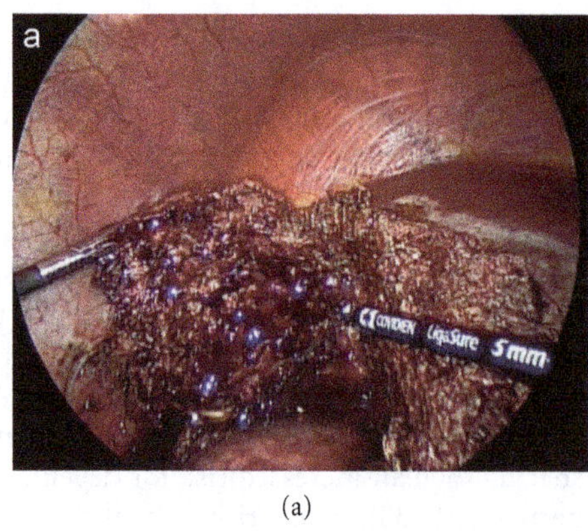

(a)

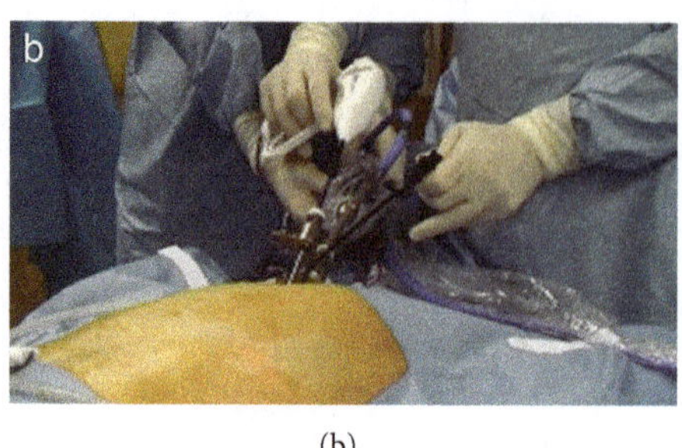

(b)

Figure 5: Other SITLLR: internal triangulation using straight disposable bipolar shears and curved reusable grasper (a), and external view (b).

a good indication for SITLLR in all the patients with well-localized lesions, whereas other authors focused on the importance of solitary tumors located on the anterolateral segments of the liver [25, 26, 28] or in the left liver lobe [21, 23] because the liver suspensory ligament helps for surgical-site exposure, and parenchymal division line remains in the same axis of the port site and instrumentations. Still, the specific technical problem created by the single caccess should not be underestimated, relying mainly on difficulties of exposure and on surgeon's and instruments' positions. Such ergonomic difficulties could lead to inadequate sections planes that could be a major concern for oncological indications, requiring safe but economic margins resection. Furthermore, other steps of SITLLR technique are limiting factors, like the frequent changes of the instruments for the surgeon's dominant hand and the use of IOUS through the single umbilical access. We agree with other authors [24] to consider limiting factors for SITLLR, patients with vascular involvement, extrahepatic disease, contraindication to laparoscopy, malignant lesions greater than 5 cm because the incision required to extract the specimen itself defeats the purpose of SITL. Other challenges in SITLLR remain technical difficulties related to massive liver dissection, access to the hilum for eventual Pringle maneuver, insertion of ultrasound probe through the single access, frequent alternation and adjustment of instruments, shifted division line, restriction by the length of the laparoscopic instrument, inappropriate placement of the drain, and control of bleeding during parenchymal dissection. Hence insertion of one or more trocars [22, 24] or conversion to open surgery [24] becomes strongly recommended. The following question relies on the identification of eventual intraoperative and early postoperative benefits of SITLLR as compared with multiport LLR. Regarding the results of LLR, even in the absence of randomized studies, several reports clearly indicated nowadays the advantages of this technique as compared with open liver resection, including less intraoperative blood losses, reduced requirements for blood transfusions [36–42], eventually associated with reduced postoperative complications rates and shorter hospital stays [38–40, 42, 43]. Short-term benefits of LLR, as compared with classical open liver resections, were strikingly observed in treatment of hepatocellular carcinoma in cirrhotic patients; in these cases, the avoidance of a subcostal incision interrupting venous portocaval shunts could be critical. Potential benefits of SITL, out of cosmetic outcomes, could be the postoperative pain, which has been considered one of the major outcome measures in the prospective randomized studies [44, 45], but a final sentence remains of concern. We achieved a non-additional use of pain medication used for LLR in this initial experience as reported [21–23, 26], allowing the patients to be discharged before the postoperative day 5. In conclusion, at this time SITLLR remains a challenging procedure. Feasibility has been reserved for highly selected cases, but it has to be performed by formed surgeons in hepatobiliary and laparoscopic surgery with skills in general SITL. Apart from its cosmetic benefits, the future of this technique will be dependent on the confirmation of significant results if compared with multiport LLR and, then, of objective advantages, such as a reduction of the global operative stress and/or an improvement of postoperative outcomes.

References

[1] M. Gagner, M. Rheault, and J. Dubuc, "Laparoscopic partial hepatectomy for liver tumor," *Surgical Endoscopy and Other Interventional Techniques*, vol. 6, article 99, 1992.

[2] J. S. Azagra, M. Goergen, E. Gilbart, and D. Jacobs, "Laparoscopic anatomical (hepatic) left lateral segmentectomy—technical aspects," *Surgical Endoscopy and Other Interventional Techniques*, vol. 10, no. 7, pp. 758–761, 1996.

[3] B. Descottes, D. Glineur, F. Lachachi et al., "Laparoscopic liver resection of benign liver tumors," *Surgical Endoscopy and Other Interventional Techniques*, vol. 17, no. 1, pp. 23–30, 2003.

[4] J. F. Gigot, D. Glineur, J. S. Azagra et al., "Laparoscopic liver resection for malignant liver tumors: preliminary results of

a multicenter European study," *Annals of Surgery*, vol. 236, no. 1, pp. 90–97, 2002.

[5] Y. S. Yoon, H. S. Han, J. Y. Cho, and K. S. Ahn, "Total laparoscopic liver resection for hepatocellular carcinoma located in all segments of the liver," *Surgical Endoscopy and Other Interventional Techniques*, vol. 24, no. 7, pp. 1630–1637, 2010.

[6] D. Cherqui, O. Soubrane, E. Husson et al., "Laparoscopic living donor hepatectomy for liver transplantation in children," *The Lancet*, vol. 359, no. 9304, pp. 392–396, 2002.

[7] P. C. Giulianotti, I. Tzvetanov, H. Jeon et al., "Robot-assisted right lobe donor hepatectomy," *Transplant International*, vol. 25, pp. e5–e9, 2012.

[8] M. A. Pelosi and M. A. Pelosi III, "Laparoscopic appendectomy using a single umbilical puncture (minilaparoscopy)," *The Journal of Reproductive Medicine*, vol. 37, no. 7, pp. 588–594, 1992.

[9] I. Ahmed and P. Paraskeva, "A clinical review of single-incision laparoscopic surgery," *Surgeon*, vol. 9, pp. 341–351, 2011.

[10] K. Shibao, A. Higure, and K. Yamaguchi, "Case report: laparoendoscopic single-site fenestration of giant hepatic cyst," *Surgical Technology International*, vol. 20, pp. 133–136, 2010.

[11] K. Sasaki, G. Watanabe, M. Matsuda, M. Hashimoto, and T. Harano, "Original method of transumbilical single-incision laparoscopic deroofing for liver cyst," *Journal of Hepato-Biliary-Pancreatic Sciences*, vol. 17, no. 5, pp. 733–734, 2010.

[12] S. Kobayashi, H. Nagano, S. Marubashi et al., "A single-incision laparoscopic hepatectomy for hepatocellular carcinoma: initial experience in a Japanese patient," *Minimally Invasive Therapy and Allied Technologies*, vol. 19, no. 6, pp. 367–371, 2010.

[13] A. G. Patel, A. P. Belgaumkar, J. James, U. P. Singh, K. A. Carswell, and B. Murgatroyd, "Single-incision laparoscopic left lateral segmentectomy of colorectal liver metastasis," *Surgical Endoscopy and Other Interventional Techniques*, vol. 25, no. 2, pp. 649–650, 2011.

[14] L. Aldrighetti, E. Guzzetti, and G. Ferla, "Laparoscopic hepatic left lateral sectionectomy using the laparoendoscopic single site approach: evolution of minimally invasive liver surgery," *Journal of Hepato-Biliary-Pancreatic Sciences*, vol. 18, no. 1, pp. 103–105, 2011.

[15] S. K. Y. Chang, M. Mayasari, I. S. Ganpathi, V. L. T. Wen, and K. Madhavan, "Single port laparoscopic liver resection for hepatocellular carcinoma: a preliminary report," *International Journal of Hepatology*, vol. 2011, pp. 579–203, 2011.

[16] G. Belli, C. Fantini, A. D'Agostino et al., "Laparoendoscopic single site liver resection for recurrent hepatocellular carcinoma in cirrhosis: first technical note," *Surgical Laparoscopy Endoscopy & Percutaneous Techniques*, vol. 21, pp. 166–168, 2011.

[17] H. Kashiwagi, K. Kumagai, and M. Nozue, "Single incision laparoscopic surgery for a life-threatening, cyst of liver," *Tokai Journal of Experimental and Clinical Medicine*, vol. 36, no. 1, pp. 13–16, 2011.

[18] M. G. Hu, G. D. Zhao, D. B. Xu, and R. Liu, "Transumbilical single-incision laparoscopic hepatectomy: an initial report," *Chinese Medical Journal*, vol. 124, no. 5, pp. 787–789, 2011.

[19] U. Barbaros, T. Demirel, O. Gozkun et al., "A new era in minimally invasive liver resection (MILR) single-incision laparoscopic liver resection (SIL-LR): the first two cases," *Surgical Technology International*, vol. 21, pp. 81–84, 2012.

[20] B. I. Rosok and B. Edwin, "Single-incision laparoscopic liver resection for colorectal metastasis through stoma site at the time of reversal of diversion ileostomy: a case report," *Minimally Invasive Surgery*, vol. 2011, Article ID 502176, 3 pages, 2011.

[21] S. Gaujoux, T. P. Kingham, W. R. Jarnagin, M. I. D'Angelica, P. J. Allen, and Y. Fong, "Single-incision laparoscopic liver resection," *Surgical Endoscopy and Other Interventional Techniques*, vol. 25, no. 5, pp. 1489–1494, 2011.

[22] G. Zhao, M. Hu, R. Liu et al., "Laparoendoscopic single-site liver resection: a preliminary report of 12 cases," *Surgical Endoscopy and Other Interventional Techniques*, vol. 25, pp. 3286–3293, 2011.

[23] F. Cipriani, M. Catena, F. Ratti, M. Paganelli, F. Ferla, and L. Aldrighetti, "LESS technique for liver resection: the progress of the mini-invasive approach: a single-centre experience," *Minimally Invasive Therapy & Allied Technologies*, vol. 21, pp. 55–58, 2012.

[24] G. S. Shetty, Y. K. You, H. J. Choi, G. H. Na, T. H. Hong, and D. G. Kim, "Extending the limitations of liver surgery: outcomes of initial human experience in a high-volume center performing single-port laparoscopic liver resection for hepatocellular carcinoma," *Surgical Endoscopy and Other Interventional Techniques*, vol. 26, pp. 1602–1608, 2012.

[25] M. Aikawa, M. Miyazawa, K. Okamoto, Y. Toshimitsu, K. Okada, and Y. Ueno, "Single-port laparoscopic hepatectomy: technique, safety, and feasibility in a clinical case series," *Surgical Endoscopy and Other Interventional Techniques*, vol. 26, pp. 1696–1701, 2012.

[26] E. K. Tan, V. T. Lee, S. K. Chang, I. S. Ganpathi, K. Madhavan, and D. Lomanto, "Laparoendoscopic single-site minor hepatectomy for liver tumors," *Surgical Endoscopy and Other Interventional Techniques*, vol. 26, pp. 2086–2091, 2012.

[27] W. Cai, J. Xu, M. Zheng, M. Qin, and H. Zhao, "Combined laparoendoscopic single-site surgery: initial experience of a single center," *Hepato-Gastroenterology*, vol. 59, pp. 986–989, 2012.

[28] M. Pan, Z. Jiang, Y. Cheng et al., "Single-incision laparoscopic hepatectomy for benign and malignant hepatopathy: initial experience in 8 chinese patients," *Surgical Innovation*. In press.

[29] S. K. Reddy, A. Tsung, and D. A. Geller, "Laparoscopic liver resection," *World Journal of Surgery*, vol. 35, pp. 1478–1486, 2011.

[30] J. F. Buell, D. Cherqui, D. A. Geller et al., "The international position on laparoscopic liver surgery: The Louisville Statement," *Annals of Surgery*, vol. 250, pp. 825–830, 2008.

[31] G. B. Hanna, T. Drew, P. Clinch, B. Hunter, and A. Cuschieri, "Computer-controlled endoscopic performance assessment system," *Surgical Endoscopy and Other Interventional Techniques*, vol. 12, no. 7, pp. 997–1000, 1998.

[32] F. Helgstrand, J. Rosenberg, and T. Bisgaard, "Trocar site hernia after laparoscopic surgery: a qualitative systematic review," *Hernia*, vol. 15, no. 2, pp. 113–121, 2011.

[33] S. A. Antoniou, R. Pointner, and F. A. Granderath, "Single-incision laparoscopic cholecystectomy: a systematic review," *Surgical Endoscopy and Other Interventional Techniques*, vol. 25, no. 2, pp. 367–377, 2011.

[34] A. Koffron, D. Geller, T. C. Gamblin, and M. Abecassis, "Laparoscopic liver surgery: shifting the management of liver tumors," *Hepatology*, vol. 44, no. 6, pp. 1694–1700, 2006.

[35] B. Gayet, D. Cavaliere, E. Vibert et al., "Totally laparoscopic right hepatectomy," *American Journal of Surgery*, vol. 194, no. 5, pp. 685–689, 2007.

[36] G. Belli, P. Limongelli, C. Fantini et al., "Laparoscopic and open treatment of hepatocellular carcinoma in patients with cirrhosis," *British Journal of Surgery*, vol. 96, no. 9, pp. 1041–1048, 2009.

[37] D. Castaing, E. Vibert, L. Ricca, D. Azoulay, R. Adam, and B. Gayet, "Oncologic results of laparoscopic versus open hepatectomy for colorectal liver metastases in two specialized centers," *Annals of Surgery*, vol. 250, no. 5, pp. 849–855, 2009.

[38] I. Dagher, N. O'Rourke, D. A. Geller et al., "Laparoscopic major hepatectomy: an evolution in standard of care," *Annals of Surgery*, vol. 250, no. 5, pp. 856–860, 2009.

[39] M. Morino, I. Morra, E. Rosso, C. Miglietta, and C. Garrone, "Laparoscopic vs open hepatic resection: a comparative study," *Surgical Endoscopy and Other Interventional Techniques*, vol. 17, no. 12, pp. 1914–1918, 2003.

[40] B. Topal, S. Fieuws, R. Aerts, H. Vandeweyer, and F. Penninckx, "Laparoscopic versus open liver resection of hepatic neoplasms: comparative analysis of short-term results," *Surgical Endoscopy and Other Interventional Techniques*, vol. 22, no. 10, pp. 2208–2213, 2008.

[41] F. M. Polignano, A. J. Quyn, R. S. M. de Figueiredo, N. A. Henderson, C. Kulli, and I. S. Tait, "Laparoscopic versus open liver segmentectomy: prospective, case-matched, intention-to-treat analysis of clinical outcomes and cost effectiveness," *Surgical Endoscopy and Other Interventional Techniques*, vol. 22, no. 12, pp. 2564–2570, 2008.

[42] M. Tsinberg, G. Tellioglu, C. H. Simpfendorfer et al., "Comparison of laparoscopic versus open liver tumor resection: a case-controlled study," *Surgical Endoscopy and Other Interventional Techniques*, vol. 23, no. 4, pp. 847–853, 2009.

[43] R. Troisi, R. Montalti, P. Smeets et al., "The value of laparoscopic liver surgery for solid benign hepatic tumors," *Surgical Endoscopy and Other Interventional Techniques*, vol. 22, no. 1, pp. 38–44, 2008.

[44] E. C. Tsimoyiannis, K. E. Tsimogiannis, G. Pappas-Gogos et al., "Different pain scores in single transumbilical incision laparoscopic cholecystectomy versus classic laparoscopic cholecystectomy: a randomized controlled trial," *Surgical Endoscopy and Other Interventional Techniques*, vol. 24, no. 8, pp. 1842–1848, 2010.

[45] P. C. Lee, C. Lo, P. S. Lai et al., "Randomized clinical trial of single-incision laparoscopic cholecystectomy versus mini-laparoscopic cholecystectomy," *British Journal of Surgery*, vol. 97, no. 7, pp. 1007–1012, 2010.

Intraoperative Fluid Excess Is a Risk Factor for Pancreatic Fistula after Partial Pancreaticoduodenectomy

Helge Bruns, Veronika Kortendieck, Hans-Rudolf Raab, and Dalibor Antolovic

Department of General and Visceral Surgery, Carl von Ossietzky University of Oldenburg, Oldenburg, Germany

Correspondence should be addressed to Helge Bruns; helge.bruns@uni-oldenburg.de

Academic Editor: Laureano Fernández-Cruz

Background. After pancreaticoduodenectomy (PD), pancreatic fistulas (PF) are a frequent complication. Infusions may compromise anastomotic integrity. This retrospective analysis evaluated associations between intraoperative fluid excess and PF. *Methods.* Data on perioperative parameters including age, sex, laboratory findings, histology, infusions, surgery time, and occurrence of grade B/C PF was collected from all PD with pancreaticojejunostomy (PJ) performed in our department from 12/2011 till 02/2015. The glomerular filtration rate (GFR), infusion rate, and the ratio of both and its association with PF were calculated. ROC analysis was employed to identify a threshold. *Results.* Complete datasets were available for 83 of 86 consecutive cases. Median age was 66 years (34–84; 60% male), GFR was 93 mL/min (IQR 78–113), and surgery time was 259 min (IQR 217–307). Intraoperatively, 13.6 mL/min (7–31) was infused. In total, $n = 18$ (21%) PF occurred. When the infusion : GFR ratio exceeded 0.15, PF increased from 11% to 34% ($p = 0.0157$). No significant association was detected for any of the other parameters. *Conclusions.* This analysis demonstrates for the first time an association between intraoperative fluid excess and PF after PD with PJ even in patients with normal renal function. A carefully patient-adopted fluid management with due regard to renal function may help to prevent postoperative PF.

1. Introduction

In high volume centers, partial pancreaticoduodenectomy (PD) can be performed with acceptable morbidity and mortality [1]. While the outcome is clearly associated with surgeon and center experience, the rate of pancreatic fistulas seems not to drop below a certain level [2, 3]. Even after thousands of PD, highly experienced surgeons in high-volume centers report an almost constant or even increasing rate of pancreatic fistulas [2]. Depending on the definition, the published rate of postoperative fistulas after PD is estimated to be 20–30% [4]. Numerous interventions and techniques have been introduced and a number of standardized anastomotic techniques exist, but there is little evidence for superiority of one anastomotic technique over the other [5–13]. Isolation of the pancreaticojejunostomy (PJ) using dual-loop reconstruction has been discussed as possible intervention to decrease the rate of pancreatic fistulas but seems not to be superior to single-loop reconstruction [1].

In multivariate analyses, some risk factors for anastomotic leakage have already been identified [14–18]. Soft pancreatic texture, a history of weight loss, intraoperative blood loss, diameter of the pancreatic duct, and decreased preoperative albumin seem to be associated with leakage. Renal insufficiency has been shown to be associated with increased complication rates after pancreatic resection [19].

In general, intraoperative fluid management aims at stabilizing the patient. For some types of abdominal surgery, a restrictive fluid regimen is considered common sense: as far as liver resection is concerned, fluid management at a low central venous pressure below 5 cm H_2O is made use of to decrease intraoperative blood loss [20–23]. Anesthesiological guidelines may vary between institutions but usually consider hemodynamic parameters, blood values, blood loss, and duration of surgery to be triggers that guide the intraoperative regimen [24]. Interstitial fluid overload due to infusion of large amounts of fluid can lead to visible edema and might compromise the anastomotic integrity [25]. For rectal resections, an increased risk of anastomotic leakage after excessive perioperative infusions has been shown [26]. In pancreatic surgery, there is evidence pointing out that the same mechanisms might be relevant. In a study focusing on normovolemic hemodilution to decrease blood loss in pancreatic surgery, no effect on blood loss was identified but an increased rate of 21.5% versus 7.7% anastomotic complications was apparent after 6250 mL versus 3900 mL of intraoperative intravenous fluid [27]. As far as postoperative fluid management is concerned, a restrictive management aiming at a fluid balance of less than 1 liter on postoperative day has been shown to be associated with decreased complication rates [28].

This study was designed to identify associations between renal function, intraoperative infusions, and occurrence of clinical relevant postoperative pancreatic fistulas after PD with PJ.

2. Methods

2.1. Patient Data. Data extraction, handling, and analysis were performed in accordance with national and institutional guidelines. All PDs with PJ performed from 12/2011 till 02/2015 were analyzed and data on patient age, indication to surgery, concomitant diseases, preoperative laboratory values, duration of surgery, blood loss, intraoperative infusions, postoperative infusions during the first 72 hours after surgery, occurrence of pancreatic fistulas, and interventions (both surgical or other) was extracted from patient folders. Glomerular filtration rate (GFR) was calculated as published elsewhere [29]. Patients with pancreaticogastrostomies were excluded. PF were considered to be clinically relevant when drainages had to be kept longer than 72 h and pancreatic enzyme levels in the drainage fluid were at least three times higher than in the serum, drainages had to be reintroduced (e.g., guided using computer tomography or ultrasound), and pancreatic enzymes were detected in the drainage fluid or patients had to undergo reoperations for complications caused by PF.

While duct diameter and pancreatic texture have been discussed as factors associated with postoperative fistula, these parameters lack clear definitions: "duct wideness" and "tissue softness" strongly depend on the individual surgeon's definition and experience. Without clear definition of both parameters prior to documentation, including this type of data in a retrospective analysis cannot be considered to be reliable. Thus, we did not include this in our analysis and have assumed an equal distribution of both parameters between groups.

2.2. Statistical Analysis. For descriptive statistics, median and interquartile range (IQR) or range are used unless stated otherwise. To determine a meaningful cutoff for the infusion rate : GFR ratio, receiver operating characteristics (ROC) were employed, and the area under the ROC curve (AUC-ROC) and Youden's J were calculated. Testing for statistical significance was performed using ANOVA and Fisher's Exact Test as appropriate. p values were two tailed and a value of $p < 0.05$ was considered statistically significant.

2.3. Surgical Technique and Postoperative Management. In our institution, PD is performed in a highly standardized fashion. Usually, single-loop reconstruction with a Warren-Cattell end-to-side PJ using poly-p-dioxanone (PDS 5.0, Johnson & Johnson Medical GmbH, Ethicon, Norderstedt, Germany) is performed. A pancreaticogastrostomy may be performed depending on the surgeon's choice. A surgical drain is routinely placed to the pancreatic anastomosis. Intraoperative and postoperative fluid management and post-operative course are routinely monitored and logged. Patients are extubated in the operating room and transferred to the intensive care unit where mobilization is started and oral fluids are introduced on the day of surgery. Solid foods are introduced depending on enteral passage. As soon as patients have been stable for at least 24 hours, they are transferred to the intermediate care ward. Drains are removed as soon as the fluid is less than 500 mL and is serous. If there is suspicion of a PF, drains are kept in place and enzyme levels are monitored in the drainage fluid.

3. Results

In total, 83 complete datasets were available from 86 consecutive PD with PJ. In total, $n = 18$ (21%) relevant pancreatic fistulas occurred (Table 1). Median age was 66 years (range 34–84 years; 60% male), GFR was 93 mL/min (IQR 78–113 mL/min; Figure 1), and surgery time was 259 min (IQR 217–307; Table 1). Intraoperatively, 13.6 mL/min (range 7–31 mL/min) was infused (Figure 2; Table 1). Crystalloids were used in all patients during surgery and during the first 72 h after surgery. Colloids were infused in 46% of patients during surgery (56% and 43% in patients with and without fistulas; $p = 0.4264$), while 24% of patients received colloids during the first 72 h after surgery (0% versus 31% in patients with and without fistulas; $p = 0.0046$; Table 1). The amount of postoperative infusions had no effect on occurrence of pancreatic fistulas (Table 1). Except for creatinine, GFR, and postoperative infusion of colloids, no statistical differences were identified between patients with or without pancreatic fistulas (Table 1). There was no correlation between the amount of intraoperatively infused volume and GFR (Figure 3). ROC analysis identified an infusion rate : GFR ratio of 0.15 as threshold for occurrence of pancreatic fistulas (Figure 4). A significant increase of pancreatic fistulas from 11% to 34% was detected for patients below and above the identified threshold ($p = 0.0157$; Table 2).

4. Discussion

Perioperative fluid management strongly depends on teamwork involving both anesthesiologists and surgeons [30]. This can be quite demanding and needs experience on the anesthesiologists' side similar to surgical experience needed when complex surgery is performed. Without a balanced and careful fluid regimen, the surgery's success is jeopardized. It is a common misconception that fluid management has little effect on surgical complication rates, although this has been demonstrated frequently [22, 23, 26–28, 31]. In abdominal surgery, restrictive fluid management has repeatedly proven to be superior over dilutive regimens.

TABLE 1: Patient characteristics.

	Postop. fistula (n = 18)		No postop. fistula (n = 65)		p
	n	%	n	%	
Sex					0.5956
Female	6	33	27	42	
Male	12	67	38	58	
	Median (IQR)		Median (IQR)		
Age [years]	65 (58.25–73)		66 (57–73)		0.8038
Creatinine [mg/dL]	0.9 (0.725–1.0)		0.8 (0.7–0.9)		**0.0074**
GFR [mL/min]	83 (61–98)		100 (79–115)		**0.0219**
Surgical duration [min]	231 (202–295)		230 (262–313)		0.5004
Intraoperative infusions					
Total [mL]	3250 (3000–4188)		3500 (3000–4000)		0.5626
Infusion rate [mL/min]	13.4 (10.7–17.0)		13.8 (10.8–16.1)		0.9634
INF : GFR	0.1688 (0.1397–0.2403)		0.1465 (0.1043–0.1743)		0.0585
Postop. infusions [mL/72 h]	12763 (11778.25–14718.75)		12500 (11548.75–14157.5)		0.8501
	n	%	n	%	
Usage of colloids					
Intraoperatively	10	56	28	43	0.4264
Postoperatively	0	0	20	31	**0.0046**

IQR: interquartile range; GFR: glomerular filtration rate; INF : GFR: infusion rate [mL/min] : GFR [mL/min] ratio.

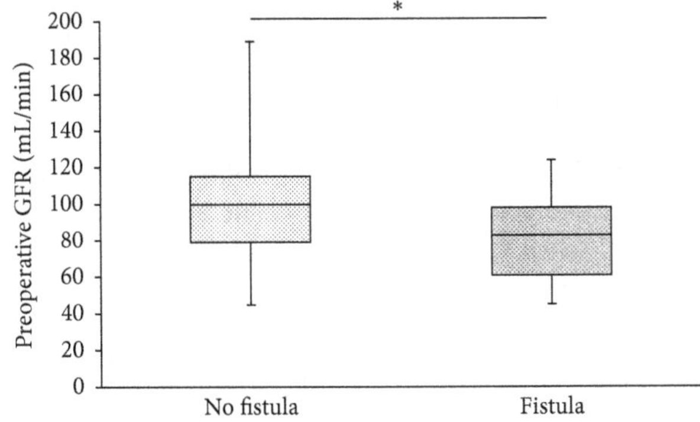

FIGURE 1: Glomerular filtration rate (GFR). In patients with postoperative pancreatic fistulas, the median GFR was 83 mL/min versus 100 mL/min in patients without fistulas ($^*p$ = 0.0219).

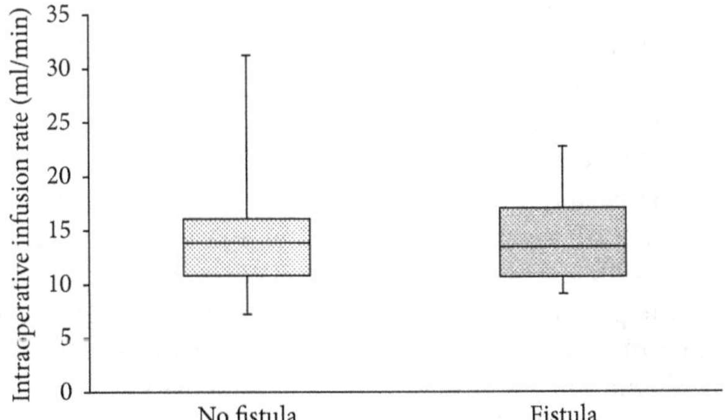

FIGURE 2: Intraoperative infusion rates (mL/min). No significant difference was detected for intraoperative infusions for patients with versus without postoperative pancreatic fistulas (p = 0.9633).

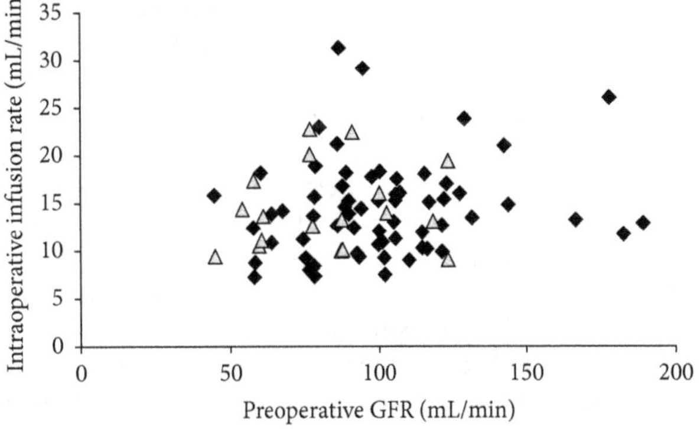

FIGURE 3: Scatterplot illustrating correlation between GFR and intraoperative infusion rate. Intraoperative infusion rates were not related to preoperative GFR (coefficient of determination: r^2 = 0.0271). Black squares: patients without fistulas. Grey triangles: patients with fistulas.

In liver resection, restrictive fluid management is used to achieve a low central venous pressure and leads to decreased intraoperative blood loss, which is known to be associated with increased morbidity [22, 23]. In rectum resection, anastomotic complications increase after perioperative fluid excess [26]. In pancreatic surgery, both intraoperative and postoperative amounts of infusions have been linked to anastomotic complications [27, 28]. Excessive (and in this context: mindless) infusion management can be linked to increased postoperative complications including impaired wound healing, pulmonary complications, and intestinal paralysis [31–35]. It seems obvious that successful fluid

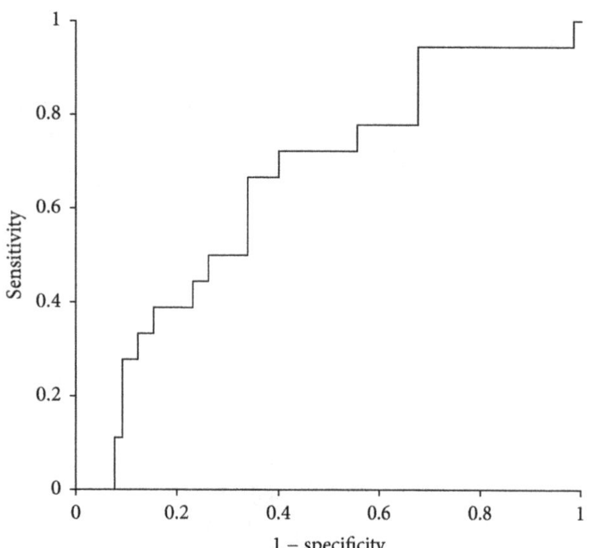

Figure 4: Receiver operating characteristics (ROC) curve for the infusion rate : GFR ratio. A threshold of 0.15 was detected using ROC analysis (ROC-AUC: 0.6564; Youden's J for 0.15: 0.3282).

Table 2: Rates of postoperative pancreatic fistulas for patients exceeding the infusion rate : GFR ratio.

	INF : GFR ≥ 0.15		INF : GFR < 0.15	
	$n = 38$	100%	$n = 45$	100%
Postoperative fistula	13	34	5	11
No postoperative fistula	25	66	40	89

INF : GFR: infusion rate [mL/min] : glomerular filtration rate [mL/min] ratio. $p = 0.0157$.

management in pancreatic surgery needs to be balanced: while excretory renal function can visually be monitored during surgery and hemodynamic parameters are constantly made use of as triggers for infusions and pharmacological interventions, renal function is usually only considered important when already compromised. Most of our patients had a normal renal function with a GFR within normal values (Table 1, Figure 1). Nonetheless, it is quite clear that even the hardest working and healthiest kidney can be overloaded by volume excess. Interstitial fluid shifting can result from generous substitution during surgery and is aggravated by increased vascular permeability [30]. In these cases, resulting edema is visible for surgeons and should be considered an alarm signal and threat to the patient, especially when risky anastomoses with known potential of fistulas need to be carried out. In the authors' opinion, this mechanism, which is supported by the findings presented in this study, seems intuitive and quite obvious. Consequently, anesthesiologists need to hand over part of the responsibility for adequate fluid management to surgeons and need to be aware that misguided fluid management can increase risk of surgical complications. The bottom line is that there is a good share of responsibility for surgical complications for the anesthesiologist and every discipline involved in the teamwork necessary to carry out complex surgical procedures needs to understand any intraoperative action contributes to success or failure.

Perioperative infusion management relies on both measurable parameters and experience. Fluid overload needs to be avoided, while fluids lost need to be replaced and hemodynamic parameters need to be manipulated to stabilize the patient during and after surgery [30]. During induction of anesthesia, a starting bolus volume is very often applied and is considered necessary to compensate for both hypovolemia of the fasting patient and vasodilatation during anesthesia or caused by epidural catheters [36–38]. This has been considered good practice for years but may be inappropriate and the foundation to postoperative complications even before surgery starts. During surgery, excessive volumes are infused to compensate loss to the third space, which has been an accepted concept for decades but may not even exist [39, 40]. Very often, sympathomimetic medication will be avoided since an impaired renal function is feared and crystalloids and colloids will be applied [41]. Intraoperatively, no significant difference was seen for the type of infusion solutions (i.e., crystalloids versus colloids) in our patients. Most interestingly, there was a striking difference in postoperative regimens: none of the patients with fistulas had received colloids during the first 72 h after surgery. Smaller volumes of colloids are needed to achieve the same effect compared to crystalloids; thus crystalloid substitution using colloids might be a worthwhile intervention, but data on this topic remains controversial [42]. It has to be remarked that in large meta-analyses no positive effect on survival and complications rates of colloids versus crystalloids could be identified; consequently, the usage of colloids has decreased over the last decade while the rate of pancreatic fistulas after PD with PJ remained unchanged [2, 43].

In a study from 2014, a threshold of 1 L positive fluid balance on postoperative day one was identified to be associated with an increased risk of complications after pancreatic surgery [28]. Since fluid balance during the first 24 h after surgery exceeded 1 L in any of our patients, this finding was not reproducible using our data.

5. Conclusion

Pancreatic surgery involves both sophisticated surgical and anesthesiological management, amongst other prerequisites [44–46]. Fluid management, which is within reach for interventions, needs to be considered as surgical and anesthesiological teamwork [30, 47]. Our analysis has demonstrated a clear association between intraoperative fluid excess and occurrence of pancreatic fistulas after PD with PJ even in patients with normal renal function. When in our patients the intraoperative infusion rate : GFR ratio exceeded 0.15, the rate of postoperative pancreatic fistulas was more than tripled. Our analysis points at an increased use of intra- and postoperative colloids as a possible intervention. High quality randomized clinical trials comparing different fluid regimens are needed to generate evidence in this important aspect of pancreatic surgery.

Competing Interests

The authors declare that they have no competing interests.

References

[1] U. Klaiber, P. Probst, P. Knebel et al., "Meta-analysis of complication rates for single-loop versus dual-loop (Roux-en-Y) with isolated pancreaticojejunostomy reconstruction after pancreaticoduodenectomy," *British Journal of Surgery*, vol. 102, pp. 331–340, 2015.

[2] J. L. Cameron and J. He, "Two thousand consecutive pancreaticoduodenectomies," *Journal of the American College of Surgeons*, vol. 220, no. 4, pp. 530–536, 2015.

[3] U. A. Wittel, F. Makowiec, O. Sick et al., "Retrospective analyses of trends in pancreatic surgery: indications, operative techniques, and postoperative outcome of 1,120 pancreatic resections," *World Journal of Surgical Oncology*, vol. 13, article 102, 2015.

[4] W. B. Pratt, M. P. Callery, and C. M. Vollmer Jr., "Risk prediction for development of pancreatic fistula using the ISGPF classification scheme," *World Journal of Surgery*, vol. 32, no. 3, pp. 419–428, 2008.

[5] C. G. Ball and T. J. Howard, "Does the type of pancreaticojejunostomy after whipple alter the leak rate?" *Advances in Surgery*, vol. 44, no. 1, pp. 131–148, 2010.

[6] L. Chen, "Applying transductal invaginational pancreaticojejunostomy to decrease pancreatic leakage after pancreaticoduodenectomy," *Hepato-Gastroenterology*, vol. 60, no. 125, pp. 1018–1020, 2013.

[7] Y. Chen, N. Ke, C. Tan et al., "Continuous versus interrupted suture techniques of pancreaticojejunostomy after pancreaticoduodenectomy," *Journal of Surgical Research*, vol. 193, no. 2, pp. 590–597, 2015.

[8] D. Hashimoto, M. Hirota, Y. Yagi, and H. Baba, "End-to-side pancreaticojejunostomy without stitches in the pancreatic stump," *Surgery Today*, vol. 43, no. 7, pp. 821–824, 2013.

[9] D. D. Karavias, D. D. Karavias, I. G. Chaveles, S. K. Kakkos, N. A. Katsiakis, and I. C. Maroulis, "'True' duct-to-mucosa pancreaticojejunostomy, with secure eversion of the enteric mucosa, in whipple operation," *Journal of Gastrointestinal Surgery*, vol. 19, no. 3, pp. 498–505, 2015.

[10] T. Keck, U. F. Wellner, M. Bahra et al., "Pancreatogastrostomy versus pancreatojejunostomy for RECOnstruction After PANCreatoduodenectomy (RECOPANC, DRKS 00000767)," *Annals of Surgery*, vol. 263, no. 3, pp. 440–449, 2015.

[11] A. Kleespies, M. Rentsch, H. Seeliger, M. Albertsmeier, K. W. Jauch, and C. J. Bruns, "Blumgart anastomosis for pancreaticojejunostomy minimizes severe complications after pancreatic head resection," *British Journal of Surgery*, vol. 96, no. 7, pp. 741–750, 2009.

[12] B. Menahem, L. Guittet, A. Mulliri, A. Alves, and J. Lubrano, "Pancreaticogastrostomy is superior to pancreaticojejunostomy for prevention of pancreatic fistula after pancreaticoduodenectomy: an updated meta-analysis of randomized controlled trials," *Annals of Surgery*, vol. 261, no. 5, pp. 882–887, 2015.

[13] N. Torer, A. Ezer, and T. Z. Nursal, "Mattress sutures for the modification of end-to-end dunking pancreaticojejunostomy," *Hepatobiliary and Pancreatic Diseases International*, vol. 12, no. 5, pp. 556–558, 2013.

[14] U. F. Wellner, G. Kayser, H. Lapshyn et al., "A simple scoring system based on clinical factors related to pancreatic texture predicts postoperative pancreatic fistula preoperatively," *HPB*, vol. 12, no. 10, pp. 696–702, 2010.

[15] T. Schnelldorfer, P. D. Mauldin, D. N. Lewin, and D. B. Adams, "Distal pancreatectomy for chronic pancreatitis: risk factors for postoperative pancreatic fistula," *Journal of Gastrointestinal Surgery*, vol. 11, no. 8, pp. 991–997, 2007.

[16] S.-J. Fu, S.-L. Shen, S.-Q. Li et al., "Risk factors and outcomes of postoperative pancreatic fistula after pancreaticoduodenectomy: an audit of 532 consecutive cases," *BMC Surgery*, vol. 15, article 34, 2015.

[17] Y. Fujiwara, H. Shiba, Y. Shirai et al., "Perioperative serum albumin correlates with postoperative pancreatic fistula after pancreaticoduodenectomy," *Anticancer Research*, vol. 35, no. 1, pp. 499–504, 2015.

[18] L. Yu, Q. Huang, F. Xie, X. Lin, and C. Liu, "Risk factors of postoperative complications of pancreatoduodenectomy," *Hepato-gastroenterology*, vol. 61, no. 135, pp. 2091–2095, 2014.

[19] M. H. Squires III, V. V. Mehta, S. B. Fisher et al., "Effect of preoperative renal insufficiency on postoperative outcomes after pancreatic resection: a single institution experience of 1,061 consecutive patients," *Journal of the American College of Surgeons*, vol. 218, no. 1, pp. 92–101, 2014.

[20] R. M. Jones, C. E. Moulton, and K. J. Hardy, "Central venous pressure and its effect on blood loss during liver resection," *British Journal of Surgery*, vol. 85, no. 8, pp. 1058–1060, 1998.

[21] Z. Li, Y.-M. Sun, F.-X. Wu, L.-Q. Yang, Z.-J. Lu, and W.-F. Yu, "Controlled low central venous pressure reduces blood loss and transfusion requirements in hepatectomy," *World Journal of Gastroenterology*, vol. 20, no. 1, pp. 303–309, 2014.

[22] P. Schemmer, H. Bruns, J. Weitz, J. Schmidt, and M. W. Büchler, "Liver transection using vascular stapler: a review," *HPB*, vol. 10, no. 4, pp. 249–252, 2008.

[23] H. Bruns, M. W. Büchler, and P. Schemmer, "Liver transection: modern procedure: technique, results and costs," *Chirurg*, vol. 86, no. 6, pp. 552–560, 2015.

[24] T. Tatara, Y. Nagao, and C. Tashiro, "The effect of duration of surgery on fluid balance during abdominal surgery: a mathematical model," *Anesthesia and Analgesia*, vol. 109, no. 1, pp. 211–216, 2009.

[25] D. N. Lobo, D. A. L. Macafee, and S. P. Allison, "How perioperative fluid balance influences postoperative outcomes," *Best Practice and Research: Clinical Anaesthesiology*, vol. 20, no. 3, pp. 439–455, 2006.

[26] A. K. Boesen, Y. Maeda, and M. Rorbæk Madsen, "Perioperative fluid infusion and its influence on anastomotic leakage after rectal cancer surgery: implications for prevention strategies," *Colorectal Disease*, vol. 15, no. 9, pp. e522–e527, 2013.

[27] M. Fischer, K. Matsuo, M. Gonen et al., "Relationship between intraoperative fluid administration and perioperative outcome after pancreaticoduodenectomy: results of a prospective randomized trial of acute normovolemic hemodilution compared with standard intraoperative management," *Annals of Surgery*, vol. 252, no. 6, pp. 952–958, 2010.

[28] L. Weinberg, D. Wong, D. Karalapillai et al., "The impact of fluid intervention on complications and length of hospital stay after pancreaticoduodenectomy (Whipple's procedure)," *BMC Anesthesiology*, vol. 14, article 35, 2014.

[29] S. Klahr, A. S. Levey, G. J. Beck et al., "The effects of dietary protein restriction and blood-pressure control on the progression of chronic renal disease. Modification of Diet in Renal Disease Study Group," *The New England Journal of Medicine*, vol. 330, no. 13, pp. 877–884, 1994.

[30] B. Brandstrup, "Fluid therapy for the surgical patient," *Best Practice and Research: Clinical Anaesthesiology*, vol. 20, no. 2, pp. 265–283, 2006.

[31] B. Brandstrup, H. Tonnesen, R. Beier-Holgersen et al., "Effects of intravenous fluid restriction on postoperative complications: comparison of two perioperative fluid regimens: a randomized assessor-blinded multicenter trial," *Annals of Surgery*, vol. 238, pp. 641–648, 2003.

[32] K. Holte, N. E. Sharrock, and H. Kehlet, "Pathophysiology and clinical implications of perioperative fluid excess," *British Journal of Anaesthesia*, vol. 89, no. 4, pp. 622–632, 2002.

[33] K. Jonsson, J. A. Jensen, W. H. Goodson III et al., "Tissue oxygenation, anemia, and perfusion in relation to wound healing in surgical patients," *Annals of Surgery*, vol. 214, no. 5, pp. 605–613, 1991.

[34] T. E. Miller, K. Raghunathan, and T. J. Gan, "State-of-the-art fluid management in the operating room," *Best Practice and Research: Clinical Anaesthesiology*, vol. 28, no. 3, pp. 261–273, 2014.

[35] D. W. Wilmore, R. J. Smith, S. T. O'Dwyer, D. O. Jacobs, T. R. Ziegler, and X.-D. Wang, "The gut: a central organ after surgical stress," *Surgery*, vol. 104, no. 5, pp. 917–923, 1988.

[36] A. F. McCrae and J. A. W. Wildsmith, "Prevention and treatment of hypotension during central neural block," *British Journal of Anaesthesia*, vol. 70, no. 6, pp. 672–680, 1993.

[37] A. M. Pouta, J. Karinen, O. J. Vuolteenaho, and T. J. Laatikainen, "Effect of intravenous fluid preload on vasoactive peptide secretion during Caesarean section under spinal anaesthesia," *Anaesthesia*, vol. 51, no. 2, pp. 128–132, 1996.

[38] G. E. Morgan, M. S. Mikhail, and M. J. Murray, *Clinical Anesthesiology*, vol. 14, Lange Medical Books/McGraw Hill, New York, NY, USA, 2006.

[39] E. A. M. Frost, "The rise and fall of the third space: appropriate intraoperative fluid management," *Journal of the Medical Association of Thailand*, vol. 96, no. 8, pp. 1001–1008, 2013.

[40] M. Jacob, D. Chappell, and M. Rehm, "The 'third space'—fact or fiction?" *Best Practice and Research: Clinical Anaesthesiology*, vol. 23, no. 2, pp. 145–157, 2009.

[41] J. W. Sear, "Kidney dysfunction in the postoperative period," *British Journal of Anaesthesia*, vol. 95, no. 1, pp. 20–32, 2005.

[42] D. Orbegozo Cortés, T. Gamarano Barros, H. Njimi, and J.-L. Vincent, "Crystalloids versus colloids: exploring differences in fluid requirements by systematic review and meta-regression," *Anesthesia & Analgesia*, vol. 120, no. 2, pp. 389–402, 2015.

[43] P. Perel, I. Roberts, and K. Ker, "Colloids versus crystalloids for fluid resuscitation in critically ill patients," *Cochrane Database of Systematic Reviews*, vol. 2, Article ID CD000567, 2013.

[44] G. Alemanno, C. Bergamini, J. Martellucci et al., "Surgical outcome of pancreaticoduodenectomy: high volume center or multidisciplinary management?" *Minerva Chirurgica*, vol. 71, no. 1, pp. 8–14, 2016.

[45] F. Gani, Y. Kim, M. J. Weiss et al., "Effect of surgeon and anesthesiologist volume on surgical outcomes," *Journal of Surgical Research*, vol. 200, no. 2, pp. 427–434, 2016.

[46] H. Bruns, N. N. Rahbari, T. Löffler et al., "Perioperative management in distal pancreatectomy: results of a survey in 23 European participating centres of the DISPACT trial and a review of literature," *Trials*, vol. 10, article 58, 2009.

[47] K. Raghunathan, M. Singh, and D. N. Lobo, "Fluid management in abdominal surgery. what, when, and when not to administer," *Anesthesiology Clinics*, vol. 33, no. 1, pp. 51–64, 2015.

The Role of Eugenol in the Prevention of Acute Pancreatitis-Induced Acute Kidney Injury: Experimental Study

Charalampos Markakis,[1] Alexandra Tsaroucha,[2] Apostolos E. Papalois,[3] Maria Lambropoulou,[4] Eleftherios Spartalis,[5] Christina Tsigalou,[2] Konstantinos Romanidis,[2] and Constantinos Simopoulos[2]

[1] *Department of Surgery, St. Georges' Hospital, Tooting SW17 0QT, UK*
[2] *Department of Surgery and Laboratory of Experimental Surgery, Faculty of Medicine, Democritus University of Thrace, 68100 Alexandroupolis, Greece*
[3] *Experimental Research Center, ELPEN Pharmaceuticals, Pikermi, 19009 Attica, Greece*
[4] *Laboratory of Histology, Faculty of Medicine, Democritus University of Thrace, 68100 Alexandroupolis, Greece*
[5] *Second Propaedeutic Department of Surgery, Thoracic Surgery Department, "Laiko" General Hospital, 11527 Athens, Greece*

Correspondence should be addressed to Charalampos Markakis; harismarkakis@hotmail.com

Academic Editor: Richard Charnley

Aim. Acute pancreatitis is an inflammatory intra-abdominal disease, which takes a severe form in 15–20% of patients and can result in high mortality especially when complicated by acute renal failure. The aim of this study is to assess the possible reduction in the extent of acute kidney injury after administration of eugenol in an experimental model of acute pancreatitis. *Materials and Methods.* 106 male Wistar rats weighing 220–350 g were divided into 3 groups: (1) Sham, with sham surgery; (2) Control, with induction of acute pancreatitis, through ligation of the biliopancreatic duct; and (3) Eugenol, with induction of acute pancreatitis and eugenol administration at a dose of 15 mg/kg. Serum urea and creatinine, histopathological changes, TNF-α, IL-6, and MPO activity in the kidneys were evaluated at predetermined time intervals. *Results.* The group that was administered eugenol showed milder histopathological changes than the Control group, TNF-α activity was milder in the Eugenol group, and there was no difference in activity for MPO and IL-6. Serum urea and creatinine levels were lower in the Eugenol group than in the Control group. *Conclusions.* Eugenol administration was protective for the kidneys in an experimental model of acute pancreatitis in rats.

1. Introduction

Acute pancreatitis is an inflammatory intra-abdominal process, which in approximately 15–20% of patients presents in a severe form, with a gradual establishment of multiple organ dysfunction or local complications, including necrosis, pseudocyst, and abscess [1]. Severe acute pancreatitis is a condition associated with high mortality, which is characterized by a complex and incompletely understood pathophysiological mechanism [2, 3].

The deficit in our understanding of the mechanism driving the inflammatory process in acute pancreatitis is a reason why our therapeutic strategy has failed to reduce mortality, despite ongoing research. The aetiology of early mortality after acute pancreatitis is multiple organ failure. When acute pancreatitis leads to the establishment of acute kidney injury, there is a 5- to 10-fold rise in mortality, which can reach 70% [4–6]. The prevention of acute kidney injury can be a useful strategy in the prevention of the morbidity and mortality associated with acute pancreatitis.

Eugenol (1-allyl-4-hydroxy-3-methoxybenzene) is a naturally occurring substance, found in the essential oil of commonly consumed spices such as clove oil as well as cinnamon, basil, and nutmeg oils [7]. It has many pharmacological properties which are mainly analgesic, anti-inflammatory, antioxidant, and vasodilatory action [7], while it has been shown to ameliorate kidney injury in a model of gentamycin-induced nephrotoxicity [8]. The aim of this study is to assess

TABLE 1: Semiquantitative scoring system.

Variable	Result	Score
Histopathological variables		
Hyperemia and dilation of renal parenchyma capillaries	None	0 = −
Hyperemia and dilation of renal corpuscles capillaries Inflammatory infiltration of renal parenchyma	Mild	1 = +
Edema	Moderate	2 = ++
Acute tubular necrosis	Severe	3 = + + +
Immunohistochemical variables		
IL-6	None	0 = −
TNF-α	Mild	1 = +
	Moderate	2 = ++
MPO	Severe	3 = + + +

the possible reduction in the extent of acute kidney injury after administration of eugenol in an experimental model of acute pancreatitis.

2. Materials and Methods

2.1. Experimental Animals. 106 male Wistar rats, aged 3-4 months and weighing 220–350 gr, were used in this study. They were housed in cages under standard laboratory conditions (12 hr light-dark cycles, 22–25°C room temperature, and 55–58% humidity), with free access to food and water. The animals were procured from the Hellenic Pasteur Institute (Athens, Greece). The experiment took place at the ELPEN Experimental Research Center (Pikermi, Greece), while the histological analysis was carried out at the Lab of Histology, Embryology, Medical School, Democritus University of Thrace. The experimental surgical procedures and the general handling of the animals conformed to the international guidelines of Directive 86/609/EEC on the protection of animals used for experimental and other scientific purposes. The animals were randomly assigned in 3 groups: Sham (N = 20), Control (N = 46), and Eugenol (N = 40).

2.2. Acute Pancreatitis Experimental Model. The animals were anaesthetized initially by being placed in a glass box containing isoflurane and then through administration of 0.25 mL of butorphanol (Dolorex; Intervet/Schering/Plough Animal Health, Boxmeer, Holland) by subcutaneous injection. The animals were intubated with a 16 G venous catheter, which was then connected to a ventilator set at 70 breaths/min and a tidal volume of 3 mL. After confirmation of the success of intubation, anaesthesia was maintained by a mixture of 93% O_2, 5% CO_2, and 2% isoflurane. Acute pancreatitis was induced according to a previously described model [9]. Briefly, after induction of anaesthesia and preparation of the surgical site, the abdomen was entered via a 3 cm midline incision under sterile conditions. The pancreas was identified and mobilized in all animals. The biliopancreatic duct was identified and ligated near the duodenal wall with a 4-0 silk sutures (in the Control and Eugenol groups, but not in the Sham group). 1 mL of normal saline and 1 mL of 5% D_5W were instilled in the abdominal cavity. The abdomen was closed with vicryl 2-0 sutures. In the Eugenol group, eugenol was administered by a nasogastric catheter in a dose of 15 mg/kg, while the Sham and Control groups received corn oil solution without eugenol.

Postoperatively, analgesia was maintained through subcutaneous administration of 2 mL/Kg butorphanol (Dolorex; Intervet/Schering/Plough Animal Health, Boxmeer, Holland). Euthanasia was performed at a predetermined time for each animal with the use of ketamine (Narcetan; Vetoquinol, Buckingham, UK) 0.3–0.6 mL and xylazine (Rompun; Bayer, Uxbridge, UK) 0.1–0.3 mL, followed by a midline laparotomy and exsanguination of the abdominal aorta. Time points for analysis were 6, 12, 24, 48, and 72 hours postoperatively. Serum samples for measurement of urea and creatinine as well as specimens from both kidneys for histopathological examination were acquired.

2.3. Preparation of Eugenol. Pure eugenol (eugenol 99%, Aldrich Chemistry, St. Louis, MO, USA) was purchased and prepared in an oily solution in the chemical laboratory of Elpen Pharmaceutical Co. Inc. (ELPEN Pharmaceutical Co. Inc., Pikermi Attica, Greece). This was achieved with the admixture of pure eugenol in a corn oil solution in a concentration of 1.5 mg eugenol/mL.

2.4. Histopathological and Immunohistochemical Evaluation. Samples were placed in 10% buffered formalin solution, and 4 μm paraffin-embedded sections were stained with hematoxylin/eosin. All specimens were evaluated by a pathologist blinded to the sequence of the biopsy specimens. Slides were evaluated with regard to 5 histopathological parameters and with the use of a semiquantitative scoring system as depicted on Table 1. The scores of each individual parameter for each slide were added and a histopathological score was obtained for each specimen.

Immunohistochemical staining was applied to detect the possible expression of inflammatory cytokines like IL-6, TNF-α, and myeloperoxidase. The following antibodies were used: myeloperoxidase (rabbit polyclonal), DAKO (A 0398), diluted 1 : 400 TNF-α (rabbit polyclonal), ABNOVA (PAB8016), diluted 1 : 1000, IL-6 (rabbit polyclonal), and Abcam (ab6672), diluted 1 : 500.

The buffers, blocking solutions, secondary antibodies, avidin-biotin complex reagents, and chromogen were supplied in a detection kit (EnVision HRP, Mouse/Rabbit detection system (K 5007), DAKO). To inhibit endogenous peroxidase, the specimens were incubated with 3% H_2O_2 (200 mL H_2O and 6 mL H_2O_2) for 15 min in a dark room. Before the primary antibody was applied, the sections were immersed in 10 mM citrate buffer (pH 6.0), rinsed in tris-buffered saline, and subsequently heated in a microwave oven (650–800 W) for three cycles of 5 min. The slides were washed with tris-buffered saline before application of the primary antibody in order to reduce nonspecific binding of antisera. Control slides were used as common negative controls for all antibody staining. Sections were then briefly counterstained with Mayer's hematoxylin, mounted, and examined under a Nikon Eclipse 50i microscope (Nikon Instruments Inc, NY, USA).

Scoring was assigned according to the proportion of cells with cytoplasmic staining. The positivity of the expression was determined by counting the number of stained cells. The average labeling index was assessed according to the proportion of positive cells, after scanning the entire section of the specimen. Sections with greater than 10% stained cells were considered as being positive. The results were graded as negative (0) for <10% of stained cells, low (1) for >10% and <30% of cells stained, moderate (2) for >30% and <70% cells stained, and high expression (3) for >70% cells stained (Table 1).

2.5. Statistical Analysis. The statistical analysis of the results was completed with the use of the 20th version of SPSS (Statistical Package for the Social Sciences, SPSS Inc., Chicago, IL, USA). We performed an analysis in which the data were treated as qualitative using Fisher's exact test (this test was preferable to x^2 because of the small number of animals in each subcategory/time point). Use of the semiquantitative scoring allowed us to also treat the data as ordinal. Evaluation of the different variables was performed to determine whether they were normally distributed (Kolmogorov-Smirnov are Shapiro-Wilk). The three different groups were then analyzed using the Kruskal-Wallis one-way analysis of variance test. Finally, the Mann-Whitney U test was further used to compare the groups in pairs. These tests were applied to the overall sample and for each individual subgroup corresponding to individual time points (6, 12, 24, 48, and 72 hours postoperatively).

3. Results

3.1. Surgical Outcomes. The operation was concluded successfully on all animals and all animals survived the operation. The animals resumed normal diet and activity with normal bowel function. Six animals died before the predetermined time point for their euthanasia. These animals were all part of the Control group. They were substituted and were not included in the statistical analysis.

3.2. Statistical Analysis. The statistical analysis showed that none of the variables followed a normal distribution. Thus, nonparametric tests were used to analyze the results.

3.3. Histological Evaluation. Eugenol administration resulted in a lower histological score in rats with acute pancreatitis. The difference between the Eugenol and Control groups is apparent at 48 and 72 hours after induction of pancreatitis (Figures 1 and 2). The histological score for these two groups is higher compared to the Sham group at 48 and 72 hours and for the whole sample.

Eugenol administration lowers hyperemia and dilation of renal parenchyma capillaries and the difference was statistically significant for the 48 and 72 hour time points and for the whole sample. The Eugenol group exhibited lower values than the Control group and both exhibited higher values than the Sham group. The same was true for hyperemia and dilation of renal corpuscles capillaries for the 48- and 72-hour time points, but not for the whole sample.

There were no inflammatory infiltrations in any of the animals in our experimental model and measurement of this factor did not produce any results.

Edema was reduced through the administration of eugenol and, again, the difference to the Control group was significant for the 48- and 72-hour time points and the whole sample. The Control group had higher values than the Sham group at 48 hours and also higher values than both the Sham and Eugenol groups at 72 hours. When values of the whole sample were considered, the Control group had higher values than the Eugenol group, which in turn had higher values than the Sham group.

Finally, eugenol did not reduce acute tubular necrosis in our experimental model. There was no statistically significant difference at any of the time points studied. Analysis of the whole sample showed only higher values for the Eugenol and Control groups when compared to the Sham group.

3.4. Immunohistochemical Evaluation. There was no clear difference regarding IL-6 expression between the different groups (Figures 3 and 4). On the contrary, TNF-α expression was attenuated through eugenol administration. There was a statistically significant difference between the Eugenol and Control groups 72 hours after induction of pancreatitis, while both groups exhibit higher TNF-α expression than the Sham group. There was no statistically significant difference between the Eugenol and Control groups for MPO expression, although there was a trend toward higher expression for the Control group after 72 hours.

3.5. Renal Function. Eugenol administration resulted in lower serum levels of urea and creatinine especially at the 48- and 72-hour time points, compared to the Control group. Urea and creatinine levels were higher for both the Eugenol and Control groups, when they were compared to the Sham group (Figure 4).

4. Discussion

The results of this study suggest that eugenol attenuates the intensity of the histopathological changes and the expression of TNF-α and MPO in the renal parenchyma, while lowering the values of serum urea and creatinine when administered in a rat acute pancreatitis experimental model.

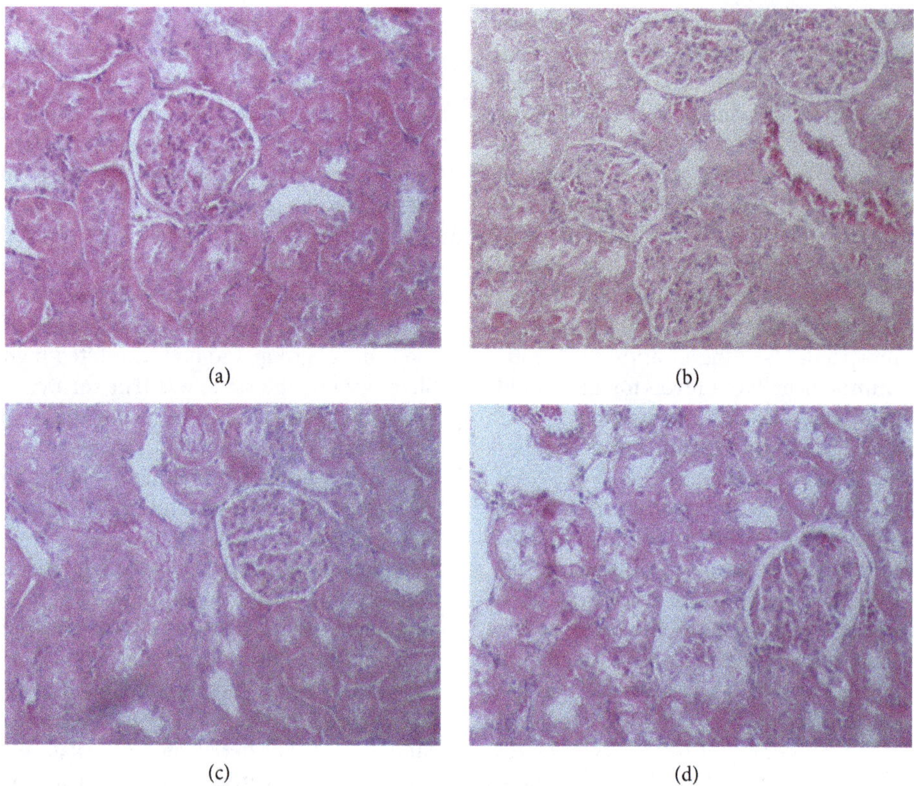

Figure 1: Different levels of inflammation and the corresponding histopathological score (H&E, ×200). (a) Sham group: score 0. (b) Control group: score 3. (c) Eugenol group: score 5.5. (d) Control group: score 9.

To evaluate the extent of kidney injury, we decided to evaluate serum urea and creatinine levels and the histopathological changes in the kidney, as well as the expression of TNF-α, IL-6, and MPO in the renal parenchyma. The role of cytokines, such as TNF-α and IL-6, in the pathophysiology of acute pancreatitis has been studied extensively and they have been found to contribute to the activation of the systematic inflammatory response process and multiorgan failure, which is a hallmark of severe acute pancreatitis and is, ultimately, correlated with the observed high mortality rates [10, 11]. The role of cytokines in acute kidney injury has been found to be equally important. The cytokine-mediated inflammatory response has a central role in the pathophysiology of acute renal failure irrespective of its cause. MPO has been used as a marker of neutrophil migration in acute pancreatitis studies and has been correlated to the severity of kidney injury [12–14].

The histopathological evaluation showed that the histologic score was lower for the Eugenol group in comparison to the Control group at 48 and 72 hours from the initiation of the inflammatory process (means: 3.75/6.5 and 4.12/7.62, resp.) and this difference was statistically significant. This difference between the two groups was also present for individual histological changes such as hyperemia and dilation of renal parenchyma and renal corpuscles capillaries and edema. The difference observed in the degree of acute tubular necrosis and inflammatory infiltration was not statistically significant.

Regarding the expression of inflammatory mediators, TNF-α levels were higher for the Control group in comparison to the Eugenol group with the difference reaching statistical significance at the 72-hour time point, while there was a trend for higher MPO expression in the Control group at 72 hours, which was, however, not statistically significant. In contrast, IL-6 levels did not show the same correlation and there were no statistically significant differences between the Eugenol and Control groups.

We chose the bile-pancreatic duct ligation model as it is a well-characterized model of acute pancreatitis, which mimics acute pancreatitis caused by biliary obstruction, which is a frequent clinical scenario and results in multiorgan failure similar to that observed in humans [15, 16]. We have previously used this experimental model and we were able to show that it generates acute pancreatitis with histopathological changes in the pancreatic tissue including hemorrhage and necrosis [17]. Out of a total of 106 animals, 6 died and the fact that they were all in the Control group could be seen as further evidence supporting the protective role of eugenol. It is possible that these animals would have exhibited signs of severe kidney injury, if they had survived until the predetermined time of euthanasia. However, since the distal bile-pancreatic duct ligation model is not usually fatal, we cannot directly attribute the death of these animals to the severity of acute pancreatitis. These animals were, therefore, excluded from the statistical analysis and were replaced.

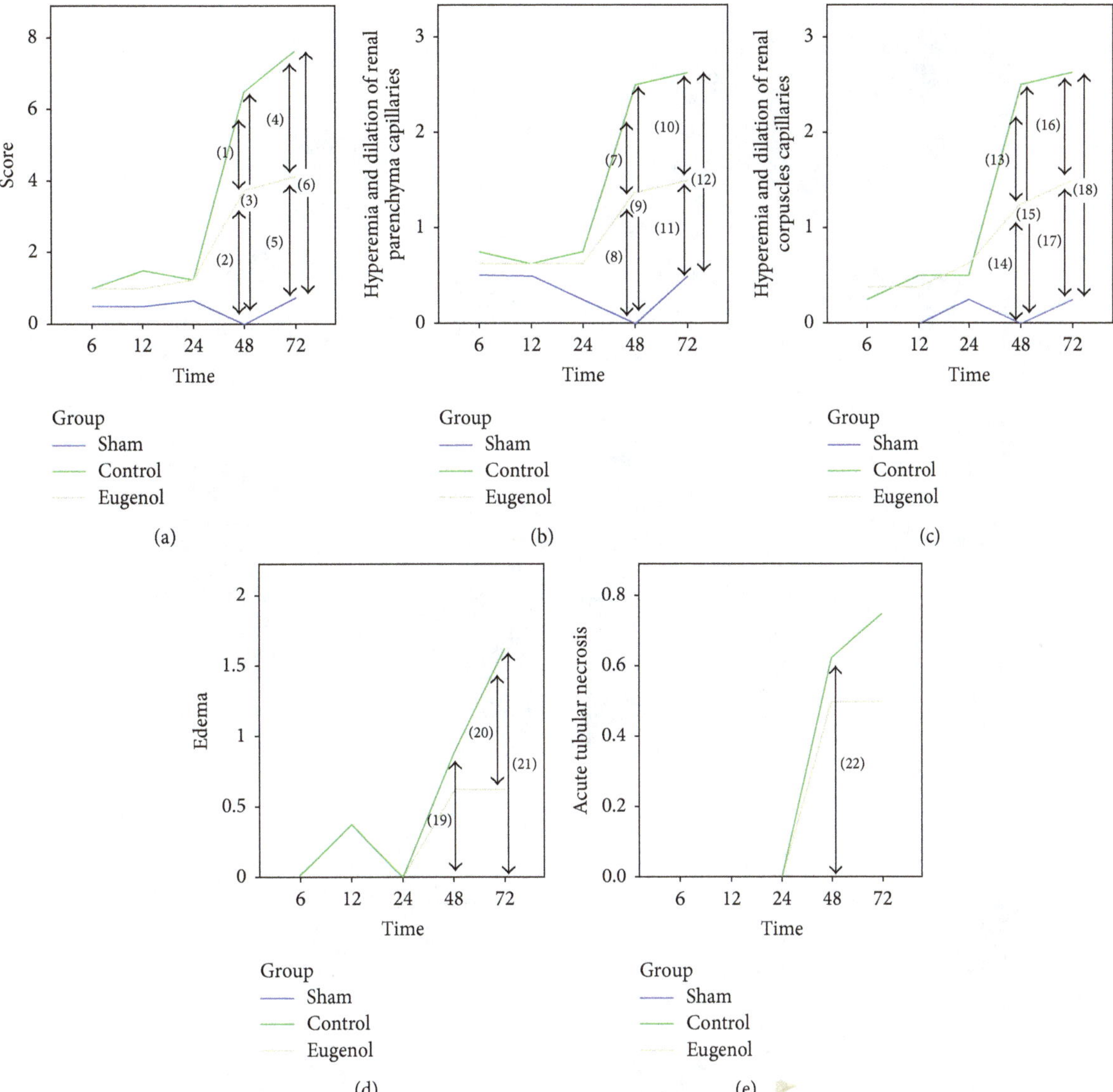

FIGURE 2: Comparative results of histopathological analysis (statistically significant differences are marked by arrows). (a) Histological score. (b) Hyperemia and dilatation of renal parenchymal capillaries. (c) Hyperemia and dilatation of renal corpuscles capillaries. (d) Edema. (e) Acute tubular necrosis. p values (Mann-Whitney test) (1): 0.002, (2): 0.004, (3): 0.004, (4): <0.001, (5): 0.004, (6): 0.004, (7): 0.005, (8): 0.004, (9): 0.004, (10): 0.005, (11): 0.048, (12): 0.004, (13): 0.002, (14): 0.004, (15): 0.004, (16): 0.005, (17): 0.016, (18): 0.004, (19): 0.048, (20): 0.007, (21): 0.004, and (22): 0.048.

Eugenol has been shown to possess a multitude of pharmacological effects [7], some of which make it a likely candidate for use in the setting of acute pancreatitis and can explain the results observed in our study. The analgesic action of eugenol has been well documented and doses in the range of 40–100 mg/kg have been shown to be effective in rat experimental models [18–20]. In addition, eugenol acts as an anti-inflammatory substance inhibiting cyclooxygenase [21] and reducing the release of proinflammatory mediators such as IL-1β, TNF-α, and PGE2 [22–24]. The antioxidative potential of eugenol has been studied in a number of, mainly in vitro, studies where it has been shown to bind to free oxygen radicals and attenuate the action of oxidative substances [25–28], while a recent study of gentamycin-induced nephrotoxicity offers insight into how eugenol can prevent kidney injury by reducing oxidative damage [8]. These combined properties of eugenol can be used to explain the observed reduction in TNF-α expression, as well as the reduction of kidney inflammation. Eugenol administration causes a dose-dependent, reversible vasodilation through its effect on the endothelial cells [29, 30], which is comparable to nifedipine [31]. The potential of eugenol to inhibit the vasoconstriction that is associated with kidney injury points to another potential mechanism for its effect in the model of acute pancreatitis.

A number of authors have proposed strategies to reduce kidney injury caused by acute pancreatitis. Zhang et al.

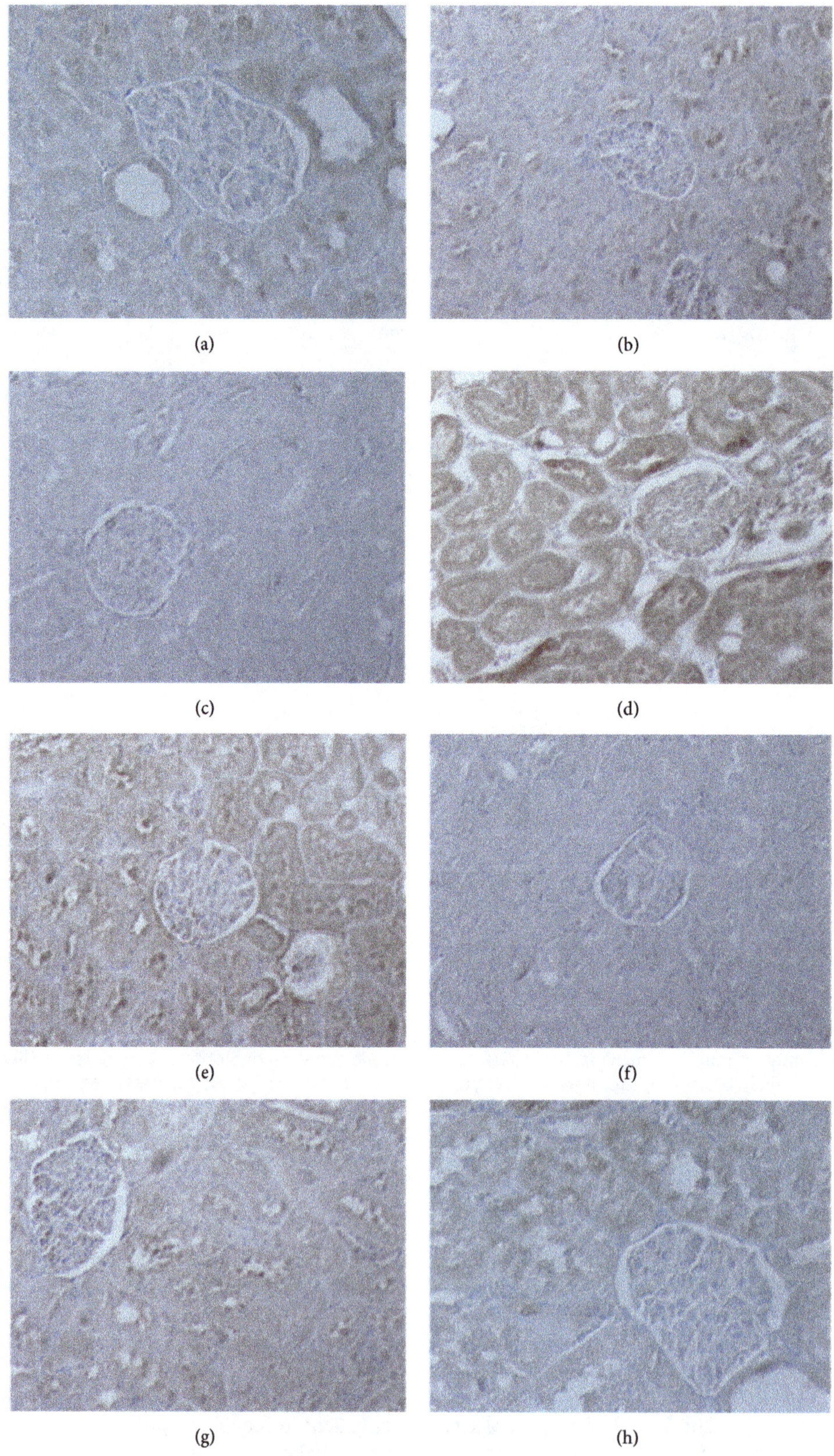

FIGURE 3: Different levels of immunohistochemical staining expression (×200). (a) Control group: mild expression of IL-6 after 72 hours. (b) Eugenol group: moderate expression of IL-6 after 72 hours. (c) Sham group: no expression of TNF-α at 72 hours. (d) Control group: moderate expression of TNF-α at 72 hours. (e) Eugenol group: mild expression of TNF-α at 72 hours. (f) Sham group: no expression of MPO at 72 hours. (g) Control group: severe expression of MPO at 72 hours. (h) Eugenol group: moderate expression of MPO at 72 hours.

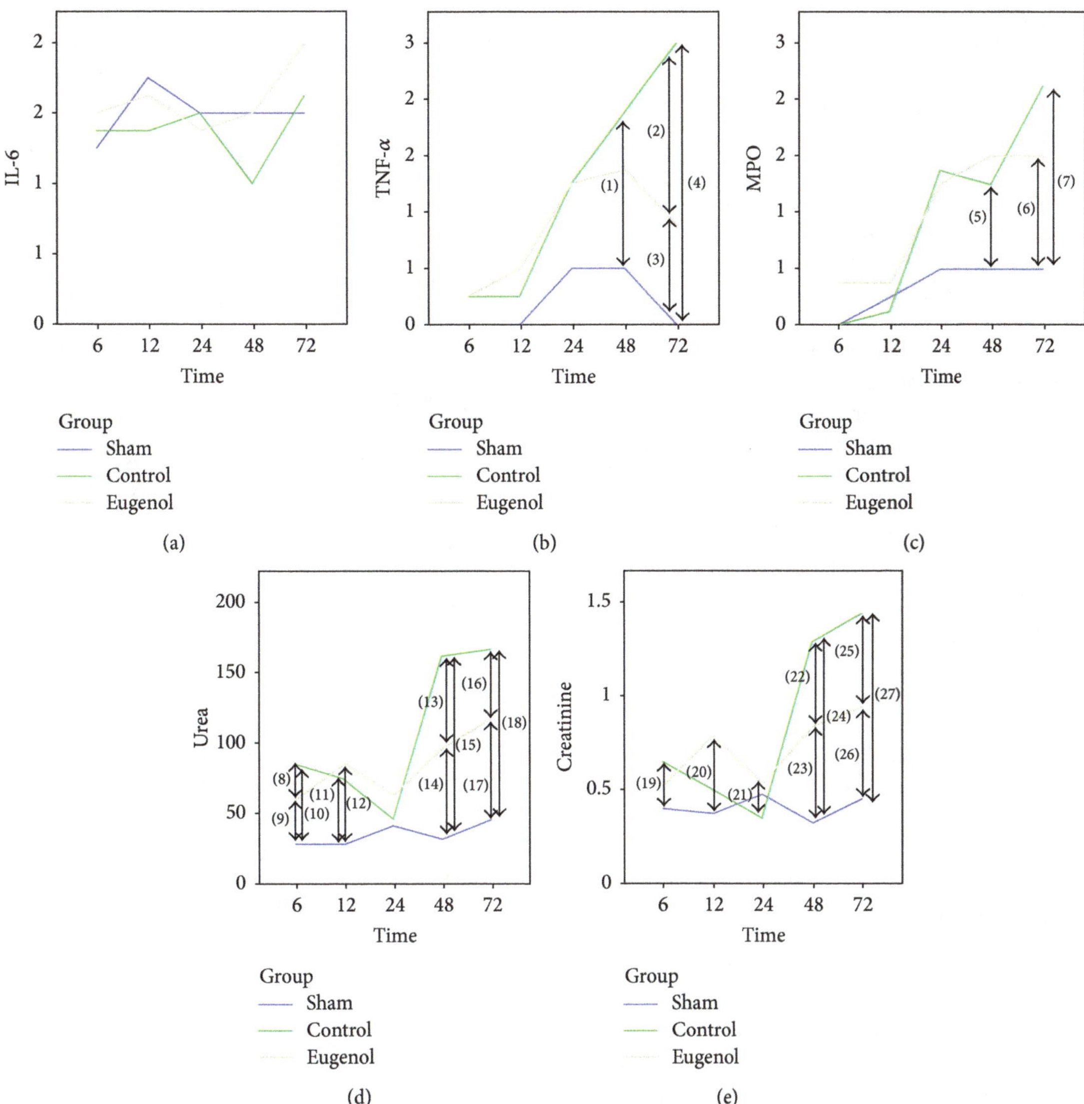

Figure 4: Serum urea and creatinine and immunohistochemical staining results (statistically significant differences are marked by arrows). (a) IL-6. (b) TNF-α. (c) MPO. (d) Urea. (e) Creatinine. p valves (Mann-Whitney test) (1): 0.008, (2): <0.001, (3): 0.016, (4): 0.004, (5): 0.048, (6): 0.008, (7): 0.048, (8): 0.050, (9): 0.004, (10): 0.004, (11): 0.004, (12): 0.004, (13): <0.001, (14): 0.004, (15): 0.004, (16): 0.001, (17): 0.004, (18): 0.004, (19): 0.008, (20): 0.028, (21): 0.001, (22): 0.040, (23): 0.004, (24): 0.004, (25): 0.002, and (26): 0.004.

have tried dexamethasone administration in an experimental model of retrograde injection of sodium taurocholate in the pancreatic duct [32]. The dexamethasone group exhibited milder congestion of the glomerular capillary, swelling of the renal tubular epithelial cells, and less inflammatory cell infiltration than that of the Control group, which was shown by the lower histological score at the 6- and 12-hour time points. The same authors found a significant difference in the serum levels of TNF-α in favor of the dexamethasone group, while expression of NF-κB in the renal tissue was more pronounced in the dexamethasone group [33]. The same model has been used to study octreotide and baicalin (5,6,7-trihydroxyflavone-7-O-D-glucuronic acid) [34]. The administration of these substances had a protective effect on the kidney and both the histological score and renal parenchyma NF-κb expression were lower in comparison to the Control group. Serum levels of urea, creatinine, TNF-α, and IL-6 were reduced compared to the Control group in another study with the same experimental protocol [35]. There have been a number of studies of plant derived substances, used in traditional Chinese medicine. Ligustrazine proved to be protective for the kidney as was demonstrated by the lower creatinine levels and the milder histopathological changes in comparison to the Control group [36]. In another study, the administration of 3 traditional Chinese medicine substances (ligustrazine, kakonein, and *Panax* notoginsenosides) resulted in reduced mortality and milder histopathological changes in the rat kidney [37]. Finally, the model of induction of acute pancreatitis through sodium taurocholate administration was used for the study of poly(ADP-ribose) polymerase inhibition, through 3-aminobenzamide (3-AB) administration. The administration of 3-AB resulted in reduced mortality and a reduction in the increase of creatinine, TNF-α, IL-1b, and IL-6, milder histopathological changes, and reduced MPO expression in the kidney [18].

There are some limitations to our experimental protocol. The half life of eugenol in the rat has been determined to be 18,3 hours [18]; therefore, at 72 hours, most of the initial dose would have been cleared from the circulation. It is possible that a repeat administration of eugenol could further increase the therapeutic result. Moreover, the time frame of our protocol reached 72 hours, which was not adequate for the complete evaluation of the effect of eugenol. Indeed, a difference in the extent of kidney injury between the Eugenol and Control groups is first observed 48 hours after the onset of acute pancreatitis and it is greater at 72 hours. Further observations at additional time points could yield even larger differences in results.

In conclusion, the administration of eugenol in a rat model of acute pancreatitis was protective for the kidneys in our experimental model. Further research is necessary to determine the possible role of eugenol in the management of acute pancreatitis.

Disclaimer

The authors alone are responsible for the content and writing of the paper.

Acknowledgments

This study was funded with a scholarship by the Experimental Research Center ELPEN Pharmaceuticals (ERCE), Athens, Greece, which also provided the research facilities for this project. The authors would like to thank A. Zacharioudaki DVM, MLAS, E. Karampela, MSc, K. Tsarea, M. Karamperi, N. Psychalakis, A. Karaiskos, S. Gerakis, and E. Gerakis, staff members of the ERCE, for their important assistance during the experiments, and Myrto Kogevina for the editing of the paper.

References

[1] E. L. Bradley III, "A clinically based classification system for acute pancreatitis: summary of the International Symposium on Acute Pancreatitis, Atlanta, Ga, September 11 through 13, 1992," *Archives of Surgery*, vol. 128, no. 5, pp. 586–590, 1993.

[2] K. I. Halonen, A. K. Leppäniemi, P. A. Puolakkainen et al., "Severe acute pancreatitis: prognostic factors in 270 consecutive patients," *Pancreas*, vol. 21, no. 3, pp. 266–271, 2000.

[3] L. Compañy, J. Sáez, J. Martínez et al., "Factors predicting mortality in severe acute pancreatitis," *Pancreatology*, vol. 3, no. 2, pp. 144–148, 2003.

[4] P. Kes, Ž. VuČIČEviĆ, I. RatkoviĆ-GusiĆ, and A. Fotivec, "Acute renal failure complicating severe acute pancreatitis," *Renal Failure*, vol. 18, no. 4, pp. 621–628, 1996.

[5] M. E. Herrera Gutiérrez, G. Seller Pérez, C. de la Rubia De Gracia, M. J. Chaparro Sánchez, and B. Nacle López, "Acute renal failure profile and prognostic value in severe acute pancreatitis," *Medicina Clinica*, vol. 115, no. 19, pp. 721–725, 2000.

[6] H. Li, Z. Qian, Z. Liu, X. Liu, X. Han, and H. Kang, "Risk factors and outcome of acute renal failure in patients with severe acute pancreatitis," *Journal of Critical Care*, vol. 25, no. 2, pp. 225–229, 2010.

[7] K. Pramod, S. H. Ansari, and J. Ali, "Eugenol: a natural compound with versatile pharmacological actions," *Natural Product Communications*, vol. 5, no. 12, pp. 1999–2006, 2010.

[8] M. M. Said, "The protective effect of eugenol against gentamicin-induced nephrotoxicity and oxidative damage in rat kidney," *Fundamental and Clinical Pharmacology*, vol. 25, no. 6, pp. 708–716, 2011.

[9] B. D. Yildiz and E. Hamaloglu, "Basic experimental pancreatitis models for beginners," *Surgical Science*, vol. 1, no. 2, pp. 31–39, 2010.

[10] M. Brady, S. Christmas, R. Sutton, J. Neoptolemos, and J. Slavin, "Cytokines and acute pancreatitis," *Baillieres Best Practice in Clinical Gastroenterology*, vol. 13, no. 2, pp. 265–289, 1999.

[11] A. C. De Beaux, A. S. Goldie, J. A. Ross, D. C. Carter, and K. C. H. Fearon, "Serum concentrations of inflammatory mediators related to organ failure in patients with acute pancreatitis," *British Journal of Surgery*, vol. 83, no. 3, pp. 349–353, 1996.

[12] C. Chen, S. Xu, W.-X. Wang et al., "Rosiglitazone attenuates the severity of sodium taurocholate-induced acute pancreatitis and pancreatitis-associated lung injury," *Archives of Medical Research*, vol. 40, no. 2, pp. 79–88, 2009.

[13] R. Mota, F. Sánchez-Bueno, J. J. Berenguer-Pina, D. Hernández-Espinosa, P. Parrilla, and J. Yélamos, "Therapeutic treatment with poly(ADP-ribose) polymerase inhibitors attenuates the severity of acute pancreatitis and associated liver and lung injury," *British Journal of Pharmacology*, vol. 151, no. 7, pp. 998–1005, 2007.

[14] M. D. Okusa, J. Linden, L. Huang, J. M. Rieger, T. L. MacDonald, and L. P. Huynh, "A_{2A} adenosine receptor-mediated inhibition of renal injury and neutrophil adhesion," *The American Journal of Physiology—Renal Physiology*, vol. 279, no. 5, pp. F809–F818, 2000.

[15] K. H. Su, C. Cuthbertson, and C. Christophi, "Review of experimental animal models of acute pancreatitis," *HPB*, vol. 8, no. 4, pp. 264–286, 2006.

[16] P. Lampropoulos, M. Lambropoulou, A. Papalois et al., "The role of apigenin in an experimental model of acute pancreatitis," *Journal of Surgical Research*, vol. 183, no. 1, pp. 129–137, 2013.

[17] R. Kurian, D. K. Arulmozhi, A. Veeranjaneyulu, and S. L. Bodhankar, "Effect of eugenol on animal models of nociception," *Indian Journal of Pharmacology*, vol. 38, no. 5, pp. 341–345, 2006.

[18] S. A. Guenette, F. Beaudry, J. F. Marier, and P. Vachon, "Pharmacokinetics and anesthetic activity of eugenol in male Sprague-Dawley rats," *Journal of Veterinary Pharmacology and Therapeutics*, vol. 29, no. 4, pp. 265–270, 2006.

[19] S. A. Guénette, A. Ross, J.-F. Marier, F. Beaudry, and P. Vachon, "Pharmacokinetics of eugenol and its effects on thermal hypersensitivity in rats," *European Journal of Pharmacology*, vol. 562, no. 1-2, pp. 60–67, 2007.

[20] D. Thompson and T. Eling, "Mechanism of inhibition of prostaglandin H synthase by eugenol and other phenolic peroxidase substrates," *Molecular Pharmacology*, vol. 36, no. 5, pp. 809–817, 1989.

[21] Y.-Y. Lee, S.-L. Hung, S.-F. Pai, Y.-H. Lee, and S.-F. Yang, "Eugenol suppressed the expression of lipopolysaccharide-induced proinflammatory mediators in human macrophages," *Journal of Endodontics*, vol. 33, no. 6, pp. 698–702, 2007.

[22] J. N. Sharma, K. C. Srivastava, and E. K. Gan, "Suppressive effects of eugenol and ginger oil on arthritic rats," *Pharmacology*, vol. 49, no. 5, pp. 314–318, 1994.

[23] T. G. Rodrigues, A. Fernandes Jr., J. P. B. Sousa, J. K. Bastos, and J. M. Sforcin, "In vitro and in vivo effects of clove on pro-inflammatory cytokines production by macrophages," *Natural Product Research*, vol. 23, no. 4, pp. 319–326, 2009.

[24] S. Fujisawa, T. Atsumi, Y. Kadoma, and H. Sakagami, "Antioxidant and prooxidant action of eugenol-related compounds and their cytotoxicity," *Toxicology*, vol. 177, no. 1, pp. 39–54, 2002.

[25] N. Vidhya and S. N. Devaraj, "Antioxidant effect of eugenol in rat intestine," *Indian Journal of Experimental Biology*, vol. 37, no. 12, pp. 1192–1195, 1999.

[26] H. Kabuto, M. Tada, and M. Kohno, "Eugenol [2-methoxy-4-(2-propenyl)phenol] prevents 6-hydroxydopamine-induced dopamine depression and lipid peroxidation inductivity in mouse striatum," *Biological and Pharmaceutical Bulletin*, vol. 30, no. 3, pp. 423–427, 2007.

[27] L. Jirovetz, G. Buchbauer, I. Stoilova, A. Stoyanova, A. Krastanov, and E. Schmidt, "Chemical composition and antioxidant properties of clove leaf essential oil," *Journal of Agricultural and Food Chemistry*, vol. 54, no. 17, pp. 6303–6307, 2006.

[28] D. N. Criddle, S. V. Frota Madeira, and R. S. De Moura, "Endothelium-dependent and -independent vasodilator effects of eugenol in the rat mesenteric vascular bed," *Journal of Pharmacy and Pharmacology*, vol. 55, no. 3, pp. 359–365, 2003.

[29] L. F. L. Interaminense, D. M. Jucá, P. J. C. Magalhães, J. H. Leal-Cardoso, G. P. Duarte, and S. Lahlou, "Pharmacological evidence of calcium-channel blockade by essential oil of *Ocimum gratissimum* and its main constituent, eugenol, in isolated aortic rings from DOCA-salt hypertensive rats," *Fundamental & Clinical Pharmacology*, vol. 21, no. 5, pp. 497–506, 2007.

[30] O. Sensch, W. Vierling, W. Brandt, and M. Reiter, "Effects of inhibition of calcium and potassium currents in guinea-pig cardiac contraction: comparison of β-caryophyllene oxide, eugenol, and nifedipine," *British Journal of Pharmacology*, vol. 131, no. 6, pp. 1089–1096, 2000.

[31] X. P. Zhang, L. Zhang, Y. Wang et al., "Study of the protective effects of dexamethasone on multiple organ injury in rats with severe acute pancreatitis," *Journal of the Pancreas*, vol. 8, no. 4, pp. 400–412, 2007.

[32] X.-P. Zhang, L. Zhang, L.-J. Chen et al., "Influence of dexamethasone on inflammatory mediators and NF-κB expression in multiple organs of rats with severe acute pancreatitis," *World Journal of Gastroenterology*, vol. 13, no. 4, pp. 548–556, 2007.

[33] Z. Xiping, Z. Jie, X. Qin et al., "Influence of baicalin and octreotide on NF-kappaB and p-selectin expression in liver and kidney of rats with severe acute pancreatitis," *Inflammation*, vol. 32, no. 1, pp. 1–11, 2009.

[34] X.-P. Zhang, H. Tian, Y.-H. Lai et al., "Protective effects and mechanisms of Baicalin and octreotide on renal injury of rats with severe acute pancreatitis," *World Journal of Gastroenterology*, vol. 13, no. 38, pp. 5079–5089, 2007.

[35] J.-X. Zhang, S.-C. Dang, J.-G. Qu, and X.-Q. Wang, "Ligustrazine alleviates acute renal injury in a rat model of acute necrotizing pancreatitis," *World Journal of Gastroenterology*, vol. 12, no. 47, pp. 7705–7709, 2006.

[36] X. P. Zhang, C. Wang, D. J. Wu, M. L. Ma, and J. M. Ou, "Protective effects of ligustrazine, kakonein and Panax notoginsenosides on multiple organs in rats with severe acute pancreatitis," *Methods and Findings in Experimental and Clinical Pharmacology*, vol. 32, no. 9, pp. 631–644, 2010.

[37] J. Yu, W. Deng, W. Wang et al., "Inhibition of poly(ADP-Ribose) polymerase attenuates acute kidney injury in sodium taurocholate-induced acute pancreatitis in rats," *Pancreas*, vol. 41, no. 8, pp. 1299–1305, 2012.

Liver Resections of Isolated Liver Metastasis in Breast Cancer: Results and Possible Prognostic Factors

Malte Weinrich,[1,2] Christel Weiß,[3] Jochen Schuld,[2] and Bettina M. Rau[1,2]

[1] *Department of General, Thoracic, Vascular and Transplantation Surgery, University Hospital Rostock, Schillingallee 35, 18057 Rostock, Germany*
[2] *Department of General, Visceral, Vascular and Paediatric Surgery, University Hospital of the Saarland, Kirrberger Straße, 66424 Homburg/Saar, Germany*
[3] *Department of Medical Statistics, Medical Faculty Mannheim, University of Heidelberg, Theodor-Kutzer-Ufer 1-3, 68167 Mannheim, Germany*

Correspondence should be addressed to Malte Weinrich; malte.weinrich@med.uni-rostock.de

Academic Editor: Attila Olah

Background. Breast cancer liver metastasis is a hematogenous spread of the primary tumour. It can, however, be the expression of an isolated recurrence. Surgical resection is often possible but controversial. *Methods.* We report on 29 female patients treated operatively due to isolated breast cancer liver metastasis over a period of six years. Prior to surgery all metastases appeared resectable. Liver metastasis had been diagnosed 55 (median, range 1–177) months after primary surgery. *Results.* Complete resection of the metastases was performed in 21 cases. The intraoperative staging did not confirm the preoperative radiological findings in 14 cases, which did not generally lead to inoperability. One-year survival rate was 86% in resected patients and 37.5% in nonresected patients. Significant prognostic factors were R0 resection, low T- and N-stages as well as a low-grade histopathology of the primary tumour, lower number of liver metastases, and a longer time interval between primary surgery and the occurrence of liver metastasis. *Conclusions.* Complete resection of metastases was possible in three-quarters of the patients. Some of the studied factors showed a prognostic value and therefore might influence indication for resection in the future.

1. Introduction

Metastasis is the most common cause of death in cancer patients [1]. Breast cancer might spread via blood stream and cause liver metastasis. This can arise simultaneously or decades after the primary tumour. Metastases are often the sole sign of recurrence of the breast cancer. References show that 2–12% of patients with breast cancer have liver metastasis [2, 3], which, however, might be isolated in some cases. In patients with resectable colorectal liver metastasis, surgical resection is the only curative approach, if an additional nonresectable extrahepatic tumour is excluded. References report 5-year survival rates of 30 to 47% in these patients [4–7]. Surgical management is therefore recommended in the German S3-guidelines for colorectal cancer [8]. In contrast to this the data on isolated liver metastasis in breast cancer patients is not as explicit.

After the release of the initial study on resection of noncolorectal nonneuroendocrine liver metastases [9], innumerous similar studies followed [10–15]. The large range of tumour entities including patients with breast cancer is the common denominator of these studies. Breast cancer, however, represents only a minor share in the tumours examined and is stated to have a comparably good prognosis [10, 12–15]. The survival rates are reported to be equivalent to those of colorectal metastases [9, 15]. Thus the logical consequence was a recent increase in the number of publications on liver resections of isolated metastases in breast cancer patients [16–30], in which however the results of case series were merely compiled, whereas probable prognostic factors were only sometimes examined.

As shown in a previous study, patients with resectable liver metastasis from gynecological cancers benefit from

TABLE 1: Histopathological T- and N-stages as well as gradings of the primary breast cancer and the number of metastases in $n = 29$ operations.

Parameter	Degree	Absolute number	Relative frequency
T-stage	T1	11	0.38
	T2	14	0.48
	T3	3	0.10
	T4	1	0.03
N-stage	N0	10	0.34
	N1	17	0.59
	N2	2	0.07
Grading	G1	0	0
	G2	16	0.59
	G3	11	0.41
	G4	0	0
	(Unknown)	2	—
Number of metastases	1	16	0.55
	2	6	0.21
	3	3	0.10
	4	1	0.03
	5	3	0.10

surgical treatment in comparison to patients who had non-resectable metastases intraoperatively [31]. The aim of the present study was to prove this survival advantage after resection of isolated liver metastasis for solely breast cancer patients and to identify pre- and intraoperative factors which might have influence on the survival rates after resection.

2. Patients and Methods

The patients treated over a six-year period (February 2001 to January 2007) were drawn from the prospectively started data bank (Access for Windows; Version 2002, © Microsoft Corporation, Redmond, WA, USA) including all patients undergoing liver surgery at the University Hospital of the Saarland. During the evaluation period, 29 operations were performed on 24 patients suffering from isolated liver metastases of breast cancer. Three patients required two surgical interventions and one patient required three. The patients were 53.3±9.3 (range 38–77) years of age and had a body mass index of 25.9±3.5 (range 18.2–32.0) kg/m^2 at the time point of liver surgery. The T- and N-stages as well as the gradings of the primary cancer and the number of metastases are compiled in Table 1.

Local resectability seemed to be possible in all patients judging by the preoperative findings in computer tomography or magnetic resonance tomography which had in part not been performed at our clinic. The usual preoperative criteria such as remaining parenchymal tissue, at least one tumour free liver vein, and no infiltration of the liver hilus were taken into consideration. A locoregional recurrence or additional distant metastasis was excluded by renewed staging prior to liver surgery: clinical examination, ultrasound, and sometimes mammography as well as bone scintigraphy and CT/MRI of the brain and thorax.

The median interval between primary surgery and liver surgery was 55 (range 1–177) months. Only two patients had a synchronic metastasis of the breast cancer. Bilobar metastases were seen in eight cases. Five cases had a recurrent liver metastasis and eight patients had a history of an operatively treated locoregional tumour recurrence. A chemotherapeutic treatment in the past was performed in 26 cases. No neoadjuvant treatment for downsizing of the metastasis prior to liver surgery was initiated in our study group. Postoperative hormone and/or chemotherapy were recommended in palliative cases following surgical exploration only. Adjuvant treatment following liver resection was determined by the gynecologist or oncologist giving further treatment.

Surgery was performed in general anesthesia and perioperative antibiotic prophylactic treatment was applied. Intraoperative ultrasonography was employed in all cases in addition to the visual and palpatory examination of the liver. Selective vascular clamping or Pringle maneuver was used to control intraoperative blood loss according to the intraoperative findings. The parenchymal tissue was resected using a dissection instrument while occluding the vascular structures and bile ducts. Postoperative monitoring in the intensive care unit was standard following liver resection.

All statistical calculations were performed with the SAS software, release 9.2 (© SAS Institute Inc., Cary, NC, USA). Survival rates were compared with the logrank test. Multiple regression analysis was performed using a Cox regression. Mortality rates of two groups at fixed time points were compared with Fisher's exact test. Test results with P values of less than 0.05 were considered statistically significant and results with P values between 0.05 and 0.10 were statistically only slightly significant.

3. Results

Resection of all metastases was possible in 21 cases (72%), and the median duration of surgery was 144 (range 28–285) minutes. Anatomical resection according to the segments of Couinaud was performed in seven cases and atypical resection in twelve. A combination of both surgical methods was employed in two patients. Extensive resection (≥3 liver segments) became necessary in six cases. Eight operations ended as explorative laparotomies due to nonresectable liver metastasis and/or peritoneal carcinosis. The intraoperative findings differed from the preoperative radiological findings in 14 cases (48%). Yet, merely 8 of these 14 patients (57%) had nonresectable tumours and/or peritoneal carcinosis; in the other cases, the divergent pattern of liver metastasis was still resectable. The median estimated blood loss was 200 (range 50–1500) mL, and seven patients required perioperative blood transfusions (24%). On average, the postoperative stay was 7 (range 3–29) days. The 30-day and the in-hospital mortality were 0%. After surgery one major complication occurred in form of biliary leakage and two cases of minor

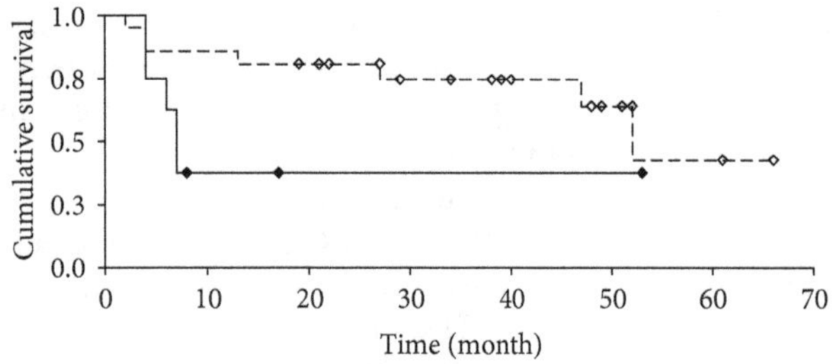

FIGURE 1: Overall survival of patients after liver resection (white) and surgical exploration only (black).

complications with urinary tract infections and cholangitis were registered. Histopathology revealed positive resection margins in three patients.

Median follow-up was 22 (range 2–65) months including 12 death events of 24 patients. The one-year survival rate was 86% in the patients who had undergone liver resection and 37.5% in patients intraoperatively estimated as unresectable. The two- and five-year survival rates were 81% and 33%, respectively, in patients with liver resection. The survival rate in both patient groups is depicted in Figure 1 in form of a Kaplan-Meier plot.

Median survival rates were 53 months for the resected patients and only 7.5 months for the patients without resection. The logrank test showed a slightly significant difference ($P = 0.0922$). The survival rates of both subgroups in comparison showed no significant difference after 6 months ($P = 0.3045$); after 12 months, however, statistically significant higher survival rates for the resected patients were registered ($P = 0.0114$) as well as after 18 and 24 months ($P = 0.0097$ and $P = 0.0183$, resp.), using Fisher's exact test.

The logrank test proved that the survival rate of the complete sample was dependent on T- ($P = 0.0444$) and N-stages ($P = 0.0090$) as well as the histopathological grading ($P = 0.0002$) of the primary tumour. The N-stage and the histopathological grading also influenced the survival in the subgroup of the resected patients significantly (N-stage: $P = 0.0505$; grading: $P = 0.0045$). Precedent locoregional recurrence ($P = 0.1279$) and chemotherapy ($P = 0.8601$) had no influence on survival rates. The patients' age ($P = 0.5991$) and body mass index ($P = 0.7346$) were not significant influencing factors. The logrank test, however, showed that the temporal interval between the resection of the primary breast cancer and the liver resection had a trend toward a significant prognostic factor ($P = 0.0628$).

R0 resection ($P = 0.0289$) and number of metastases ($P = 0.0306$) were furthermore significant influencing factors. Bilobar metastases ($P = 0.3544$), deviating but still resectable metastatic distribution intraoperatively ($P = 0.8393$), and extent of the resection ($P = 0.4557$) did not show significant influence. Even perioperative blood transfusion had no influence on the survival rate ($P = 0.3795$).

Multiple Cox regression analysis revealed that the survival rate depended mainly on the grading of the primary breast cancer (hazard ratio 19.763, $P = 0.0059$) and slightly on the preoperatively determined number of metastases (hazard ratio 1.503, $P = 0.0592$), whereas the other variables had no additional significant influence.

4. Discussion

Complete resection of the metastases was possible in three-fourth of our patients without mortality and with a low morbidity rate. The high number of solely surgical explorations was due to additional metastases or peritoneal carcinosis found intraoperatively not known from preoperative diagnostics leading to nonresectable metastasis. This is a common phenomenon in liver surgery; most references merely report on the resection of liver metastases. Consequent use of modern imaging techniques such as multislice CT or contrast-enhanced MRI should be mandatory to minimize the risk for surgical exploration only nowadays, which was not standard in our study population. In accordance with our results, there is one reference in which a 66% resection rate is stated [16]. In another study, a liver metastasis resection with curative intention was only possible in nine out of ninety breast cancer patients (10%). However, this series was obtained without preoperative selection of suitable patients [19]. The intraoperative deviation of metastasis distribution (in 48% of the cases in the present study) does not exclude resectability in general. A complete metastasis resection was still possible in nearly half of these patients. In addition to the routine use of up-to-date imaging techniques, staging laparoscopy combined with intraoperative ultrasound should be considered for a further reduction of the risk for surgical exploration only even in patients with breast cancer liver metastasis as stated recently [32].

The 1-, 2-, and 5-year survival rates of 86%, 81%, and 33% in our resected patients correlate well to those published on surgically treated liver metastasis in breast cancer for 1-, 2-, and 5-year survival rates over a period of the last 20 years: 77–100% [20, 28–30, 33], 50–86% [16, 20, 24, 33], and 9–61% [10, 12–14, 16, 19, 21–24, 26, 28–30, 33, 34], respectively. Survival rates for liver metastasis of colorectal cancer are comparable [35]. The mean overall survival rate in the present patient collective also coincides with that stated in references on liver metastasis resection in noncolorectal nonneuroendocrine tumours of 32–45 months including breast cancers [9, 12, 15] and breast cancer of 26–63 months [16, 23–27, 29, 33, 34, 36, 37]. A postoperative benefit following resection of breast cancer liver metastasis might be better reflected by the disease free survival. The lack of this end point is a limitation of the present study due to incomplete data in a retrospective analysis. Recent studies reported on mean disease free survival rates of 14–34 months with corresponding overall survival rates of 43–58 months [33, 34, 36, 37].

The present series of R0 resected patients showed a significantly higher survival rate compared to the patients with surgical exploration only. This was also observed in studies on noncolorectal nonneuroendocrine tumours including breast cancers [9–12, 14] and breast cancer [16, 17, 26, 30]. Overall, this is not surprising due to different tumour masses before and after the resection/exploration only. A recent review of the literature has shown a benefit of resection in breast cancer liver metastasis with a median survival of 38 months compared to 18 months in patients with chemotherapy alone [38]. The major limitation of this review consists in selected patients in the resection population as well. A prospective randomized controlled study regarding this aspect is missing yet. In general, the prognosis of patients with breast cancer liver metastasis with a median survival of 6–14 months is poor [13, 39].

The median time interval between surgery of the primary breast cancer and resection of liver metastasis was 55 months in our patients and therewith again correlates well with the known references reporting 36–41 months in patients with noncolorectal nonneuroendocrine tumours including breast cancers [9, 11] and 19–75 months in patients with breast cancer [14, 17, 25, 29]. The span of this interval as such is a slightly significant prognostic factor in our patients in accordance with the known data on breast cancer [19–21, 36, 40] and noncolorectal nonneuroendocrine tumours including breast cancer [11, 12, 15] and colorectal cancer [35], even though this aspect was not described in some of the references quoted above [14, 29, 30, 34]. In accordance, the prognosis of local recurrence in breast cancer is also influenced by this time interval [41].

Further significant influencing factors on the survival rate in this study were the T- and N-stages of the primary breast cancer. However, data on the primary tumour stages are controversially discussed in the references [19, 21, 29, 30, 34, 36]. On the one hand, a good histopathological grading of the primary cancer proved to be statistically the most favorable prognostic factor as shown herein, which had already been observed in examinations of locoregional recurrence in breast cancer [41]. On the other hand, there are references in which the grading of the primary breast cancer was stated to be irrelevant in liver metastasis [29, 30].

The hormone receptor status of the primary breast cancer seems to be relevant in some studies [23, 27, 29, 33, 37], whereas other authors are refusing it [30, 36]. Unfortunately, we cannot answer this question for our study group. Our limited data at this point result from treatment of the primary breast cancer at different institutions and an interval between primary surgery and liver surgery of up to 17 years. Although the survival of patients with breast cancer liver metastasis is influenced by the breast cancer subtype with the shortest for patients with triple negative breast cancer [40], the receptor status of the primary breast cancer is not necessarily the same in the metastases. Receptor conversion is relatively uncommon but does occur especially in liver metastasis [42]. The receptor status of breast cancer patients developing liver metastasis is therefore not a good indicator to select candidates for liver resection. Furthermore, diverse expression patterns with different immunohistochemical phenotypes depending on the site of breast cancer metastasis exist [43, 44]. On the other hand, breast cancer biological subtypes have a tendency to give rise to first distant metastases at certain body sites [45].

The number of metastases proved to be a prognostically relevant factor in our study. Reports on the influence of number and size of metastases are controversial [11, 14, 23, 27, 29, 30, 33, 34, 40]. The extent of resection and the intraoperatively deviating metastasis distribution had no prognostic relevance in our patients if resection was possible. Some references state the exact opposite as regards the extent of resection for colorectal surgery [12, 21, 27, 29, 30, 34–36]. Perioperative blood transfusion was of no prognostic significance in our study and also in one further study [29].

Whereas a history of local recurrence made no difference in the prognosis of our patients in accordance with a previous study [30], it has also been shown to be derogatory to the prognosis [17]. There are, however, subgroups in patients with local recurrence of breast cancer with a more favorable prognosis [41], so that a selection of patients in the present study is likely. On whole, the 3- and 5-year survival rates of patients with local recurrence are 67 and 42%, respectively, and 57% of these patients develop metastases [41]. Contrary to our study results, recurrence of liver metastasis was described as a negative prognostic factor previously [26, 30].

A general problem in all studies dealing with that topic is the inhomogeneous and small study groups limiting strong messages as in our results. Different tumour biologies of the underlying cancers, differing medical histories and time intervals between primary breast cancer and liver metastasis including variation in preceding endocrine treatment as well as chemotherapy, and different surgical approaches lead to an inevitable inhomogeneity. There are studies—as well—stating that response to chemotherapy before metastasectomy is the major prognostic factor defining favorable outcome [33, 37]. The percentage of patients with R1/2 resections varies in the references. In one study with a high percentage of these patients up to 33% recurrence of liver metastasis was stated [26]. The above-mentioned problem with inhomogeneous and small study populations progresses further when taking alternative treatments such as transarterial chemoembolisation and radiofrequency ablation into account [46–48].

In an ongoing debate, breast cancer is usually considered as a systemic disease [49], which explains the reserved position of gynecologists and oncologists regarding a local treatment. Improved survival rates of selected patients after resection of isolated liver metastases of breast cancer compared to chemotherapy alone commend this line of treatment. In combination with adjuvant treatment following liver resection, the results are comparable to those found in colorectal cancer liver metastasis [18]. In this context, it is important to mention that the mean survival rate of patients with breast cancer liver metastases is 6–14 months [13, 39]. It is therefore our opinion that in cases of suspected recurrence of breast cancer a renewed staging should focus on the liver considering that tumour recurrence may be expected [16] and an operative treatment might be indicated.

The results of this study show that a selected group of patients with isolated breast cancer liver metastasis benefits from complete surgical resection. This benefit was obtained with a low morbidity rate and no mortality. Beyond this several prognostic factors were identified. To our knowledge the grading of the primary breast cancer is shown to be a strong prognostic factor in isolated liver metastasis for the first time.

5. Conclusion

Resection of breast cancer liver metastasis is feasible and safe in selected patients. Within our study group we could find several pre- and intraoperative prognostic factors for a favorable outcome. Some of these are concomitant and some contrary to those stated before, but achieving R0 resection is the only well-documented consistent prognostic factor. There are no specific limits regarding number and size of breast cancer liver metastasis or features of the primary breast cancer taken into consideration if R0 resection seems achievable. Liver resection should be part in a multimodal treatment of selected patients with breast cancer liver metastasis due to a better outcome compared to patients with chemotherapy alone despite the fact that a prospective randomized evaluation is still pending. Neoadjuvant as well as adjuvant hormone and/or chemotherapy should be discussed in the setting of a planned operation for further improvement of outcome.

Authors' Contribution

Malte Weinrich and Christel Weiß contributed equally to this work.

Acknowledgment

The authors' thanks go to Mrs. B. Kopp (Department of General, Visceral, Vascular and Pediatric Surgery, University Hospital of the Saarland, Homburg/Saar, Germany) for updating of the liver data bank.

References

[1] A. Jemal, R. Siegel, E. Ward, T. Murray, J. Xu, and M. J. Thun, "Cancer statistics, 2007," *Ca-A Cancer Journal for Clinicians*, vol. 57, no. 1, pp. 43–66, 2007.

[2] E. Viadana, I. D. Bross, and J. W. Pickren, "An autopsy study of some routes of dissemination of cancer of the breast," *British Journal of Cancer*, vol. 27, no. 4, pp. 336–340, 1973.

[3] Y. T. N. Lee, "Breast carcinoma: pattern of metastasis at autopsy," *Journal of Surgical Oncology*, vol. 23, no. 3, pp. 175–180, 1983.

[4] A. Sjövall, V. Järv, L. Blomqvist et al., "The potential for improved outcome in patients with hepatic metastases from colon cancer: a population-based study," *European Journal of Surgical Oncology*, vol. 30, no. 8, pp. 834–841, 2004.

[5] J. Leporrier, J. Maurel, L. Chiche, S. Bara, P. Segol, and G. Launoy, "A population-based study of the incidence, management and prognosis of hepatic metastases from colorectal cancer," *British Journal of Surgery*, vol. 93, no. 4, pp. 465–474, 2006.

[6] P. C. Simmonds, J. N. Primrose, J. L. Colquitt, O. J. Garden, G. J. Poston, and M. Rees, "Surgical resection of hepatic metastases from colorectal cancer: a systematic review of published studies," *British Journal of Cancer*, vol. 94, no. 7, pp. 982–999, 2006.

[7] A. C. Wei, P. D. Greig, D. Grant, B. Taylor, B. Langer, and S. Gallinger, "Survival after hepatic resection for colorectal metastases: a 10-year experience," *Annals of Surgical Oncology*, vol. 13, no. 5, pp. 668–676, 2006.

[8] C. Pox, S. Aretz, S. C. Bischoff, U. Graeven, M. Hass, and P. Heußner, "S3-guideline colorectal cancer version 1.0," *Zeitschrift für Gastroenterologie*, vol. 51, pp. 753–854, 2013.

[9] L. E. Harrison, M. F. Brennan, E. Newman et al., "Hepatic resection for noncolorectal, nonneuroendocrine metastases: a fifteen-year experience with ninety-six patients," *Surgery*, vol. 121, no. 6, pp. 625–632, 1997.

[10] G. Ercolani, G. L. Grazi, M. Ravaioli et al., "The role of liver resections for noncolorectal, nonneuroendocrine metastases: experience with 142 observed cases," *Annals of Surgical Oncology*, vol. 12, no. 6, pp. 459–466, 2005.

[11] J. Weitz, L. H. Blumgart, Y. Fong et al., "Partial hepatectomy for metastases from noncolorectal, nonneuroendocrine carcinoma," *Annals of Surgery*, vol. 241, no. 2, pp. 269–276, 2005.

[12] R. Adam, L. Chiche, T. Aloia et al., "Hepatic resection for noncolorectal nonendocrine liver metastases: analysis of 1452 patients and development of a prognostic model," *Annals of Surgery*, vol. 244, no. 4, pp. 524–533, 2006.

[13] M. S. Metcalfe, E. J. Mullin, and G. J. Maddern, "Hepatectomy for metastatic noncolorectal gastrointestinal, breast and testicular tumours," *ANZ Journal of Surgery*, vol. 76, no. 4, pp. 246–250, 2006.

[14] J. Lendoire, M. Moro, O. Andriani et al., "Liver resection for non-colorectal, non-neuroendocrine metastases: analysis of a multicenter study from Argentina," *HPB*, vol. 9, no. 6, pp. 435–439, 2007.

[15] S. K. Reddy, A. S. Barbas, C. E. Marroquin, M. A. Morse, P. C. Kuo, and B. M. Clary, "Resection of noncolorectal nonneuroendocrine liver metastases: a comparative analysis," *Journal of the American College of Surgeons*, vol. 204, no. 3, pp. 372–382, 2007.

[16] D. Elias, P. H. Lasser, D. Montrucolli, S. Bonvallot, and M. Spielmann, "Hepatectomy for liver metastases from breast cancer," *European Journal of Surgical Oncology*, vol. 21, no. 5, pp. 510–513, 1995.

[17] R. Raab, K.-T. Nussbaum, M. Behrend, and A. Weimann, "Liver metastases of breast cancer: results of liver resection," *Anticancer Research*, vol. 18, no. 3, pp. 2231–2233, 1998.

[18] S. Kondo, H. Katoh, M. Omi et al., "Hepatectomy for metastases from breast cancer offers the survival benefit similar to that in hepatic metastases from colorectal cancer," *Hepato-Gastroenterology*, vol. 47, no. 36, pp. 1501–1503, 2000.

[19] S.-M. Maksan, T. Lehnert, G. Bastert, and C. Herfarth, "Curative liver resection for metastatic breast cancer," *European Journal of Surgical Oncology*, vol. 26, no. 3, pp. 209–212, 2000.

[20] M. Pocard, P. Pouillart, B. Asselain, and R.-J. Salmon, "Hepatic resection in metastatic breast cancer: results and prognostic factors," *European Journal of Surgical Oncology*, vol. 26, no. 2, pp. 155–159, 2000.

[21] M. Selzner, M. A. Morse, J. J. Vredenburgh, W. C. Meyers, and P.-A. Clavien, "Liver metastases from breast cancer: long-term survival after curative resection," *Surgery*, vol. 127, no. 4, pp. 383–389, 2000.

[22] M. Carlini, M. T. Lonardo, F. Carboni et al., "Liver metastases from breast cancer. Results of surgical resection," *Hepato-Gastroenterology*, vol. 49, no. 48, pp. 1597–1601, 2002.

[23] D. Elias, F. Maisonnette, M. Druet-Cabanac et al., "An attempt to clarify indications for hepatectomy for liver metastases from

breast cancer," *American Journal of Surgery*, vol. 185, no. 2, pp. 158–164, 2003.

[24] G. Vlastos, D. L. Smith, S. E. Singletary et al., "Long-term survival after an aggressive surgical approach in patients with breast cancer hepatic metastases," *Annals of Surgical Oncology*, vol. 11, no. 9, pp. 869–874, 2004.

[25] Y. Sakamoto, J. Yamamoto, M. Yoshimoto et al., "Hepatic resection for metastatic breast cancer: prognostic analysis of 34 patients," *World Journal of Surgery*, vol. 29, no. 4, pp. 524–527, 2005.

[26] R. Adam, T. Aloia, J. Krissat et al., "Is liver resection justified for patients with hepatic metastases from breast cancer?" *Annals of Surgery*, vol. 244, no. 6, pp. 897–907, 2006.

[27] S. R. Martinez, S. E. Young, A. E. Giuliano, and A. J. Bilchik, "The utility of estrogen receptor, progesterone receptor, and Her-2/neu status to predict survival in patients undergoing hepatic resection for breast cancer metastases," *American Journal of Surgery*, vol. 191, no. 2, pp. 281–283, 2006.

[28] M. Caralt, I. Bilbao, J. Cortés et al., "Hepatic resection for liver metastases as part of the "oncosurgical" treatment of metastatic breast cancer," *Annals of Surgical Oncology*, vol. 15, no. 10, pp. 2804–2810, 2008.

[29] J. Lubrano, H. Roman, S. Tarrab, B. Resch, L. Marpeau, and M. Scotté, "Liver resection for breast cancer metastasis: does it improve survival?" *Surgery Today*, vol. 38, no. 4, pp. 293–299, 2008.

[30] A. Thelen, C. Benckert, S. Jonas et al., "Liver resection for metastases from breast cancer," *Journal of Surgical Oncology*, vol. 97, no. 1, pp. 25–29, 2008.

[31] O. Kollmar, M. R. Moussavian, S. Richter, M. Bolli, and M. K. Schilling, "Surgery of liver metastasis in gynecological cancer—indication and results," *Onkologie*, vol. 31, no. 7, pp. 375–379, 2008.

[32] M. A. Cassera, C. W. Hammill, M. B. Ujiki, R. F. Wolf, L. L. Swanström, and P. D. Hansen, "Surgical management of breast cancer liver metastases," *HPB*, vol. 13, no. 4, pp. 272–276, 2011.

[33] D. V. Kostov, G. L. Kobakov, and D. V. Yankov, "Prognostic factors related to surgical outcome of liver metastases of breast cancer," *Journal of Breast Cancer*, vol. 16, pp. 184–192, 2013.

[34] G. A. M. van Walsum, J. A. M. de Ridder, C. Verhoef, K. Bosscha, T. M. van Gulik, and E. J. Hesselink, "Resection of liver metastases in patients with breast cancer: survival and prognostic factors," *European Journal of Surgical Oncology*, vol. 38, pp. 910–917, 2012.

[35] Y. Fong, J. Fortner, R. L. Sun, M. F. Brennan, and L. H. Blumgart, "Clinical score for predicting recurrence after hepatic resection for metastatic colorectal cancer: analysis of 1001 consecutive cases," *Annals of Surgery*, vol. 230, no. 3, pp. 309–321, 1999.

[36] K. Hoffmann, C. Franz, U. Hinz et al., "Liver resection for multimodal treatment of breast cancer metastases: identification of prognostic factors," *Annals of Surgical Oncology*, vol. 17, no. 6, pp. 1546–1554, 2010.

[37] D. E. Abbott, A. Brouquet, E. A. Mittendorf et al., "Resection of liver metastases from breast cancer: estrogen receptor status and response to chemotherapy before metastasectomy define outcome," *Surgery*, vol. 151, no. 5, pp. 710–716, 2012.

[38] S. Rodes Brown and R. C. Martin, "Management of liver dominant metastatic breast cancer: surgery, chemotherapy, or hepatic arterial therapy—benefits and limitations," *Minerva Chirurgica*, vol. 67, pp. 297–308, 2012.

[39] R. Largillier, J.-M. Ferrero, J. Doyen et al., "Prognostic factors in 1038 women with metastatic breast cancer," *Annals of Oncology*, vol. 19, no. 12, pp. 2012–2019, 2008.

[40] X. F. Duan, N. N. Dong, T. Zhang, and Q. Li, "The prognostic analysis of clinical breast cancer subtypes among patients with liver metastases from breast cancer," *International Journal of Clinical Oncology*, vol. 18, pp. 26–32, 2013.

[41] J. Willner, I. C. Kiricuta, and O. Kölbl, "Locoregional recurrence of breast cancer following mastectomy: always a fatal event? Results of univariate and multivariate analysis," *International Journal of Radiation Oncology Biology Physics*, vol. 37, no. 4, pp. 853–863, 1997.

[42] L. D. C. Hoefnagel, M. J. van de Vijver, H.-J. van Slooten et al., "Receptor conversion in distant breast cancer metastases," *Breast Cancer Research*, vol. 12, no. 5, article R75, 2010.

[43] J. S. Koo, W. Jung, and J. Jeong, "Metastatic breast cancer shows different immunohistochemical phenotype according to metastatic site," *Tumori*, vol. 96, no. 3, pp. 424–432, 2010.

[44] N. Cabioglu, A. A. Sahin, P. Morandi et al., "Chemokine receptors in advanced breast cancer: differential expression in metastatic disease sites with diagnostic and therapeutic implications," *Annals of Oncology*, vol. 20, no. 6, pp. 1013–1019, 2009.

[45] H. Sihto, J. Lundin, M. Lundin et al., "Breast cancer biological subtypes and protein expression predict for the preferential distant metastasis sites: a nationwide cohort study," *Breast Cancer Research*, vol. 13, no. 5, article no. R87, 2011.

[46] X. F. Duan, N. N. Dong, T. Zhang, and Q. Li, "Treatment outcome of patients with liver-only metastases from breast cancer after mastectomy: a retrospective analysis," *Journal of Cancer Research and Clinical Oncology*, vol. 137, no. 9, pp. 1363–1370, 2011.

[47] X.-P. Li, Z.-Q. Meng, W.-J. Guo, and J. Li, "Treatment for liver metastases from breast cancer: results and prognostic factors," *World Journal of Gastroenterology*, vol. 11, no. 24, pp. 3782–3787, 2005.

[48] C. T. Sofocleous, R. G. Nascimento, M. Gonen et al., "Radiofrequency ablation in the management of liver metastases from breast cancer," *American Journal of Roentgenology*, vol. 189, no. 4, pp. 883–889, 2007.

[49] P. D. Beitsch and E. Clifford, "Detection of carcinoma cells in the blood of breast cancer patients," *American Journal of Surgery*, vol. 180, no. 6, pp. 446–449, 2000.

23

Proposal of Two Prognostic Models for the Prediction of 10-Year Survival after Liver Resection for Colorectal Metastases

Ulf Kulik [1] **Mareike Plohmann-Meyer,** [2] **Jill Gwiasda,** [2] **Joline Kolb,** [1] **Daniel Meyer,** [2] **Alexander Kaltenborn** [2] **Frank Lehner** [1] **Jürgen Klempnauer** [1] **and Harald Schrem** [1,2]

[1] *General, Visceral and Transplantation Surgery, Hannover Medical School, Germany*
[2] *Core Facility Quality Management & Health Technology Assessment in Transplantation, Integrated Research and Treatment Center Transplantation (IFB-Tx), Hannover Medical School, Germany*

Correspondence should be addressed to Ulf Kulik; kulik.ulf@mh-hannover.de

Academic Editor: Attila Olah

Background. One-third of 5-year survivors after liver resection for colorectal liver metastases (CLM) develop recurrence or tumor-related death. Therefore 10-year survival appears more adequate in defining permanent cure. The aim of this study was to develop prognostic models for the prediction of 10-year survival after liver resection for colorectal liver metastases. *Methods.* N=965 cases of liver resection for CLM were retrospectively analyzed using univariable and multivariable regression analyses. Receiver operating curve analyses were used to assess the sensitivity and specificity of developed prognostic models and their potential clinical usefulness. *Results.* The 10-year survival rate was 15.2%. Age at liver resection, application of chemotherapies of the primary tumor, preoperative Quick's value, hemoglobin level, and grading of the primary colorectal tumor were independent significant predictors for 10-year patient survival. The generated formula to predict 10-year survival based on these preoperative factors displayed an area under the receiver operating curve (AUROC) of 0.716. In regard to perioperative variables, the distance of resection margins and performance of right segmental liver resection were additional independent predictors for 10-year survival. The logit link formula generated with pre- and perioperative variables showed an AUROC of 0.761. *Conclusion.* Both prognostic models are potentially clinically useful (AUROCs >0.700) for the prediction of 10-year survival. External validation is required prior to the introduction of these models in clinical patient counselling.

1. Introduction

Colorectal liver metastases (CLM) are one of the most common indications for hepatic surgery worldwide. In contrast to interventional treatment methods like radiofrequency ablation (RFA) the surgical treatment remains the only therapeutic option providing histological proven complete resection and mean 5-year survival rates of up to 50% [1–3]. Despite these encouraging results 5-year survival does not equate a permanent cure of the disease; several studies report that one-third of 5-year survivors appear to experience recurrence or tumor-related death [4–6]. Therefore, it seems more likely that 10-year survival after hepatic resection for CLM appears more qualified to be associated with permanent cure. A meta-analysis by Abbas et al. in 2011 reported 12-36% for 10-year survival rate; another study described a 10-year survival rate of 24% [7, 8]. In those reports, presence of positive resection margins clearly excluded patients from 10-year long-term survival. Furthermore extrahepatic disease and a high clinical risk score (CRS) derived from factors like carcinoembryonic antigen (CEA) levels, number and size of hepatic lesions, and the primary lymph node status were associated with reduced probability of long-term survival [7, 8]. Nevertheless, the estimation of individual prediction of long-term survival and especially a possible permanent cure is difficult and not well described in recent literature.

However, throughout the last decades several prognostic factors that influence overall survival (OS) after liver resection for CLM were reported. Size of CLM >50 mm, >1 lesion, age >70 years at liver resection, preoperative anemia, and other factors have been reported to be associated with negative impact on OS [9]. Some variables have been associated with a beneficial effect on OS, i.e., clear resection margins and the performance of only minor hepatic resections [10]. Additionally, the resection-severity-index (RSI) was recently introduced by our group as a new independent prognostic factor for survival after liver resection for CLM [11]. All those factors have usually been analyzed as regards the overall outcome after hepatic surgery for CLM while it remains unclear whether long-term survival of more than 10 years can be predicted with a prognostic model. Therefore the aim of this study was to analyze cases after hepatic surgery for CLM in a large German tertiary referral center for hepatobiliary surgery to determine patterns of pre- and perioperative factors that enable the prediction of long-term survival of ≥10 years.

2. Patients and Methods

2.1. Data Collection. This is a single center retrospective analysis. The setting of this study is a German tertiary referral center for hepatobiliary surgery and liver transplantation. The postoperative observational period ended on 27.07.2015. Descriptive statistics comparing patients with survival <10 years and survival ≥10 years are summarized in Supplementary Table 1 for preoperative variables and in Supplementary Table 2 for perioperative variables.

2.2. Inclusion and Exclusion Criteria. All consecutive primary liver resections for colorectal metastases performed at our institution between 01.01.1994 and 31.12.2014 (n=1155) were included. Excluded were all cases with lack of sufficient follow-up data (n=23). Furthermore all survivors with less than 10 years of follow-up (n=167) were excluded. Compliant with the STARD guidelines the analytical flow chart of the analyzed study cohort is illustrated in Figure 1 [12].

2.3. Ethical Considerations. The Ethics Committee of Hannover Medical School approved of this retrospective study (approval decision number 3233-2016). Patients provided informed consent that their data may be used for scientific purposes at the time of hospital admission which is the general policy of our institution. Patient records and patient data were anonymized and deidentified prior to analysis.

2.4. Study End-Points. The primary study end-point was observed as 10-year patient survival after liver resection (Figure 1). Patients with survival but follow-up less than 10 years cannot be included in this analysis, because we do not know whether they actually survived for 10 years or less.

2.5. Statistical Methods. Risk factors for patients' mortality within ten years after liver resection were analyzed with univariable and multivariable regression analyses.

Two risk-adjusted multivariable logistic regression models were developed using purposeful selection of preoperative covariates and pre-, intra-, and early postoperative covariates with p values in univariable regression ≤0.200 with the goal of avoiding overfitting and facilitating the detection of potential factor interactions based on the recommendations as published by Hosmer et al. [13]. Principal component analysis was used to identify two-sided variable correlations ≥ |0.500| to trigger a clinically informed decision on the exclusion of one of two highly correlated variables from multivariable regression in order to avoid collinearity in regression.

For all statistical tests a p value <0.05 was defined as significant. Binary variables and their influence on 10-year survival (yes/no) were analyzed with Chi^2 tests while the influence of continuous variables on 10-year survival (yes/no) was analyzed with the Wilcoxon test.

Receiver operating characteristic curve (ROC-curve) analyses were used to assess the sensitivity and specificity of predictions derived from the final multivariable regression models and their potential usefulness as prognostic models.

The software package JMP Pro 13.0.0 (SAS Institute, Cary, NC, USA) was used to perform all statistical analyses.

3. Results

3.1. 10-Year Survival. Out of the N=965 cases finally included in the study, N=147 cases experienced long-term survival of ≥10 years (15.2%).

3.2. Preoperative Risk Factors for 10-Year Survival after Liver Resection. Univariable logistic regression analysis revealed that the age at operation of the primary colorectal tumor, the age at liver resection in years, the localization of the primary tumor in the colon sigmoideum (yes/no), the pT staging of the primary tumor, the pN staging of the primary tumor, the grading of the primary tumor, UICC staging of the primary tumor, chemotherapy and/or radiotherapy of the primary tumor prior to liver resection (yes/no), and the preoperative Quick's value in % all had a significant influence on 10-year survival after liver resection (Table 1).

3.3. Intra- and Early Postoperative Risk Factors for 10-Year Survival after Liver Resection. Univariable logistic regression analysis demonstrated that bilateral atypical liver resection, right segmental liver resection, the duration of Pringle's procedure in min, postoperative complications during hospital stay (yes/no), the size of largest metastases in mm, and the distance of the resection margin in mm to the tumor all had a significant influence on 10-year survival after liver resection (Table 2).

3.4. Results of Principal Component Analysis. Principal component analysis of variables with p values <0.200 in univariable logistic regression analysis demonstrated two-sided factor correlations R > |0.500| for age at operation of the primary colorectal tumor and age at liver resection in years (R=0.979), localization of the primary tumor in the colon sigmoideum (yes/no) and the rectum (yes/no) (R=0.522), UICC staging of the primary tumor and pN staging of the primary tumor (R=0.592), UICC staging of the primary tumor and the M1 stage of the primary tumor (yes/no) (R=0.761), the weight of resected liver specimen in kg, and the size of the largest metastasis in mm (R=0.584). All other

TABLE 1: Shown are the results of univariable binary logistic regression to determine the influence of each *preoperative* variable on 10-year survival after liver resection. Odds ratios greater than 1 with a significant p value ($p<0.05$) indicate variables that increase the risk of mortality within 10 years significantly whereas odds ratios smaller than 1 with a significant p value indicate variables that decrease the risk of mortality within 10 years.

Variables			Odds Ratio	95%-Confidence interval	p-value
Pre-operative variables	Female gender (yes/no)		0.986	0.687 – 1.416	0.941
	Male gender (yes/no)		1.014	0.706 – 1.455	0.941
	Age at operation of primary tumor (years)		1.029	1.013 – 1.046	**<0.001**
	Age at liver resection (years)		1.028	1.012 – 1.045	**<0.001**
	Time between resection of primary tumor and resection of metastases (days)		1.000	0.999 – 1.000	0.900
	Localization of primary tumor	Coecum (yes/no)	2.119	0.902 – 4.980	**0.058**
		Colon ascendens (Yes/no)	0.895	0.528 – 1.517	0.683
		Colon transversum (yes/no)	1.061	0.438 – 2.570	0.895
		Colon descendens (yes/no)	1.136	0.568 – 2.269	0.715
		Colon sigmoideum (yes/no)	0.659	0.462 – 0.941	**0.023**
		Rectum (yes/no)	1.314	0.891 – 1.939	**0.162**
	Stage and grading of primary tumor	pT1-4 (ordinal scale)		not determined	**0.004**
		pT1 vs. pT2	0.965	0.375 – 2.478	0.940
		pT1 vs. pT3	0.610	0.255 – 1.454	0.264
		pT1 vs. pT4	0.214	0.069 – 0.670	**0.008**
		pN0-2b (ordinal scale)		not determined	**0.034**
		pN0 vs. pN1	0.587	0.380 – 0.906	**0.016**
		pN0 vs. pN2a	0.551	0.335 – 0.907	**0.019**
		pN0 vs. pN2b	0.912	0.385 – 2.158	0.834
		M1 (yes/no)	1.489	1.017 – 2.181	**0.038**
		Grading G1-3 (ordinal scale)		not determined	**0.012**
		Grading G1 vs. G2	0.324	0.140 – 0.750	**0.009**
		Grading G1 vs. G3	0.162	0.054 – 0.481	**0.001**
		UICC I-IV (ordinal scale)		not determined	**0.016**
		UICC I vs. IIa	0.438	0.227 – 0.844	**0.014**
		UICC I vs. IIb	0.206	0.025 – 1.687	**0.141**
		UICC I vs. IIIa	0.452	0.166 – 1.235	**0.122**
		UICC I vs. IIIb	0.312	0.154 – 0.633	**0.001**
		UICC I vs. IIIc	0.422	0.207 – 0.862	**0.018**
		UICC I vs. IV	0.318	0.178 – 0.567	**<0.001**
	Chemotherapy of primary tumor (yes/no)		1.831	1.281 – 2.618	**<0.001**
	Radiotherapy of primary tumor (yes/no)		1.847	0.991 – 3.444	**0.039**
	Local recurrence of primary tumor (yes/no)		1.229	0.617 – 2.447	0.549
	Simultaneous resection of primary tumor and liver metastases (yes/no)		0.979	0.502 – 1.909	0.950
	Multiple resection of metastases (yes/no)		1.131	0.624 – 2.048	0.682
	Leukocytes Tsd/μl		1.035	0.954 – 1.124	0.397
	Platelets Tsd/μl		0.999	0.997 – 1.000	**0.155**
	Hemoglobin g/dl		0.891	0.789 – 1.007	**0.062**
	Quick's value %		0.979	0.966 - 0.992	**0.002**

TABLE 2: Shown are the results of univariable binary logistic regression to determine the influence of each *intraoperative* variable on 10-year survival after liver resection. Odds ratios greater than 1 with a significant p value ($p<0.05$) indicate variables that increase the risk of mortality within 10 years significantly whereas odds ratios smaller than 1 with a significant p value indicate variables that decrease the risk of mortality within 10 years.

	Variables		Odds Ratio	95%-Confidence interval	p-value
Intra-operative variables	Left atypical liver resection	1 point	1.155	0.537 – 2.488	0.708
	Right atypical liver resection		0.947	0.621 – 1.444	0.801
	Bilateral atypical liver resection	2 points	2.448	1.165 – 5.142	**0.008**
	Left segmental liver resection		0.764	0.397 – 1.468	0.430
	Right segmental liver resection		0.352	0.192 – 0.645	**0.002**
	Left hemihepatectomy	3 points	2.477	0.883 – 6.951	0.512
	Right hemihepatectomy	4 points	0.781	0.521 – 1.171	0.238
	Extended left hepatectomy	5 points	1.114	0.645 – 1.922	0.696
	Left hepatectomy and right atypical liver resection	6 points	-	-	-
	Extended right hepatectomy		1.145	0.475 – 2.759	0.760
	Right hepatectomy and left atypical liver resection	7 points	1.034	0.352 – 3.035	0.951
	Extent of resection (ordinal scale)		not determined		0.455
	Extent of resection 1 point vs. 2 points		1.084	0.668 – 1.760	0.745
	Extent of resection 1 point vs. 3 points		0.418	0.143 – 1.217	**0.110**
	Extent of resection 1 point vs. 4 points		1.202	0.741 – 1.949	0.455
	Extent of resection 1 point vs. 5 points		0.905	0.491 – 1.668	0.749
	Extent of resection 1 point vs. 6 points		0.707	0.284 – 1.760	0.456
	Extent of resection 1 point vs. 7 points		0.963	0.316 – 2.930	0.947
	Operative duration in min		1.001	0.999 – 1.002	0.568
	Duration of Pringle's procedure in min		0.983	0.973 – 0.994	**0.003**
	Complications yes/no		1.734	1.028 – 2.925	**0.030**
	Intraoperative transfusion of units of packed red blood cells		1.078	1.001 – 1.161	**0.031**
	Size of largest metastasis in mm		1.005	1.000 – 1.011	**0.039**
	Weight of liver specimen in kg		1.297	0.868 – 1.939	**0.188**
	Distance to resection margin in mm		0.972	0.960 – 0.986	**<0.001**
	Grading G1-G3 (ordinal scale)		not determined		**0.173**
	Grading G1 vs. G2		1.873	0.238 – 14.749	0.551
	Grading G1 vs. G3		0.732	0.069 – 7.799	0.796
	R-status R0 (yes/no)		0.363	0.086 – 1.537	**0.111**

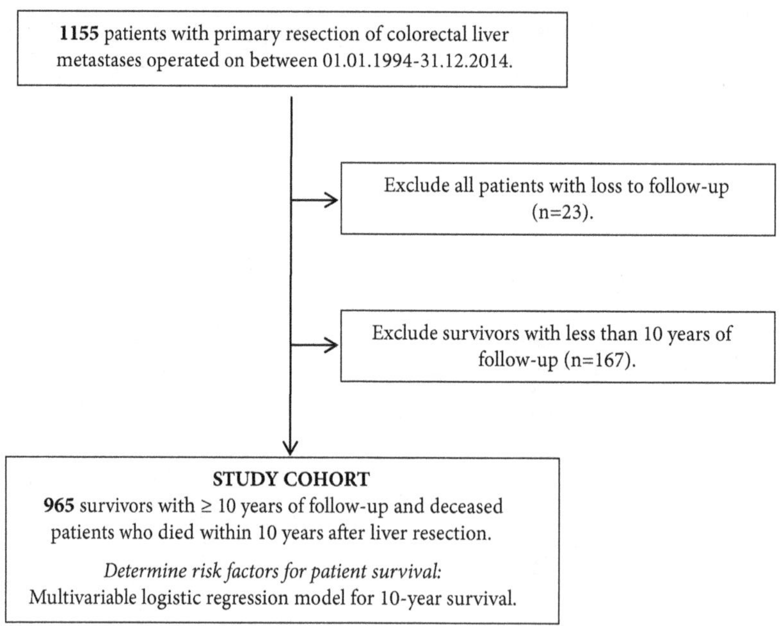

FIGURE 1: Depicted is the study flow chart of analyzed patients.

variables demonstrated low two-sided factor correlations $R < |0.500|$.

These results lead to the decision to include the variables age at resection of liver metastases, localization of the primary tumor in the colon sigmoideum (yes/no), UICC staging of the primary tumor, and the size of the largest metastasis in mm into multivariable logistic regression analysis and to exclude the variables age at resection of primary tumor, localization of the primary tumor in the rectum, pN staging of the primary tumor, M1 stage of the primary tumor (yes/no), and the weight of resected liver specimen (kg).

3.5. Independent Preoperative Risk Factors for 10-Year Survival after Liver Resection. The finally determined logistic regression model demonstrated that age at liver resection (years), chemotherapy of the primary tumor, preoperative Quick's value in %, and hemoglobin in g/dl as well as the grading of the primary colorectal tumor were independent significant risk factors for 10-year patient survival (Table 3(a)). This model exhibited an area under the receiver operating curve (AUROC) >0.700 indicating a potential prognostic model for the prediction of 10-year survival (AUROC = 0.716) (Figure 2(a)).

This model with preoperative variables resulted in the following logit link formula:

> y = 2.893 + (0.038 ∗ age at resection of metastases in years) + (0.755 ∗ grading of the primary tumor, G1-3) + (-0.444, if no chemotherapy of the primary tumor was given—otherwise 0) + (0.444, if chemotherapy of the primary tumor was given—otherwise 0) + (-0.209 ∗ preoperative hemoglobin in g/dl) + (-0.022 ∗ preoperative Quick's value in %)

The formula for the calculation of the predicted 10-year mortality risk in % after liver resection using the logit link formula described above for preoperative variables is as follows:

$$\text{10-year mortality risk (\%)} = 1/(1 + \text{Exp}_{(-y)})$$

3.6. Independent Pre-, Intra-, and Early Postoperative Risk Factors for 10-Year Survival after Liver Resection. The finally determined logistic regression model demonstrated that the age at liver resection in years, the distance of the tumor to resection margin in mm, chemotherapy of the primary tumor, right segmental liver resection (yes/no), preoperative Quick's value in % and hemoglobin in g/dl, grading of the primary colorectal tumor (G1-3), and pT1-4 stage of the primary colorectal carcinoma were independent significant risk factors for 10-year patient survival (Table 3(b)). This model exhibited an area under the receiver operating curve (AUROC) >0.700 indicating a potential prognostic model for the prediction of 10-year survival (AUROC = 0.761) (Figure 2(b)).

This model with pre-, intra-, and early postoperative variables resulted in the following logit link formula:

> y = 1.391 + (0.043 ∗ age at resection of metastases in years) + (0.3502 ∗ pT stage of the primary tumor, pT1-4) + (0.723 ∗ grading of the primary tumor, G1-3) + (-0.387, if no chemotherapy of the primary tumor was given—otherwise 0) + (0.387, if chemotherapy of the primary tumor was given—otherwise 0) + (-0.204 ∗ preoperative hemoglobin in g/dl) + (-0.021 ∗ preoperative Quick's value in %) + (0.575, if no right segmental liver resection was performed—otherwise 0) + (-0.575, if right segmental liver resection was performed—otherwise 0) + (-0.033 ∗ distance of liver metastasis to resection margin in mm)

Table 3

(a) Shown is the final multivariable model with *preoperative* risk factors only for 10-year survival after liver resection. Odds ratios greater than 1 with a significant p value ($p<0.05$) indicate variables that increase the risk of mortality within 10 years independently and significantly whereas odds ratios smaller than 1 with a significant p value indicate variables that decrease the risk of mortality within 10 years independently and significantly

Variables	Odds Ratio	95%-Confidence interval	p-value
Chemotherapy of primary tumor (yes/no)	2.432	1.570 – 3.770	**<0.001**
Age at liver resection (years)	1.039	1.019 – 1.060	**<0.001**
Quick's value %	0.979	0.964 – 0.993	**0.005**
Hemoglobin g/dl	0.811	0.698 – 0.943	**0.006**
Grading of primary tumor G1-3 (ordinal scale)	2.127	1.108 – 4.081	**0.019**

(b) Shown is the final multivariable model with *preoperative and perioperative* risk factors for 10-year survival after liver resection. Odds ratios greater than 1 with a significant p value ($p<0.05$) indicate variables that increase the risk of mortality within 10 years independently and significantly whereas odds ratios smaller than 1 with a significant p value indicate variables that decrease the risk of mortality within 10 years independently and significantly

Variables	Odds Ratio	95%-Confidence interval	p-value
Age at liver resection (years)	1.044	1.022 – 1.066	**<0.001**
Distance to resection margin in mm	0.968	0.950 – 0.986	**<0.001**
Chemotherapy of primary tumor (yes/no)	2.168	1.368 – 3.435	**<0.001**
Right segmental liver resection	0.317	0.152 – 0.661	**0.003**
Quick's value %	0.980	0.964 – 0.994	**0.006**
Hemoglobin g/dl	0.815	0.700 – 0.955	**0.010**
Grading of primary tumor G1-3 (ordinal scale)	2.060	1.050 – 4.037	**0.031**
pT1-4 primary tumor (ordinal scale)	1.420	1.013 – 1.990	**0.044**

Calculation of the predicted 10-year mortality risk in % after liver resection using the logit link formula described above for pre-, intra-, and early postoperative variables is as follows:

$$\text{10-year mortality risk (\%)} = 1/(1 + \mathrm{Exp}_{(-y)})$$

4. Discussion

This study identified factors with an independent significant influence on long-term survival of ≥10 years after hepatic surgery for CLM in a large collective including 147 patients who survived at least 10 years. Two prognostic models for the prediction of the probability of experiencing that long-term survival are proposed. The proposed models are specific to estimate 10-year survival after liver resection. The first model is based on preoperative factors and offers the chance to estimate possible 10-year survival before performance of the liver surgery, for example, when meeting a patient in the outpatient clinic (Figure 2(a)). The second model includes factors from the surgery and the early postoperative course and opens a more detailed view based on the specific liver surgery that was performed and the results of the histopathology (Figure 2(b)). That model might enable a more elaborated design of the medical aftercare. Up to now, no prognostic model was available to estimate the odds for long-term survival of ≥10 years after liver resection for CLM. Most recently published studies only aimed for the assessment of long-term survival rates and risk factors that generally influence long-term or overall survival. The 10-years survival rate of 15.2% found in our study matches the range of long-term survival reported in that current literature [7, 8].

Based on the first preoperative model the odds for 10-year survival are better when the patients are younger, showed a low primary tumor grading, did not receive a chemotherapy of the primary tumor, and displayed higher Hb-values and Quick values preoperatively (Table 3(a)). We believe that an as accurate as possible prediction of the likelihood of 10-year survival before liver surgery may play a role for many patients to understand the chances of cure after surgery. The influence of the patients' age on overall survival is well described; various studies reported limited overall survival in elderly patients. Nevertheless outcome is still far better than without surgical treatment of CLM [9, 14, 15]. Similar findings were repeatedly published as regards the primary tumor grading; a G3-grading is usually associated with decreased survival [16, 17]. Likewise, a lower Hb-value was recently reported by our center as negative predictor for survival [18]. Furthermore, a lower Hb-value might cause an increased need for perioperative blood transfusion, lately reported to impair disease-free and overall survival [19, 20]. The Quick's value in % was not described previously as prognostic factor in liver resection for colorectal liver metastases but it appears logical that a higher value correlates with a better synthetic function of the organ and a more stable function of the liver remnant after resection.

The negative influence of chemotherapies applied in the context of the primary tumor appears more surprising. It can be speculated that patients who received chemotherapies showed an initially higher UICC-stage and displayed synchronous, possibly nonresectable liver metastases. Hence, the chemotherapy might be considered as a surrogate parameter for a more advanced disease with corresponding impaired

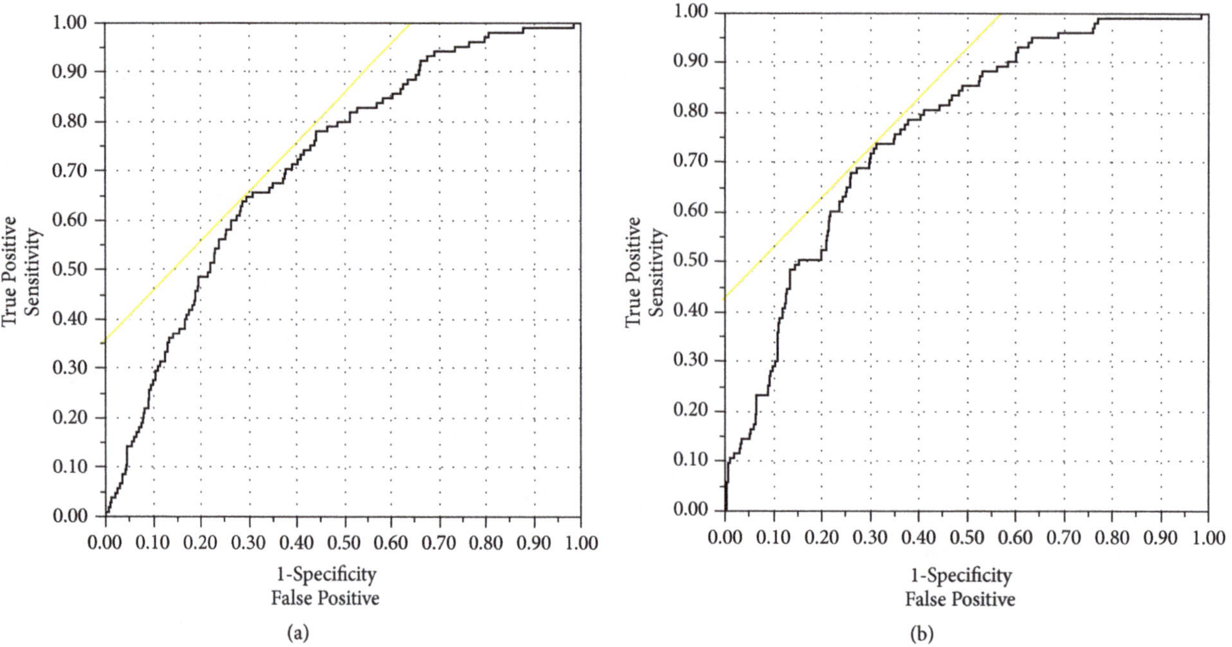

FIGURE 2: (a) Shown is the result of ROC-curve analysis of the final multivariable regression model with *preoperative* risk factors for 10-year survival (AUROC = 0.716). (b) Shown is the result of ROC-curve analysis of the final multivariable regression model with *preoperative and perioperative* risk factors for 10-year survival (AUROC = 0.761).

outcome. In contrast to this notion, the correlation of chemotherapy for the primary tumor with more advanced disease stages of the primary tumor was low in this study ($R < |0.500|$). Unfortunately, the heterogeneity of chemotherapy protocols given over the study period and the different approaches (neoadjuvant, adjuvant, or initially palliative as regards synchronous nonresectable CLM) limits the statistically convincing analysis; therefore a deeper analysis in our cohort was disregarded. Of note, chemotherapy of primary tumor in this study defines chemotherapy with any purpose that was delivered before liver resection. This may have created to some degree a bias in the results of this investigation.

Nevertheless, another group reported an inferior outcome after resection for CLM in these cases with chemotherapeutical treatment prior to liver resection. In this study a chemotherapy was significantly more often applied when synchronous liver metastases or more than three liver lesions were diagnosed [21]. Furthermore, over the last years chemotherapies are more frequently used as regards downsizing liver lesions and to converse initially nonresectable into resectable CLM (conversion chemotherapy). For instance, following the use of fluorouracil, leucovorin, oxaliplatin, and irinotecan regimes (FOLFOXIRI) a secondary resectability of CLM of 36% was described [22]. Reasonable outcome was reported with 2-year survival of 83% and 5-year survival rate of 33-50% after a conversion therapy and secondary liver resection [23–25]. In all these studies the majority of patients displayed synchronous liver metastases; therefore those chemotherapies might be considered as adjuvant or with initial palliative intent as regards the primary tumor. Furthermore, the negative impact of chemotherapies on long-term survival might be related to chemotherapy associated liver damage (CALI). Various agents drive several mechanisms of hepatic injury; e.g., oxaliplatin is associated with the sinusoidal obstruction syndrome (SOS), 5-fluorouracil is known to cause steatosis, and irinotecan may induce steatohepatitis [26]. Those toxicities might be linked to increased postoperative morbidity after liver resection [27, 28]. Taken together, the association of chemotherapy with inferior odds for 10-year survival is most likely related to advanced primary disease and may be a possible consequence of chemotherapy induced liver damage. However, it can be assumed that such cases with advanced diseases would be most likely associated with an even worse prognosis without chemotherapy of the primary tumor.

The second model is expanded by parameters of the surgical resection and the histopathology. Basically in addition to the preoperative model the odds for 10-year survival are better in case of a right segmental resection and wider distance of liver metastasis to the resection margin (Table 3(b)). As preluded, positive resection margins were previously identified as risk factor with negative influence on long-term survival [7]. The same effect was repeatedly reported regarding the overall survival: A positive resection margin or a distance of <1 mm to the metastasis was associated with inferior 5-year survival or overall outcome [29–31]. In our cohort no definite benefit of a R0 resection in comparison to R1 resection was observed in the univariable analyses but in the multivariable model wider distance of metastasis to the resection margins is clearly associated with better outcome. Further research to define possible cut-off values of margin width that are associated with poorer outcome or no more benefit on survival is needed. Nevertheless, the strong effect on long-term survival is presumably related to higher rates of tumor recurrence limiting subsequent treatment options.

As regards the beneficial effect of right segmental resections the interpretation is more difficult. It has been previously described that minor liver resections are associated with a better outcome, possibly because of a larger liver remnant with more stable liver function and the technical possibility of future resections in case of recurrence [10, 32]. On the other hand, what favors a right segmental resection in contrast to other minor resections, like nonanatomic right/left or a left segmental resection, is unclear. In that context, one older study showed no influence on overall survival in comparison of nonanatomical and anatomical minor liver resections [33]. Nevertheless, the right liver appears to be more commonly affected by CLM than the left liver, probably due to the more right oriented portal vein flow [34]. Speculatively, in case of a right segmental resection the chances that the metastasis there is truly the only lesion and no other occult nodes are present in the left lobe and that possible subdetectable lesions in the same segment are also removed might be better than in case of a nonanatomical resection with subsequent higher odds for long-term survival of >10 years.

In summary, this work proposes prognostic models for the prediction of the likelihood of long-term survival of >10 years after liver resection for CLM based on easy to access pre- and perioperative factors. Of course the retrospective approach and the single-center nature of this study limit the generalizability of the findings. Therefore the results need to be reevaluated by others to exclude a center-bias. The proposed prognostic models warrant external model validation.

Authors' Contributions

Both the authors Ulf Kulik and Mareike Plohmann-Meyer contributed equally.

Acknowledgments

This work was supported by a grant from the German Federal Ministry of Education and Research (reference number: 01EO1302).

References

[1] J. N. Primrose, "Treatment of colorectal metastases: Surgery, cryotherapy, or radiofrequency ablation," *Gut*, vol. 50, no. 1, pp. 1-5, 2002.

[2] P. C. Simmonds, J. N. Primrose, J. L. Colquitt, O. J. Garden, G. J. Poston, and M. Rees, "Surgical resection of hepatic metastases from colorectal cancer: A systematic review of published studies," *British Journal of Cancer*, vol. 94, no. 7, pp. 982–999, 2006.

[3] H. Z. Malik, K. R. Prasad, K. J. Halazun et al., "Preoperative prognostic score for predicting survival after hepatic resection for colorectal liver metastases," *Annals of Surgery*, vol. 246, no. 5, pp. 806–814, 2007.

[4] C. Pulitanó, F. Castillo, L. Aldrighetti et al., "What defines 'cure' after liver resection for colorectal metastases? Results after 10 years of follow-up," *HPB*, vol. 12, no. 4, pp. 244–249, 2010.

[5] K. J. Roberts, A. White, A. Cockbain et al., "Performance of prognostic scores in predicting long-term outcome following resection of colorectal liver metastases," *British Journal of Surgery*, vol. 101, no. 7, pp. 856–866, 2014.

[6] N. Bouviez, Z. Lakkis, J. Lubrano et al., "Liver resection for colorectal metastases: results and prognostic factors with 10-year follow-up," *Langenbeck's Archives of Surgery*, vol. 399, no. 8, pp. 1031–1038, 2014.

[7] S. Abbas, V. Lam, and M. Hollands, "Ten-year survival after liver resection for colorectalmetastases: systematic review and meta-analysis," *ISRN Oncology*, vol. 2011, Article ID 763245, 11 pages, 2011.

[8] J. M. Creasy, E. Sadot, B. G. Koerkamp et al., "Actual 10-year survival after hepatic resection of colorectal liver metastases: What factors preclude cure?" *Surgery*, 2018.

[9] U. Kulik, T. Framke, A. Grosshennig et al., "Liver resection of colorectal liver metastases in elderly patients," *World Journal of Surgery*, vol. 35, no. 9, pp. 2063–2072, 2011.

[10] U. Kulik, H. Bektas, J. Klempnauer, and F. Lehner, "Repeat liver resection for colorectal metastases.," *British Journal of Surgery*, vol. 100, no. 7, pp. 926–932, 2013.

[11] J. Gwiasda, H. Schrem, A. Kaltenborn et al., "Introduction of the resection severity index as independent risk factor limiting survival after resection of colorectal liver metastases," *Surgical Oncology*, vol. 26, no. 4, pp. 382–388, 2017.

[12] P. M. Bossuyt, J. F. Cohen, C. A. Gatsonis, and D. A. Korevaar, "STARD 2015: Updated reporting guidelines for all diagnostic accuracy studies," *Annals of Translational Medicine*, vol. 4, no. 85, 2016.

[13] D. W. Hosmer, S. Lemeshow, and R. X. Sturdivant, *Applied Logistic Regression*, Wiley, Hoboken, NJ, USA, 3rd edition, 2013.

[14] R. Adam, A. Frilling, D. Elias et al., "Liver resection of colorectal metastases in elderly patients," *British Journal of Surgery*, vol. 97, no. 3, pp. 366–376, 2010.

[15] B. Nardo, S. Serafini, M. Ruggiero et al., "Liver resection for metastases from colorectal cancer in very elderly patients: New surgical horizons," *International Journal of Surgery*, vol. 33, pp. S135–S141, 2016.

[16] M. Rees, P. P. Tekkis, F. K. S. Welsh, T. O'Rourke, and T. G. John, "Evaluation of long-term survival after hepatic resection for metastatic colorectal cancer: A multifactorial model of 929 patients," *Annals of Surgery*, vol. 247, no. 1, pp. 125–135, 2008.

[17] J. Scheele, A. Altendorf-Hofmann, T. Grube, W. Hohenberger, R. Stangl, and K. Schmidt, "Resection of colorectal liver metas-

tases. What prognostic factors determine patient selection?" *Der Chirurg*, vol. 72, no. 5, pp. 547–560, 2001.

[18] U. Kulik, H. Schrem, H. Bektas, J. Klempnauer, and F. Lehner, "Prognostic relevance of hematological profile before resection for colorectal liver metastases," *Journal of Surgical Research*, vol. 206, no. 2, pp. 498–506, 2016.

[19] X. Lyu, W. Qiao, D. Li, and Y. Leng, "Impact of perioperative blood transfusion on clinical outcomes in patients with colorectal liver metastasis after hepatectomy: A meta-analysis," *Oncotarget* , vol. 8, no. 25, pp. 41740–41748, 2017.

[20] T. S. Schiergens, M. Rentsch, M. S. Kasparek, K. Frenes, K.-W. Jauch, and W. E. Thasler, "Impact of perioperative allogeneic red blood cell transfusion on recurrence and overall survival after resection of colorectal liver metastases," *Diseases of the Colon & Rectum*, vol. 58, no. 1, pp. 74–82, 2015.

[21] U. Settmacher, Y. Dittmar, T. Knösel et al., "Predictors of long-term survival in patients with colorectal liver metastases: A single center study and review of the literature," *International Journal of Colorectal Disease*, vol. 26, no. 8, pp. 967–981, 2011.

[22] A. Falcone, S. Ricci, and I. Brunetti, "Phase III trial of infusional fluorouracil, leucovorin, oxaliplatin, and irinotecan (FOLFOXIRI) compared with infusional fluorouracil, leucovorin, and irinotecan (FOLFIRI) as first-line treatment for metastatic colorectal cancer: the Gruppo Oncologico Nor," *Journal of Clinical Oncology*, vol. 25, no. 13, pp. 1670–1676, 2007.

[23] R. Adam, D. A. Wicherts, R. De Haas et al., "Patients with initially unresectable colorectal liver metastases: Is there a possibility of cure?" *Journal of Clinical Oncology*, vol. 27, no. 11, pp. 1829–1835, 2009.

[24] S. Giacchetti, M. Itzhaki, G. Gruia et al., "Long-term survival of patients with unresectable colorectal cancer liver metastases following infusional chemotherapy with 5-fluorouracil, leucovorin, oxaliplatin and surgery," *Annals of Oncology*, vol. 10, no. 6, pp. 663–669, 1999.

[25] M. Ychou, F. Viret, A. Kramar et al., "Tritherapy with fluorouracil/leucovorin, irinotecan and oxaliplatin (FOLFIRINOX): A phase II study in colorectal cancer patients with non-resectable liver metastases," *Cancer Chemotherapy and Pharmacology*, vol. 62, no. 2, pp. 195–201, 2008.

[26] G. Duwe, S. Knitter, S. Pesthy et al., "Hepatotoxicity following systemic therapy for colorectal liver metastases and the impact of chemotherapy-associated liver injury on outcomes after curative liver resection," *European Journal of Surgical Oncology*, vol. 43, no. 9, pp. 1668–1681, 2017.

[27] S. M. Robinson, C. H. Wilson, A. D. Burt, D. M. Manas, and S. A. White, "Chemotherapy-associated liver injury in patients with colorectal liver metastases: A systematic review and meta-analysis," *Annals of Surgical Oncology*, vol. 19, no. 13, pp. 4287–4299, 2012.

[28] J. Zhao, K. M. C. van Mierlo, J. Gómez-Ramírez et al., "Systematic review of the influence of chemotherapy-associated liver injury on outcome after partial hepatectomy for colorectal liver metastases," *British Journal of Surgery*, vol. 104, no. 8, pp. 990–1002, 2017.

[29] F. Makowiec, P. Bronsert, A. Klock, U. T. Hopt, and H. P. Neeff, "Prognostic influence of hepatic margin after resection of colorectal liver metastasis: role of modern preoperative chemotherapy," *International Journal of Colorectal Disease*, vol. 33, no. 1, pp. 71–78, 2018.

[30] R. Mao, J. Zhao, X. Bi et al., "Interaction of margin status and tumour burden determines survival after resection of colorectal liver metastases: A retrospective cohort study," *International Journal of Surgery*, vol. 53, pp. 371–377, 2018.

[31] J. Wang, G. A. Margonis, N. Amini et al., "The prognostic value of varying definitions of positive resection margin in patients with colorectal cancer liver metastases," *Journal of Gastrointestinal Surgery*, vol. 22, no. 8, pp. 1350–1357, 2018.

[32] K. Tanaka, H. Shimada, C. Matsumoto et al., "Impact of the degree of liver resection on survival for patients with multiple liver metastases from colorectal cancer," *World Journal of Surgery*, vol. 32, no. 9, pp. 2057–2069, 2008.

[33] E. Guzzetti, C. Pulitanò, M. Catena et al., "Impact of type of liver resection on the outcome of colorectal liver metastases: A case-matched analysis," *Journal of Surgical Oncology*, vol. 97, no. 6, pp. 503–507, 2008.

[34] R. F. Holbrook, M. A. Rodriguez-Bigas, K. Ramakrishnan, L. Blumenson, and N. J. Petrelli, "Patterns of colorectal liver metastases according to Couinaud's segments," *Diseases of the Colon & Rectum*, vol. 38, no. 3, pp. 245–248, 1995.

Child-Pugh Parameters and Platelet Count as an Alternative to ICG Test for Assessing Liver Function for Major Hepatectomy

Kin-Pan Au, See-Ching Chan, Kenneth Siu-Ho Chok, Albert Chi-Yan Chan, Tan-To Cheung, Kelvin Kwok-Chai Ng, and Chung-Mau Lo

Department of Surgery, The University of Hong Kong, Hong Kong

Correspondence should be addressed to See-Ching Chan; seechingchan@gmail.com

Academic Editor: Dahmen Uta

Objective. To study the correlations and discrepancies between Child-Pugh system and indocyanine green (ICG) clearance test in assessing liver function reserve and explore the possibility of combining two systems to gain an overall liver function assessment. *Design.* Retrospective analysis of 2832 hepatocellular carcinoma (HCC) patients graded as Child-Pugh A and Child-Pugh B with ICG clearance test being performed was conducted. *Results.* ICG retention rate at 15 minutes (ICG15) correlates with Child-Pugh score, however, with a large variance. Platelet count improves the correlation between Child-Pugh score and ICG15. ICG15 can be estimated using the following regression formula: estimated ICG15 (eICG15) = 45.1 + 0.435 × bilirubin − 0.917 × albumin + 0.491 × prothrombin time − 0.0283 × platelet (R^2 = 0.455). Patients with eICG15 >20.0% who underwent major hepatectomy had a tendency towards more posthepatectomy liver failure (4.1% versus 8.0%, p = 0.09) and higher in-hospital mortality (3.7% versus 8.0%, p = 0.052). They also had shorter median overall survival (5.10 ± 0.553 versus 3.01 ± 0.878 years, p = 0.015) and disease-free survival (1.37 ± 0.215 versus 0.707 ± 0.183 years, p = 0.018). *Conclusion.* eICG15 can be predicted from Child-Pugh parameters and platelet count. eICG15 correlates with in-hospital mortality after major hepatectomy and predicts long-term survival.

1. Introduction

Pugh's [1] gut feeling prompted the modification of the classification devised by Child [2] in the assessment of liver function reserve. Child-Pugh's [3] classification has stood the test of time in guiding treatment decisions and prognostication of patients with hepatocellular carcinoma (HCC) in the west [4]. The five variables are bilirubin, albumin, prothrombin time, ascites, and presence of hepatic encephalopathy. Application of these five factors was the judgment made by very experienced clinicians. It was subsequently validated by numerous clinical series in a recursive manner [5, 6]. Excretory function of the liver is expressed by the serum bilirubin level. Synthetic functions are assessed by the serum albumin level and prothrombin time. Detoxification failure leads to hepatic encephalopathy. Development of ascites is a consequence of poor synthetic function and portal hypertension. Child-Pugh A and certain Child-Pugh B patients are candidates for major hepatectomy [7].

Quantitative assessment by indocyanine green (ICG) clearance test is more commonly used in the East [8]. ICG is a water-soluble fluorescent cyanine dye. In vivo it is exclusively excreted by the liver into the bile without metabolism or enterohepatic circulation [9]. The ICG retention is an indirect assessment of functional hepatic blood flow [10]. Cirrhotic liver decreases hepatic blood flow and results in an increase in total splanchnic sequestration [11]. In the trauma model, it is used to assess splanchnic haemodynamics [12]. An ICG retention rate at 15 minutes (ICG15) of no more than 14.0% has been validated as a minimal requirement for major hepatectomy [13], as defined by resection of 4 or more Couinaud segments [14]. ICG15 is however not used in most centres in the west [15], and reliance is rather on Child-Pugh score and grade [7].

Though ICG clearance test is a step further to assess liver functional reserve, it is an additional test. The facilities to measure ICG15 are not readily available in some centres. In this study, we looked into the correlation between ICG retention rate with Child-Pugh score and grade in a consecutive series of patients in our centre. Discrepancy between the two systems is just as important. The aim was to better apply the two systems and to explore the possibility of combining and complementing the advantages of the two systems. In our study, the unique role of platelet count in associating Child-Pugh score and ICG15 has been highlighted. Thrombocytopenia is a constant phenomenon of portal hypertension [16]. Clinically, it is associated with increased posthepatectomy liver failure and operative mortality [17]. However, it has not been routinely considered during preoperative liver function assessment. In this study, we investigated the additional role of platelet count when combined with preexisting liver function assessment.

2. Methods

2.1. Patients. From May 1989 to December 2015, 3466 HCC patients graded A or B by Child-Pugh system underwent ICG clearance test to evaluate for liver resection in the Department of Surgery, Queen Mary Hospital, the University of Hong Kong. 634 patients with alkaline phosphatase (ALP) or gamma-glutamyl transferase (GGT) levels higher than 2 times upper limit of normal were excluded, as their ICG15 could have been affected by ductal obstruction. The remaining 2832 patients formed the basis of this retrospective study. 848 patients who underwent major hepatectomy were included for survival analysis. The number of patients analysed in each step of this study was summarized in Figure 1.

All patients were regularly followed up at our outpatient clinic and were prospectively monitored for recurrence by serum alpha-fetoprotein level and contrast computed tomography (CT) scan, together with chest X-ray, every 3 to 6 months. A computerized database has been established since 1989 for prospective collection of patient data. Any postoperative recurrence was entered into the database immediately upon diagnosis.

2.2. ICG Clearance Test. ICG clearance test was performed by rapid intravenous injection of 0.5 mg/kg body weight of ICG. After a 15-minute interval, blood was drawn from the contralateral cubital vein and read with a spectrophotometer. ICG retention was expressed as a percentage of the fluorescent dye retained at 15 minutes.

2.3. Statistics. Factors affecting ICG15 were identified with univariate and multivariate linear regressions. ICG15 was plotted against Child-Pugh score with their standard deviations denoted by error bars. Patients who received surgical resection were further analysed for survival with Kaplan-Meier curve and compared with log-rank test. Their baseline characteristics were compared, with t-test for continuous variables and chi-square test for discrete variables. Statistic calculations were computed with Statistical Product and Service Solution (SPSS) 16.0.

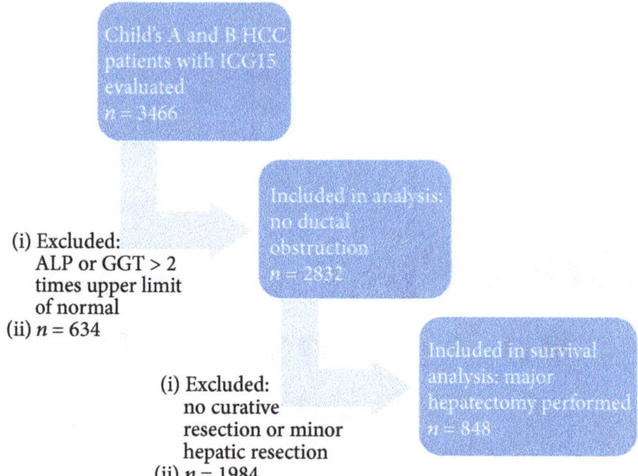

FIGURE 1: Flow diagram of this study.

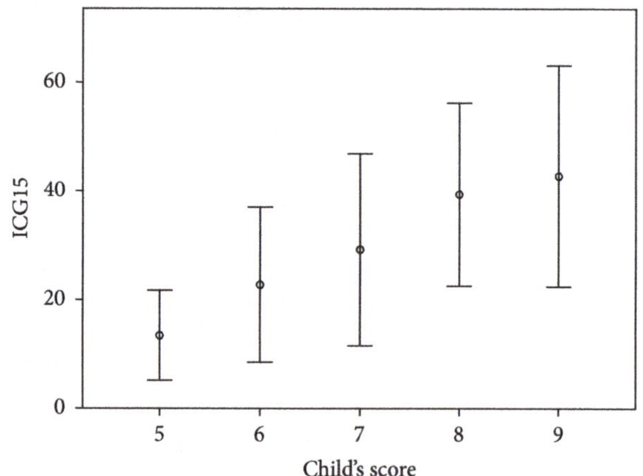

FIGURE 2: Correlation between ICG15 and Child-Pugh score. A linear relationship is expressed by ICG15 = −27.4 + 8.21 × Child-Pugh score (R^2 = 0.264). Error bars: ±1 SD.

3. Results

3.1. Relation between ICG15 and Child-Pugh Score. There is an almost linear correlation between ICG15 and the Child-Pugh score (Figure 2). The low R^2 value (0.264) of this linear relationship and the large deviance of ICG15 (standard deviation 8.30–20.3) reflect heterogeneity among patients with same Child-Pugh score. This is of great importance, as patients with prolonged ICG retention are at risk of liver failure after major hepatectomy. Using local ablative therapy extensively for multiple lesions may result in hepatic dysfunction.

3.2. Factors Affecting ICG15. The Child-Pugh score comprises fiver parameters: ascites, hepatic encephalopathy, bilirubin, albumin, and prothrombin time. Linear regression analysis (Table 1) shows that bilirubin level (OR 1.63, 95% CI 1.49–1.78, $p < 0.001$), albumin level (OR 0.461, 95% CI 0.381–0.556, $p < 0.001$), and prothrombin time (OR 2.28, 95% CI 1.18–4.40, $p = 0.014$) predict ICG15. Ascites and grading

TABLE 1: Univariate and multivariate analysis for factors associated with ICG15.

	Univariate analysis		Multivariate analysis	
	OR (95% CI)	p-value	OR (95% CI)	p value
Ascites	16 (804–14191)	<0.001	0.98 (0.0660–14.4)	0.99
HE	10.3 (0.0433–2453)	0.40		
Bilirubin	1.90 (1.82–1.98)	<0.001	1.63 (1.49–1.78)	<0.001
ALT/SGPT	1.02 (1.02–1.03)	<0.001	1.01 (0.987–1.03)	0.53
GGT	1.04 (1.00–1.08)	0.038	1.02 (0.993–1.05)	0.15
Albumin	0.298 (0.276–0.321)	<0.001	0.461 (0.381–0.556)	<0.001
PT	12.9 (10.0–16.7)	<0.001	2.28 (1.18–4.40)	0.014
Platelet	0.956 (0.951–0.960)	<0.001	0.973 (0.963–0.983)	<0.001
Heamoglobin	0.28 (0.221–0.355)	<0.001	0.720 (0.439–1.18)	0.19

TABLE 2: ICG15 of patients with various Child-Pugh score stratified by platelet count.

Child-Pugh		Platelet $\geq 150 \times 10^9$/L				Platelet $< 150 \times 10^9$/L			
		ICG15 (mean ± SD)		Number/%		ICG15 (mean ± SD)		Number/%	
5	A	11.7 ± 6.57	12.4 ± 7.39	1264	44.6%	16.2 ± 9.81	19.2 ± 12.4	827	29.2%
6		16.1 ± 10.1		231	8.16%	28.9 ± 14.8		254	8.97%
7	B	18.7 ± 12.8	21.0 ± 14.0	77	2.72%	38.4 ± 16.3	42.0 ± 16.4	89	3.14%
8		29.5 ± 17.6		20	0.71%	44.3 ± 14.3		40	1.41%
9		22.2 ± 8.78		10	0.35%	53.7 ± 15.6		20	0.71%

of hepatic encephalopathy do not affect ICG clearance rate. Liver enzymes including alanine aminotransferase (ALT) and gamma-glutamyl transferase (GGT) do not affect ICG15.

Thrombocytopenia is a constant phenomenon of portal hypertension [16]. Low platelet count is associated with increased posthepatectomy liver failure and operative mortality [17]. The question of this being a confounding factor of the above five, or an additional parameter to assess liver function reserve, is worth investigating. In our series, platelet count remains a robust independent predictor of ICG15 (OR 0.973, 95% CI 0.963–0.983, $p < 0.001$). In Table 2, when patients in each category of Child-Pugh score are subdivided into two groups based on the platelet count equal to or above 150×10^9/L, that is, normal and those below normal, the ICG15 of the patients in this series diverted in a predictable manner. As shown in Figure 3, incorporation of platelet count improves the correlation between ICG15 and Child-Pugh score. Patients with thrombocytopenia consistently have slower ICG clearance across all Child-Pugh groups. It is worth noting that patients with normal platelet count constantly outperform their counterparts with lower Child-Pugh scores. For example, Child-Pugh score 7 patients with normal platelet count have better ICG15 (18.7 ± 12.8) than Child-Pugh score 6 patients with thrombocytopenia (28.9 ± 14.8). Child-Pugh score 8 patients with normal platelet count have lower ICG15 (29.5 ± 17.6) as those who scored 7 but with thrombocytopenia (38.4 ± 16.3) (Table 2 and Figure 3). This highlighted the role of platelet count in correlating the two systems.

Table 3 summarizes the differences between patients with normal and low platelet counts. Minimal numbers of hepatic encephalopathy [2 (0.125%) versus 3 (0.244%), $p = 0.66$] were found in both groups, of which its presence would preclude surgical treatment in most situations. As expected, patients with normal platelet count had fewer numbers of ascites [66 (4.12%) versus 78 (6.34%), $p = 0.001$], as both thrombocytopenia and ascites result from portal hypertension. Patients

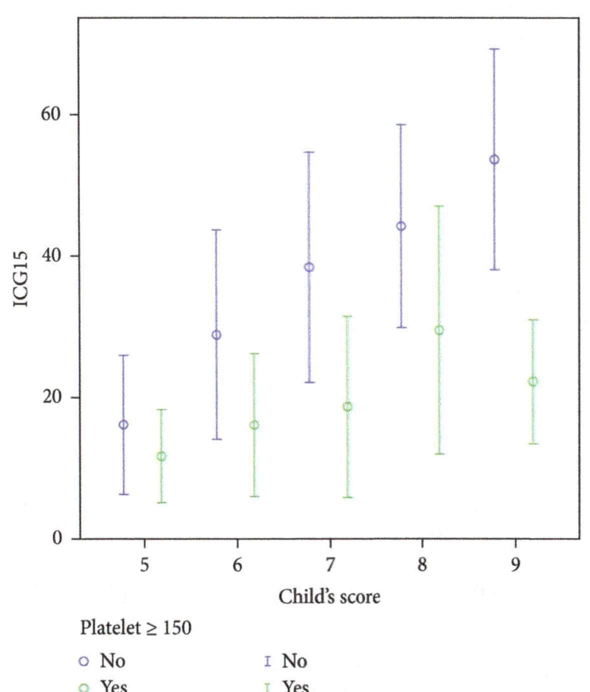

FIGURE 3: Correlation between ICG15 and Child-Pugh score stratified by platelet count. Error bars: ±1 SD.

TABLE 3: Characteristics of patients stratified by platelet count.

	Platelet ≥ 150 × 10^9/L	Platelet < 150 × 10^9/L	p value
Total number	1602 (56.6%)	1230 (43.4%)	
Age	56.9 ± 12.8	60.2 ± 10.7	<0.001
Gender (M/F)	1313/289	986/244	0.23
Hepatic encephalopathy			0.66
No	1600 (100%)	1227 (99.8%)	
Grades 1-2	2 (0.125%)	3 (0.244%)	
Grades 3-4	0 (0%)	0 (0%)	
Ascites			0.001
No	1536 (96%)	1152 (93.7%)	
Mild	47 (2.93%)	70 (5.69%)	
Moderate	9 (0.562%)	5 (0.407%)	
Gross	10 (0.624%)	3 (0.244%)	
Bilirubin (μmol/L)	12.8 ± 7.67	17.7 ± 11.4	<0.001
Albumin (g/L)	40.0 ± 5.03	38.4 ± 5.28	<0.001
Prothrombin time (sec)	12.3 ± 1.65	13.1 ± 1.65	<0.001
ICG15 (%)	13.0 ± 8.29	21.9 ± 14.9	<0.001
Platelet (×10^9/L)	231 ± 78.9	103 ± 31.5	<0.001

with normal platelet count also have lower level of bilirubin (12.8±7.67 versus 17.7±11.4 μmol/L, $p < 0.001$), higher level of albumin (40.0 ± 5.03 versus 38.4 ± 5.28 g/L, $p < 0.001$), and less prolonged prothrombin time (12.3 ± 1.65 versus 13.1 ± 1.65, $p < 0.001$). These differences, though statistically significant, were hardly clinically evident. By contrast, the normal platelet group performed remarkably better in terms of ICG clearance (ICG15 13.0 ± 8.29 versus 21.9 ± 14.9%, $p < 0.001$). This reemphasizes the unique importance of platelet count as the missing link between Child-Pugh score and ICG retention test.

3.3. Prediction of ICG15 from Child-Pugh Parameters and Platelet Count. We investigated the possibility of estimating ICG15 from objective Child-Pugh parameters and platelet count. Ascites and hepatic encephalopathy are not included for analysis, because clinical assessment of their grading could be subjective and because of the paucity of positive samples. In our series, numbers of patients with ascites or hepatic encephalopathy were few; therefore, their inclusion is unlikely to yield meaningful results.

By stepwise multiple linear regression analysis, the relation between ICG15 with bilirubin, albumin, prothrombin time, and platelet count was tested. The following formula is derived:

$$\begin{aligned}\text{Estimated ICG15 (eICG15)} \\ &= 45.1 + 0.435 \times \text{Bilirubin} - 0.917 \times \text{Albumin} \\ &+ 0.491 \times \text{Prothrombin time} - 0.0283 \times \text{Platelet} \\ &\left(R^2 = 0.455\right).\end{aligned} \quad (1)$$

Mean eICG15 from this formula was plotted against ICG15 on Figure 4. The linear correlation is stronger while ICG15 is relatively small, that is, less than 30%. Figure 5 plotted the mean error of this estimation against measured ICG15. The formula performs best when ICG15 is 15%, close to the value of 14% which is of clinical interest. Estimation becomes less accurate when ICG15 is large, that is, higher than 30%.

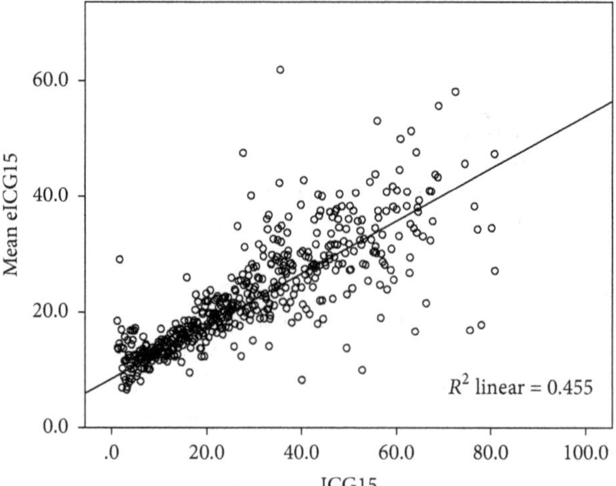

FIGURE 4: Relation between mean eICG15 and ICG15.

Receiver operating characteristic curve (Figure 6, area under curve = 0.804) shows that a cut-off of eICG15 >20.0% predicts ICG15 >14.0% by a specificity of 90.7%. Numbers of patients with measured ICG15 ≤14% are plotted against eICG15 in Figure 7. Patients in the shaded area have an eICG15 higher than 20.0%, and among them less than 9.3% would have an ICG15 less than or equal to 14%, that is, agreeable to major hepatectomy.

3.4. Clinical Implications of eICG15. In our series, 848 patients underwent major hepatectomy. 761 (89.7%) of them had an eICG15 ≤20.0%, while 87 (10.3%) of them had a

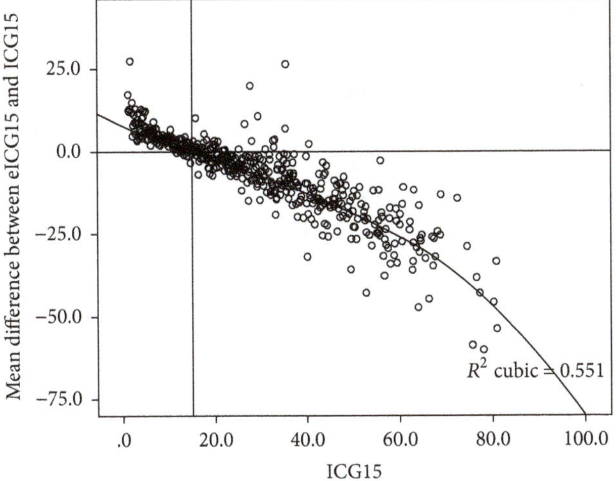

FIGURE 5: Mean error of eICG15 against ICG15.

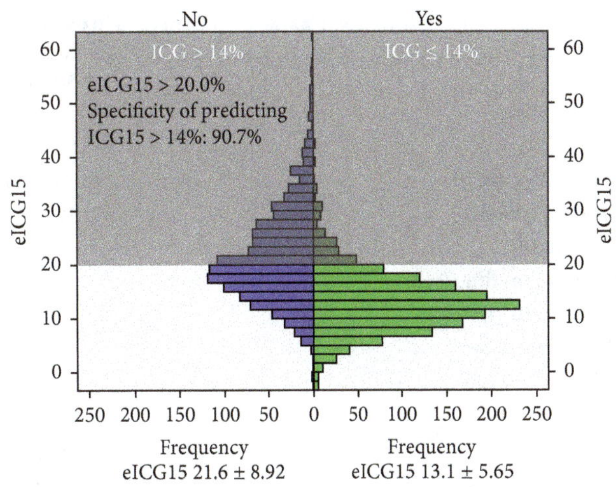

FIGURE 7: Distribution of patients with ICG15 >14% by eICG15.

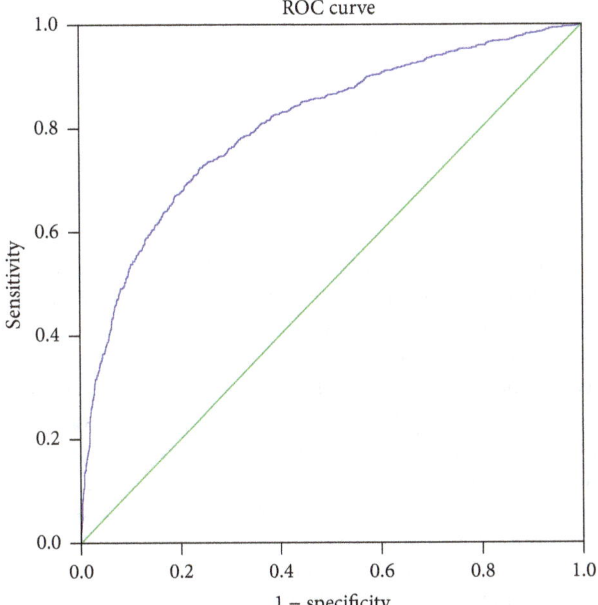

FIGURE 6: Receiver operating characteristic curve determining cut-off point of eICG15 to predict ICG15 ≤14%. Area under curve = 0.804. Diagonal segments are produced by ties.

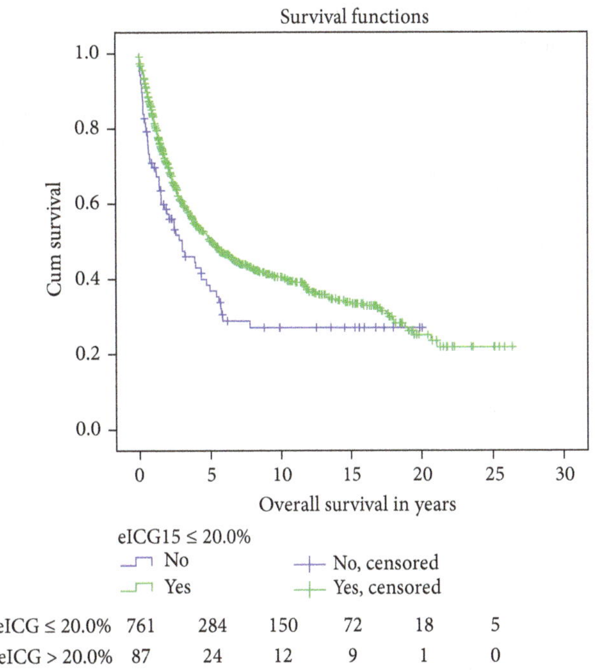

FIGURE 8: Overall survival after major hepatectomy, stratified by eICG15. Median overall survival 5.10 ± 0.553 versus 3.01 ± 0.878 years, $p = 0.015$.

level higher than that (Table 4). Patients with eICG15 ≤20.0% had clinically observable differences in terms of Child-Pugh parameters. They had lower level of bilirubin (10.9 ± 4.45 versus 20.9 ± 12.2 μmol/L, $p < 0.001$), higher level of albumin (41.2 ± 3.95 versus 34.1 ± 4.40 g/L, $p < 0.001$), and less prolonged prothrombin time (12.1 ± 1.16 versus 13.3 ± 2.44, $p < 0.001$). They also had higher platelet counts (209 ± 81 versus 175 ± 67, $p < 0.001$).

There is a trend towards more posthepatectomy liver failure in patients with eICG15 >20.0% [31 (4.1%) versus 7 (8.0%), $p = 0.09$]. eICG15 > 20.0% also predicted higher in-hospital mortality after major hepatectomy [28 (3.7%) versus 7 (8.0%), $p = 0.052$].

In long term, eICG15 > 20.0% indicated inferior oncological outcomes. Both groups of patients have comparable tumour size (6.97 ± 3.72 versus 8.23 ± 4.42 cm, $p = 0.13$). Despite having fewer tumours with portal venous invasion (5.3% versus 1.5%, $p = 0.04$), patients with eICG15 >20% had shorter median overall survival (5.10 ± 0.553 versus 3.01 ± 0.878 years, $p = 0.015$) (Figure 8) and disease-free survival (1.37 ± 0.215 versus 0.707 ± 0.183 years, $p = 0.018$) (Figure 9).

4. Discussion

Assessing the degree of functional impairment of the liver from cirrhosis is pivotal to the choice of treatment of HCC,

TABLE 4: Characteristics of patients who underwent major hepatectomy, stratified by eICG15.

	eICG15 ≤ 20.0	eICG15 > 20.0	p value
Total number	761 (89.7%)	87 (10.3%)	
Age	55.7 ± 11.7	58.7 ± 10.6	<0.001
Gender M/F (% M)	615/146 (80.8%)	75/12 (86.2%)	0.22
Bilirubin (μmol/L)	10.9 ± 4.49	20.9 ± 12.2	<0.001
Albumin (g/L)	41.2 ± 3.95	34.1 ± 4.40	<0.001
Prothrombin time (sec)	12.1 ± 1.16	13.3 ± 2.44	<0.001
Platelet ($\times 10^9$/L)	209 ± 81	175 ± 67	<0.001
Child-Pugh score			<0.001
5	678 (89.1%)	25 (28.7%)	
6	73 (9.6%)	45 (51.7%)	
7	10 (1.3%)	15 (17.2%)	
8	0 (0.0%)	1 (1.1%)	
9	0 (0.0%)	1 (1.1%)	
ICG15 (%)	10.7 ± 5.59	15.0 ± 7.33	<0.001
Tumour size (cm)	6.97 ± 3.72	8.23 ± 4.42	0.13
Portal venous invasion	42 (5.3%)	10 (1.5%)	0.04
Posthepatectomy liver failure	31 (4.1%)	7 (8.0%)	0.09
In-hospital mortality	28 (3.7%)	7 (8.0%)	0.052
Median overall survival (year)	5.10 ± 0.553	3.01 ± 0.878	0.015
Median disease free survival (year)	1.37 ± 0.215	0.707 ± 0.183	0.018

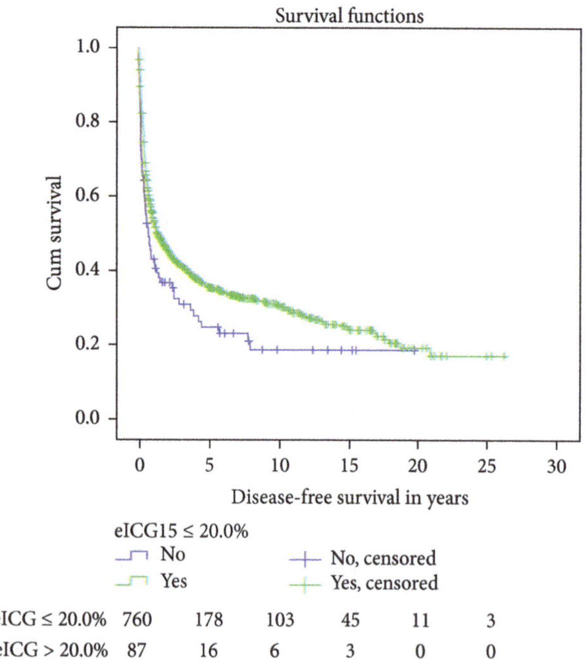

FIGURE 9: Disease-free survival after major hepatectomy, stratified by eICG15. Median disease-free survival 1.37 ± 0.215 versus 0.707 ± 0.183 years, $p = 0.018$.

as various treatment modalities inflict various extent of insult to the cirrhotic liver. The advantage of the Child-Pugh score and grade is that a comprehensive assessment of liver function could be readily determined from routine blood tests and careful clinical assessment. ICG15 provides a more gradated evaluation over the ordinal scale, however, at the expense of additional invasiveness and cost. ICG contains sodium iodide and ICG clearance test is contraindicated for patients allergic to iodide. Adverse reactions occur in 0.7% of patients receiving intravenous ICG injection [18]. Additional labour and equipment, that is, spectrometer, are required. Platelet count improves the correlation between the two systems (Figure 3). It is constantly an important parameter in assessing liver function [16] and reflects the prognosis of HCC patients [19, 20]. Our regression formula combines Child-Pugh parameters and platelet count to achieve a quantitative assessment as with ICG15, so that the simplicity of Child-Pugh system and the agility of ICG15 are incorporated. Using a cut-off value of 20.0%, eICG15 identifies patients with higher operative risk (in-hospital mortality after major hepatectomy 3.7% versus 8.0%, $p = 0.052$) and inferior oncological outcomes (median overall survival 5.10 ± 0.553 versus 3.01 ± 0.878 years, $p = 0.015$). These figures should be considered before major hepatectomy is offered (Figure 10).

The standard deviation of ICG when plotted against Child-Pugh score was large (8.30–20.3). Thus, whether Child-Pugh score may replace ICG15 is questioned. Correlation is improved when patients were stratified by their platelet counts (Figure 3). The fact that patients with normal platelet have better ICG15 compared to their counterparts with lower Child-Pugh scores indicates the necessity of taking platelet count into consideration when relating the two systems. Using platelet count and objective Child-Pugh parameters, our regression formula gives an equally simple yet more gradated estimation of liver function reserve comparing to

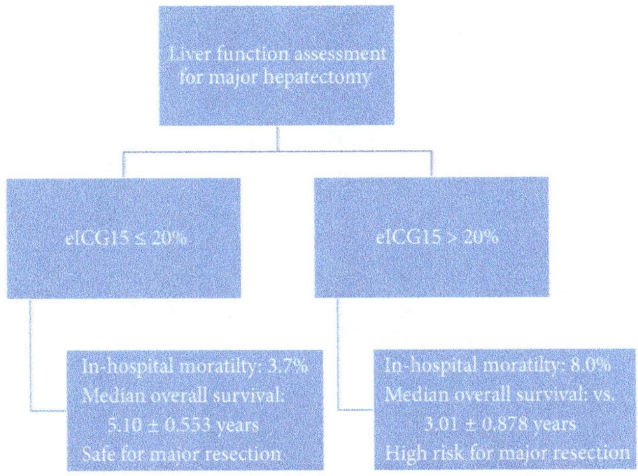

Figure 10: Algorithm for interpreting eICG15.

Child-Pugh score. The formula provides reliable estimation when the ICG15 is closed to the clinically interested value of 14% (Figure 5).

Though the Child-Pugh system and ICG clearance test have been employed in parallel in the west and the East for a quarter of century, literature describing their relation was scarce. This study delineates the correlation and discrepancies between them. We are first to emphasize the role of platelet count in associating the two systems and to correlate both using a regression formula. The implications of this formula have been emphasized by its prediction of both operative and oncological outcomes. The greatest limitation of this study is its retrospective nature. Further validation of this formula would be with prospective data that would allow us to overcome this weakness. ICG clearance test was performed for potential surgical candidates and patients who were obviously not candidate for surgery; that is, Child-Pugh C liver function were not included. When the subset of operated patients was compared stratified by their eICG15, the two groups differed in terms of extent of surgery. Nevertheless, the sample in this series resembled the actual patients of which surgery is contemplated. This study presents a simple liver function reserve assessment to guide clinicians in treatment decision and prognosis for HCC patients.

Abbreviations

ALP: Alkaline phosphatase
CT: Computed tomography
eICG15: Estimated indocyanine green retention rate at 15 minutes
GGT: Gamma-glutamyl transferase
HCC: Hepatocellular carcinoma
ICG: Indocyanine green
ICG15: Indocyanine green retention rate at 15 minutes
MELD: Model of end-stage liver disease
SPSS: Statistical Product and Service Solution.

References

[1] R. N. H. Pugh, "Pugh's grading in the classification of liver decompensation," *Gut*, vol. 33, no. 11, p. 1583, 1992.

[2] K. F. Bader, "Thoracic Ileopexy for Portal Hypertension," *Archives of Surgery*, vol. 89, no. 1, p. 228, 1964.

[3] R. N. H. Pugh, I. M. Murray Lyon, and J. L. Dawson, "Transection of the oesophagus for bleeding oesophageal varices," *The British Journal of Surgery*, vol. 60, no. 8, pp. 646–649, 1973.

[4] J. M. Llovet, J. Bruix, and G. J. Gores, "Surgical resection versus transplantation for early hepatocellular carcinoma: Clues for the best strategy," *Hepatology*, vol. 31, no. 4, pp. 1019–1021, 2000.

[5] E. Christensen, P. Schlichting, L. Fauerholdt et al., "Prognostic value of child-turcotte criteria in medically treated cirrhosis," *Hepatology*, vol. 4, no. 3, pp. 430–435, 1984.

[6] J. M. Llovet, C. Brú, and J. Bruix, "Prognosis of hepatocellular carcinoma: the BCLC staging classification," *Seminars in Liver Disease*, vol. 19, no. 3, pp. 329–338, 1999.

[7] J. M. Llovet, J. Fuster, and J. Bruix, "The Barcelona approach: Diagnosis, staging, and treatment of hepatocellular carcinoma," *Liver Transplantation*, vol. 10, no. 2, pp. S115–S120, 2004.

[8] H. Lau, K. Man, S.-T. Fan, W.-C. Yu, C.-M. Lo, and J. Wong, "Evaluation of preoperative hepatic function in patients with hepatocellular carcinoma undergoing hepatectomy," *British Journal of Surgery*, vol. 84, no. 9, pp. 1255–1259, 1997.

[9] G. Cherrick, S. Stein, C. Leevy, and C. Davidson, "Indocyanine green: observations on its physical properties, plasma decay, and hepatic extraction," *The Journal of Clinical Investigation*, vol. 39, pp. 592–600, 1960.

[10] M. Teranaka and W. G. Schenk Jr., "Hepatic blood flow measurement. A comparison of the indocyanine green and electromagnetic techniques in normal and abnormal flow states in the dog," *Annals of Surgery*, vol. 185, no. 1, pp. 58–63, 1977.

[11] H. H. Stone, W. D. Long, R. B. Smith III, and C. D. Haynes, "Physiologic considerations in major hepatic resections," *The American Journal of Surgery*, vol. 117, no. 1, pp. 78–84, 1969.

[12] M. E. Gottlieb, I. James Sarfeh, H. Stratton, M. L. Goldman, J. C. Newell, and D. M. Shah, "Hepatic perfusion and splanchnic oxygen consumption in patients postinjury," *Journal of Trauma - Injury, Infection and Critical Care*, vol. 23, no. 9, pp. 836–843, 1983.

[13] S.-T. Fan, E. C. S. Lai, C.-M. Lo, I. O. L. Ng, and J. Wong, "Hospital mortality of major hepatectomy for hepatocellular carcinoma associated with *Cirrhosis*," *Archives of Surgery*, vol. 130, no. 2, pp. 198–203, 1995.

[14] F. Sutherland and J. Harris, "Claude Couinaud," *Archives of Surgery*, vol. 137, no. 11, 2002.

[15] Y. Fong, R. L. Sun, W. Jarnagin, and L. H. Blumgart, "An analysis of 412 cases of hepatocellular carcinoma at a Western center," *Annals of Surgery*, vol. 229, no. 6, pp. 790–800, 1999.

[16] M. Peck-Radosavljevic, "Thrombocytopenia in liver disease," *Canadian Journal of Gastroenterology*, vol. 14, Supplement D, pp. 60D–66D, 2000.

[17] S. K. Maithel, P. J. Kneuertz, D. A. Kooby et al., "Importance of low preoperative platelet count in selecting patients for resection of hepatocellular carcinoma: A multi-institutional

analysis," *Journal of the American College of Surgeons*, vol. 212, no. 4, pp. 638–648, 2011.

[18] M. Hope-Ross, L. A. Yannuzzi, E. S. Gragoudas et al., "Adverse reactions due to indocyanine green," *Ophthalmology*, vol. 101, no. 3, pp. 529–533, 1994.

[19] E. G. Giannini and V. Savarino, "Platelet count and survival of patients with compensated cirrhosis and small hepatocellular carcinoma treated with surgery," *Hepatology*, vol. 59, no. 4, pp. 1649-1649, 2014.

[20] Q. Pang, K. Qu, J.-Y. Zhang et al., "The prognostic value of platelet count in patients with hepatocellular carcinoma: a systematic review and meta-analysis," *Medicine*, vol. 94, no. 37, p. e1431, 2015.

The Role of Normothermic Perfusion in Liver Transplantation (TRaNsIT Study): A Systematic Review of Preliminary Studies

Kumar Jayant,[1] Isabella Reccia,[1] Francesco Virdis,[2] and A. M. James Shapiro[3]

[1]*Department of Surgery and Cancer, Imperial College London, London, UK*
[2]*Department of Surgery, Kings College, London, UK*
[3]*Department of Surgery, University of Alberta, Edmonton, Canada*

Correspondence should be addressed to Kumar Jayant; jkumar@ic.ac.uk

Academic Editor: Shu-Sen Zheng

Introduction. The success of liver transplantation has been limited by the unavailability of suitable donor livers. The current organ preservation technique, i.e., static cold storage (SCS), is not suitable for marginal organs. Alternatively, normothermic machine perfusion (NMP) promises to recreate the physiological environment and hence holds promise for the better organ preservation. The objective of this systematic review is to provide an overview of the safety, benefits, and insight into the other potential useful parameters of NMP in the liver preservation. *Material and Methods.* We searched the current literature following registration in the International Prospective Register of Systematic Reviews (PROSPERO) with registration number CRD42018086034 for prospective trials comparing the role of NMP device to SCS in liver transplant by searching the PubMed, EMBASE, Cochrane, BIOSIS, Crossref, and Scopus databases and clinical trial registry. *Results.* The literature search identified five prospective clinical trials (four being early phase single institutional and single randomized multi-institutional) comparing 187 donor livers on NMP device to 273 donor livers on SCS. The primary outcome of interest was to assess the safety and graft survival at day 30 after transplant following NMP of the donor liver. Secondary outcomes included were early allograft dysfunction (EAD) in the first seven days; serum measures of liver functions as bilirubin, aspartate aminotransferase (AST), alanine amino transferase (ALT), alkaline phosphatase (ALP), and international normalized ratio (INR) on days 1–7; major complications as defined by a Clavien-Dindo score ≥ 3; and patient and graft survival and biliary complications at six months. The peaked median AST level between days 1 and 7 in the five trials was 417–1252 U/L (range 84–15009 U/L) while on NMP and 839–1474 U/L (range 153–8786 U/L) in SCS group. The median bilirubin level on day 7 ranged within 25–79 μmol/L (range 8–344 μmol/l) and 30–47.53 μmol/l (range 9–340 μmol/l) in NMP and SCS groups, respectively. A single case of PNF was reported in NMP group in the randomized trial while none of the other preliminary studies reported any in either group. There was intertrial variability in EAD which ranged within 15–56% in NMP group while being within 23–37% in SCS group. Biliary complications observed in NMP group ranged from 0 to 20%. Single device malfunction was reported in randomized controlled trial leading to renouncement of transplant while none of the other trials reported any machine failure, although two user related device errors inadvertent were reported. *Conclusion.* This review outlines that NMP not only demonstrated safety and efficacy but also provided the favourable environment of organ preservation, repair, and viability assessment to donor liver prior to the transplantation with low rate of posttransplantation complication as PNF, EAD, and biliary complication; however further studies are needed to broaden our horizon.

1. Introduction

Liver transplantation is established as the treatment of choice for patients with the end-stage liver disease. While the success of liver transplantation is unquestioned, the scarcity of donor organs limits the delivery of this therapy in a sufficiently timely manner to prevent deaths on the waiting list. Despite the rise in organ donation, the potential requirement of liver transplantation still far exceeds demand, and patients may have compromised outcomes as they end up being transplanted with high model of end-stage liver disease (MELD) scores and in a severely deconditioned state [1, 2]. The United States Organ Procurement and Transplantation Network 2016 national data found that 1,104 patients died while waiting

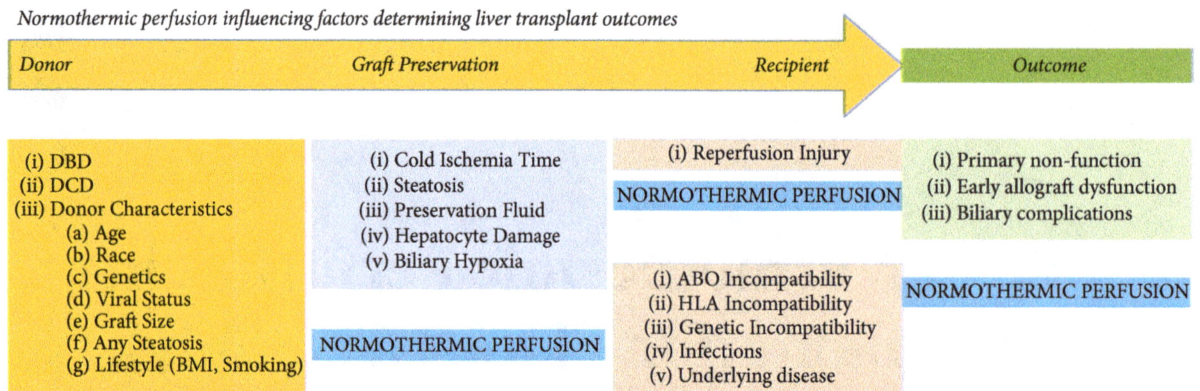

Figure 1: Factors modified by normothermic perfusion during liver transplantation.

for a liver transplant and a further 1,317 were removed from the list as they became too sick to transplant [3]. The global escalating shortage of organ donors has driven centres to use extended criteria donors (ECD), including elderly people, steatotic liver, and donation after cardiac death (DCD), as well as recently using donors that are actively infected with hepatitis C virus. However, inadequate liver preservation and extensive ischemic injury in ECD grafts have been recognized as key factors associated with primary non function (PNF), early allograft dysfunction (EAD), and biliary complications [4, 5]. If more marginal and ECD livers could be preserved with a system that could protect and reverse hepatocyte and biliary injury, without excess risk in transplanting, then potentially the supply and demand for liver transplantation could become more manageable (Figure 1) [1, 6].

The acute termination of oxygenated blood supply during liver procurement initiates a cascade of injury and inflammation, triggered initially by hypoxic anaerobic metabolism, nutrient, cofactor, and adenosine triphosphate (ATP) depletion, with lactic acid accumulation. These injurious processes are further exaggerated during static cold storage (SCS). Disruption of sodium-potassium membrane pumps leads to disruption of electrolyte cell membrane gradients, resulting in cellular edema, influx of free calcium, and subsequent activation of proteolytic enzymes terminating with cell death. Accumulation of xanthine oxide following ATP breakdown generates free radical upon restoration of circulation. These free radicals lead to lipid peroxidation and cellular destruction known as ischemia-reperfusion injury [7–9].

The traditional method of organ preservation involves flushing of cold preservation solution following complete dissection and interruption of blood supply to the donor organ. Cold preservation works on the principle of diminishing cellular metabolism with a decrease in temperature (the Q10 effect), which limits need for ATP [10]. However, anaerobic metabolism continues albeit slowly down to temperatures of +1°C, which can lead to continual depletion of ATP reserve and accumulation of metabolic waste. These insults are exaggerated in marginal livers, increasing risk of initial poor function (IPF), primary nonfunction (PNF), and biliary complications including ischemic cholangiopathy (IC) in comparison to standard criteria donors [11–13]. The increasing level of societal obesity and associated steatosis pose their own additional challenges, as such livers already have increased risk of IPF [14, 15]. Such marginal livers are especially vulnerable to ischemia-reperfusion injury [16, 17]. Hence, graft reperfusion may induce acute metabolic stress and give rise to hemodynamic instability known as "postreperfusion syndrome (PRS)" [18, 19]. PRS is defined as a decrease in the mean arterial pressure (MAP) of more than 30% from baseline measure recorded during the anhepatic phase, lasting for more than one minute, within the first five minutes of the reestablishment of graft perfusion [20]. The incidence of PRS varies between 25 and 50% and is associated with increased risk of acute kidney injury and increased risk of death [21–23].

The possibility of avoiding cold ischemic injury altogether in marginal grafts has recently become possible with the introduction of the new technology of ex vivo normothermic liver perfusion (NMP). The concept of normothermic perfusion is simple, in that maintaining an entirely physiological milieu for the liver during transport should diminish risk of ischemic injury within the liver, and ischemia-reperfusion has already occurred on the device, thereby reducing risk of PRS in the recipient [24]. It remains to be seen, however, if elimination of the cold ischemic phase in DCD and other marginal grafts can protect against IC and other biliary complications through application of NMP [25–27]. If reliable predictive markers of posttransplant function can be established during the NMP phase, then livers at highest risk of PNF and IPF could be eliminated before exposing a recipient to a higher risk of demise. By selecting an increasing number of livers based on ex situ function and eliminating those at demonstrably higher risk, the ceiling for extended criteria liver donors could be raised considerably. The added advantage of having a donor liver function physiologically ex situ is that protective supplements may be added to the circuit with potential to stabilize, reverse, and even repair preexisting injury. Furthermore, immunological manipulation of liver grafts could mitigate need for potent antirejection therapies in the recipient if HLA Class II expression and other donor antigens could be modified. Livers could be loaded with protective cells such as regulatory T cells (Tregs) or mesenchymal stem cells (MSCs) that also have immunoregulatory and anti-inflammatory properties (Figure 1) [28–30]. NMP has already been shown to be highly effective in lung transplantation and is currently in early developmental testing in kidney and whole pancreas transplantation [31, 32].

Based upon extensive promising results in preclinical large animal studies in NMP porcine or rodent models [33–36], at least three commercial normothermic perfusion devices have emerged in early clinical trials till date. Each NMP technology works on similar principles but differs in terms of portability, degree of automation, substrate type and delivery, pressure and pulsatility of the recirculating perfusate, and hepatic arterial and portal vein flow targets [37, 38]. The first technology to reach the clinic was the Metra device developed by Peter Friend and colleagues in a partnership between the University of Oxford and a spin-off company (OrganOx Ltd.). The Metra is a fully automated, portable device, perfusing livers at 37°C with whole blood supplemented with plasma expander (Gelofusine), bile salts, parenteral nutrition solution, heparin, insulin, and prostacyclin through a closed perfusion, continuous, nonpulsatile portal vein, and hepatic arterial flow technique [39]. The Organ Care System (OCS) liver was developed by TransMedics (Andover, MA) is also a fully automated portable device, and follows similar principles of NMP [40]. Organ Assist (Groningen, Netherlands) developed a semiautomated device but with only limited portability which allows liver perfusion at temperatures ranging from 8°C to 37°C. The arterial and portal pressures can be modulated to adjust vascular flow [41]. The importance of device portability remains an open question presently. Provision of on-board oxygen generation and a need to transport heavy, complex equipment great distances by road or plane pose their own unique challenges and markedly escalate the cost of the technology. Some institutes are now exploring the more limited intervention of perfusing the liver once it has arrived at the recipient centre. While this may not completely protect against hepatocyte injury and IC, it still offers a promising role in confirming that a liver will function before it is transplanted and offers the added advantage of being able to be more flexible to schedule liver transplantation surgeries during daylight hours.

In the present systematic review, we provide a detailed analysis of all available human liver NMP studies that assess safety, feasibility, and reliability of this new technology and where possible available evidence reflecting the clinical effectiveness of NMP as an alternative to SCS in patients undergoing liver transplantation is summated. Finally, we explored potential directions for future research and translation of NMP technique into clinical practice.

2. Material and Methods

2.1. Search Strategy. A comprehensive systematic literature review was performed according to the Preferred Reporting Items for Systematic reviews and Meta-Analyses for Protocols 2015 (PRISMA-P 2015) [46], following registration in the International Prospective Register of Systematic Reviews (PROSPERO) [47], at https://www.crd.york.ac.uk/prospero with registration number CRD42018086034. An extensive search of all the published literature describing the role with NMP based device in liver transplantation as an alternative to SCS was made on National Library of Medicine Database, EMBASE, Cochrane, BIOSIS, Crossref, and Scopus databases and clinical trial registry on 10 October 2017. The search covered the period from May 2016 (the year of the first reported clinical trial of NMP based device) to 18 April 2018 and search was last carried out on 18 April 2018 [39]. Our search strategy comprised compiling keywords as "Normothermic Perfusion", "OrganOx", "Organ Assist", "Organ Care System", "Graft Rejection", "Graft Survival", and "Liver Transplantation" from all the salient articles and broad literature searches on the given databases.

Table 1: Criteria for the inclusion of studies.

Study design	Prospective study design with a well-defined study population
Study group	Liver transplant
Study size	Any
Length of follow-up	Any
Source	Peer-reviewed journals
Language	Any
Outcome measure	Patient safety, adverse events, graft function, Graft & patient survival and perfusion machine logistics.

2.2. Inclusion and Exclusion Criteria. Only studies which systematically and quantitatively assessed the graft safety, functioning, and graft survival on NMP based devices including the OrganOx (Metra), the Organ Assist (Liver Assist), and TransMedics (OCS) in different clinical studies were analyzed. All other publications as editorials, reviews, and letters were excluded. The primary outcome of interest was to assess the safety and graft survival at day 30 after transplant following NMP of the donor liver. Secondary outcomes included were early allograft dysfunction (EAD) on the first seven days; serum measures of liver functions as bilirubin, aspartate aminotransferase (AST), alanine amino transferase (ALT), alkaline phosphatase (ALP), and international normalized ratio (INR) on days 1–7; major complications as defined by a Clavien-Dindo score ≥ 3; and patient and graft survival and biliary complications at six months (Table 1).

2.3. Data Extraction. Two separate physician reviewers, KJ and IR, employed a two-stage method to conduct study screening independently. At the first stage, titles and abstracts were scrutinized for excluding obviously ineligible studies. At the second stage, the full text was read carefully for further excluding ineligible studies. Disagreements were resolved via consensus and discussion with chief author AMJS. We analyzed literature with empirical studies using a standardized quality assessment tool and prespecified inclusion and exclusion criteria. The present systematic review was performed using the Preferred Reporting Items for Systematic Reviews and Meta-Analyses (PRISMA) guidelines and registered in the PROSPERO, an international database of prospectively registered systematic reviews (Figure 2).

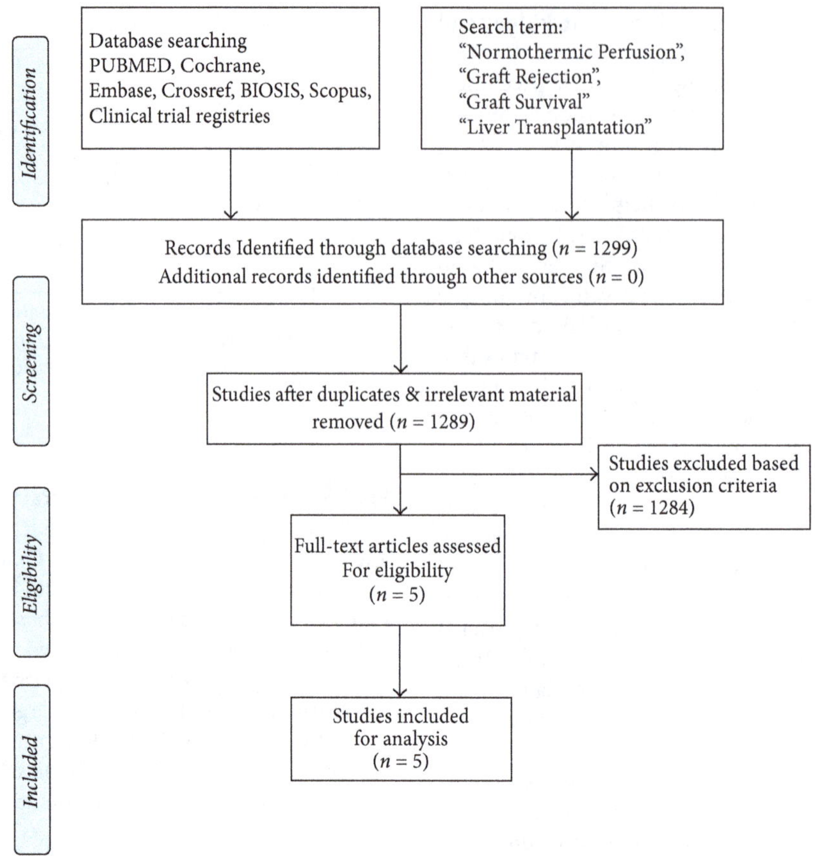

FIGURE 2: Search strategy and study selection used in this systematic review as per PRISMA protocol.

2.4. Quality Testing. The QUADAS-II (quality assessment of diagnostic accuracy studies-II) based analysis was done to assess the internal validity of prespecified inclusion and exclusion criteria of the various studies. QUADAS-II is an evidence-based bias assessment tool to evaluate the quality of diagnostic accuracy studies in a systematic review. Each study was reviewed comprehensively and data extracted to assess the earlier outlined parameters (Table 2).

2.5. Publication Bias. Publication bias is formally assessed through funnel plots, but that requires at least ten trials; unfortunately present systematic review involved only five trials, so we could not have assessed publication bias.

3. Results

Our literature search yielded a total of 1299 manuscripts using keywords listed above. After screening titles and abstracts, 5 studies (4 full articles and single poster with limited data) were included in present review analysis, data extraction of four of which involved Metra device and single with OCS (TransMedics) [39, 42–45] (Table 2). Two studies, published insofar with Organ Assist (Liver Assist) device, were not included because one of them was done at temperature of 20°C while the other did not have any control group [48, 49]. However, we did include the safety issues outlined in the article [49]. Four included studies were single institutional, nonrandomized prospective phase 1 clinical trials [39, 42–44], while study by Nasralla et al. was multi-institutional randomized study [45, 50].

The detailed data related to study characteristics in terms of perioperative and normothermic perfusion, clinical outcomes, safety, adverse events, and survival were summarized in Tables 2–6.

3.1. Donor and Recipient Perioperative Characteristics. A total of 460 patients were included in the five trials; we have outlined the demographic and clinical data of patients undergoing liver transplantation following organ preservation by NMP or SCS. NMP based organ preservation was done in 187 cases, while the conventional method of cold storage was used in 273 cases. Nasralla et al. reported that 48 donor livers were discarded (16 (11.7%) NMP, 32 (24.1%) SCS; $P = 0.004$) owing to presence of significant steatosis, increasing lactate level, cirrhosis in donor liver, WIT > 30 mins, incidental malignancy (colon and lung cancer), and device related errors [45]. The median patient age was outlined in four trials within 48.0–58.0 years (range 14–85) in NMP group and 46.0–58.5 years (range 20–86) in SCS group. The median MELD score reported in four trials ranged within 12–21 (range 6–40) and

TABLE 2: Pretransplant and perioperative characteristics of included studies.

Study	Sample Size (NMP vs Control)	Donor Age (years) (NMP vs Control)	MELD Score (NMP vs Control)	NMP Time vs Control SCS in minutes [median (range)]	DCD (NMP vs Control)
Ravikumar et al. [39] (May 2016)	20 vs 40	58.0 (21–85) vs 58.5 (21–82) ($P = 0.93$)	12.0 (7–27) vs 14.0 (6–25) ($P = 0.55$)	558 (210–1170) vs 534 (242–684) ($P = 0.63$)	4 vs 4
Selzner et al. [42] (October 2016)	10 vs 30	48.0 (17–75) vs 46.0 (22–68) ($P = 0.56$)	21.0 (8–40) vs 23.0 (7–37) ($P = 0.85$)	586 (221–731) vs 634 (523–783) ($P = 0.11$)	2 vs 6
Bral et al. [43] (Nov 2017)	10 vs 30	56.0 (14–71) vs 52.0 (20–77) ($P = 0.91$)	13.0 (9–32) vs 19.0 (7–34) ($P = 0.37$)	786 (304–1631) vs 235 (64–890) ($P = 0.001$)	4 vs 8
Liu et al. [44] (May 2017)	10 vs 40	NA ($P > 0.05$)	NA ($P > 0.05$)	(240–472) vs NA ($P > 0.05$)	2 vs 8
Nasralla et al. [45] (Apr 2018)	137 vs 133	56.0 (16–84) vs 56.0 (20–86) ($P > 0.05$)	13.0 (6–35) vs 14.0 (9–18) (P = NA)	714 (258–1527) vs 465 (223–967) ($P < 0.000$)	34 vs 21

MELD: model for end-stage liver disease; DCD: donation after circulatory death; NMP: normothermic machine perfusion; WIT: warm ischemia time; SCS: static cold storage; NA: not available.

14–23 (range 6–37), respectively, in NMP and SCS group. The range of DCD donor sources in NMP and SCS groups ranged between 20–40% and 10–27%, respectively (Table 2).

The reported median NMP time in trials varied considerably, from 558 to 786 minutes (range 210–1631 minutes) while median CIT on cold storage was 235–634 minutes (range 64–967 minutes). There was no significant difference in organ preservation time in the study by Ravikumar et al., Selzner et al., and Liu et al. [39, 42, 44]. However, Bral et al. noted a significantly more prolonged total liver preservation time (786 minutes NMP versus 235 minutes SCS, $P < 0.001$) between study groups [43]. They further commented in supplementary data that they extended NMP duration to enhance operating room logistics, apparently without compromising clinical outcomes for the liver. Similarly, Nasralla et al. did report significantly prolonged total liver preservation time (714 minutes NMP versus 465, $P < 0.000$) [45] (Table 2).

The attributes to assess donor liver functioning while on NMP such as hepatic transaminases, INR, pH, lactate level, bile production, hepatic artery, and portal vein flow were found normal in all the reviewed trials. The perfusate used in all studies was blood based using ABO-blood group O packed red blood cells; however, in the studies by Ravikumar et al., Bral et al., and Nasralla et al., the circuit and liver were additionally primed with gelatin-based plasma expander (Gelofusine™, B. Braun, Melsungen, Germany), whereas in the study by Selzner et al. Steen solution was used instead (Table 3).

3.2. Clinical and Laboratory Outcomes of Normothermic Ex Vivo Perfusion (NMP) and Static Cold Storage Liver (SCS). The peak median AST level between days 1 and 7 in the five trials was 417–1252 U/L (range 84–15009 U/L) while on NMP and 839–1474 U/L (range 153–8786 U/L) in SCS group.

Three trials reported data with median INR value, on day 7, in NMP group being 1.05–1.1 (range 0.88–1.6) and 1.03–1.1 (range 0.90–2.2) in SCS group. The median bilirubin level on day 7 was 25–79 μmol/L (range 8–344 μmol/L) and 30–48 μmol/L (range 9–340 μmol/L) in NMP and SCS groups, respectively. Only three trials outlined day 7 median ALP level, 139–245 U/L (range 40–626 U/L) in NMP group while being 147–243 U/L (range 58–743 U/L) in SCS group (Table 4).

3.3. Post-Liver Transplant Outcomes. The PNF was observed in a single recipient in the randomized study done by Nasralla et al. in NMP group while none of the other trials reported such event in either groups. There was intertrial variability in EAD which ranged from 10 to 56% in NMP group while being within 23–30% in SCS group. Nasralla et al. reported 93% less likelihood of developing EAD in DCD liver while on NMP rather than SCS [45]. In the randomized trial by Nasralla et al. the occurrence of PRS was reported less frequently in NMP group (15 cases) than the SCS (32 cases) which gives credence to the earlier trial of Bral et al. [43, 45].

The median intensive care unit (ICU) stay was 3–16 days (range 1–65 days) in NMP group while in SCS group the median was 3-4 days (range 0–41 days). The median hospital stay in NMP and SCS was 12–45 days (range 6–114 days) and 13–25 days (range 7–89 days), respectively. Between 10–22% and 22–37% recipients developed Clavien-Dindo score ≥ 3 in NMP and SCS groups, respectively. Biliary complications 6 months after transplant were observed in NMP group ranging from 0 to 20%. The trial by Bral et al. evidenced lower 6 months' biliary stricture in NMP group (0%) compared to 14.8% in SCS; however a recent randomized study published by Nasralla et al. did not observe any statistical difference in occurrence of nonanastomotic biliary stricture in either groups [43, 45] (Table 5).

3.4. Post-Liver Transplant Survival Outcomes. During follow-up, 30 days' graft survival reported by three trials was between 90 and 100% in NMP group and 97.5 and 100% in SCS group [39, 43, 45]. Furthermore, 30 days' mortality ranged within 2.5–11% and within 0–2.5% in NMP and SCS group, respectively (Table 6).

3.5. Safety, Feasibility, and Logistics. None of the earlier four preliminary trials reported any issues related to device failure;

Table 3: Characteristics during normothermic ex vivo liver perfusion of included studies.

Study	Perfusate	Peak AST (U/L)	Peak ALT (U/L)	Final lactate (mmol/L)	pH	Bile production (mL/hr)	Hepatic artery flow (mL/minutes)	Portal venous flow (mL/minutes)	Device failure	Major Technical Complication
Ravikumar et al. [39]	Gelofusine + 3-unit donor cross-matched PRBC	NA	NA	NA	NA (7.2–7.4)	NA	NA	NA	0	**0**
Selzner et al. [42]	Steen Solution + 3-unit PRBC	1647 (227–9200)	444 (152–1460)	1.46 (0.56–1.74)	7.26 (7.13–7.33)	7.6 (2.4–15.1)	300 (200–400)	1250 (1200–1300)	0	0
Bral et al. [43]	Gelofusine + 3-unit type "O" PRBC	NA	NA	NA	NA	6.2 (1.9–32.2)	NA	NA	0	1 (Single liver discarded due to portal vein twist)
Liu et al. [44]	Plasma + matched PRBC	NA	NA	NA	NA	NA (1–13)	NA	NA	0	0
Nasralla et al. [45]	Gelofusine + 3-unit donor cross-matched PRBC	NA	NA	NA	NA	NA	NA	NA	1 (Single liver discarded due to the pinch valve mis-calibration causing hepatic artery hypoper-fusion)	2

PRBC: packed red blood cells; AST: aspartate aminotransferase; ALT: alanine amino transferase; NA: not available.

TABLE 4: Clinical outcomes following normothermic ex vivo perfusion (NMP) of included studies.

Study	Peak AST, days 1-7, U/L, median (range) (NMP vs Control)	INR 1 week, median (range) (NMP vs Control)	Bilirubin 1 week, μmol/L, median (range) (NMP vs Control)	ALP 1 week, U/L, median (range) (NMP vs Control)
Ravikumar et al. [39]	417 (84–4681) vs 902 (218–8786) ($P = 0.03$)	1.05 (0.88–1.40) vs 1.03 (0.90–2.22) ($P = 0.92$)	25 (8–211) vs 30 (9–221) ($P = 0.20$)	245 (81–568) vs 243 (76–743) ($P = 0.79$)
Selzner et al. [42]	619 (55–2858) vs 949 (233–3073) ($P = 0.55$)	1.1 (1–1.56) vs 1.1 (1–1.3) ($P = 0.47$)	25.6 (17.1–131.6) vs 47.53 (6.8–256.5) ($P = 0.20$)	202 (96–452) vs 147 (87–456) ($P = 0.21$)
Bral et al. [43]	1252 (383 to >2600) vs 839 (153 to >2600) ($P = 0.52$)	1.1 (1.1–1.6) vs 1.1 (0.9–1.5) ($P = 0.44$)	79 (17–344) vs 53 (8–340) ($P = 0.35$)	139 (40–626) vs 187 (58–524) ($P = 0.62$)
Liu et al. [44]	NA ($P = 0.001$)	NA	NA ($P > 0.05$)	NA
Nasralla et al. [45]	488.1 (408.9–582.8) vs 964.9 (794.5–1172.0) ($P < 0.000$)	1.24 (1.15–1.38) vs 1.24 (1.16–1.39) ($P = 0.64$)	38.5 (21.0–73.2) vs 49.1 (26.0–85.5) ($P = 0.02$)	NA

AST: aspartate aminotransferase; ALT: alanine amino transferase; ALP: alkaline phosphatase; NA: not available.

however Nasralla et al. in a recent randomized trial (2018) did report single event of graft loss following device malfunction and two user related device errors [45]. Previously, Bral et al. reported loss of marginal DCD graft following unrecognized twist above the portal bifurcation led to initial perfusion failure [43]. Another technical complication, an airlock in the fluid sensing system encountered during transportation, was reported in the study by Ravikumar et al., necessitating transient stop for rectification [39] (Table 2). The study by Bral et al. observed a markedly prolonged ICU stay in the NMP group but attributed that largely to patient selection bias with greater preexisting comorbidities in the NMP group [43]. However, the authors could not discount the possibility that the NMP technology could have contributed in some manner, especially since they deliberately pushed the boundaries of perfusion times to the outer limits in some cases (up to 23 hours). Since all studies reported significantly lower reperfusion transaminases with NMP, one would anticipate that healthier livers with lower ICU stay; however, none of studies observed any difference in terms of ICU stay (Table 2).

4. Discussion

With the increasing incidence of the liver disease, the number of transplants required has been outpaced by the number of transplants performed. This disparity between liver transplant candidates and the availability of donor liver has led to an increase in mortality while waiting for transplantation. In order to meet the ever-increasing demand, transplant centres have started exploring the probability for utilization of marginal donor organs. However, the equilibrium has never been achieved owing to the compromised quality of such organs. Recent data from the Organ Procurement and Transplantation Network (OPTN) in the United States reveal that almost 22% of procured livers are discarded before transplantation, and likely many more are never offered as they are considered to have too high risk for cold storage. Currently, SCS technique is the mainstay of organ preservation. However this method works well for livers from healthy donors, achieving acceptable rates of EAD, PNF, and biliary complications [51, 52]. It does not hold true for marginal livers. Increasing evidence suggests that normothermic machine perfusion attempts to recreate the physiological environment by delivering oxygen, temperature, and nutrition. NMP has paved its way for the continuation of aerobic metabolism during the period of organ preservation by minimizing the effects of ischemia/reperfusion injury and PRS [53–56].

The efficacy of normothermic perfusion for liver preservation has not been fully described by clinical studies. In the present review, we have compiled all the evidence and shortcomings illustrated in the studies done so far. These trials were primarily done to assess the safety of NMP; however, data related to functioning and viability of organ were also included [39, 42, 43]. We note that there are very few clinical studies available to date, and thus far virtually all have been limited to safety and feasibility. Since the target population has generally been low-risk, more extensive studies in higher risk subjects will be needed to better define the full potential of this technology to enhance clinical outcomes and make unusable livers more usable for transplantation. Only future studies that focus on more marginal grafts will be able to define this potential more clearly.

4.1. NMP and Safety Issues. The primary aim of this review was to assess the safety of NMP by combining analyses of all available early phase clinical trials. The most frequently cited impediments to broader clinical significance of NMP include the unproven benefit and risk of this new technology, the potential substantial costs associated with complex portable machinery, complex procedures, and additional personnel required to tether and maintain liver stability during ex situ perfusion, risk of microbial contamination, and risk that good livers could be destroyed by exposure to instant warm anoxia if a device were to fail during transportation.

Table 5: Posttransplant outcomes of included studies.

Study	PNF n (%) (NMP vs Control)	EAD n (%) (NMP vs Control)	ICU stay days [median (range)] (NMP vs Control)	Hospital stay days [median (range)] (NMP vs Control)	Major Complications (Clavien-Dindo ≥ 3b) n (%) (NMP vs Control)	Biliary Complications (6 months) NMP n (%)
Ravikumar et al. [39]	0 (0) vs 0 (0) (P = 1.0)	3 (15) vs 9 (22.5) (P = 0.73)	3.0 (1–8) vs 3 (1–41) (P = 0.45)	12.0 (6–34) vs 14.0 (8–88) (P = 0.10)	NA	4 (20)
Selzner et al. [42]	0 (0) vs 0 (0) (P = 1.0)	NA	1.0 (0–8) vs 2 (0–23) (P = 0.54)	11.0 (8–17) vs 13.0 (7–89) (P = 0.23)	1 (10) vs 7 (23) (P = 0.5)	0 (0)
Bral et al. [43]	0 (0) vs 0 (0) (P = 1.0)	5 (55.5) vs 8 (29.6) (P = 0.23)	16.0 (2–65) vs 4 (1–29) (P = 0.004)	11.0 (8–17) vs 13.0 (7–89) (P = 0.23)	2 (22) vs 10 (37) (P = 0.6)	0 (0)
Liu et al. [44]	NA	1 (10%) vs 15 (36.8%) (P = 0.13)	NA	NA	NA	NA
Nasralla et al. [45]	1 (0.8) vs 0 (0) (P = NA)	12 (10.1%) vs 29 (29.9%) (P = 0.000)	4 (2–7) vs 4 (3–7) (P = 0.339)	15 (10–24) vs 15 (11–24) (P = 0.926)	21 (16.4) vs 36 (22) (P = NA)	13 (10.1)

PNF: primary nonfunction; EAD: early graft dysfunction; ICU: intensive care unit; NA: not available.

TABLE 6: Posttransplant survival outcomes of included studies.

Study	30 days of graft survival n (%)	3 months of graft survival n (%)	6 months of graft survival n (%)	Mortality n (%)
Ravikumar et al. [39]	20 (100) vs 39 (97.5) ($P = 1.0$)	NA	20 (100) vs 39 (97.5) ($P = 1.0$)	0 (0) vs 1 (2.5) ($P = 1.0$)
Selzner et al. [42]	NA	10 (100) vs 30 (100) ($P = 1.0$)	NA	0 (0) vs 0 (0) ($P =$ NA)
Bral et al. [43]	9 (90) vs 30 (100) ($P = 0.25$)	9 (90) vs 30 (100) ($P = 0.25$)	8 (80) vs 30 (100) ($P = 0.06$)	2 (11) vs 0 (0) ($P = 0.25$)
Liu et al. [44]	NA	NA	NA	NA
Nasralla et al. [45]	116 (95.86) vs 99 (98.01) ($P = 0.46$)	NA	(95) vs (96) ($P = 0.69$)	NA

NA: not available.

Inadvertent incidents as graft loss following single event of unrecognized twist in portal vein or catheter occlusion in hepatic vein and bile duct or other user related errors could be a part learning curve associated with new technology and may get minimized with the greater cumulative team experience [43, 45, 49]. The real need for device portability remains undefined in clinical studies presently. Adequately powered randomized controlled head-to-head trials are needed to address many of these concerns. Portability allows for direct delivery of NMP at the donor centre with curtailment of cold ischemic exposure but substantially raises the complexity of moving large, heavy machinery by road or air transportation and requires additional technical staff to travel with the donor team. This would require engagement of additional or larger planes for transportation in donor centres that are more remote from the recipient transplant centre. The possibility of perfusing the procured liver once it arrives in the recipient centre (so-called "back-to-base") could still potentially deliver many of the potential benefits of NMP but with far less cost and complexity. NMP technology does not eliminate reperfusion injury but rather brings that process ex situ such that, with appropriate predictive tools to assess function, the transplant surgeon may more accurately assess likelihood that a more marginal liver would work adequately in a particular recipient, before that recipient is exposed to that added risk. As more DCD livers are employed in clinical practice to address the acute liver donor shortage, balancing acute recipient need against potential escalating risk becomes critical. It remains to be seen whether NMP in its current form can protect against ischemic cholangiopathy (IC) in DCD donation. Since NMP does not prevent ischemic-reperfusion injury and biliary epithelial integrity cannot be readily assessed acutely based on currently available testing, we suspect that NMP will not eliminate risk of IC. Potentially, addition of antioxidants, caspase inhibitors, or other cellular protectants could ultimately protect human livers from such risk when added to NMP circuits, but this remains undefined presently.

The loss of clinically usable livers remains of potential concern if more centres are to face the learning curve of a more complex technology for liver preservation than the standard cold storage solution box, which is cheap, efficient, and of proven and known quantum over the past 40 years. It is possible that reporting bias may underreport technical errors in early studies.

A large body of large animal preclinical and now preliminary clinical data demonstrates that ex situ NMP based liver perfusion is generally safe, in most but not all cases lowers early transaminase levels in the recipient, and can accommodate a much prolonged storage phase than could safely be contemplated with SCS. However, adequately powered larger randomized studies are eagerly awaited to more fully define the risk-benefit balance, and until then the exact technique for this exciting new technology remains to be defined.

4.2. NMP and Prediction of the Viability of Donor's Liver. At present, the viability of any particular donor liver can only be assessed following the transplantation into a recipient, which could potentially prove disastrous when extreme marginal donor livers are transplanted, with elevated risk of PNF, EAD, or other detrimental effects of ischemic-reperfusion injuries, including PRS leading to acute renal injury [57–60].

NMP may help overcome such risks by allowing liver function assessment before implantation of the organ into a recipient. The benefits of NMP have been tested in numerous studies and suggest that the viability of donor organ can be predicted by a combination of hemodynamic, metabolic, and synthetic parameters derived during the ex situ perfusion phase, providing a functional assessment of the donor liver, which heretofore was not possible with SCS [34, 61]. The parameters assessed include bile production, stability of hepatic artery and portal flow and/or pressure, and other metabolic parameters as AST and ALT [39, 42, 43, 45]. The most potent predictors of adequate liver function posttransplant thus far are lactate clearance, pH stability, and need for repeated bicarbonate correction during NMP [33, 34, 62]. Mergental et al. suggested criteria including perfusate lactate < 2.5 mmol/l, bile production within 2 hours of initiation of NMP, pH > 7.3, hepatic artery flow > 150 ml/min, portal vein flow > 500 ml/min, and homogenous graft perfusion with soft parenchymal consistency fulfilled within 3 hours of initiation of NMP. Not all groups agree with this data, and one has to interpret any potential criterion within the context of which type of NMP or subnormothermic system they were developed within and within the constraints of which perfusates and additives were given, as it is likely that such

Table 7: Mergental et al. viability criterion to define suitability of liver for transplantation.

Essential Parameters	Lactate < 2.5 mmol/L	OR	Bile Production
	Any two of the following three criterions		
Perfusate pH > 7.3	Stable HA flow > 150 ml/min & PV flow > 500 ml/min		Homogenous graft perfusion with soft parenchymal consistency

criteria will not be universal across technologies (Table 7). Clearly, more detailed and extensive studies will be needed to cross validate such criteria.

4.3. NMP and Posttransplant Complications. Currently, up to one-third of the total pool of marginal livers are made up of DCD donor livers, even though such livers carry added risk [63–66]. While experimentally in porcine models the data is compelling that application of NMP can mitigate most of the added risk of the DCD donor, such data is currently lacking in clinical practice [64, 65]. Brockmann et al. found that NMP-perfused porcine DCD liver grafts have superior function and better survival compared with SCS [66]. Fondevila et al. found that porcine DCD livers exposed to a WIT up to 120 mins had 100% survival with NMP but 100% mortality with SCS [67]. The subsequent clinical trials published by Ravikumar, Selzner, Bral, and Nasralla et al. used 20%, 20%, 40%, and 24.8% DCD liver, respectively, and demonstrated similar outcomes to SCS controls in DCD grafts. Recent study by Nasralla et al. (2018) outlined better outcome with DCD livers preserved with NMP in comparison to SCS group; however further studies are required to strengthen this outcome owing to limitations of inadequately powered subgroup analysis [45].

Bral et al. did not show significant improvement in opening transaminase levels in the recipients, likely due to their increased proportion of DCD donors and prolonged cold ischemia time while a relatively higher proportion of replaced and accessory hepatic arteries were reconstructed on the back table, and their NMP duration was extended to outer limits often while their small surgical team rested overnight or were engaged in other hepatobiliary surgeries [43]. The primary safety outcomes were similar in the NMP group to SCS controls, and long term outcomes up to six months were comparable, suggesting potential benefit from NMP.

4.4. NMP and Posttransplant Primary Nonfunction (PNF). Although SCS is considered as the gold standard method for liver preservation, the injurious impacts upon hepatocyte and biliary epithelial survival are well described [68, 69]. The combination of prolonged cold storage with a marginal liver graft may provide an insurmountable risk for a recipient [70–75]. PNF occurs in up to 5–8% of liver transplants and will result in recipient death if prompt retransplantation is not possible [76, 77]. Though PNF may be caused by technical failure resulting in inadequate blood flow through the graft [70], the association between excess donor risk factors and PNF suggests that it is likely multifactorial [71, 72]. None of the early phase NMP trials have thus far been associated with PNF.

4.5. NMP and Posttransplant Early Allograft Dysfunction (EAD). Early allograft dysfunction (EAD) reflected by elevated recipient transaminase levels within the first postoperative week also poses increased risk for the recipient [78–80]. In the present systematic review EAD of clinical trials ranged from 10 to 55.5% with NMP. There were four incidents of EAD in Bral et al. study of these 2/3 that occurred in DCD grafts [39, 42–44]. All of these livers functioned well at the end and transaminase level returned to the baseline levels. In a recently completed randomized trial Nasralla et al. reported 93% less likelihood of developing EAD in DCD liver and improved graft functioning with NMP [45, 50].

4.6. NMP and Posttransplant Biliary Complication. Anastomotic biliary strictures or more diffuse IC are one of the most feared complications of DCD liver transplantation. The incidence of biliary strictures ranges between 4 and 15% following DBD liver transplantation while being within 30–40% after DCD [14, 74]. Injury to the peribiliary glands (PBG) following formation of microthrombi in peribiliary vascular plexus (PVP) at the time of ischemia-reperfusion or a circulatory phase of DCD has been implicated in biliary stricture formation [75, 81]. Later, Seal et al. reported that administration of a thrombolytic agent, tissue plasminogen factor (tPA), into hepatic artery dissolved thrombi in microcirculations and prevented any occurrence of thrombus and hence biliary strictures [82].

Op Den Dries et al. and Boehnert et al. reported significantly fewer bile duct related complications following NMP in the porcine model [25, 69]. Liu et al. demonstrated that biliary epithelium regeneration and differentiation of multipotent stem cells present in PBG into cholangiocytes after NMP in porcine model could prevent biliary strictures [83, 84].

However, subsequent clinical trials showed varied results as Bral et al. and Selzner et al. did not observe any late biliary complications despite the high number of DCD donors (40% and 20%, resp.), while Ravikumar et al. did report anastomotic strictures in 4 cases (20%) in the NMP group [39, 42, 43]. A recent randomized trial published by Nasralla et al. (2018) encountered similar rate of nonanastomotic strictures for DCD livers in NMP group 11.1% versus SCS 26.3% ($P = 0.180$). However, further research is warranted with NMP and DCD donation to more fully define risk and protection to the biliary epithelium.

4.7. NMP and Duration of Organ Preservation. Currently, the current median liver preservation time in the US is approximately 8 hours [85]. There are potential practical benefits if the preservation period can be more safely extended. Recently Vogel et al. showed successful liver transplantation after 48 hours of preservation on NMP device in their porcine model [78, 79]. The OrganOx Metra is currently licensed for clinical experimental study to preserve livers for up to 24 hours. In the study conducted by Ravikumar et al. one liver was perfused for 18.5 hours before being successfully transplanted [39]. Similarly, Bral et al. reported a DCD liver being successfully maintained for 22.5 hours on NMP before safe transplantation, although it should be noted in this case that the recipient sustained a prolonged period of cholestasis before eventual full recovery [43]. In a study by Nasralla et al. (2018) they observed significantly prolonged preservation in NMP group and reported significantly better early graft functioning with peak AST (NMP: 485 IU/L versus SCS: 974 IU/L; $P < 0.0001$) and EAD (NMP: 12.6% versus SCS: 29.9%; $P = 0.002$) [45, 50]. Hence, extended duration of preservation provides a more structured and orderly proposition for liver transplantation by promoting the judicious allocation of logistics as an assessing viability, operating room, staffing, and if required facilitating the preoperative optimization of the recipient. Additionally, there is potential that NMP could provide a window for introducing therapeutic interventions to further improve graft quality, and this requires more detailed study.

4.8. NMP in Liver Steatosis. Steatotic livers constitute a proportion of ECD grafts but have traditionally been discarded before transplantation due to their known increased risk for PNF [62, 80]. Spitzer et al. reported a 71% increased risk of 1-year graft loss with >30% macrosteatosis compared to controls with <15% steatosis [85]. Others have shown successful outcomes despite macrosteatosis > 30% provided that donor age is <40 years, CIT is < 11 hours, and donors were not DCD-derived [86–89]. Jamieson et al. (2011) reported substantial improvement in grade of steatosis in NMP perfusion of rat livers [30]. Others have demonstrated reduction in macrovascular steatosis with NMP alone or in association with defatting solutions [62, 90]. Nagrath et al. (2009) promoted the role of a "defatting cocktail" to esterify hepatic triglycerides and oxidation in steatotic rat livers with 65% reduction in hepatic triglyceride content [91]. However, Jamieson et al. found no evident reduction in NMP-perfused steatotic human livers, explained in part on the basis of inherent interspecies differences, fat solidification during obligate periods of cold storage, and total duration of perfusion (24 and 48 hours) [30, 91]. Further studies are required to clarify this issue and to optimize the role of defatting agents.

There are certain limitations to the present systematic review owing to a small number of studies available in the literature which might influence the interpretation of related outcomes. Despite these limitations, this systematic review has outlined the advantages of NMP over SCS in organ preservation and safety issues associated with its usage; however further randomized trials are much warranted to confirm these findings.

5. Conclusions

Over the past 40 years, SCS with refined cold preservation solutions has served the field well and has led to outstanding short and long term outcomes with clinical liver transplantation. As a result, liver transplantation remains a life-saving standard of care for all forms of acute, irreversible, and progressive chronic liver disease. The established success of this therapy and propagation of societal diseases such as hepatitis B, hepatitis C, and now widespread nonalcoholic steatohepatitis (NASH) had placed escalating pressure on transplant lists, driven supply-demand imbalance, and unacceptable rates of waiting list mortality. This situation has warranted a reevaluation of the methodology of storage and transportation of organs, as higher risk livers are used to attempt to match demand. Emerging evidence advocates that NMP may extend the safe utilization of the more marginal spectrum of liver donor grafts, but this remains to be proven in practice. This exciting technology has demonstrated safety and efficacy in preliminary clinical studies, and ongoing trials will continue to explore the full potential of NMP technologies, will determine the need for portability, and will more completely define the cost-benefit balance.

Abbreviations

ATP: Adenosine triphosphate
ALP: Alkaline phosphatase
ALT: Alanine aminotransferase
AST: Aspartate aminotransferase
INR: International normalized ratio
CIT: Cold ischemia time
DBD: Donors after brain death
DCD: Donor after circulatory death
ECD: Extended criteria donor
HA: Hepatic artery
IC: Ischemic cholangiopathy
IPF: Initial poor function
PNF: Primary nonfunction
PV: Portal vein
MAP: Mean arterial pressure
MELD: Model for End-Stage Disease
MSCs: Mesenchymal stem cells
NMP: Normothermic machine perfusion
PBG: Peribiliary gland
PVP: Peribiliary vascular plexus
PRS: Postreperfusion syndrome
SCS: Static cold storage
TPT: Total preservation time
Tregs: Regulatory T cells
WIT: Warm ischemia time.

Disclosure

This research was not funded by any internal or external agency.

Authors' Contributions

Kumar Jayant and Isabella Reccia developed concept and design of the study. Kumar Jayant, Isabella Reccia, and A. M. James Shapiro screened the abstract and full text, extracted data, and assessed studies. Kumar Jayant, Isabella Reccia, and Francesco Virdis wrote the manuscript. A. M. James Shapiro critically revised the manuscript. All authors read and approved the final version of the manuscript.

References

[1] R. M. Merion, D. E. Schaubel, D. M. Dykstra, R. B. Freeman, F. K. Port, and R. A. Wolfe, "The survival benefit of liver transplantation," *American Journal of Transplantation*, vol. 5, no. 2, pp. 307–313, 2005.

[2] J. C. Lai, S. Feng, N. A. Terrault, B. Lizaola, H. Hayssen, and K. Covinsky, "Frailty predicts waitlist mortality in liver transplant candidates," *American Journal of Transplantation*, vol. 14, no. 8, pp. 1870–1879, 2014.

[3] OPTN, https://optn.transplant.hrsa.gov/data/view-data-reports/national-data/, 2016; December.

[4] S. C. Rayhill, Y. M. Wu, D. A. Katz et al., "Older donor livers show early severe histological activity, fibrosis, and graft failure after liver transplantation for hepatitis C," *Transplantation*, vol. 84, no. 3, pp. 331–339, 2007.

[5] A. R. Mueller, K.-P. Platz, and B. Kremer, "Early postoperative complications following liver transplantation," *Best Practice & Research Clinical Gastroenterology*, vol. 18, no. 5, pp. 881–900, 2004.

[6] F. Su, L. Yu, K. Berry et al., "Aging of liver transplant registrants and recipients: trends and impact on waitlist outcomes, post-transplantation outcomes, and transplant-related survival benefit," *Gastroenterology*, vol. 150, no. 2, pp. 441–453e6, 2016.

[7] H. Jaeschke, "Molecular mechanisms of hepatic ischemia-reperfusion injury and preconditioning," *American Journal of Physiology-Gastrointestinal and Liver Physiology*, vol. 284, no. 1, pp. G15–G26, 2003.

[8] A. Amador, L. Grande, J. Martí et al., "Ischemic pre-conditioning in deceased donor liver transplantation: a prospective randomized clinical trial," *American Journal of Transplantation*, vol. 7, no. 9, pp. 2180–2189, 2007.

[9] W. Jassem, S. Fuggle, R. Thompson et al., "Effect of ischemic preconditioning on the genomic response to reperfusion injury in deceased donor liver transplantation," *Liver Transplantation*, vol. 15, no. 12, pp. 1750–1765, 2009.

[10] F. O. Belzer and J. H. Southard, "Principles of solid-organ preservation by cold storage," *Transplantation*, vol. 45, no. 4, pp. 673–676, 1988.

[11] U. Rauen and H. De Groot, "New insights into the cellular and molecular mechanisms of cold storage injury," *Journal of Investigative Medicine*, vol. 52, no. 5, pp. 299–309, 2004.

[12] X.-N. Feng, X. Xu, and S.-S. Zheng, "Current status and perspective of liver preservation solutions," *Hepatobiliary & Pancreatic Diseases International*, vol. 5, no. 4, pp. 490–494, 2006.

[13] E. E. Guibert, A. Y. Petrenko, C. L. Balaban, A. Y. Somov, J. V. Rodriguez, and B. J. Fuller, "Organ preservation: current concepts and new strategies for the next decade," *Transfusion Medicine and Hemotherapy*, vol. 38, no. 2, pp. 125–142, 2011.

[14] S. Op Den Dries, M. E. Sutton, T. Lisman, and R. J. Porte, "Protection of bile ducts in liver transplantation: looking beyond ischemia," *Transplantation*, vol. 92, no. 4, pp. 373–379, 2011.

[15] S. Op Den Dries, M. E. Sutton, N. Karimian et al., "Hypothermic oxygenated machine perfusion prevents arteriolonecrosis of the peribiliary plexus in pig livers donated after circulatory death," *PLoS ONE*, vol. 9, no. 2, Article ID e88521, 2014.

[16] Y. Zhai, H. Petrowsky, J. C. Hong, R. W. Busuttil, and J. W. Kupiec-Weglinski, "Ischaemia-reperfusion injury in liver transplantation-from bench to bedside," *Nature Reviews Gastroenterology & Hepatology*, vol. 10, no. 2, pp. 79–89, 2013.

[17] J. Gracia-Sancho, A. Casillas-Ramírez, and C. Peralta, "Molecular pathways in protecting the liver from ischaemia/reperfusion injury: a 2015 update," *Clinical Science*, vol. 129, no. 4, pp. 345–362, 2015.

[18] Z.-D. Xu, H.-T. Xu, H.-B. Yuan et al., "Postreperfusion syndrome during orthotopic liver transplantation: a single-center experience," *Hepatobiliary & Pancreatic Diseases International*, vol. 11, no. 1, pp. 34–39, 2012.

[19] I. Hilmi, C. N. Horton, R. M. Planinsic et al., "The impact of postreperfusion syndrome on short-term patient and liver allograft outcome in patients undergoing orthotopic liver transplantation," *Liver Transplantation*, vol. 14, no. 4, pp. 504–508, 2008.

[20] S. Aggarwal, Y. Kang, J. A. Freeman, F. L. Fortunato Jr., and M. R. Pinsky, "Postreperfusion syndrome: Hypotension after reperfusion of the transplanted liver," *Journal of Critical Care*, vol. 8, no. 3, pp. 154–160, 1993.

[21] H. O. Ayanoglu, S. Ulukaya, and Y. Tokat, "Causes of postreperfusion syndrome in living or cadaveric donor liver transplantations," *Transplantation Proceedings*, vol. 35, no. 4, pp. 1442–1444, 2003.

[22] B. Bukowicka, R. A. Akar, A. Olszewska, P. Smoter, and M. Krawczyk, "The occurrence of postreperfusion syndrome in orthotopic liver transplantation and its significance in terms of complications and short-term survival," *Annals of Transplantation*, vol. 16, no. 2, pp. 26–30, 2011.

[23] K. Fukazawa, Y. Yamada, E. Gologorsky, K. L. Arheart, and E. A. Pretto, "Hemodynamic recovery following postreperfusion syndrome in liver transplantation," *Journal of Cardiothoracic and Vascular Anesthesia*, vol. 28, no. 4, pp. 994–1002, 2014.

[24] A. Schlegel, O. D. Rougemont, R. Graf, P.-A. Clavien, and P. Dutkowski, "Protective mechanisms of end-ischemic cold machine perfusion in DCD liver grafts," *Journal of Hepatology*, vol. 58, no. 2, pp. 278–286, 2013.

[25] S. Op Den Dries, N. Karimian, A. C. Westerkamp et al., "Normothermic machine perfusion reduces bile duct injury and improves biliary epithelial function in rat donor livers," *Liver Transplantation*, vol. 22, no. 7, pp. 994–1005, 2016.

[26] G. Warnecke, J. Moradiellos, I. Tudorache et al., "Normothermic perfusion of donor lungs for preservation and assessment with the organ care system lung before bilateral transplantation: a pilot study of 12 patients," *The Lancet*, vol. 380, no. 9856, pp. 1851–1858, 2012.

[27] M. Cypel, M. Rubacha, J. Yeung et al., "Normothermic Ex Vivo perfusion prevents lung injury compared to extended cold preservation for transplantation," *American Journal of Transplantation*, vol. 9, no. 10, pp. 2262–2269, 2009.

[28] E. S. Baskin-Bey, K. Washburn, S. Feng et al., "Clinical trial of the pan-caspase inhibitor, IDN-6556, in human liver preservation injury," *American Journal of Transplantation*, vol. 7, no. 1, pp. 218–225, 2007.

[29] R. W. Busuttil, G. S. Lipshutz, J. W. Kupiec-Weglinski et al., "RPSGL-Ig for improvement of early liver allograft function: a double-blind, placebo-controlled, single-center phase II study," *American Journal of Transplantation*, vol. 11, no. 4, pp. 786–797, 2011.

[30] R. W. Jamieson, M. Zilvetti, D. Roy et al., "Hepatic steatosis and normothermic perfusion-preliminary experiments in a porcine model," *Transplantation*, vol. 92, no. 3, pp. 289–295, 2011.

[31] S. A. Hosgood, "Renal transplantation after ex vivo normothermic perfusion: the first clinical study," *American Journal of Transplantation*, vol. 13, no. 5, pp. 1246–1252, 2013.

[32] M. L. Nicholson and S. A. Hosgood, "Renal transplantation, after ex-vivo normothermic perfusion: the first clinical series," *Transplant International*, vol. 24, no. 94, 2011.

[33] M. E. Sutton, S. Op Den Dries, N. Karimian et al., "Criteria for viability assessment of discarded human donor livers during ex vivo normothermic machine perfusion," *PLoS ONE*, vol. 9, no. 11, Article ID e110642, 2014.

[34] S. Op Den Dries, N. Karimian, M. E. Sutton et al., "Ex vivo normothermic machine perfusion and viability testing of discarded human donor livers," *American Journal of Transplantation*, vol. 13, no. 5, pp. 1327–1335, 2013.

[35] M. J. Yska, C. I. Buis, D. Monbaliu et al., "The role of bile salt toxicity in the pathogenesis of bile duct injury after non-heart-beating porcine liver transplantation," *Transplantation*, vol. 85, no. 11, pp. 1625–1631, 2008.

[36] J. A. Graham and J. V. Guarrera, "'Resuscitation' of marginal liver allografts for transplantation with machine perfusion technology," *Journal of Hepatology*, vol. 61, no. 2, pp. 418–431, 2014.

[37] H. Mergental and G. R. Roll, "Normothermic machine perfusion of the liver," *Clinical Liver Disease*, vol. 10, no. 4, pp. 97–99, 2017.

[38] T. Vogel, J. G. Brockmann, and P. J. Friend, "Ex-vivo normothermic liver perfusion: An update," *Current Opinion in Organ Transplantation*, vol. 15, no. 2, pp. 167–172, 2010.

[39] R. Ravikumar, W. Jassem, H. Mergental et al., "Liver transplantation after ex vivo normothermic machine preservation: a phase 1 (first-in-man) clinical trial," *American Journal of Transplantation*, vol. 16, no. 6, pp. 1779–1787, 2016.

[40] "Transmedics. Liver Preservation," http://www.transmed-ics.com/wt/page/ocsliverintro_med; 2014.

[41] T. Minor, P. Efferz, M. Fox, J. Wohlschlaeger, and B. Lüer, "Controlled oxygenated rewarming of cold stored liver grafts by thermally graduated machine perfusion prior to reperfusion," *American Journal of Transplantation*, vol. 13, no. 6, pp. 1450–1460, 2013.

[42] M. Selzner, N. Goldaracena, J. Echeverri et al., "Normothermic ex vivo liver perfusion using steen solution as perfusate for human liver transplantation: first North American results," *Liver Transplantation*, vol. 22, no. 11, pp. 1501–1508, 2016.

[43] M. Bral, B. Gala-Lopez, D. Bigam et al., "Preliminary single-center canadian experience of human normothermic ex vivo liver perfusion: results of a clinical trial," *American Journal of Transplantation*, vol. 17, no. 4, pp. 1071–1080, 2017.

[44] Q. Liu, B. Soliman, G. Iuppa et al., "First report of human liver transplantation after normothermic machine perfusion (NMP) in the United States," *American Journal of Transplantation*, vol. 17, supplement 3, 2017.

[45] D. Nasralla, C. C. Coussios, H. Mergental, M. Z. Akhtar, A. J. Butler, C. D. L. Ceresa et al., "A randomized trial of normothermic preservation in liver transplantation," *Nature*, 2018.

[46] L. Shamseer, D. Moher, M. Clarke et al., "Preferred reporting items for systematic review and meta-analysis protocols (prisma-p) 2015: elaboration and explanation," *British Medical Journal*, vol. 349, Article ID g7647, 2015.

[47] P. F. W. Chien, K. S. Khan, and D. Siassakos, "Registration of systematic reviews: PROSPERO," *BJOG: An International Journal of Obstetrics & Gynaecology*, vol. 119, no. 8, pp. 903–905, 2012.

[48] D. P. Hoyer, Z. Mathé, A. Gallinat et al., "Controlled oxygenated rewarming of cold stored livers prior to transplantation: first clinical application of a new concept," *Transplantation*, vol. 100, no. 1, pp. 147–152, 2016.

[49] C. J. E. Watson, V. Kosmoliaptsis, L. V. Randle et al., "Normothermic perfusion in the assessment and preservation of declined livers before transplantation: hyperoxia and vasoplegia-important lessons from the first 12 cases," *Transplantation*, vol. 101, no. 5, pp. 1084–1098, 2017.

[50] D. Nasralla, Consortium for Organ Preservation in Europe Liver Research Group, R. Ploeg, C. Coussios, and P. Friend, "Outcomes from a multinational randomised controlled trial comparing normothermic machine perfusion with static cold storage in human liver transplantation," *American Journal of Transplantation*, supplement 3, 2017.

[51] L. Sanchez-Urdazpal, G. J. Gores, E. M. Ward et al., "Ischemic-type biliary complications after orthotopic liver transplantation," *Hepatology*, vol. 16, no. 1, pp. 49–53, 1992.

[52] R. Carini, M. G. De Cesaris, G. Bellomo, and E. Albano, "Intracellular Na^+ accumulation and hepatocyte injury during cold storage," *Transplantation*, vol. 68, no. 2, pp. 294–297, 1999.

[53] H. Xu, T. Berendsen, K. Kim et al., "Excorporeal normothermic machine perfusion resuscitates pig DCD livers with extended warm ischemia," *Journal of Surgical Research*, vol. 173, no. 2, pp. e83–e88, 2012.

[54] H. Tolboom, J. M. Milwid, M. L. Izamis, K. Uygun, F. Berthiaume, and M. L. Yarmush, "Sequential cold storage and normothermic perfusion of the ischemic rat liver," *Transplantation Proceedings*, vol. 40, no. 5, pp. 1306–1309, 2008.

[55] X. Tillou, R. Thuret, and A. Doerfler, "Ischemia/Reperfusion during normothermic perfusion," *Progrès en Urologie*, vol. 24, no. 1, pp. S51–S55, 2014.

[56] R. Angelico, M. T. Perera, R. Ravikumar et al., "Normothermic machine perfusion of deceased donor liver grafts is associated with improved postreperfusion hemodynamics," *Transplantation Direct*, vol. 2, no. 9, p. e97, 2016.

[57] M. Vairetti, A. Ferrigno, V. Rizzo et al., "Subnormothermic machine perfusion protects against rat liver preservation injury: a comparative evaluation with conventional cold storage," *Transplantation Proceedings*, vol. 39, no. 6, pp. 1765–1767, 2007.

[58] A. Ferrigno, V. Rizzo, E. Boncompagni et al., "Machine perfusion at 20°C reduces preservation damage to livers from non-heart beating donors," *Cryobiology*, vol. 62, no. 2, pp. 152–158, 2011.

[59] C. J. Imber, S. D. St. Peter, I. Lopez de Cenarruzabeitia et al., "Advantages of normothermic perfusion over cold storage in liver preservation," *Transplantation*, vol. 73, no. 5, pp. 701–709, 2002.

[60] M. Bessems, B. M. Doorschodt, J. L. P. Kolkert et al., "Preservation of steatotic livers: a comparison between cold storage and machine perfusion preservation," *Liver Transplantation*, vol. 13, no. 4, pp. 497–504, 2007.

[61] S. M. Black, B. A. Whitson, and M. Velayutham, "EPR spectroscopy as a predictive tool for the assessment of marginal

donor livers perfused on a normothermic ex vivo perfusion circuit," *Medical Hypotheses*, vol. 82, no. 5, pp. 627–630, 2014.

[62] B. Banan, R. Watson, M. Xu, Y. Lin, and W. Chapman, "Development of a normothermic extracorporeal liver perfusion system toward improving viability and function of human extended criteria donor livers," *Liver Transplantation*, vol. 22, no. 7, pp. 979–993, 2016.

[63] W. R. Kim, J. R. Lake, and J. M. Smith, "OPTN/SRTR 2015 annual data report: liver," *American Journal of Transplantation*, vol. 17, no. S1, pp. 174–251, 2017.

[64] B. Banan, H. Chung, Z. Xiao et al., "Normothermic extracorporeal liver perfusion for donation after cardiac death (DCD) livers," *Surgery*, vol. 158, no. 6, pp. 1642–1650, 2015.

[65] P. N. A. Martins, "Normothermic machine preservation as an approach to decrease biliary complications of DCD liver grafts," *American Journal of Transplantation*, vol. 13, no. 12, pp. 3287-3288, 2013.

[66] J. Brockmann, S. Reddy, C. Coussios et al., "Normothermic perfusion: a new paradigm for organ preservation," *Annals of Surgery*, vol. 250, no. 1, pp. 1–6, 2009.

[67] C. Fondevila, A. J. Hessheimer, M.-H. J. Maathuis et al., "Superior preservation of DCD livers with continuous normothermic perfusion," *Annals of Surgery*, vol. 254, no. 6, pp. 1000–1007, 2011.

[68] L. Russo, J. Gracia-Sancho, H. García-Calderó et al., "Addition of simvastatin to cold storage solution prevents endothelial dysfunction in explanted rat livers," *Hepatology*, vol. 55, no. 3, pp. 921–930, 2012.

[69] M. U. Boehnert, J. C. Yeung, F. Bazerbachi et al., "Normothermic acellular ex vivo liver perfusion reduces liver and bile duct injury of pig livers retrieved after cardiac death," *American Journal of Transplantation*, vol. 13, no. 6, pp. 1441–1449, 2013.

[70] E. Pareja, M. Cortes, R. Navarro, F. Sanjuan, R. López, and J. Mir, "Vascular complications after orthotopic liver transplantation: hepatic artery thrombosis," *Transplantation Proceedings*, vol. 42, no. 8, pp. 2970–2972, 2010.

[71] G. Varotti, G. L. Grazi, G. Vetrone et al., "Causes of early acute graft failure after liver transplantation: analysis of a 17-year single-centre experience," *Clinical Transplantation*, vol. 19, no. 4, pp. 492–500, 2005.

[72] W. Bernal, A. Hyyrylainen, A. Gera et al., "Lessons from look-back in acute liver failure? A single centre experience of 3300 patients," *Journal of Hepatology*, vol. 59, no. 1, pp. 74–80, 2013.

[73] K. M. Olthoff, L. Kulik, B. Samstein et al., "Validation of a current definition of early allograft dysfunction in liver transplant recipients and analysis of risk factors," *Liver Transplantation*, vol. 16, no. 8, pp. 943–949, 2010.

[74] C. L. Jay, V. Lyuksemburg, D. P. Ladner et al., "Ischemic cholangiopathy after controlled donation after cardiac death liver transplantation: a meta-analysis," *Annals of Surgery*, vol. 253, no. 2, pp. 259–264, 2011.

[75] S. Op Den Dries, A. C. Westerkamp, N. Karimian et al., "Injury to peribiliary glands and vascular plexus before liver transplantation predicts formation of non-anastomotic biliary strictures," *Journal of Hepatology*, vol. 60, no. 6, pp. 1172–1179, 2014.

[76] J. P. Duffy, J. C. Hong, D. G. Farmer et al., "Vascular complications of orthotopic liver transplantation: experience in more than 4,200 patients," *Journal of the American College of Surgeons*, vol. 208, no. 5, pp. 896–903, 2009.

[77] J. Briceño and R. Ciria, "Early Graft Dysfunction After Liver Transplantation," *Transplantation Proceedings*, vol. 42, no. 2, pp. 631–633, 2010.

[78] T. Vogel, J. G. Brockmann, D. Pigott et al., "Successful transplantation of porcine liver grafts following 48-hour normothermic preservation," *PLoS ONE*, vol. 12, no. 11, Article ID e0188494, 2017.

[79] T. A. Churchill, "Organ preservation for transplantation," in *Functional Metabolism: Regulation and Adaptation*, K. B. Storey, Ed., Wiley Liss, New Jersey, NJ, USA, 2004.

[80] P. Angulo, "Nonalcoholic fatty liver disease and liver transplantation," *Liver Transplantation*, vol. 12, no. 4, pp. 525–534, 2006.

[81] K. Hashimoto, B. Eghtesad, G. Gunasekaran et al., "Use of tissue plasminogen activator in liver transplantation from donation after cardiac death donors," *American Journal of Transplantation*, vol. 10, no. 12, pp. 2665–2672, 2010.

[82] J. B. Seal, H. Bohorquez, T. Reichman et al., "Thrombolytic protocol minimizes ischemic-type biliary complications in liver transplantation from donation after circulatory death donors," *Liver Transplantation*, vol. 21, no. 3, pp. 321–328, 2015.

[83] Q. Liu, A. Nassar, K. Farias et al., "Sanguineous normothermic machine perfusion improves hemodynamics and biliary epithelial regeneration in donation after cardiac death porcine livers," *Liver Transplantation*, vol. 20, no. 8, pp. 987–999, 2014.

[84] A. Nassart, Q. Liu, K. Farias, C. Tom, A. Bennett, G. DAmico et al., "The effect of normothermic machine perfusion (NMP) using various perfusates on the hepatocellular and biliary epithelial integrity in porcine donation after cardiac death (DCD) models," *Liver Transplantation*, vol. 19, no. 6, 2013.

[85] A. L. Spitzer, O. B. Lao, A. A. S. Dick et al., "The biopsied donor liver: incorporating macrosteatosis into high-risk donor assessment," *Liver Transplantation*, vol. 16, no. 7, pp. 874–884, 2010.

[86] M. K. Angele, M. Rentsch, W. H. Hartl et al., "Effect of graft steatosis on liver function and organ survival after liver transplantation," *The American Journal of Surgery*, vol. 195, no. 2, pp. 214–220, 2008.

[87] J. A. Perez-Daga, J. Santoyo, M. A. Suárez et al., "Influence of degree of hepatic steatosis on graft function and postoperative complications of liver transplantation," *Transplantation Proceedings*, vol. 38, no. 8, pp. 2468–2470, 2006.

[88] J. Li, B. Liu, L.-N. Yan et al., "Reversal of graft steatosis after liver transplantation: prospective study," *Transplantation Proceedings*, vol. 41, no. 9, pp. 3560–3563, 2009.

[89] A. C. Westerkamp, M. T. De Boer, A. P. Van Den Berg, A. S. H. Gouw, and R. J. Porte, "Similar outcome after transplantation of moderate macrovesicular steatotic and nonsteatotic livers when the cold ischemia time is kept very short," *Transplant International*, vol. 28, no. 3, pp. 319–329, 2015.

[90] T. Vogel, J. G. Brockmann, A. Quaglia et al., "The 24-hour normothermic machine perfusion of discarded human liver grafts," *Liver Transplantation*, vol. 23, no. 2, pp. 207–220, 2017.

[91] D. Nagrath, H. Xu, Y. Tanimura et al., "Metabolic preconditioning of donor organs: defatting fatty livers by normothermic perfusion ex vivo," *Metabolic Engineering*, vol. 11, no. 4-5, pp. 274–283, 2009.

26

Primary Leiomyoma of the Liver: A Review of a Rare Tumour

Ayodeji Oluwarotimi Omiyale

Department of General Surgery, Royal Shrewsbury Hospital, Shrewsbury SY3 8XQ, UK

Correspondence should be addressed to Ayodeji Oluwarotimi Omiyale; ayodejiomiyale@yahoo.com

Academic Editor: Shuji Isaji

Context. Primary leiomyoma of the liver is a rare tumour with uncertain pathogenesis with similar presentation with other tumours of the liver. Little is known about its clinical course. *Objectives.* To review the literature for case reports of primary leiomyoma of the liver. *Methods.* Extensive literature search was carried out for case reports of primary leiomyoma of the liver. *Results.* A total of 36 cases of primary leiomyoma of the liver were reviewed. The mean age of presentation is 43 years with slight female sex affectation; females accounted for 55.6% of the cases reported in the literature. The average size of the tumour is 8.7 cm. 34.4% of the cases reviewed were incidental finding with the mean follow-up time of 33 months with most cases reporting no evidence of disease. *Conclusions.* Primary leiomyoma of the liver is very rare tumour with complex pathogenesis which remains largely unknown. Imaging of the tumour does not allow for a tissue specific diagnosis; hence histological review of the tissue specimen and immunohistochemical stains are imperative for diagnosis. Surgical resection is both diagnostic and curative. The diagnosis of primary leiomyoma of the liver should be considered as a differential in the management of liver tumours.

1. Introduction

Leiomyoma is a benign smooth muscle neoplasm of mesenchymal origin which commonly occurs in the genitourinary system and the gastrointestinal tract of the body but which rarely occurs in the liver [1, 2]. The first case report of primary leiomyoma of the liver was first described in a 42-year-old woman by Demel in 1926 [3].

This paper seeks to review primary leiomyoma of the liver in the literature because of its rarity, unclear pathogenesis, and the diagnostic challenges it poses in clinical practice.

2. Methods

Case reports and case series of primary leiomyoma of the liver were retrieved by extensive literature search of PubMed, Ovid SP, Cochrane database of systematic reviews, Embase, and Clinical Evidence Online. Further search of the literature was carried out by manually searching the relevant references of the studies retrieved. The inclusive criteria include relevant publications of primary leiomyoma of the liver and hence studies with coexisting leiomyoma in other parts of the body were excluded.

Epidemiologic, pathologic, clinical, imaging, and prognostic data were retrieved and assessed for all studies. The search keywords include primary hepatic leiomyoma, primary leiomyoma of the liver, primary benign lesions of the liver, and primary tumours of the liver.

3. Results

The clinical and pathologic characteristics of the 35 cases reviewed with the treatment and the clinical outcome are outlined in Table 1.

4. Discussion

Primary leiomyomas of the liver are very rare tumours. Eighty-seven years after the first case of primary leiomyoma of the liver was reported, to the best knowledge of the author, 36 cases of primary leiomyoma of the liver have so far been reported in the literature.

Hawkins et al. [4] in 1980 proposed criteria that must be met for the diagnosis of primary liver leiomyoma. The tumour must be composed of leiomyocytes. Secondly, the presence of leiomyoma in other sites of the body like uterus and

Table 1: Clinical and pathologic features of the reviewed cases of primary leiomyoma of the liver.

Cases	Age	Sex	Clinical features	Size (cm)	Location	EBV status	Mitosis	Immunosuppression	Necrosis	Tx	F/U (Mths)	Outcome
Perini et al. [19]	45	M	Epigastric pain	4.3	LL	Positive	Nr	Yes	nr	sectionectomy	4	ned
Davidoff et al. [18]	5	M	Incidental	15	RL	Positive	Low	Yes	nr	R trisegmentectomy	10	ned
Cheuk et al. [22]	37	M	Abdominal discomfort	3.5	LL	Positive	Nr	Yes	nr	conservative	nr	nr
Prevot et al. [10]	33	M	Incidental (autopsy)	2	RL	Positive	None	Yes	None	no surgical tx	0	D
Sclabas et al. [20]	30	F	Epigastric pain	4.4, 0.6	LL	Positive	Low	Yes	nr	LL hepatectomy	30	ned
Luo et al. [2]	48	M	RUQ pain	4.9	LL	Negative	Low	Yes	nr	LL hepatectomy	24	ned
Raber et al. [23]	46	F	Incidental	2.8	RL	Nr	None	Yes	nr	conservative	84	ned
Doyle et al. [24]	5	F	Incidental	3	LL	Nr	Low	Yes	Yes	LL segmentectomy	8	ned
Ha et al. [25]	9	M	Incidental	5.6	LL	Nr	Nr	Yes	Yes	LL hepatectomy	nr	ned
Yoon et al. [34]	41	F	RUQ mass	19	RL	Nr	Nr	None	nr	RL hepatectomy	nr	nr
Yanase et al. [6]	59	F	Liver dysfunction	13	RL	Nr	Low	None	None	RL hepatectomy	21	ned
Beuzen et al. [5]	36	F	RUQ pain	5	LL	Nr	None	None	None	Bi segmentectomy	108	ned
Santos et al. [13]	28	F	RUQ pain	5.5	RL	None	None	None	None	segmentectomy	36	ned
Urizono et al. [8]	71	M	Incidental	3	RL	Nr	None	None	nr	caudate lobectomy	nr	ned
Perini et al. [19]	45	F	RUQ pain	20	RL	Nr	None	None	Yes	segmentectomy	72	ned
Marin et al. [39]	64	F	Incidental	3	RL	Nr	None	None	nr	R hepatectomy	12	ned
Belli et al. [12]	67	F	Abdominal mass	30	RL	Nr	Low	None	nr	ER hepatectomy	48	ned
Sousa et al. [36]	61	F	Dyspepsia	9.5	LL	Nr	None	None	nr	LL hepatectomy	16	ned
Hollands et al. [11]	17	M	Epigastric pain	9	LL	Nr	None	None	nr	LL hepatectomy	12	ned
Kanazawa et al. [37]	31	M	Incidental	3.5	LL	Nr	None	None	nr	LL segmentectomy	nr	nr
Reinertson et al. [1]	32	F	RUQ pain	10	LL	Nr	None	None	nr	LL hepatectomy	24	ned
kalil et al. [7]	44	F	RUQ mass	7	RL	Nr	Nr	None	nr	atypical resection	nr	nr
Imasato et al. [9]	61	F	Incidental	4.5	RL	Nr	Nr	None	nr	RL hepatectomy	nr	nr
Hawkins et al. [4]	66	M	Abdominal mass	13	LL	Nr	Low	Nr	nr	LL hepatectomy	48	ned
Herzberg et al. [31]	30	F	RUQ pain	19	RL	Nr	Nr	Nr	nr	R hepatectomy	nr	nr
Ishak and Rabin [35]	64	M	Abdominal mass	Nr	RL	Nr	Nr	Nr	nr	laparotomy	nr	nr
Demel [3]	42	F	RUQ pain	12	RL	Nr	Nr	Nr	nr	laparotomy	nr	nr
Mesenas et al. [48]	59	M	Incidental	3.6	RL	Nr	Nr	Nr	nr	segmentectomy	nr	nr
Rummeny et al. [33]	46	F	RUQ pain	Nr	Nr	Nr	Nr	Nr	nr	nr	nr	nr
Tan et al. [38]	31	F	Nr	Nr	Nr	Nr	None	None	nr	hepatic resection	nr	nr
Tan et al. [38]	42	M	Nr	Nr	Nr	Nr	None	None	nr	hepatic resection	nr	nr
Tan et al. [38]	69	M	Nr	Nr	Nr	Nr	None	None	nr	hepatic resection	nr	nr
Sadler et al. [21]	36	M	Abdominal pain	Nr	LL	Nr	Low	Yes	None	hepatic resection	nr	nr
Sadler et al. [21]	36	M	Abdominal pain	Nr	LL	Nr	Nr	Yes	nr	conservative	nr	nr
Bartoli et al. [49]	34	F	Incidental	Nr	RL	Nr	Nr	Nr	nr	RL hepatectomy	nr	nr
Rios-Dalenz [32]	87	F	RUQ pain	Nr	LL	Nr	Nr	Nr	nr	no surgical tx	nr	nr

Nr: not reported; ned: no evidence of disease.

the gastrointestinal tract must be excluded. If the uterus is surgically absent, the diagnosis of primary leiomyoma of the liver must not be made without the review of the report and sections from the hysterectomy.

4.1. Epidemiology. Primary leiomyomas of the liver have been reported in both paediatric and adult populations. There are reports in the literature to suggest the incidence of the tumour in both immunocompetent and immunosuppressed patients. The mean age of presentation is 43 years (range 4.6–87). Primary leiomyomas of the liver have been reported to have female sex predilection [2, 5–7]. Luo et al. suggested that the observed female preponderance may be partly due to the activity of the smooth muscle cells in female urogenital tissue in carcinogenesis [2]. However this view seems to contradict one of the main diagnostic criteria for primary leiomyoma of the liver as proposed by Hawkins et al. [4] which seeks to exclude leiomyoma in other parts of the body especially in the urogenital tissue.

This review of 36 cases however demonstrates slight female sex affectation with females accounting for 55.6% of the cases. Familial predispositions have not been reported. The distribution of the lesion is equal in both right and left lobes of the liver with two cases involving the caudate lobe of the liver [8, 9].

4.2. Pathogenesis. The pathogenesis of primary leiomyoma of the liver is not clear and largely unknown. Some theories have emerged as to the possible pathogenesis of these tumours. Proliferations of smooth muscle of the hepatic vessels or the biliary tree have been suggested as a possible origin [2, 10–13]. However the argument against origin from the bile ducts is that large extra hepatic ducts have very few smooth cells [11, 14].

Immunosuppressive states which include either post-transplant patients on immunosuppressive therapy or patients with human immunodeficiency virus (HIV) have been suggested as a possible causal factor in primary leiomyoma of the liver. Increased risks of de novo neoplasia after transplantation are well documented in the literature [15–17].

Possible explanations for the susceptibility of immunocompromised patients to neoplasms include the disruption of the immunosurveillance ability of the host with the subsequent development of the tumours that would otherwise have been suppressed by a normal immune system [18]. The incidence of primary leiomyoma of the liver within the setting of immunosuppression in this review which accounts for 39.3% of the cases appears to be in support of this theory [2, 10, 18–25]. Immunosuppression alone does not totally explain the pathogenesis of this tumour because of the incidence of the tumour in immunocompetent individuals.

The theory of the possible role of viral induced oncogenesis has been suggested. This is because of the evidence that implicates some DNA viruses in the aetiology of some neoplasms particularly Epstein-Barr virus in smooth muscle tumours [16, 18]. This theory is further supported by the observation that patients with immunosuppression are at high risks of developing virus-associated neoplasms although the exact mechanism is not known [18, 26].

A possible explanation is a multistep theory of viral oncogenesis which suggests that virus infected cells undergo an uncontrolled polyclonal proliferation in the setting of the reduced immune surveillance of the viral transformed cells. Further cytogenetic events alter the growth regulation of a subset of cells, leading to a monoclonal expansion of tumour cells [18]. In support of this theory is the observation that 5 cases were reported to be positive for EBV in this review and the 5 cases were also in the setting of immunosuppression [10, 18–20, 22]. The fact that other case reports in this review were not associated with Epstein-Barr virus suggests a rather complex pathogenesis for primary leiomyoma of the liver. Epstein-Barr viral oncogenesis alone does not explain the pathogenesis. Virus associated tumours have been observed to exhibit different range of differentiation from well differentiated to poorly differentiated and some may show features suggestive of leiomyosarcomas [27]. The risk of other cancers in patients with immunosuppression not linked to viruses is also increased [28–30].

4.3. Clinical Features. The clinical presentation of primary leiomyoma of the liver is similar to the presentation of other liver neoplasms. The most common clinical symptom in this review is abdominal, epigastric, or right upper quadrant pain which accounts for 42.4% of cases reported [1–3, 5, 11, 13, 19–21, 31–33]. 33.3% of the cases were incidental with one of them an incidental finding at autopsy [10]. Other clinical features include abdominal mass [4, 7, 12, 34, 35], abdominal discomfort [22], dyspepsia [36], and liver dysfunction [6].

Primary leiomyoma of the liver may rarely present as a composite tumour. Yanase et al. reported the case of a 59-year-old lady with $13 \times 10 \times 9$ cm firm tumour with mainly a solid tissue portion and interconnected multilocular cystic lesions. Histologic diagnosis of primary leiomyoma of the liver encasing hepatobiliary cystadenoma was made [6].

Screening for tumour markers alpha fetoprotein, carbohydrate antigen 19-9 and carcinoembryonic antigen are usually negative [11, 12, 19]. Serological testing for EBV combined with in situ hybridization indicates the tumour cells positive for EBV encoded small RNA (Figure 1) [2, 10, 18, 20]. In situ hybridization is the gold standard for the detection and localization of latent EBV in tissues [2].

4.4. Imaging. Imaging alone does not show tissue specific diagnosis and cannot reliably differentiate between primary leiomyoma and other differential diagnosis like leiomyosarcoma, hepatocellular adenoma, hepatocellular carcinoma, angiomyolipoma, and hypervascular metastatic lesions [36, 37]. There is no notable difference in the imaging of patients with or without immunosuppression [19].

4.5. CT. CT findings in leiomyoma of the liver have been variously reported in the cases reviewed as hypodense lesions with strong enhancement in both arterial and portal phase [5, 11, 13, 21, 23, 36, 38] with some reports describing peripheral rim enhancement [8, 37]. An increased enhancement in the arterial phase and a sustained homogeneous enhancement in both hepatic venous and equilibrium phases have also been reported [39] (Figure 2).

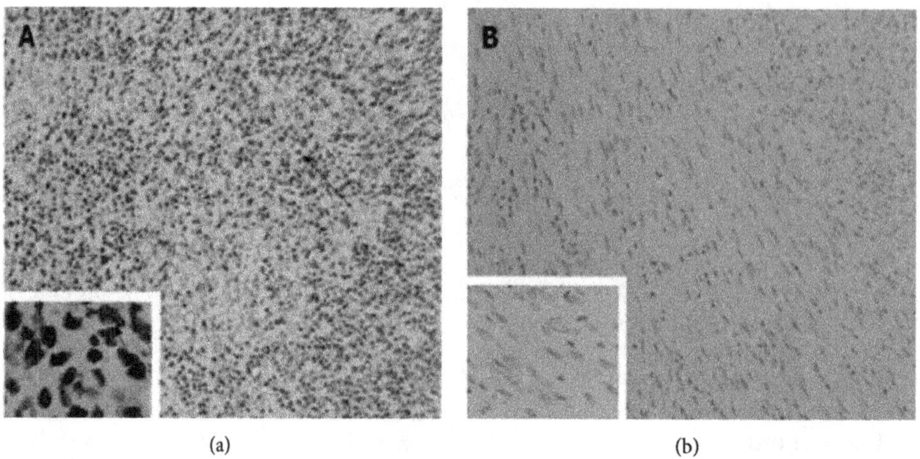

FIGURE 1: Tumour cells stained positive by *in situ* hybridization with Epstein-Barr virus-encoded small RNA. (a) Positive control staining ×200, ×1000; (b) tumour cell staining ×200, ×1000. Arrows indicate positive staining of the nuclei. Reprinted from [2] with the permission of the Director, Editorial Office of the World Journal of Gastroenterology.

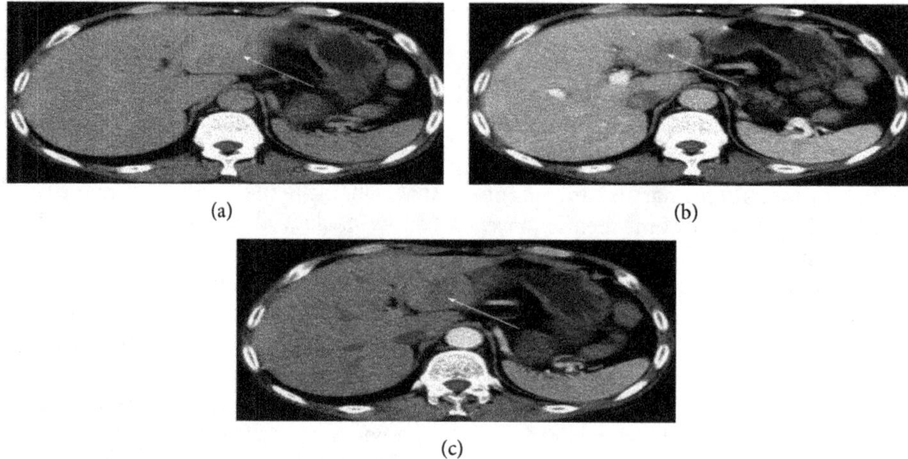

FIGURE 2: CT Abdomen with a mass in segment III of the liver in the hepatic equilibrium (a), portal venous (b), and hepatic arterial phase (c). Reprinted from [2] with the permission of the Director, Editorial Office of the World Journal of Gastroenterology.

4.6. Ultrasound. Ultrasound findings in primary leiomyoma of the liver in the literature have been described as hypoechoic lesions with varying degrees of heterogeneity [5, 8, 11, 36, 37]. Perini et al. reported heterogeneous mass displacing the inferior vena cava (IVC) and the right kidney medially across the midline [19].

4.7. MRI. MRI findings from several studies suggest hypointense lesions on T1-weighted MRI images with hyperintense lesions on T2-weighted sequences with inhomogeneous contrast uptake [8, 19, 20, 37]. However hypointense lesions in the T2-weighted MRI images have also been reported which the authors associated with the dense fusocellular nature of the tumour [36].

The development of liver specific MR contrast agents which includes reticuloendothelial system specific contrast agents and hepatocytes specific contrast agents have been shown to potentially improve the detection and characterization of liver lesions by providing functional and morphologic information of the liver simultaneously [39–41]. Gadobenate dimeglumine is a gadolinium-based contrast agent that is partially taken up by functioning liver cells and excreted without biotransformation through the biliary duct system. Gadobenate dimeglumine shows a vascular-interstitial distribution in the first minutes after bolus injection. Normal liver and benign liver lesions show increased signal intensity on T1-weighted MR images during the delayed liver-specific phase because of active contrast uptake by functioning hepatocytes. The absence of contrast retention during the liver-specific phase is believed to be indicative of malignant liver lesions [39].

It has also been suggested that liver specific MR contrast agents may be misleading in the diagnosis of primary leiomyoma of the liver. The absence of contrast retention during the liver specific contrast enhanced MRI, in the case report, led them to suspect a malignant lesion of the liver but it turned out to be a primary leiomyoma on histology after surgical resection [39]. This finding is consistent with earlier reports in the literature that demonstrated equivocal appearance of primary leiomyoma of the liver after the administration of liver specific contrast agents [36, 41].

4.8. Angiography. Angiography has been reported to demonstrate irregular [37], marginal [8], or diffuse [5] hypervascularity. Hawkins also reported a selective angiogram through the left hepatic artery which demonstrated abnormal mass effect, stretching of the feeding vessels, and scattered pooling throughout the tumour. The authors concluded that the angiography study was nondiagnostic [4].

4.9. Preoperative Diagnosis. Attempts have been made to make a preoperative diagnosis of this tumour so as to prevent unwarranted diagnostic surgical procedures. CT guided fine needle biopsy had reportedly failed to determine the nature of the mass despite the fact that the primary leiomyoma of the liver in this case was the largest ever reported in the literature with a size of 30 cm. The patient underwent extended right hepatectomy. No extra-hepatic lesions were seen at surgery and the uterus was normal [12]. Percutaneous biopsy was attempted with mixed outcomes in the two cases reported by Sadler et al. [21]. One reported "well differentiated smooth muscle neoplasm consistent with hepatic leiomyoma" while multiple attempts at percutaneous biopsy were not successful in the second case [21].

Sousa et al. initially performed a US-guided fine needle aspiration (FNA) which was inconclusive because of because of insufficient sample which included only a small group of normal looking hepatocytes [36]. The histological review of the 18G Trucut biopsy sample taken by Sousa et al. proved to be accurate in the diagnosis of leiomyoma of the liver which was further confirmed after surgical resection [36]. This accurate preoperative diagnosis from biopsy sample is consistent with other reports in the literature [24, 25].

The inconclusive FNA report from the case reported by Sousa et al. is consistent with the series reported by Guy et al. who further reiterated the difficulty of getting adequate sample in 10% of cases where FNA was used in the diagnosis of spindle cell lesions of the liver [42]. Hence FNA does not seem appropriate and adequate for the diagnosis of primary leiomyoma of the liver.

4.10. Macroscopic Features. The average size of the tumour in this review is 8.7 cm (range 2–30). The largest size of this tumour in the literature, 30 cm, was reported by Belli et al. in a 67-year-old woman who presented with abdominal mass [12]. Primary Leiomyoma of the liver has been described in the literature as a solitary firm, white, fasciculate, and well demarcated tumour which is consistent with the findings of this review [4, 10, 19, 39]. One author reported a case of primary leiomyoma of the liver with two sharply delineated tumours [20] but other cases in the review have been reported as solitary tumours. The shape has been reported to be roughly spherical [20] to oval [19] (Figure 3(a)).

4.11. Microscopic Features. Histological review of tissue sections and specimens is absolutely important because the distinction between benign and malignant smooth muscle tumours of the gastrointestinal tract on imaging is not very clear [12].

The cellular architecture has been variably described as multiple interlacing bundles of uniform spindle cells [39] homogeneous pattern of interlacing bundles of uniform elongate cells with a plump spindle shaped [4], whirling bundles of well differentiated regular spindle shaped smooth muscle cells [2, 12], and highly cellular population of spindle cells arranged in interwoven fascicles (Figure 3(b)). Cells have slightly eosinophilic [20] to abundant eosinophilic cytoplasm [10, 24]. High density reticular fibres with a peripheral collagen rich zone which indicates expanding growth have been reported [20, 24]. Electron microscopy findings suggest tumour cells with well-defined basement membrane, scattered electron dense condensations in the plasma membrane, abundant glycogen, and pinocytotic vesicles and cytoplasmic filaments [24].

Central [19, 25] and focal [24] areas of necrosis have been described in the case reports. However it was not stated in the case reports if the necrosis were coagulative in nature.

Primary leiomyomas of the liver have been largely reported without evidence of mitotic changes except for few case reports which variously reported scarce, low, and rare mitoses [2, 4, 6, 12, 18, 20, 21, 24]. Histological features suggestive of malignancy include prominent cellular atypia with nuclear pleomorphism, large size, presence of infiltration, dense cellularity, degenerative changes, areas of coagulative necrosis, and increased mitotic rates (more than 1/10 HPF) [1, 12, 18, 19].

Mitotic index as defined by the number of mitoses per specified high power field was not documented for some of the case reports [2, 12, 21]. Doyle et al. [24] and Hawkins et al. [4] reported mitotic count of less than 1/10 HPF (high power field). Davidoff et al. [18] and Sclabas et al. [20] reported a mitotic count of 1/50 HPF and less than 1/20 HPF, respectively. Various mitotic indexes have been suggested as a cut off criteria for leiomyosarcoma in nonuterine smooth muscle tumours. Ranchod and Kempson [43] suggested five or more mitoses/10 HPF while between 5–10/50 HPF has been suggested by some authors [44–46]. The use of mitotic index in a uniform manner for all cases reported in the future is needful to ensure unequivocal diagnosis especially in a case reported with mild cellular atypia in the presence of mitoses [21] which may suggest a distinct possibility of malignancy.

4.12. Immunohistochemistry. The cells in the case reports reviewed have been reported to be positive to alpha smooth muscle actin (Figure 3(c)). Some of the cells also stained positive to Desmin (Figure 3(d)) [2, 24] and Vimentin [12]. There is lack of expression of CD 34 [20, 39], CD 68, Vimentin [10] HMB-45, S100 [19, 20], CD 117, and DOG1 [2]. Ultrastructural studies have been reported to show filaments, some dense bodies, and a few pinocytic vesicles [4]. The immunohistochemical stains are useful in ruling out possible differential diagnosis. CD 117, CD34, and DOG1 are markers of gastrointestinal stromal tumours (GIST) and HMB-45 reactivity suggests angiomyolipoma [5, 36, 47].

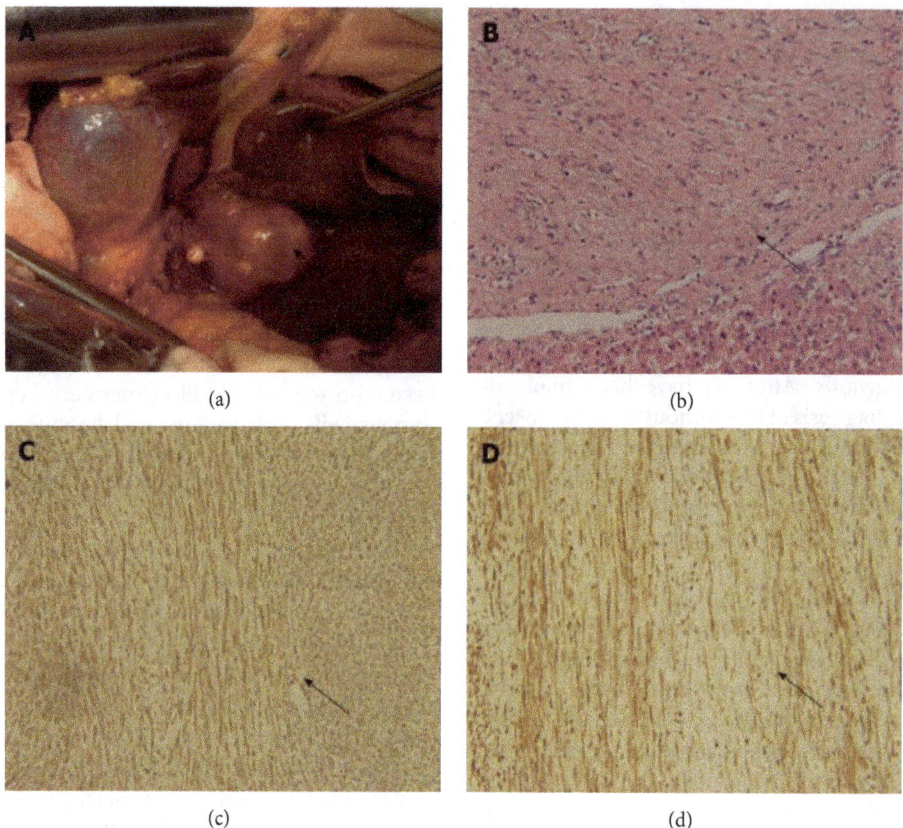

(a) (b) (c) (d)

FIGURE 3: Pathologic features. (a) Intraoperative feature of primary leiomyoma of the liver. (b) Tumour (arrow) and normal liver tissue, H&E staining, ×200; (c) α-smooth muscle actin staining (arrow) of tumour tissues, immunohistochemical staining, ×200; (d) Desmin staining (arrow) of tumour tissues, immunohistochemical staining, ×200. Reprinted from [2] with the permission of the Director, Editorial Office of the World Journal of Gastroenterology.

4.13. Treatment. Primary leiomyoma of the liver is amenable to surgery. Surgical resection of the tumour appears to be both diagnostic and curative in this review of the literature. The prognosis of this tumour appears to be excellent without evidence of disease during the follow-up of the cases. The average follow-up of the cases in this review is 33 months (range 4–108).

5. Conclusion

This paper to the best of the knowledge of the author is the largest review of case reports of primary leiomyoma of the liver in the literature. Primary leiomyoma of the liver is a very rare tumour with a complex pathogenesis which remains largely unknown. The diagnosis of the primary leiomyoma of the liver must meet a set of diagnostic criteria proposed by Hawkins et al. which ensures the cells are leiomyocytes and the exclusion of coexisting leiomyoma from other sites of the body. Metastatic workup to exclude occult leiomyoma elsewhere should be undertaken. This should include investigations like oesophagogastroduodenoscopy, colonoscopy, imaging techniques like CT scans and MRI, and a thorough exploration during surgery.

Primary leiomyoma of the liver should be considered as a differential diagnosis of liver lesions with or without immunosuppression. Multiple imaging techniques do not allow for a tissue specific diagnosis; hence histological review of the tissue specimen and immunohistochemical stains are imperative for diagnosis. Surgical resection is both diagnostic and curative.

Acknowledgment

Many thanks to the Director, Editorial Office of the World Journal of Gastroenterology for the kind permission to use the slides reprinted from [2].

References

[1] T. E. Reinertson, J. B. Fortune, J. C. Peters, I. Pagnotta, and J. A. Balint, "Primary leiomyoma of the liver. A case report and review of the literature," *Digestive Diseases and Sciences*, vol. 37, no. 4, pp. 622–627, 1992.

[2] X.-Z. Luo, C.-S. Ming, X.-P. Chen, and N.-Q. Gong, "Epstein-Barr virus negative primary hepatic leiomyoma: case report and

literature review," *World Journal of Gastroenterology*, vol. 19, no. 25, pp. 4094–4098, 2013.

[3] R. Demel, "Ein operierter fall von leber-myom," *Virchows Archiv für Pathologische Anatomie und Physiologie und für Klinische Medizin*, vol. 261, no. 3, pp. 881–884, 1926.

[4] E. P. Hawkins, G. L. Jordan, and M. H. McGavran, "Primary leiomyoma of the liver. Successful treatment by lobectomy and presentation of criteria for diagnosis," *The American Journal of Surgical Pathology*, vol. 4, no. 3, pp. 301–304, 1980.

[5] F. Beuzen, J. Roudie, I. Moali, S. Maitre, P. Barthelemy, and C. Smadja, "Primary leiomyoma of the liver: a rare benign tumor," *Gastroenterologie Clinique et Biologique*, vol. 28, no. 11, pp. 1169–1172, 2004.

[6] M. Yanase, H. Ikeda, I. Ogata et al., "Primary smooth muscle tumor of the liver encasing hepatobiliary cystadenoma without mesenchymal stroma," *The American Journal of Surgical Pathology*, vol. 23, no. 7, pp. 854–859, 1999.

[7] A. N. Kalil, M. T. Ferreira, F. Ressler, and C. Zettler, "Hepatic leyomioma in an immunocompetent patient," *Revista do Colegio Brasileiro de Cirurgioes*, vol. 36, no. 4, pp. 362–363, 2009.

[8] Y. Urizono, S. Ko, H. Kanehiro et al., "Primary leiomyoma of the liver: report of a case," *Surgery Today*, vol. 36, no. 7, pp. 629–632, 2006.

[9] M. Imasato, T. Tono, T. Kano et al., "Primary leiomyoma of the liver: a case report," *Nippon Geka Gakkai Zasshi*, vol. 106, no. 11, pp. 725–729, 2005.

[10] S. Prevot, J. Neris, and P. P. de Saint Maur, "Detection of Epstein Barr virus in an hepatic leiomyomatous neoplasm in an adult human immunodeficiency virus 1-infected patient," *Virchows Archiv*, vol. 425, no. 3, pp. 321–325, 1994.

[11] M. J. Hollands, R. Jaworski, K. P. Wong, and J. M. Little, "A leiomyoma of the liver," *HPB Surgery*, vol. 1, no. 4, pp. 337–343, 1989.

[12] G. Belli, F. Ciciliano, A. Iannelli, and I. Marano, "Hepatic resection for primary giant leiomyoma of the liver," *HPB*, vol. 3, no. 1, pp. 11–12, 2001.

[13] I. Santos, C. Valls, D. Leiva, T. Serrano, L. Martinez, and S. Ruiz, "Primary hepatic leiomyoma: case report," *Abdominal Imaging*, vol. 36, no. 3, pp. 315–317, 2011.

[14] G. H. Mahour, K. G. Wakim, E. H. Soule, and D. O. Ferris, "Structure of the common bile duct in man: presence or absence of smooth muscle," *Annals of Surgery*, vol. 166, no. 1, pp. 91–94, 1967.

[15] I. Penn, "Malignancies associated with immunosuppressive or cytotoxic therapy," *Surgery*, vol. 83, no. 5, pp. 492–502, 1978.

[16] E. S. Lee, J. Locker, M. Nalesnik et al., "The association of Epstein-Barr virus with smooth-muscle tumors occurring after organ transplantation," *The New England Journal of Medicine*, vol. 332, no. 1, pp. 19–25, 1995.

[17] T. E. Starzl, M. A. Nalesnik, K. A. Porter et al., "Reversibility of lymphomas and lymphoproliferative lesions developing under cyclosporin-steroid therapy," *The Lancet*, vol. 1, no. 8377, pp. 583–587, 1984.

[18] A. M. Davidoff, A. Hebra, B. J. Clark III et al., "Epstein-Barr virus-associated hepatic smooth muscle neoplasm in a cardiac transplant recipient," *Transplantation*, vol. 61, no. 3, pp. 515–517, 1996.

[19] M. V. Perini, M. A. Fink, D. A. Yeo et al., "Primary liver leiomyoma: a review of this unusual tumour," *ANZ Journal of Surgery*, vol. 83, no. 4, pp. 230–233, 2013.

[20] G. M. Sclabas, C. A. Maurer, M. N. Wente, A. Zimmermann, and M. W. Büchler, "Case report: hepatic leiomyoma in a renal transplant recipient," *Transplantation Proceedings*, vol. 34, no. 8, pp. 3200–3202, 2002.

[21] M. Sadler, W. L. Mays, P. Albert, and B. Javors, "Hepatic leiomyomas in two adult patients with aids: intravenous contrast-enhanced CT and MR imaging," *Emergency Radiology*, vol. 9, no. 3, pp. 175–177, 2002.

[22] W. Cheuk, P. C. K. Li, and J. K. C. Chan, "Epstein-Barr virus-associated smooth muscle tumour: a distinctive mesenchymal tumour of immunocompromised individuals," *Pathology*, vol. 34, no. 3, pp. 245–249, 2002.

[23] E. L. Raber, A.-L. Cheng, W.-F. Dong, and F. Sutherland, "Primary hepatic leiomyoma in a transplant patient: characterization with magnetic resonance imaging," *Transplantation*, vol. 93, no. 2, pp. e4–e5, 2012.

[24] H. Doyle, A. G. Tzakis, E. Yunis, and T. E. Starzl, "Smooth muscle tumor arising de novo in a liver allograft: a case report," *Clinical Transplantation*, vol. 5, no. 1, pp. 60–62, 1991.

[25] C. Ha, J. O. Haller, and N. K. Rollins, "Smooth muscle tumors in immunocompromised (HIV negative) children," *Pediatric Radiology*, vol. 23, no. 5, pp. 413–414, 1993.

[26] B. Safai, B. Diaz, and J. Schwartz, "Malignant neoplasms associated with human immunodeficiency virus infection," *A Cancer Journal for Clinicians*, vol. 42, no. 2, pp. 74–95, 1992.

[27] H. Chelimilla, K. Badipatla, A. Ihimoyan, and M. Niazi, "A rare occurrence of primary hepatic leiomyosarcoma associated with Epstein Barr virus infection in an AIDs patient," *Case Reports in Gastrointestinal Medicine*, vol. 2013, Article ID 691862, 5 pages, 2013.

[28] N. J. London, S. M. Farmery, E. J. Will, A. M. Davison, and J. P. A. Lodge, "Risk of neoplasia in renal transplant patients," *The Lancet*, vol. 346, no. 8972, pp. 403–406, 1995.

[29] G. Buccianti, B. Ravasi, D. Cresseri, P. Maisonneuve, P. Boyle, and F. Locatelli, "Cancer in patients on renal replacement therapy in Lombardy, Italy," *The Lancet*, vol. 347, no. 8993, pp. 59–60, 1996.

[30] J. Dantal, M. Hourmant, D. Cantarovich et al., "Effect of long-term immunosuppression in kidney-graft recipients on cancer incidence: randomised comparison of two cyclosporin regimens," *The Lancet*, vol. 351, no. 9103, pp. 623–628, 1998.

[31] A. J. Herzberg, J. A. MacDonald, J. A. Tucker, P. A. Humphrey, and W. C. Meyers, "Primary leiomyoma of the liver," *American Journal of Gastroenterology*, vol. 85, no. 12, pp. 1642–1645, 1990.

[32] J. L. Rios-Dalenz, "Leiomyoma of the liver," *Archives of Pathology*, vol. 79, pp. 54–56, 1965.

[33] E. Rummeny, R. Weissleder, D. D. Stark et al., "Primary liver tumors: diagnosis by MR imaging," *The American Journal of Roentgenology*, vol. 152, no. 1, pp. 63–72, 1989.

[34] G. S. Yoon, G. H. Kang, and O. J. Kim, "Primary myxoid leiomyoma of the liver," *Archives of Pathology and Laboratory Medicine*, vol. 122, no. 12, pp. 1112–1115, 1998.

[35] K. G. Ishak and L. Rabin, "Benign tumors of the liver," *Medical Clinics of North America*, vol. 59, no. 4, pp. 995–1013, 1975.

[36] H. T. Sousa, F. Portela, L. Semedo et al., "Primary leiomyoma of the liver: accurate preoperative diagnosis on liver biopsy," *BMJ Case Reports*, 2009.

[37] N. Kanazawa, N. Izumi, K. Tsuchiya et al., "A case of primary leiomyoma of the liver in a patient without evidence of immunosuppression," *Hepatology Research*, vol. 24, no. 1, pp. 80–88, 2002.

[38] W. Tan, G. Wu, and C. Zheng, "Imaging findings of primary hepatic leiomyoma," *Chinese-German Journal of Clinical Oncology*, vol. 8, no. 3, pp. 134–136, 2009.

[39] D. Marin, C. Catalano, M. Rossi et al., "Gadobenate dimeglumine-enhanced magnetic resonance imaging of primary leiomyoma of the liver," *Journal of Magnetic Resonance Imaging*, vol. 28, no. 3, pp. 755–758, 2008.

[40] R. C. Semelka and T. K. G. Helmberger, "Contrast agents for mr imaging of the liver," *Radiology*, vol. 218, no. 1, pp. 27–38, 2001.

[41] S. N. Gandhi, M. A. Brown, J. G. Wong, D. A. Aguirre, and C. B. Sirlin, "MR contrast agents for liver imaging: what, when, how?" *Radiographics*, vol. 26, no. 6, pp. 1621-1636, 2006.

[42] C. D. Guy, S. Yuan, and M. S. Ballo, "Spindle-cell lesions of the liver: diagnosis by fine-needle aspiration biopsy," *Diagnostic Cytopathology*, vol. 25, no. 2, pp. 94–100, 2001.

[43] M. Ranchod and R. L. Kempson, "Smooth muscle tumors of the gastrointestinal tract and retroperitoneum: a pathologic analysis of 100 cases," *Cancer*, vol. 39, no. 1, pp. 255–262, 1977.

[44] B. K. Morgan, C. Compton, M. Talbert, W. J. Gallagher, and W. C. Wood, "Benign smooth muscle tumors of the gastrointestinal tract. A 24-year experience," *Annals of Surgery*, vol. 211, no. 1, pp. 63–66, 1990.

[45] H. D. Appelman, "Smooth muscle tumours of the GI Tract: what we know that Stout didn't know," *The American Journal of Surgical Pathology*, vol. 10, pp. 83–99, 1986.

[46] O. E. Akwari, R. R. Dozois, L. H. Weiland, and O. H. Beahrs, "Leiomyosarcoma of the small and large bowel," *Cancer*, vol. 42, no. 3, pp. 1375–1384, 1978.

[47] H. R. Makhlouf, H. E. Remotti, and K. G. Ishak, "Expression of KIT (CD117) in angiomyolipoma," *The American Journal of Surgical Pathology*, vol. 26, no. 4, pp. 493–497, 2002.

[48] S. J. Mesenas, K. Y. Ng, P. Raj, J. M. S. Ho, and H. S. Ng, "Primary leiomyoma of the liver," *Singapore Medical Journal*, vol. 41, no. 3, pp. 129–131, 2000.

[49] S. Bartoli, P. Alo, P. Leporelli, E. Puce, U. Di Tondo, and A. Thau, "Primary leiomyoma of the liveer," *Minerva Chirurgica*, vol. 46, no. 13-14, pp. 777–779, 1991.

Laparoscopic versus Open Liver Resection: Differences in Intraoperative and Early Postoperative Outcome among Cirrhotic Patients with Hepatocellular Carcinoma—A Retrospective Observational Study

Antonio Siniscalchi,[1] Giorgio Ercolani,[2] Giulia Tarozzi,[1] Lorenzo Gamberini,[1] Lucia Cipolat,[1] Antonio D. Pinna,[2] and Stefano Faenza[1]

[1]*Division of Anesthesiology, Alma Mater Studiorum University of Bologna, Policlinico S. Orsola-Malpighi, Via Massarenti 9, 40138 Bologna, Italy*
[2]*Division of Surgery and Transplantation, Policlinico S. Orsola-Malpighi, University of Bologna, Via Massarenti 9, 40138 Bologna, Italy*

Correspondence should be addressed to Lorenzo Gamberini; gambero6891@hotmail.it

Academic Editor: Christos G. Dervenis

Introduction. Laparoscopic liver resection is considered risky in cirrhotic patients, even if minor surgical trauma of laparoscopy could be useful to prevent deterioration of a compromised liver function. This study aimed to identify the differences in terms of perioperative complications and early outcome in cirrhotic patients undergoing minor hepatic resection for hepatocellular carcinoma with open or laparoscopic technique. *Methods.* In this retrospective study, 156 cirrhotic patients undergoing liver resection for hepatocellular carcinoma were divided into two groups according to type of surgical approach: laparoscopy (LS group: 23 patients) or laparotomy (LT group: 133 patients). Perioperative data, mortality, and length of hospital stay were recorded. *Results.* Groups were matched for type of resection, median number of nodules, and median diameter of largest lesions. Groups were also homogeneous for preoperative liver and renal function tests. Intraoperative haemoglobin decrease and transfusions of red blood cells and fresh frozen plasma were significantly lower in LS group. MELD score lasted stable after laparoscopic resection, while it increased in laparotomic group. Postoperative liver and renal failure and mortality were all lower in LS group. *Conclusions.* Lower morbidity and mortality, maintenance of liver function, and shorter hospital stay suggest the safety and benefit of laparoscopic approach.

1. Introduction

Hepatocellular carcinoma (HCC) is one of the most common malignancies of western countries with an increased incidence in patients with chronic liver disease, especially those with HCV and HBV related cirrhosis [1, 2]. Hepatic resection is certainly one of the most important treatment options and surgery can be carried out with open or laparoscopic technique; among advantages of laparoscopic surgery there are reduction of perioperative bleeding, lower hemodynamic impact, shorter hospital stay, lower postoperative pain, and earlier return to normal activities [3]. However, laparoscopy is considered risky in cirrhotic patients because of the presence of complications related to the disease such as hyperdynamic circulation, coagulopathy, renal failure, and increased intra-abdominal pressure, so its use is widely debated; moreover, some studies report a greater impairment of oncologic integrity, uncontrollable bleeding, and risk of embolism [4]. This study aimed to identify the differences in terms of intraoperative and postoperative complications and early outcome in cirrhotic patients undergoing minor hepatic resection for hepatocellular carcinoma with open or laparoscopic technique.

2. Methods

2.1. Study Design. After Institutional Review Board approval (Protocol Code: LAPARO2011), this retrospective observational study included a total of 194 cirrhotic patients, undergoing minor hepatic resection for HCC between 2005 and 2010 at the Department of Surgery and Transplantation of the University of Bologna, divided into two groups on the basis of the kind of surgery carried out: laparotomic (LT group) or laparoscopic (LS group) liver resection.

Liver resections were defined according to the Brisbane 2000 classification. Atypical resections were generally reserved for small peripheral lesions, whereas anatomical resections were performed when it was deemed that hepatic functional reserve was sufficient [2, 5].

Indications for liver laparoscopic resection were patients with small number of lesions (≤3), 5 cm or less, located in liver segments 2 to 6 [6].

Patients with tumors which were either large (>5 cm), central, bilateral, or connected with liver hilum, major hepatic veins, or the inferior vena cava were not accepted as candidates for laparoscopic resection (modified from Louisville Statement [7]).

Patients whose lesion characteristics were incompatible with a laparoscopic approach were excluded from the open group.

(i) LS Group. It involved 33 patients operated on between 2006 and 2010. Five patients were subsequently excluded for lack of data and other 5 for the conversion into open technique. Causes of conversion were uncontrolled bleeding (2), hepatomegaly (1), and inability to view or isolate the tumor due to technical reasons (2).

The final number of patients included in this group was 23.

For lesions located in the left lobe requiring left lateral lobectomy or wedge resection, the standard three-trocar technique was used.

For lesions located in the other hepatic segments, a four-trocar technique was applied. In all cases, intraoperative laparoscopic ultrasound was applied to confirm the number, size, and location of nodules and guide the extension of the partial hepatectomy. Parenchymal dissection was performed by harmonic scalpel. The main vascular and biliary pedicles were secured with EndoGIA; smaller pedicles were closed by the use of haemoclip. Pringle maneuver was never applied in this series. A closed system suction drain was left in place for 2 days if no major bleeding or postoperative biliary fistula appeared. Fascial closure was attempted only at the umbilical cannula site. If the tumor size was larger than 3 cm, a Pfannenstiel incision was used to take out the piece.

(ii) LT Group. It included 161 patients. Twenty-eight of these were later excluded because they underwent major liver resection such as right hepatectomy (9), left hepatectomy (11), enlarged left hepatectomy (4), mesohepatectomy (1), and trisegmentectomy (3).

The final number of patients included in this group was 133.

The right subcostal incision extended to the xiphoid process along the middle line ("J shape incision") is our standard laparotomy for hepatobiliary surgery. Parenchymal transaction was carried out by harmonic scalpel (similar to the laparoscopic technique) or traditional Kellyclasia technique (based on single surgeon's preference). Vascular clamping was usually applied when excessive bleeding was encountered during transaction; type of clamping was arbitrarily chosen by the operator. Precise detailes about our surgical technique have been already reported [8].

Intraoperative ultrasound was performed to guide all types of liver resections. One or two closed system suction drains were left in place for 48 hours.

Patients in both groups underwent minor liver resection: wedge resection, segmentectomy, bisegmentectomy, or left lobectomy (Table 1), according to IHPBA classification [9].

2.2. Anesthesiologic Management. In both groups, induction was performed by intravenous infusion of propofol (1–1.5 mg kg^{-1}), fentanyl (3 mcg kg^{-1}), midazolam (0.05 mg kg^{-1}), and atracurium (0.1 mg kg^{-1}) at 100% of FiO_2. After intubation, maintenance was achieved with sevoflurane (0.8–1.2%), fentanyl, and vecuronium. Mechanical ventilation was performed by setting the tidal volume to 8–10 mL kg^{-1} with 8–12 breaths per minute and a FiO_2 of 40–50%. In all patients, radial artery and right internal jugular vein were cannulated for monitoring and rapid infusion of liquids. From incision to complete resection, fluid infusions were restricted in order to maintain low central venous pressure values to avoid excessive bleeding during resection.

2.3. Statistical Analysis. Statistical analysis was performed using Microsoft Excel 2011 and SPSS 17.0. Preoperative and postoperative variables were compared using t-test for numeral variables, Fisher exact test for dichotomous nominal variables, Pearson chi-square test for multicategorical nominal variables, and Mann-Whitney test for ordinal variables. For the analysis of intraoperative variables, we used a two-level linear model for repeated measures using the group membership as a factor between the subjects. All the results with $P < 0.05$ were considered statistically significant. Numeral variables are expressed as mean ± standard deviation (SD), while nominal or ordinals are expressed as a percentage and an absolute value.

3. Collected Data

3.1. Preoperative Phase. Clinical and biochemical variables recorded in all patients were age, gender, aetiology of cirrhosis (alcohol, HCV, HBV, and HDV), presence of comorbidities (HIV, diabetes) or complications related to cirrhosis (preoperative ascites, esophageal varices), necessity of drug treatment, or portal vein embolization (PVE).

TABLE 1: The two groups (laparoscopic versus open resection) were matched based on type of resection and median number and diameter of nodules.

Variables	LS group (23)		LT group (133)		
	Mean	SD	Mean	SD	P
		Preoperative data			
Number of lesions	1.23 (1–3)	0.56	1.26 (1–6)	0.68	0.898
Diameter of the lesion (cm)	3.21 (1.9–8)	1.04	3.6 (1–9)	1.64	0.074
	Number	%	Number	%	P
		Type of resection			
Wedge (n)	10	43.5%	90	67.7%	0.165
Segmentectomy (n)	8	34.8%	27	20.3%	
Bisegmentectomy (n)	2	8.7%	8	6.0%	
Left lobectomy (n)	3	13%	8	6.0%	

We also evaluated renal and liver function tests, cell blood count and biochemical parameters.

The severity of cirrhosis was assessed by calculating the "Model of End Stage Liver Disease" (MELD) score and Child-Pugh-Turcotte score (CPT), using the latest laboratory data prior to surgery. We also evaluated the total number of HCC nodules (HCC) radiologically detected, the diameter of the lesion (cm), the number of liver segments treated, and any associated procedures.

The two groups were matched based on type of resection (all patients included in the study received minor hepatectomies) and on median number and median diameter of largest nodule. As reported in Table 1, the two groups were comparable for type of resection and tumor characteristics.

3.2. Intraoperative Phase. Blood gas analyses were carried out in all patients from the beginning to the end of the resection. We considered for each patient only the baseline and intraoperative worst values. Blood gas parameters recorded, corrected for body temperature and FiO_2, were as follows.

(i) Respiratory parameters: oxygen partial pressure (PaO_2) and carbon dioxide partial pressure ($PaCO_2$).

(ii) Metabolic parameters: pH, bicarbonate ions concentration (HCO_3^-), bases excess (BE), and haemoglobin (Hb). Other intraoperative variables recorded were amount of blood red cells and fresh frozen plasma transfusions and number of patients transfused, volume of fluids infused (crystalloids, colloids), amount of albumin administered, need for correction of metabolic acidosis with sodium bicarbonate ($NaHCO_3$), and hypotensive episodes (systolic blood pressure under 80 mmHg) and their duration. For patients undergoing open resection, we also collected data on the type of clamping and its duration, while length of pneumoperitoneum was recorded for patients undergoing laparoscopic resection.

3.3. Postoperative Phase. We recorded worst levels of creatinine, bilirubin, and INR in the first 7 days after surgery, to recalculate MELD score. We recorded also the occurrence of postoperative ascites, bilirubin levels above 3 mg dL^{-1}, 50-50 criterion (bilirubin > 50 mmol L^{-1} (>3 mg dL^{-1}) and PT < 50%) [10], postoperative coagulopathy (INR > 1.50 or PT < 50% requiring correction with plasma), postoperative renal failure (creatinine > 2 mg dL^{-1}, urea > 200 mg dL^{-1}), progressive liver failure that caused patient death or needed liver transplantation (OLT), other morbidities, overall mortality and cause of death, and hospital stay (calculated from the first day after surgery until date of discharge).

4. Results

Clinical variables, comorbidities, and complications related to cirrhosis are recorded in Table 2; LT patients were significantly older and presented a lower incidence of alcoholic cirrhosis.

Preoperative data are recoded in Table 2; LS group had significantly higher mean INR values and lower alanine aminotransferase (ALT), platelets, and haematocrit, and MELD score was comparable between the two groups. Intraoperative respiratory and metabolic parameters are recoded in Table 3; among metabolic parameters, only Base Excess (BE) showed no significant differences between the two groups ($P = 0.595$) while the other parameters such as pCO_2 and pH were statistically significant but not clinically salient because they reasonably derived from pneumoperitoneum physiopathology. Operative time was slightly superior in the laparoscopic group.

Intraoperative values of haemoglobin (Hb) also revealed significant differences between the two groups ($P < 0.001$); in fact, haemoglobin remained stable during laparoscopy while it decreased during open resections (Table 3).

There were not any red blood cells (RBC) transfusions in LS group while 27.4% of patients that underwent open resection needed blood transfusions ($P = 0.002$). With regard to transfusions of fresh frozen plasma (FFP), LS group received an average of 0.22 ± 0.52 units of plasma versus 0.68 ± 1.08 units in control group ($P = 0.02$).

Duration of vascular pedicle clamping during laparotomic liver resections was 5–63 minutes; pneumoperitoneum during laparoscopic resections ranged from a minimum of 55 minutes to a maximum of 230 minutes.

Table 2: Preoperative data, clinical variables, comorbidities, and complications related to cirrhosis divided according to type of resection.

Variables	LS group (23)		LT group (133)		
	Mean	SD	Mean	SD	P
Age (n)	57.91 (30–73)	10.92	63.26 (41–77)	7.89	0.033*
Male/female	15/8		104/29		0.19
	Number	%	Number	%	P
		Pathologies			
Alcohol (n)	5	21.7%	6	4.5%	0.011*
HCV (n)	17	73.9%	88	67.6%	1
HBV (n)	6	26.1%	35	26.5%	1
HDV (n)	1	4.3%	5	3.8%	1
HIV (n)	3	13%	19	14.4%	1
Diabetes (n)	4	17.4%	36	27.3%	0.441
Preoperative ascites (n)	3	13%	8	6.1%	0.211
Esophageal varices (n)	13	56.6%	40	34.8%	0.062
	Mean	SD	Mean	SD	P
		Preoperative data			
Serum urea (g/L)	0.37	0.12	0.4	0.17	0.521
Serum creatinine (mg/dL)	0.9	0.2	0.98	0.29	0.197
Proteins (g/dL)	7.59	0.71	7.57	0.6	0.878
Albumin (g/dL)	3.91	0.39	3.73	0.41	0.139
Bilirubin (mg/dL)	1.45	1.18	0.98	0.51	0.074
ALP (U/L)	305.5	103.65	281.55	108.28	0.597
AST (U/L)	60	30.84	86.78	77.08	0.103
ALT (U/L)	55.48	43.38	87.76	72.41	0.04*
INR	1.25	0.17	1.16	0.11	0.015*
MELD	10.09 (7–18)	3.04	8.95 (6–15)	1.82	0.096
Na^+ (mmol/L)	140.65	3.5	138.8	2.67	0.023*
WBC (U/mL)	5272.61	2125.79	5389.83	1728.14	0.772
Hb (g/dL)	13.36	1.74	13.9	1.47	0.119
HCT (%)	39.2	4.37	41.17	4	0.035*
PLT (U/mL)	111 217	60 336	138 439	59 880	0.046*

*$P < 0.05$.

Pathologic characteristics of the tumor and the rate of curative resection were comparable between the two groups as reported in Table 4.

Postoperative data are recorded in Table 5.

Worst postoperative serum creatinine was statistically different ($P < 0.0001$) and so also postoperative MELD scores ($P = 0.035$). In 8 patients (34.8%) belonging to the LS group, the 50-50 criterion were fulfilled, while only 25 (12.9%) of the patients in LT group had this criterion satisfied ($P = 0.014$).

Treatment for postoperative liver failure, consisting essentially of liver transplantation (OLT), was applied in 2,3% of patients of LT group and none in LS group ($P = 0.475$).

Although hospital stay was not statistically different ($P = 0.339$), it was smaller in LS group, with a range of 3–29 days and an average duration of 7.61 days, while it was greater in LT group with a mean value of 14.38 days and a range of 4–166 days.

Postoperative mortality was lower in LS group (none), while it reached a value of 7.5% (10 patients) in LT group ($P = 0.36$) (Table 5). The largest part of deaths was caused by progressive liver failure (11 patients) and acute myocardial infarction (2 patients).

5. Discussion

To date, no randomized clinical trial evaluating laparoscopic against laparotomic liver resection has still been performed, but case series and prospective studies assessed its safety in terms of oncological integrity and the possibility to reduce postoperative hospital stay [11]. This study focused on perioperative period of cirrhotic patients undergoing minor liver resection and its results are in line with literature [12]; interestingly we found a lower incidence of acute kidney

Table 3: Intraoperative respiratory and metabolic parameters, transfusions, and operative time divided in two groups according to type of surgical approach; RBC: red blood cells; FFP: fresh frozen plasma; PT RBC/FFP: patients transfused with units of RBC/FFP.

Variables	LS group (23)		LT group (133)		
			Intraoperative data		
	Mean	SD	Mean	SD	P
Basal PaO_2 (mmHg)	253.02	109.88	227.29	66.57	<0.001*
Worst PaO_2 (mmHg)	181.53	75.86	235.29	68.77	<0.001*
Basal $PaCO_2$ (mmHg)	34.94	5.07	35.74	4.8	<0.001*
Worst $PaCO_2$ (mmHg)	43.75	8.56	35.96	4.65	<0.001*
Basal pH	7.44	0.04	7.43	0.05	<0.001*
Worst pH	7.35	0.07	7.39	0.06	<0.001*
Basal HCO_3^- (mmol/L)	23.38	2.46	24.04	1.73	<0.001*
Worst HCO_3^- (mmol/L)	23.65	2.37	21.93	1.97	<0.001*
Basal BE (mmol/L)	−0.49	2.05	−0.61	2.06	0.595
Worst BE (mmol/L)	−2.3	2.53	−2.69	2.56	0.595
Basal Hb (g/dL)	11.96	1.62	12.23	1.58	<0.001*
Worst Hb (g/dL)	12.11	1.84	11.21	1.7	<0.001*
RBC (U)	0	0	0.58	1.1	<0.001*
FFP (U)	0.22	0.52	0.68	1.07	0.002*
	Number	%	Number	%	P
PT RBC	0	0%	36	27.4%	0.002*
PT FFP	4	17.4%	45	34.2%	0.143
Acidosis correction ($NaHCO_3$)	2	8.7%	16	19%	0.35
	Min	SD	Min	SD	P
Operative time	175	91	165	80	0.588

$^*P < 0.05$.

Table 4: Pathologic tumor characteristics and curative resection based on laparoscopic versus open resection.

Variables	LS group (23)		LT group (133)		P
	Number	%	Number	%	
Edmonds on grades I-II	8	34.8%	42	31.6%	0.951
Edmonds on grades III-IV	15	65.2%	91	68.4%	
Microvascular invasion (yes)	13	56.5	71	53.4	0.958
Microvascular invasion (no)	10	43.5	62	46.6	
Curative resection (R0)	22	95.6%	129	97.0%	0.761

injury and postoperative liver failure which could account for the lower hospital stay underlined in other studies [13].

Minor surgical trauma and a more precise haemostasis, associated with the effect of hydrostatic pressure of pneumoperitoneum on the surface of dissected parenchyma, justify the maintenance of haemoglobin almost constant during surgery, resulting in a reduced necessity for transfusion of blood products. This is an important aspect since bleeding and consequently blood transfusions are associated with a higher postoperative morbidity in cirrhotic patients [11, 13, 14].

In this series we have applied Harmonic scalpel as our basic transaction technique; in the case of laparoscopic major hepatectomies we have used ultrasonic dissector. Anyway, Gobardhan et al. [15] have recently reported that no single method for parenchymal transaction has proven to be better than the other one. Based on single surgeon's experience, ultrasound dissector or ultrasound scissors (such as Harmonic scalpel or Thunderbeat) are mainly used together with monopolar or bipolar coagulators. Stappler technique has been also reported as alternative technique [16].

Postoperative values of MELD scores, expression of an increased risk of hepatic injury [17], were significantly lower after surgery in patients undergoing laparoscopic resection.

Postoperative ascites had a lower incidence in the LS group, and even if this parameter is not statistically significant, it may be an important aspect of postoperative trend. Ascites, in fact, represents a frequent complication of liver resection. Reduction of its incidence in patients undergoing laparoscopic resection can be attributed to the type of surgical approach [18]. This phenomenon could be due to the preservation of collateral circulation in the abdomen, avoiding long incisions and reducing the damage to muscle and round ligament, which may contain important

Table 5: Postoperative data: hepatic and renal functions, coagulopathies, other morbidities, mortality, and hospital stay divided in two groups according to type of surgical approach.

Variables	LS group (23)		LT group (133)		
			Postoperative data		
	Mean	SD	Mean	SD	P
Worse creatinine (mg/dL)	0.84	0.18	1.18	0.44	<0.001*
Worse bilirubin (mg/dL)	2.48	1.45	2.17	3.43	0.673
Worse INR	1.33	0.18	1.33	0.19	0.987
Worse MELD	10.6 (5–17)	3.58	12.6 (5–29)	4.24	0.035*
	Number	%	Number	%	P
PO ascites	3	13%	34	25.8%	0.288
PO jaundice	10	43.5%	30	22.7%	0.067
50-50 criterion	8	34.8%	17	12.9%	0.014*
PO coagulopathy	5	21.7%	25	18.9%	0.777
PO renal failure	0	0%	9	6.8%	0.357
POLF	0	0%	9	6.8%	0.357
Treatment of POLF	0	0%	3	2.3%	0.475
Morbidity	5	21.7%	47	35.6%	0.237
Status (dead/alive)	0/23	0/100%	10/123	7.5/92.5%	0.36
	Mean	SD	Mean	SD	P
Hospital stay (n)	7.61 (3–29)	5.5	14.38 (4–166)	21.78	0.339

$^{*}P < 0.05$.

collateral vessels. Other mechanisms that could be part of this phenomenon are the smaller mobilization and manipulation of the liver parenchyma, which reduces the trauma [18], the reduced section of lymph vessels, and minor demand for intraoperative fluids.

Due to these reasons, a reduced incidence of postoperative ascites in resected patients by laparoscopic approach has been reported in particular in F4-liver cirrhosis [19]; similar results have been confirmed in a recent meta-analysis regarding laparoscopic versus open approach for HCC and including 550 patients [20].

Absence of postoperative liver failure in LS group could also be traced in part to this type of mechanisms. This last parameter is an important result; liver failure in fact is one of the most severe postoperative complications, especially in cirrhotic patients, in which this is still more common [21].

The group undergoing laparoscopic liver resection did not develop renal failure. This finding, not underlined from other studies, could be related to lower incidence of ascites [20] and absence of liver failure, which allowed the maintenance of adequate renal function; on the other hand LT group had an incidence of postoperative renal failure of 6.8%.

The reduced incidence of postoperative complications after laparoscopic liver resection for HCC compared to conventional approach has been clearly reported in the literature both by single-center experience and by meta-analysis [13, 19, 20, 22]; we think the reduced functional reserve of cirrhotic patients considered in this study could rapidly impair under intense surgical insults as open surgery.

We have also to underline the conversion rate of laparoscopy (17,9%), which is in line with data found in literature [1]. The main causes of conversion were excessive bleeding and the inability to view/isolate the lesion, in particular at the beginning of our experience. This reflects the fact that laparoscopic liver resection techniques are not a completely solved problem, especially in cirrhotic patients [1]. Certainly, as stated by many authors [11, 14, 23], this procedure should be practiced by experienced surgeons, with an extensive experience in both types of resection and advanced laparoscopy in specialized centres.

Limitations of this study are the important difference in sample size between the two groups and its retrospective nature; another possible limitation could be represented by a significant difference in the average age of the two groups, lower in the LS group. However, homogeneity of the sample in relation to the type of resection, tumor characteristics, underlying liver disease, and other comorbidities, such as diabetes, HIV, preoperative ascites, and esophageal varices, can make this difference less significant.

6. Conclusions

Our study showed that intraoperative bleeding and transfusion requirements were significantly lower in the group undergoing laparoscopic liver resection.

Laparoscopic approach, opposed to open surgery, has not led to the development of hepatic or renal failure and mortality, morbidity, and postoperative hospital stay were lower.

The advantages of laparoscopic liver resection compared to traditional technique are several, especially if laparoscopic approach is used in patients with a higher MELD score and with a potentially increased risk of perioperative complications.

References

[1] D. Cherqui, A. Laurent, C. Tayar et al., "Laparoscopic liver resection for peripheral hepatocellular carcinoma in patients with chronic liver disease: midterm results and perspectives," *Annals of Surgery*, vol. 243, no. 4, pp. 499–506, 2006.

[2] G. Belli, C. Fantini, A. Belli, and P. Limongelli, "Laparoscopic liver resection for hepatocellular carcinoma in cirrhosis: long-term outcomes," *Digestive Surgery*, vol. 28, no. 2, pp. 134–140, 2011.

[3] K. T. Nguyen, T. C. Gamblin, and D. A. Geller, "Laparoscopic liver resection for cancer," *Future Oncology*, vol. 4, no. 5, pp. 661–671, 2008.

[4] K. A. Carswell, F. G. Sagias, B. Murgatroyd, M. Rela, N. Heaton, and A. G. Patel, "Laparoscopic versus open left lateral segmentectomy," *BMC Surgery*, vol. 9, no. 1, article 14, 2009.

[5] A. Cucchetti, M. Cescon, F. Trevisani, and A. D. Pinna, "Current concepts in hepatic resection for hepatocellular carcinoma in cirrhotic patients," *World Journal of Gastroenterology*, vol. 18, no. 44, pp. 6398–6408, 2012.

[6] M. D. Kluger and D. Cherqui, "Laparoscopic resection of hepatocellular carcinoma," in *Multidisciplinary Treatment of Hepatocellular Carcinoma*, J.-N. Vauthey and A. Brouquet, Eds., vol. 190 of *Recent Results in Cancer Research*, pp. 111–126, Springer, Berlin, Germany, 2013.

[7] J. F. Buell, D. Cherqui, D. A. Geller et al., "Position on laparoscopic liver surgery," *Annals of Surgery*, vol. 250, no. 5, pp. 825–830, 2009.

[8] A. Mazziotti, A. Cavallari, and J. Belghiti, *Techniques in Liver Surgery*, p. 370, Greenwich Medical Media, 1997.

[9] S. M. Strasberg, "Nomenclature of hepatic anatomy and resections: a review of the Brisbane 2000 system," *Journal of Hepato-Biliary-Pancreatic Surgery*, vol. 12, no. 5, pp. 351–355, 2005.

[10] S. Balzan, J. Belghiti, O. Farges et al., "The "50-50 criteria" on postoperative day 5: an accurate predictor of liver failure and death after hepatectomy," *Annals of Surgery*, vol. 242, no. 6, pp. 824–829, 2005.

[11] K. T. Nguyen and D. A. Geller, "Is laparoscopic liver resection safe and comparable to open liver resection for hepatocellular carcinoma?" *Annals of Surgical Oncology*, vol. 16, no. 7, pp. 1765–1767, 2009.

[12] F. M. Polignano, A. J. Quyn, R. S. M. de Figueiredo, N. A. Henderson, C. Kulli, and I. S. Tait, "Laparoscopic versus open liver segmentectomy: prospective, case-matched, intention-to-treat analysis of clinical outcomes and cost effectiveness," *Surgical Endoscopy*, vol. 22, no. 12, pp. 2564–2570, 2008.

[13] T. T. Cheung, R. T. Poon, W. K. Yuen et al., "Long-term survival analysis of pure laparoscopic versus open hepatectomy for hepatocellular carcinoma in patients with cirrhosis: a single-center experience," *Annals of Surgery*, vol. 257, no. 3, pp. 506–511, 2013.

[14] C. H. C. Pilgrim, H. To, V. Usatoff, and P. M. Evans, "Laparoscopic hepatectomy is a safe procedure for cancer patients," *HPB*, vol. 11, no. 3, pp. 247–251, 2009.

[15] P. D. Gobardhan, D. Subar, and B. Gayet, "Laparoscopic liver surgery: an overview of the literature and experiences of a single centre," *Best Practice & Research: Clinical Gastroenterology*, vol. 28, no. 1, pp. 111–121, 2014.

[16] J. F. Buell, B. Gayet, H.-S. Han et al., "Evaluation of stapler hepatectomy during a laparoscopic liver resection," *HPB*, vol. 15, no. 11, pp. 845–850, 2013.

[17] A. Cucchetti, A. Siniscalchi, G. Ercolani et al., "Modification of acid-base balance in cirrhotic patients undergoing liver resection for hepatocellular carcinoma," *Annals of Surgery*, vol. 245, no. 6, pp. 902–908, 2007.

[18] A. Laurent, D. Cherqui, M. Lesurtel et al., "Laparoscopic liver resection for subcapsular hepatocellular carcinoma complicating chronic liver disease," *Archives of Surgery*, vol. 138, no. 7, pp. 763–769, 2003.

[19] A. Kanazawa, T. Tsukamoto, S. Shimizu et al., "Impact of laparoscopic liver resection for hepatocellular carcinoma with F4-liver cirrhosis," *Surgical Endoscopy and Other Interventional Techniques*, vol. 27, no. 7, pp. 2592–2597, 2013.

[20] J.-J. Xiong, K. Altaf, M. A. Javed et al., "Meta-analysis of laparoscopic vs open liver resection for hepatocellular carcinoma," *World Journal of Gastroenterology*, vol. 18, no. 45, pp. 6657–6668, 2012.

[21] S. G. Delis, A. Bakoyiannis, I. Biliatis, K. Athanassiou, N. Tassopoulos, and C. Dervenis, "Model for end-stage liver disease (MELD) score, as a prognostic factor for post-operative morbidity and mortality in cirrhotic patients, undergoing hepatectomy for hepatocellular carcinoma," *HPB*, vol. 11, no. 4, pp. 351–357, 2009.

[22] Z. Yin, X. Fan, H. Ye, D. Yin, and J. Wang, "Short- and long-term outcomes after laparoscopic and open hepatectomy for hepatocellular carcinoma: a global systematic review and meta-analysis," *Annals of Surgical Oncology*, vol. 20, no. 4, pp. 1203–1215, 2013.

[23] I. S. Kwon, S. S. Yun, D. S. Lee, and H. J. Kim, "Laparoscopic liver resection for malignant liver tumors, why not more?" *Journal of the Korean Surgical Society*, vol. 83, no. 1, pp. 30–35, 2012.

Nonoperative Management May Be a Viable Approach to Plexiform Neurofibroma of the Porta Hepatis in Patients with Neurofibromatosis-1

Natesh Yepuri,[1] **Rana Naous**,[2] **Camille Richards**,[1] **Dilip Kittur**,[1] **Ajay Jain**,[1] **and Mashaal Dhir**[1]

[1]*Department of Surgery, SUNY Upstate Medical University, Syracuse, NY 13210, USA*
[2]*Department of Pathology, SUNY Upstate Medical University, Syracuse, NY 13210, USA*

Correspondence should be addressed to Mashaal Dhir; dhirm@upstate.edu

Academic Editor: Shusen Zheng

Background. Plexiform neurofibroma (PNF) in the porta hepatis (PH) is an unusual manifestation of neurofibromatosis-1 (NF-1). Resection is often recommended given the risk of malignant transformation. We encountered a challenging case in clinical practice which prompted us to report our findings and perform a systematic review on the management of these tumors. *Methods.* We reported the case of a 31-year-old woman with NF-1 and PNF of the PH. PRISMA 2009 guidelines were followed for systematic review. *Results.* Our patient was found to have unresectable disease at exploration. After >5 years of follow-up, she continued to have stable disease on imaging. We identified 12 studies/case reports including 10 adult and 6 pediatric patients with PNF of PH. None of the 7 adult patients with NF-1 and PNF of PH underwent a successful tumor resection. All pediatric patients were managed with surveillance alone. All but one pediatric patient had NF-1. None of the reported cases of PNF of PH had malignant transformation. *Conclusion.* Our findings suggest that PNFs of PH in the setting of NF-1 are often unresectable and may have an indolent course. Surveillance alone may be a reasonable option in some patients; however, further studies are needed.

1. Introduction

Neurofibromatosis-1 (NF-1) is a progressive multisystem neurocutaneous genetic disorder with an autosomal dominant inheritance [1]. NF-1 is caused by mutations in the NF-1 gene and affects both genders equally, with an incidence of one in 2500–3000 births [1–3]. NF-1 gene mutations can lead to dysregulation of RAS/MAP kinase and mammalian target of rapamycin (mTOR) signaling pathways which can lead to development of several types of neoplasms [1, 2]. Almost half of these mutations occur de novo in patients with no family history [1, 2] and there are several genotype-phenotype variations [1, 2]. Given the complex underlying genetics, diagnosis is often based on clinical features such as café-au-lait spots, Lisch nodules (iris hamartomas), and neurofibromas [1–3]. Neurofibromas are one of the most common and characteristic clinical manifestations of NF-1. These tumors can be located superficially in the skin or internally in the entire body including mediastinum, retroperitoneum, or GI tract. Plexiform neurofibromas (PNFs) are noncutaneous neurofibromas which are pathognomonic of NF-1 and overall one of the most challenging neoplasms to manage in NF-1.

PNFs are usually slow growing and affect 15–30% patients with NF-1. Clinical presentation of PNF is variable based on the organ of involvement, that is, mediastinum, retroperitoneum or GI tract, and so on [4]. In contrast to cutaneous neurofibromas which grow intraneurally, PNFs can involve an entire plexus of nerves and demonstrate an infiltrative pattern. Although PNFs are benign they have the potential to transform into malignant peripheral nerve sheath tumors which demonstrate aggressive behavior. Many experts recommend resection given the underlying malignant potential. However, locally infiltrative pattern can make these resections quite difficult.

We encountered a challenging case of PNF of Porta hepatis (PH) in clinical practice which prompted us to report our findings. PNFs of the PH are extremely rare and even

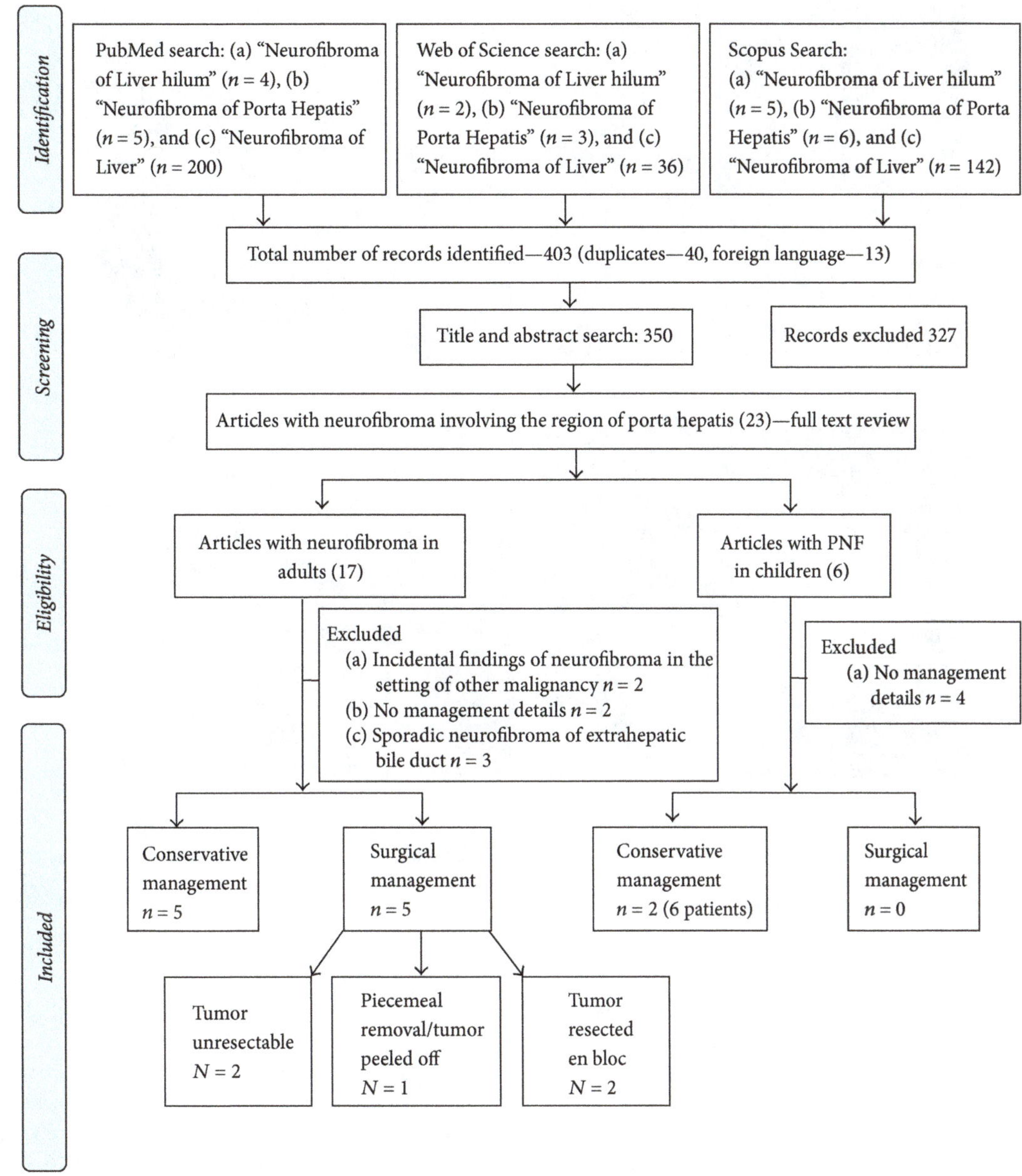

FIGURE 1: Study flow diagram and selection strategy.

more technically challenging to resect given the location and close relationship with the biliary and vascular inflow to the liver. There is no consensus on the management of these tumors given the rarity of clinical presentation. We hereby present the findings of our case. Additionally, we performed a systematic review of the literature to summarize the current evidence on the management of PNFs involving the PH.

2. Methodology

2.1. Systematic Review: Plexiform Neurofibroma of Porta Hepatis. A literature search was performed using the PubMed, Scopus, and Web of Science databases. Final search was conducted in 10/2017. Following search criteria were utilized: (a) "Neurofibroma of Liver hilum," (b) "Neurofibroma of Porta Hepatis," and (c) "Neurofibroma of Liver." For data extraction, first author (N. Y.) and senior author (M. D.) selected the studies and assessed for eligibility. A total of 403 articles were identified. Duplicates ($n = 40$) and articles in foreign languages ($n = 13$) were excluded. Title and abstract review were conducted for the remaining 350 articles. Inclusion criteria included case reports/series of neurofibroma in the region of porta hepatis with intent to include only PNF in the region of PH in the final qualitative synthesis. Full texts were reviewed for 23 articles. A backward search was also performed using cross references from the bibliographies of relevant articles and review articles to ensure a comprehensive search. Articles discussing imaging findings only without clinical management were excluded. Nineteen studies were included in the final qualitative synthesis. Studies reporting on adults (Age ≥ 18 years) and children (<18 years) were summarized separately. Figure 1 summarizes

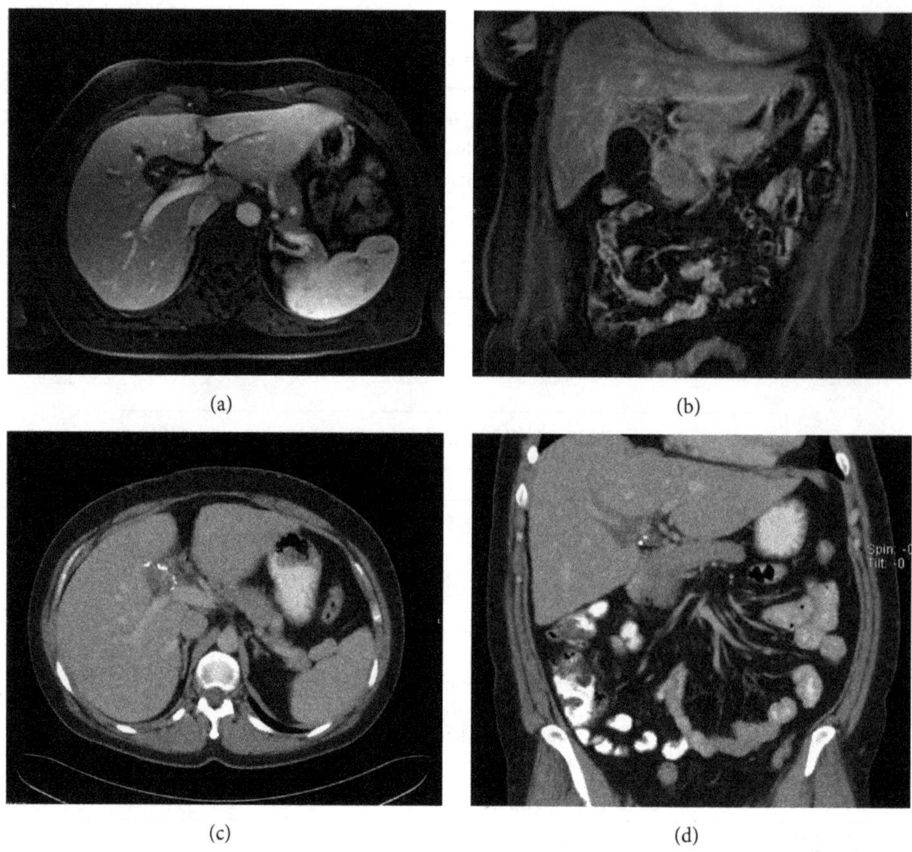

FIGURE 2: (a and b) Representative axial and coronal images from contrast enhanced preoperative MRI of the patient. Encasement of hepatic artery with extension of the mass predominantly towards the right side is noted in GB fossa. (c & d) Follow-up postoperative CT scans 5 years later depicting almost stable appearance of the mass.

the search strategy and inclusion/exclusion criteria per the PRISMA 2009 guidelines for systematic reviews.

3. Results

3.1. Case Presentation. A 31-year-old woman previously diagnosed with NF-1 presented to the emergency department with RUQ pain. Physical examination, liver function tests, and blood chemistries were unremarkable. Abdominal ultrasound (US) revealed a lobulated hypoechoic mass in the gallbladder fossa. A subsequent MRI scan noted a T1 hypointense and heterogeneously T2 hyperintense mass encasing the hepatic artery and portal vein within the PH (Figures 2(a) and 2(b)). There was no loss of signal on the out-of-phase images. The preoperative diagnosis for this mass was felt to be a neurofibroma. Given the symptomatic nature of the mass, decision was made to proceed with resection.

During laparotomy a cholecystectomy was performed as the gallbladder was closely adherent to the mass. Further dissection revealed that mass was infiltrating the entire PH. There was intrahepatic extension along the right posterior, right anterior, and left portal pedicles. Given the intraoperative extent of the disease it was decided to abort surgical resection. Surgical pathology revealed plexiform neurofibroma involving the gallbladder without any evidence of malignant transformation. Figure 3 highlights the gross and histopathologic features of PNF.

The patient's postoperative course was uneventful; however, the patient had neuropathic pain which was successfully managed with celiac plexus block and oral pain medications. The patient has been followed with serial MRIs and more recently with yearly CT scans of abdomen and pelvis. Over a period of six years the mass has remained stable. Figure 2 shows the preoperative and postoperative representative images of the PNF along with gross and histopathologic images. Our patient has one of the longest reported follow-ups for PNF of the PH.

3.2. Systematic Review. We identified twenty-three studies/case reports on neurofibroma involving the region of PH. Seventeen studies included adult patients whereas six studies were on pediatric patients. Among the seventeen studies with adult patients 3 studies/cases were excluded as they reported on sporadic neurofibroma involving the bile ducts [5–7]. All three of these patients underwent successful resection of the sporadic neurofibroma. Two required roux-en-Y hepaticojejunostomy and one underwent a pancreaticoduodenectomy. Two studies reported on cases with incidentally found nonplexiform hepatic neurofibromas in the setting of other malignancies such as angiosarcoma and cholangiocarcinoma

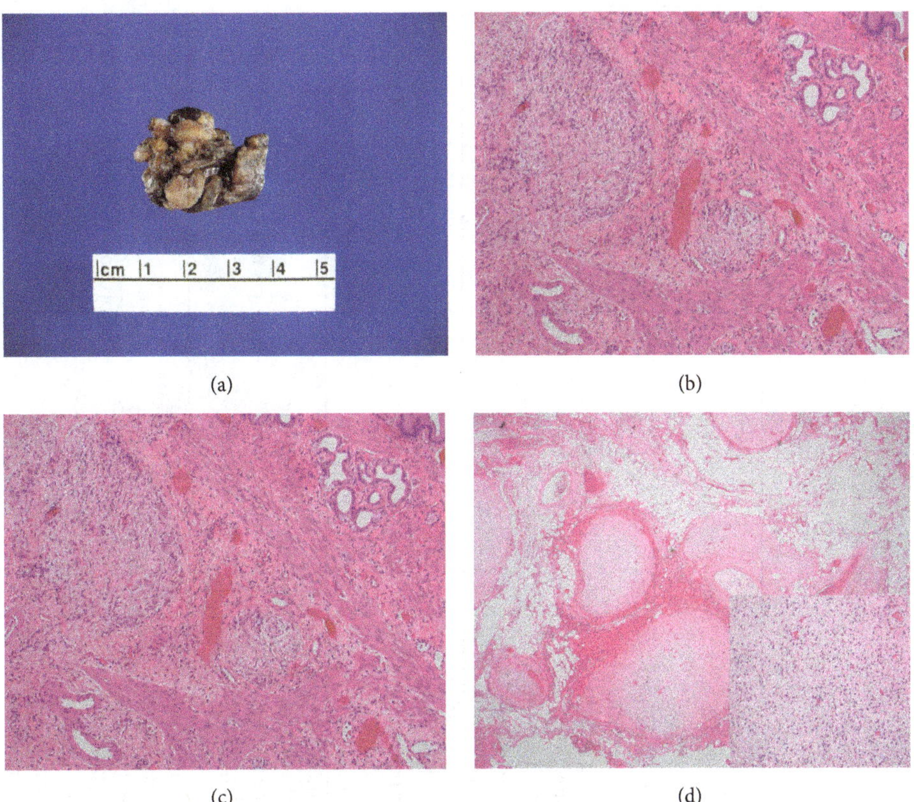

FIGURE 3: (a) Gross morphology of "Mass in Gallbladder." Note the lobulated and nodular overall surface resembling a "bag of worms." The mass measured in total 3.2 × 2.2 × 1.3 cm. (b) Plexiform neurofibroma involving the muscularis propria of the gallbladder wall (H&E, 200x). (c) Higher magnification highlights the loosely arranged spindle shaped cells of plexiform neurofibroma with peripheral entrapment of native ganglion cells (H&E, 400x). (d) Plexiform neurofibroma residing within the fibrofatty tissue adjacent to the gallbladder. (H&E, 200x) (inset) plexiform neurofibroma showing typical histologic findings with loosely arranged comma-shaped nuclei in a myxoid stroma (H&E, 600x).

[8, 9]. These studies were excluded. Two other studies were excluded as one discussed imaging findings only and the other did not provide details on the management of the case [10, 11].

Ten adult patients with PNF of the PH were identified (Table 1) [4, 12–20]. Seven patients had NF-1 [4, 12, 14, 15, 17, 19, 20], 2 had PNF without NF-1, and status of NF-1 was unknown in one patient [13, 16, 18]. Five out of 10 patients underwent conservative management [4, 12, 13, 19, 20]. Resection was attempted in other 5 but only 2 underwent successful en bloc resection [16, 18]. Tumor was removed piecemeal in one patient [15] and found to be unresectable in the other two [14, 17]. Among the 7 patients with PNF of PH and NF-1, resection was not attempted in 4 due to imaging features suggestive of unresectability. Among the remaining 3 patients, tumor was found to be unresectable at exploration in two [14, 17] and could only be removed piecemeal in one patient [15].

We identified 6 articles with PNF of PH in patients < 18 years of age [21–26]. Four studies did not provide management details and were excluded [23–26]. Scheurkogel et al. reported a case of healthy 9-year-old male who underwent a renal ultrasound for intermittent low back pain and was found to have a periportal mass [21]. CT and MRI confirmed a mass in the PH extending into the liver and along the celiac axis. Probable diagnosis was PNF but given absence of family history and other clinical features of NF-1 diagnosis could not be confirmed without a biopsy. An open biopsy was then performed which confirmed PNF without transformation on final pathology (Figure 2). This PNF was thought to be unresectable on imaging and conservative management was appropriately chosen [21]. The largest series of PNF involving PH was reported by Delgado et al. [22]. PNF involving the PH was noted in 5/161 (3.1%) patients with NF-1. These authors suggested that periportal infiltration was the hallmark of PNF involving the liver. Imaging features of pediatric PNF are similar to those in adults. Age of patients varied from 4.1 to 17.8 years with a follow-up of 3 months–8.8 years. All patients were managed conservatively and underwent surveillance as tumors were very extensive and there was no evidence of transformation on MRI [22].

4. Discussion

Abdominal involvement in NF-1 occurs in the form of sporadic neurofibromas versus PNFs which can involve the liver [17, 24], mesentery [25, 27, 28], retroperitoneum [29], and gastrointestinal (GI) tract [30]. The GI involvement occurs in 10–25% of patients with NF-1 presenting as solitary or multiple neurofibromas, leiomyomas, and rarely PNF [30].

Table 1: Summary of case reports of management of PNF involving Porta Hepatis in adults.

S. number	Author	Year	Age (Y)	Gender	NF-1	Clinical presentation	MRI/CT if MRI not available	Treatment approach	Path	Follow-up
(1)	Lee et al.	2016	49	M	Yes	Asymptomatic, incidental findings of portal hypertension on EGD and US	Hypointense T1 lesion and low attenuating mass-like lesion with weak enhancement on T2 images	Medical management with beta-blockers for portal hypertension. Mass thought to be unresectable due to extension into hepatic hilum and lesser omentum	-	-
(2)	Poon et al.	2008	40	M	No	4-5-year history of intermittent upper abdominal pain with nausea and vomiting	T1 hypointense and in homogenously T2 hyperintense	Tumor resected en-bloc	Neurofibroma	1 year
(3)	Ghalib et al.	1995	30	F	Yes	Intermittent right upper quadrant pain	Low attenuating mass encasing the left portal vein, extending into the liver, extending into the gastrohepatic ligament, encasement of hepatic artery up to celiac axis	Exploratory laparotomy. Mass found to be unresectable	Plexiform neurofibroma	-
(4)	Rastogi	2008	35	M	Yes	6-month history of vague abdominal pain	Multiple hypoattenuating masses in the liver, porta hepatis, peripancreatic region and retroperitoneum	Nonsurgical management	-	4 months
(5)	Malagari et al.	2001	24	M	Yes	Asymptomatic, incidentally found on US	7 cm well defined lesion in left hepatic lobe extending into porta hepatis and encasing the hepatic artery and celiac trunk	Exploratory laparotomy. Mass found to be unresectable	Plexiform neurofibroma	-
(6)	Hoshimoto et al.	2009	24	F	Yes	Intermittent abdominal pain	T2 hyperintense tumor involving hepatoduodenal ligament and hepatic hilum, extending along intrahepatic Glisson's sheath	The tumor was resected, leaving behind the intrahepatic extension	Plexiform neurofibroma	3 years
(7)	Ji et al.	2017	54	M	No	3-month history of abdominal pain and weight loss of 3 months	3.6 × 1.7 cm homogenous low-attenuation mass at the porta hepatis with irregular infiltrative margins, encasing and spreading along hepatic artery	Tumor resected; tumor was gradually peeled off from the hepatic artery along the arterial sheath	Plexiform neurofibroma	18 months

Table 1: Continued.

S. number	Author	Year	Age (Y)	Gender	NF-1	Clinical presentation	MRI/CT if MRI not available	Treatment approach	Path	Follow-up
(8)	Gallego et al.	1998	50	M	Unknown	Unknown symptoms. Isolated neurofibromas in the liver, mediastinum, celiac axis and mesentery	Anomalous mesenteric and retroperitoneal tissue extending through hepatoduodenal ligament in to interhepatic periportal spaces. T1 hypointense and T2 hyperintense	Nonsurgical management	Plexiform neurofibroma	2 years
(9)	Rodríguez et al.	1993	24	M	Yes	Vague abdominal complaints	T1 hypointense and T2 hyperintense. Well defined mass around the porta hepatis and its peripheral branches.	Nonsurgical management		5 months
(10)	Chen et al.	1991	18	M	Yes	Presented with PNF of the skull. Liver PNF incidental	Retroperitoneal neurofibroma with extension into the liver along the portal vein	Nonsurgical management	-	3 months

In the GI tract, neurofibromas are most commonly located in the ileum, followed by the jejunum, duodenum, and stomach [30]. Hepatic neurofibroma is a rare entity often associated with extensive abdominal and retroperitoneal involvement. It was reported that the prevalence of intrahepatic lesions was 2.3% of all PNFs involving the abdomen and pelvis [18]. Only a few cases of patients with intra-abdominal PNFs have been reported in the literature [22, 31, 32]. We encountered a challenging case of PNF involving the PH in the clinic and this prompted us to report our findings and review the literature on this rare but complex clinical entity.

PNFs are nonencapsulated tumors which have an interdigitating pattern of growth and can involve the entire plexus [32]. Histologically, neurofibromas are characterized by Schwann cells, perineural-like cells, and fibroblasts, with ovoid-to-spindle-shaped nuclei [31]. PNFs of the PH are extremely rare in incidence [4, 6, 18, 22, 24–26]. Clinical symptoms of PNF at PH are caused by compression of nerves derived from the left vagal trunk and sympathetic plexus causing visceral pain and ductal obstruction [22]. Most often these lesions are discovered incidentally during workup of vague abdominal symptoms. Imaging plays a key role in diagnosis of these tumors. On CT imaging, PNFs appear as multilobulated low-attenuation masses within a major nerve distribution [33]. This low attenuation is due to myxoid and mucinous stroma within these tumors [34]. On MRI, these tumors appear hypointense on T1 weighted images and heterogeneously hyperintense on T2 weighted images. Some of these tumors have a central hypointense region giving a "target sign" type appearance on T2 weighted images [22]. However, definitive diagnosis requires a biopsy.

Grossly, plexiform neurofibromas are large lesions that affect large segments of a nerve and contort it into its characteristic appearance of "bag of worms." Microscopically, it consists of a tortuous mass of enlarged nerve branches which are seen in various planes of cut section. Early stages are characterized by expansion of the endoneurium by myxoid ground substance. With continued growth, spillage of lesional cells occur creating a backdrop of neurofibromatous tissue characterized by interlacing bundles of elongated cells with wavy nuclei intimately associated with wire-like strands of collagen that is separated by small to moderate amounts of mucoid material. The cellular components of neurofibroma consist of varying proportions of Schwann cells, fibroblasts, and peripheral perineural cells with scattered mast cells, lymphocytes, and rare xanthoma cells. Lesions with increased cellularity, atypia, or mitotic figures are at an increased risk for malignant transformation [35].

Currently, there are no specific guidelines for management of PNF involving PH. The most common cause of early death in NF-1 patients is malignant peripheral nerve sheath tumors (MPNST) which most often occur in preexisting PNFs. MPNST have a poor prognosis as they do not respond well to chemotherapy or radiation therapy [36]. Though it was reported that the lifetime risk of malignant transformation to a MPST is 7–13%, the actual transformation rate for intra-abdominal PNFs has not been well described [37]. Given the malignant potential of PNFs, a complete resection is often recommended. This can be achieved in many of the superficially located tumors but not always feasible for tumors located in PH. It is unknown if, extensive resection of deeply situated PNFs is beneficial due to the infiltrating nature and high rate of tumor regrowth [38, 39].

Our findings suggest that in adult patients with NF-1 who have PNF involving PH most of the times the tumor is unresectable on imaging. Even if the tumor appears resectable on imaging, intraoperatively these tumors are found to be unresectable due to intrahepatic extension and extension along the celiac axis. Biopsies can be taken in such instances to rule out transformation. However, it remains unknown if aborted resection with intraoperative biopsies offers any advantage over serial follow-up with MRIs which can help detect transformation as well. Therefore, given the high incidence of intraoperative unresectability in apparently resectable PNF of PH in patients with NF-1, surveillance alone may be a reasonable alternative. Conversely, sporadic PNFs which occur in the absence of NF-1 appear to be more amenable to resection. It can be speculated that the tumors are less extensive in patients with sporadic PNFs compared to those with NF-1 syndrome. PNFs occur as isolated tumors in sporadic cases compared to multiple tumors in those with NF-1. Patients with NF-1 are also at risk for several other malignancies which can prove to be fatal before PNF.

Given the slow growing nature of PNF in general, unknown rate of transformation to malignancy, and high rate of unresectability at exploration, consideration should be given to surveillance alone to assess for growth or development of symptoms. Supporting this approach, Lee et al. reported a case of PNF which infiltrated the lesser sac and hepatic hilum, causing portal hypertension. This patient was treated symptomatically with beta blockers and followed with serial imaging [4]. Delgado et al. have the largest reported experience with PNF of PH. In their series of 5 patients (age < 18 years), all patients were managed conservatively. These lesions remained stable over long-term follow-up (max 8.8 years) [22]. There were no mortalities due to malignant transformation although follow-up is still limited.

In a nice review on malignant peripheral nerve sheath tumors (MPNST), James et al. highlighted the utility of combining PET/CT with CT and MRI to assess for malignant changes [37]. These authors suggested using a SUV max cut-off of 6.1 g/ml (sensitivity 94% and specificity 91%) to differentiate between MPNST and benign nerve sheath tumors [37]. However, none of the studies in the current review used PET/CT for follow-up or surgical decision making. In the opinion of the authors and based on the review of James et al. PET/CT should be part of the radiologic evaluation if surveillance is chosen.

The current study is not without limitations. PNF of PH is a rare condition in general which speaks for the limited number of studies identified. Most of the studies are isolated case reports. An extensive forward search of several databases (PubMed, Scopus, and Web of Science) and backward search from the references of the relevant studies was performed to identify all relevant studies. There are no reports of long-term survival in patients with PNF of PH. This also makes it challenging to assess the risk of malignant transformation at a later time point. Despite the limitations this is the first systematic review focusing on the management of PNF involving the PH

In conclusion, PNFs of the PH are challenging neoplasms. When found in the setting of NF-1 these tumors are often unresectable on imaging. A high incidence of unresectability can be expected at the time of exploration. Given the low or unknown rate of transformation and high incidence of unresectability, surveillance alone can be offered to a subset of patients. The data summarized in the current study can be used to counsel patients at the time of informed consent. If exploration is attempted and unresectability is noted intraoperatively, multiple biopsies can be performed prior to aborting to confirm the diagnosis and rule out transformation. If surveillance is chosen then PET/CT should be combined with CT and MRI to get the most information regarding the biologic behavior of these tumors. Sporadic PNFs of the PH are more likely to be amenable to complete resection. Multidisciplinary management of these tumors should be pursued. We hope that the current study will encourage more authors to report their findings with PNF involving the PH and stimulate further research on these tumors. More studies are needed to evaluate the risk of transformation in these tumors. Given the limited data, a lifelong close follow-up is still recommended. Surveillance alone should be weighed against high incidence of unresectability prior to embarking on surgical management.

References

[1] J. Kresak and M. Walsh, "Neurofibromatosis: A Review of NF1, NF2, and Schwannomatosis," *Journal of Pediatric Genetics*, vol. 05, no. 02, pp. 098–104, 2016.

[2] M.-J. Lee and D. A. Stephenson, "Recent developments in neurofibromatosis type 1," *Current Opinion in Neurology*, vol. 20, no. 2, pp. 135–141, 2007.

[3] K. DeBella, J. Szudek, and J. M. Friedman, "Use of the National Institutes of Health criteria for diagnosis of neurofibromatosis 1 in children," *Pediatrics*, vol. 105, no. 3, pp. 608–614, 2000.

[4] K. H. Lee, S. H. Yoo, G. T. Noh et al., "A case of portal hypertension by presumed as plexiform neurofibroma at the hepatic hilum," *Clinical and Molecular Hepatology*, vol. 22, no. 2, pp. 276–280, 2016.

[5] A. De Rosa, D. Gomez, A. Zaitoun, and I. Cameron, "Neurofibroma of the bile duct: a rare cause of obstructive jaundice," *The Annals of The Royal College of Surgeons of England*, vol. 95, no. 2, pp. e14–e16, 2013.

[6] H. Guo, L. Chen, Z. Wang et al., "Hilar biliary neurofibroma without neurofibromatosis: case report with contrast-enhanced ultrasound findings," *Journal of Medical Ultrasonics*, vol. 43, no. 4, pp. 537–543, 2016.

[7] L. Jiang, L. Yan, N. Cheng, and L. Jiang, "Obstructive jaundice due to primary neurofibroma of the common bile duct," *Digestive and Liver Disease*, vol. 43, no. 1, pp. 85-85, 2011.

[8] S. M. Lederman, E. C. Martin, K. T. Laffey, and J. H. Lefkowitch, "Hepatic neurofibromatosis, malignant schwannoma, and angiosarcoma in von Recklinghausen's disease," *Gastroenterology*, vol. 92, no. 1, pp. 234–239, 1987.

[9] T. L. T. A. Jansen, J. W. R. Meijer, F. O. H. W. Kesselring, and C. J. J. Mulder, "Synchronous hepatic tumours 60 years after diagnostic thorotrast use," *European Journal of Gastroenterology & Hepatology*, vol. 4, no. 9, pp. 753–755, 1992.

[10] E. Salazar, F. Escoto, and L. Salazar, "Necrotizing pancreatitis presenting with hepatic portal venous gas and pneumatosis intestinalis," *International Journal of Hepatobiliary and Pancreatic Diseases*, vol. 4, p. 45, 2014.

[11] M. Sato, H. Ishida, K. Konno et al., "Abdominal involvement in neurofibromatosis 1: Sonographic findings," *Abdominal Imaging*, vol. 25, no. 5, pp. 517–522, 2000.

[12] C. T. Chen, R. W. Kuo, Y. C. Chai, and K. H. Juan, "Huge plexiform neurofibroma of the head and liver–case report," *Gaoxiong Yi Xue Ke Xue Za Zhi*, vol. 7, pp. 650–655, 1991.

[13] J. C. Gallego, P. Galindo, I. Suarez, and J. F. Garcia-Rodriguez, "MR of hepatic plexiform neurofibroma [1]," *Clinical Radiology*, vol. 53, no. 5, pp. 389-390, 1998.

[14] R. Ghalib, T. Howard, J. Lowell et al., "Plexiform neurofibromatosis of the liver: Case report and review of the literature," *Hepatology*, vol. 22, no. 4, pp. 1154–1157, 1995.

[15] S. Hoshimoto, Z. Morise, C. Takeura et al., "Plexiform Neurofibroma in the Hepatic Hilum Associated with Neurofibromatosis Type 1: A Case Report," *Rare Tumors*, vol. 1, no. 1, pp. 44–46, 2009.

[16] G. Ji, K. Wang, C. Jiao, Z. Lu, and X. Li, "Solitary Plexiform Neurofibroma of the Hepatic Artery," *Journal of Gastrointestinal Surgery*, pp. 1-2, 2017.

[17] K. Malagari, S. Drakopoulos, E. Brountzos et al., "Plexiform neurofibroma of the liver: Findings on MR imaging, angiography, and CT portography," *American Journal of Roentgenology*, vol. 176, no. 2, pp. 493–495, 2001.

[18] J. C. Poon, T. Ogilvie, and E. Dixon, "Neurofibroma of the porta hepatis," *Journal of Hepato-Biliary-Pancreatic Sciences*, vol. 15, no. 3, pp. 327–329, 2008.

[19] R. Rastogi, "Intra-abdominal manifestations of von Recklinghausen's neurofibromatosis," *Saudi Journal of Gastroenterology*, vol. 14, no. 2, pp. 80–82, 2008.

[20] E. Rodríguez, F. Pombo, I. Rodríguez, J. L. Vázquez Iglesias, and I. Galed, "Diffuse intrahepatic periportal plexiform neurofibroma," *European Journal of Radiology*, vol. 16, no. 2, pp. 151–153, 1993.

[21] M. Scheurkogel, J. Koshy, K. Cohen, T. Huisman, and T. Bosemani, "Diagnosis and Management of an Isolated Pediatric Plexiform Neurofibroma Involving the Hepatic and Celiac Plexus Using Multimodality Approach: Problem Solving with Diffusion-Weighted Magnetic Resonance Imaging," *European Journal of Pediatric Surgery Reports*, vol. 01, no. 01, pp. 005–008, 2013.

[22] J. Delgado, D. Jaramillo, V. Ho-Fung, M. J. Fisher, and S. A. Anupindi, "MRI features of plexiform neurofibromas involving the liver and pancreas in children with neurofibromatosis type 1," *Clinical Radiology*, vol. 69, no. 6, pp. e280–e284, 2014.

[23] I. Vilas-Ferrol, M. Hernandez-Gimenez, M. I. Moya-Garcia, M. A. Menargues-Irles, C. Munoz-Nunez, and E. Poblet-Martinez, "Intrahepatic plexiform neurofibroma in neurofibromatosis 1," *Pediatric Radiology*, vol. 28, no. 9, p. 733, 1998.

[24] J. S. Partin, B. P. Lane, J. C. Partin, L. R. Edelstein, and C. J. Priebe, "Plexiform neurofibromatosis of the liver and mesentery in a child," *Hepatology*, vol. 12, no. 3, pp. 559–564, 1990.

[25] L. Z. Fenton, N. Foreman, and J. Wyatt-Ashmead, "Diffuse, retroperitoneal mesenteric and intrahepatic periportal plexiform neurofibroma in a 5-year-old boy," *Pediatric Radiology*, vol. 31, no. 9, pp. 637–639, 2001.

[26] Y. Kakitsubata, S. Kakitsubata, T. Sonoda, and K. Watanabe, "Neurofibromatosis type 1 involving the liver: Ultrasound and CT manifestations," *Pediatric Radiology*, vol. 24, no. 1, pp. 66-67, 1994.

[27] K. Matsuki, Y. Kakitsubata, K. Watanabe, H. Tsukino, and K. Nakajima, "Mesenteric plexiform neurofibroma associated with Recklinghausen's disease," *Pediatric Radiology*, vol. 27, no. 3, pp. 255-256, 1997.

[28] J. Park, "Mesenteric plexiform neurofibroma in an 11-year-old boy with von Recklinghausen disease," *Journal of Pediatric Surgery*, vol. 42, no. 6, pp. e15–e18, 2007.

[29] N. Kalra, O. Vijayanadh, A. Lal, N. Khandelwal, K. K. Mukherjee, and S. Suri, "Retroperitoneal plexiform neurofibroma mimicking psoas abscesses," *Journal of Medical Imaging and Radiation Oncology*, vol. 49, no. 4, pp. 330–332, 2005.

[30] F. H. Hochberg, A. B. Dasilva, J. Galdabini, and E. P. Richardson, "Gastrointestinal involvement in von recklinghausen's neurofibromatosis," *Neurology*, vol. 24, no. 12, pp. 1144–1151, 1974.

[31] I. Sucandy, D. Sharma, G. Dalencourt, and D. Bertsch, "Gallbladder neurofibroma presenting as chronic epigastric pain - Case report and review of the literature," *North American Journal of Medical Sciences*, pp. 496–498, 2010.

[32] G. Cavallaro, U. Basile, A. Polistena et al., "Surgical management of abdominal manifestations of type 1 neurofibromatosis: experience of a single center," *The American Surgeon*, vol. 76, no. 4, pp. 389–396, 2010.

[33] S. H. Tirumani, A. K. P. Shanbhogue, R. Vikram, S. R. Prasad, and C. O. Menias, "Imaging of the porta hepatis: Spectrum of disease," *RadioGraphics*, vol. 34, no. 1, pp. 73–92, 2014.

[34] A. M. Halefoglu, "Neurofibromatosis type 1 presenting with plexiform neurofibromas in two patients: MRI features," *Case Reports in Medicine*, vol. 2012, Article ID 498518, 2012.

[35] J. Goldblum. R, Folpe. L. A., Weiss. W. S., Enzinger. M. F., and Weiss. S. W., *Benign Tumors of Peripheral Nerves*, Saunders/Elsevier, Philadelphia, 2014, 798-804.

[36] B. R. Korf, "Malignancy in neurofibromatosis type 1," *The Oncologist*, vol. 5, no. 6, pp. 477–485, 2000.

[37] A. W. James, E. Shurell, A. Singh, S. M. Dry, and F. C. Eilber, "Malignant Peripheral Nerve Sheath Tumor," *Surgical Oncology Clinics of North America*, vol. 25, no. 4, pp. 789–802, 2016.

[38] M. N. Needle, A. Cnaan, and J. Dattilo, "Prognostic signs in the surgical management of plexiform neurofibroma: the children's hospital of Philadelphia experience, 1974–1994," *Journal of Pediatrics*, vol. 131, no. 5, pp. 678–682, 1997.

[39] R. Nguyen, C. Ibrahim, R. E. Friedrich, M. Westphal, M. Schuhmann, and V.-F. Mautner, "Growth behavior of plexiform neurofibromas after surgery," *Genetics in Medicine*, vol. 15, no. 9, pp. 691–696, 2013.

29

Gallbladder Carcinoma in the United States: A Population Based Clinical Outcomes Study Involving 22,343 Patients from the Surveillance, Epidemiology, and End Result Database (1973–2013)

Christine S. M. Lau,[1,2] **Aleksander Zywot,**[1,2] **Krishnaraj Mahendraraj,**[1] **and Ronald S. Chamberlain**[1,2,3,4]

[1] *Department of Surgery, Saint Barnabas Medical Center, Livingston, NJ, USA*
[2] *School of Medicine, Saint George's University, True Blue, Grenada*
[3] *Department of Surgery, Banner MD Anderson Cancer Center, Gilbert, AZ, USA*
[4] *Department of Surgery, New Jersey Medical School, Rutgers University, Newark, NJ, USA*

Correspondence should be addressed to Ronald S. Chamberlain; ronald.chamberlain@bannerhealth.com

Academic Editor: Attila Olah

Introduction. Gallbladder carcinoma (GBC) is the most common malignancy of the biliary tract and the third most common gastrointestinal tract malignancy. This study examines a large cohort of GBC patients in the United States in an effort to define demographics, clinical, and pathologic features impacting clinical outcomes. *Methods.* Demographic and clinical data on 22,343 GBC patients was abstracted from the SEER database (1973–2013). *Results.* GBC was presented most often among Caucasian (63.9%) females (70.7%) as poorly or moderately differentiated (42.5% and 38.2%) tumors, with lymph node involvement (88.2%). Surgery alone was the most common treatment modality for GBC patients (55.0%). Combination surgery and radiation (10.6%) achieved significantly longer survival rates compared to surgery alone (4.0 ± 0.2 versus 3.7 ± 0.1 years, $p = 0.004$). Overall mortality was 87.0% and cancer-specific mortality was 75.4%. *Conclusions.* GBC is an uncommon malignancy that presents most often among females in their 8th decade of life, with over a third of cases presenting with distant metastasis. The incidence of GBC has doubled in the last decade concurrent with increases in cholecystectomy rates attributable in part to improved histopathological detection, as well as laparoscopic advances and enhanced endoscopic techniques. Surgical resection confers significant survival benefit in GBC patients.

1. Introduction

Gallbladder carcinoma (GBC) is the most common malignancy of the biliary tract and third most common gastrointestinal tract malignancy [1, 2]. While a majority of patients are asymptomatic and are diagnosed incidentally following cholecystectomy for gallstones, some patients present with advanced disease with vague abdominal symptoms including abdominal pain and discomfort [2–6]. The incidence of GBC is especially high among South America, affecting 27 per 100,000 people [1]. The high rates of GBC in South America and Asia including Pakistan, Korea, and Japan have been attributed to high rates of cholecystitis and salmonella infection, both of which are known risk factors for GBC [7, 8]. Although gallbladder carcinoma is much less prevalent in North America compared to Asia, it is still associated with an extremely poor prognosis [5, 6].

Given the low rates of GBC in North American, most existing knowledge regarding GBC is derived primarily from studies conducting in South America and Asia. This study examines a large cohort of gallbladder carcinoma patients in the United States (US) in an effort to define the demographics, clinical, and pathologic features impacting clinical outcomes in American GBC patients.

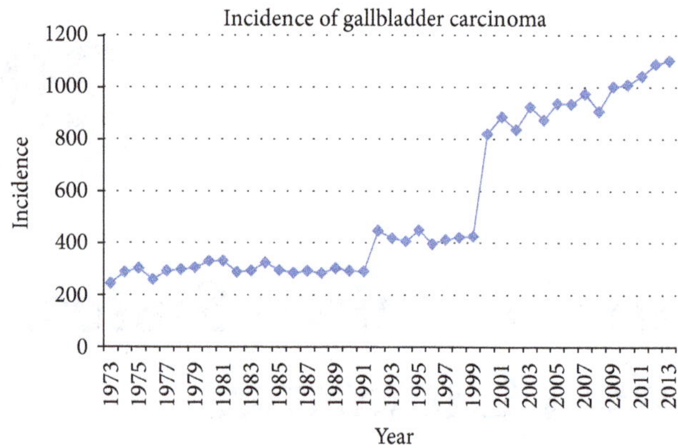

FIGURE 1: Annual cases of gallbladder carcinoma from the Surveillance, Epidemiology, and End Result (SEER) database (1973–2013).

2. Methods

Data for the current study was extracted from the Surveillance, Epidemiology, and End Result (SEER) database provided by the National Cancer Institute between 1973 and 2013. SEER Stat software version 8.0.4 was utilized to extract data from 18 SEER registries (Alaska Native Tumor Registry, Arizona Indians, Cherokee Nation, Connecticut, Detroit, Georgia Center for Cancer Statistics, Greater Bay Area Cancer Registry, Greater California, Hawaii, Iowa, Kentucky, Los Angeles, Louisiana, New Jersey, New Mexico, Seattle-Puget Sound, and Utah).

22,343 patients with GBC were identified using the SEER International Classification of Disease for Oncology (ICD-O-3) codes C23.9 [9]. Demographic and clinical data extracted included age, gender, race, tumor grade, lymph node involvement, and type of treatment received (surgery, radiation, both, or unknown/no treatment) [9]. Outcomes examined included mortality and cancer-specific mortality. *Chi*-square test was used to compare categorical data, and Student's t-test and analysis of variance (ANOVA) were used for continuous data. Multivariate analysis was performed and odds ratios (OR) were calculated to determine independent factors affecting survival. Long-term actuarial survival between groups was compared using Kaplan Meier analysis. Data was analyzed using IBM SPSS®v23 and statistical significance was accepted at the level of $p < 0.05$ [10].

3. Results

3.1. Demographic Data. A total of 22,343 cases of GBC were reported in the SEER database from 1973 to 2013. The number of GBC cases increased from approximately 200 cases per year in the 1970s to >1,000 cases per year after 2010, with a significant spike in 2000 (Table 1 and Figure 1). The average age at diagnosis was 71.2 ± 12.5 years (Table 2). GBC was significantly more common among females (70.7% versus 29.3%), with a female-to-male ratio of 2.41 : 1. A majority of GBC cases occurred among Caucasians (63.9%), followed by Hispanics (16.8%), African Americans (9.2%), and Asian/Pacific Islanders (1.7%). Most of the reported cases occurred in the Pacific Coast (43.0%), followed by the East (29.9%), Northern Plains (18.9%), Southwest (8.0%), and Alaska region (0.2%).

TABLE 1: Annual cases of gallbladder carcinoma from the Surveillance, Epidemiology, and End Result (SEER) database (1973–2013).

Year	New cases
1973	246
1974	289
1975	304
1976	261
1977	294
1978	299
1979	306
1980	331
1981	332
1982	289
1983	294
1984	325
1985	296
1986	287
1987	294
1988	285
1989	304
1990	294
1991	292
1992	447
1993	419
1994	407
1995	449
1996	397
1997	414
1998	422
1999	426
2000	820
2001	886
2002	837
2003	924
2004	874
2005	937
2006	935
2007	975
2008	907
2009	1,002
2010	1,009
2011	1,042
2012	1,089
2013	1,103

3.2. Tumor Characteristics. Most cases of GBC presented as poorly differentiated tumors (42.5%), followed by moderately differentiated (38.2%), well differentiated (15.3%),

TABLE 2: Demographics and clinical profile of 22,343 patients with gallbladder carcinoma from the Surveillance, Epidemiology, and End Result (SEER) database (1973–2013).

Variables	Frequency (%)
N	22,343
Age, years (mean ± SD)	71.17 ± 12.534
Gender, N (%)	
Male	6,549 (29.3%)
Female	15,794 (70.7%)
Region, N (%)	
Alaska	46 (0.2%)
East	6,684 (29.9%)
Northern Plains	4,230 (18.9%)
Pacific Coast	9,605 (43.0%)
Southwest	1,778 (8.0%)
Race, N (%)**	
Caucasian	14,280 (64.0%)
African American	2,056 (9.2%)
Hispanic	3,740 (16.8%)
Asian/Pacific Islander	1,861 (8.3%)
American Indian/Alaska Native	375 (1.7%)
Grade, N (%)**	
Well differentiated	2,252 (15.3%)
Moderately differentiated	5,619 (38.2%)
Poorly differentiated	6,238 (42.5%)
Undifferentiated	592 (4.0%)
Lymph node involvement, N (%)**	
Yes	15,791 (88.2%)
No	2,105 (11.8%)
Treatment received, N (%)**	
No treatment	6,811 (31.8%)
Surgery only	11,769 (55.0%)
Radiation only	545 (2.6%)
Both surgery and radiation	2,269 (10.6%)
Actuarial survival, years (mean ± SE)	2.715 ± 0.061
Actuarial survival by treatment, years (mean ± SE)	
No treatment	0.618 ± 0.049
Surgery only	3.685 ± 0.093
Radiation only	0.815 ± 0.075
Both surgery and radiation	4.029 ± 0.184
Actuarial survival by grade, years (mean ± SE)	
Well differentiated	5.926 ± 0.266
Moderately differentiated	3.720 ± 0.151
Poorly differentiated	1.664 ± 0.073
Undifferentiated	1.293 ± 0.167
Overall mortality, N (%)	19,439 (87.0%)
Cancer specific mortality, N (%)	16,856 (75.4%)
Cumulative survival, %	
3-month	66%
6-month	50%
9-month	41%
1-year	34%
2-year	22%
3-year	17%

TABLE 2: Continued.

Variables	Frequency (%)
4-year	14%
5-year	13%

N = number; SD = standard deviation; SE = standard error; ** data presented for patients with available information only.

TABLE 3: Survival outcomes of 22,343 patients with gallbladder carcinoma from the Surveillance, Epidemiology, and End Result (SEER) database (1973–2013).

	Overall	Surgery alone	Radiation alone	Both surgery and radiation	Neither
Actuarial survival by treatment, years (mean ± SE)	2.715 ± 0.061	3.685 ± 0.093	0.815 ± 0.075	4.029 ± 0.184	0.618 ± 0.049
Cumulative survival, %					
3-month	66%	75%	76%	96%	42%
6-month	50%	61%	50%	84%	23%
9-month	41%	51%	32%	72%	14%
1-year	34%	44%	29%	60%	10%
2-year	22%	31%	21%	35%	5%
3-year	17%	24%	6%	26%	3%
4-year	14%	21%	3%	21%	2%
5-year	13%	18%	2%	18%	2%

SE = standard error.

and undifferentiated (4.0%) tumors. Most patients presented with lymph node involvement (88.2%).

3.3. *Treatment.* Surgical resection alone was the most common treatment modality (55.0%). Surgical resection and adjuvant radiation were utilized by 10.6%, while radiation alone was used in 2.6% of patients. 31.8% of patients received neither surgery nor radiation. The number of GBC treated with surgery increased in the 1980s, with a concomitant decrease in patients receiving no treatment (Figure 2).

3.4. *Outcomes.* Overall survival was 2.72 ± 0.06 years. Surgical resection was associated with significantly improved survival (3.69 ± 0.09 years) compared to patients receiving no treatment (0.62 ± 0.05 years) or radiation alone (0.82 ± 0.08 years) (Table 3). Surgical resection and adjuvant radiation were associated with a slightly longer survival compared to surgical resection alone (4.03 ± 0.18 years versus 3.69 ± 0.09 years, $p < 0.01$). Kaplan Meier estimates also demonstrated prolonged survival for patients receiving surgical resection with or without adjuvant radiation (Figure 3).

When stratified by tumor grade, well differentiated tumors had the longest survival (5.93 ± 0.27 years), followed by moderately differentiated (3.72 ± 0.15 years), poorly differentiated (1.66 ± 0.07 years), and undifferentiated (1.29 ± 0.17 years) tumors.

Overall mortality was 87.0% and cancer-specific mortality was 75.4%. Cumulative survival remained low, and 1-, 2-, and 5-year survival were 34%, 22%, and 13%, respectively.

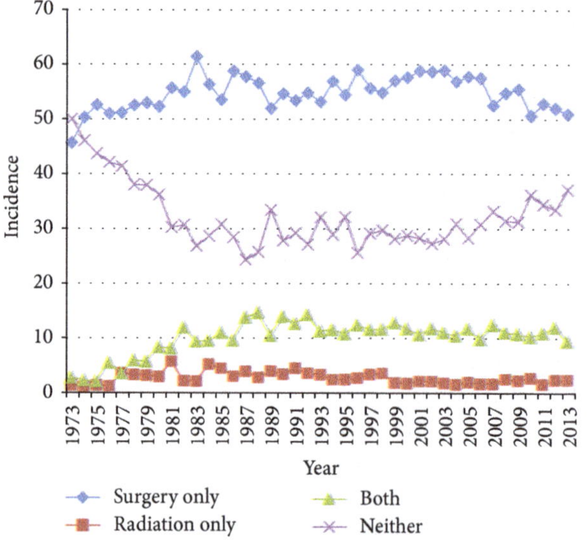

FIGURE 2: Trends in the treatment modalities utilized for gallbladder carcinoma from the Surveillance, Epidemiology, and End Result (SEER) database (1973–2013).

3.5. *Multivariate Analysis.* Multivariate analysis identified moderately differentiated (OR 1.43; 95% CI, 1.27–1.61), poorly differentiated (OR 3.10; 95% CI, 2.72–3.54), and undifferentiated (OR 3.10; 95% CI, 2.26–4.25) tumors as independently associated with increased mortality, $p < 0.05$. Conversely, surgical resection (OR 0.406; 95% CI, 0.311–0.529) and combined surgery and radiation (OR 0.321; 95% CI, 0.242–0.426) were associated with reduced mortality, $p < 0.05$.

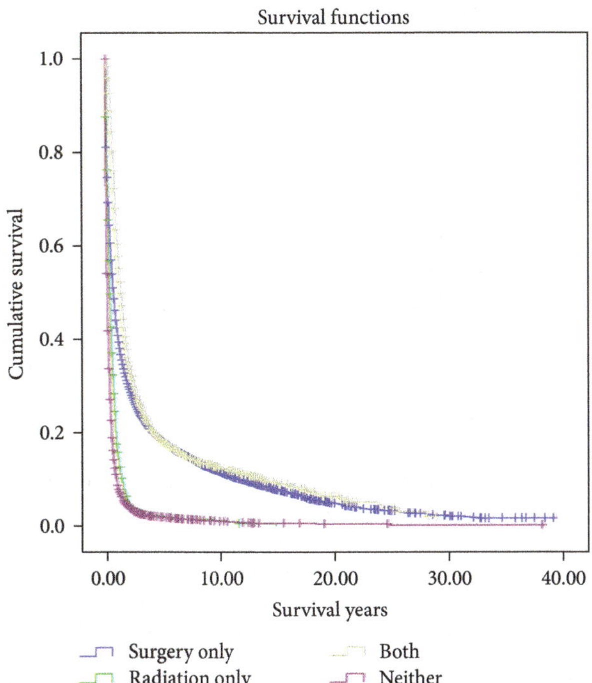

FIGURE 3: Kaplan Meier curves illustrating actuarial survival for patients with gallbladder carcinoma from the Surveillance, Epidemiology, and End Results database (1973–2013).

4. Discussion

GBC is an aggressive malignancy associated with multiple etiologies and high mortality [1, 8]. Despite being the most common biliary tract malignancy and the fifth most common gastrointestinal cancer, GBC is rare [2]. The overall incidence of GBC worldwide varies greatly from 1.5 per 100,000 in North America to as high as 27 per 100,000 in South America [1].

The large variation in incidence worldwide is due to a combination of exposure to environmental risk factors and heritable genetic traits [1, 3]. The incidence of GBC increases with age, ranging from 1.47 per 100,000 people aged 50–64 years to 4.91 per 100,000 people aged 65–74 years, and 8.69 per 100,000 people over 75 years [3]. In this study, the mean age at diagnosis was 71.2 ± 12.6 years, mirroring previous studies with a mean age of 64–69.4 years [2, 3, 11].

Female gender increases the risk of GBC by twofold to sixfold [12]. In the current study, GBC was significantly more common among females with a female-to-male ratio of 2.41 : 1. Although, female gender is associated with a higher risk of GBC, its effect varies based on ethnicity and geographies [1]. The female-to-male ratio of GBC has been reported to be as high as 3.0 : 1 among Hispanics, compared to 1.28 : 1 in African American populations [1]. Early studies on GBC have also noted increased incidence in multiparous females, suggesting a link between GBC and hormone levels [8]. Further studies have found estrogen and progestin receptors in GBC [3].

The most significant risk factor for GBC is gallstones (relative risk (RR) = 3.0–23.8) and is present in the majority (69–85%) of patients [3, 13]. Stones irritate gallbladder mucosa resulting in inflammation, which may eventually results in carcinogenesis [3]. Patients with chronic gallstones, defined as present for 20 or more years, have an increased risk of GBC (OR = 6.2–12.1) [3]. Stone size has also been shown to contribute to an increased risk of GBC, with stones larger than 3 cm increasing risk by over ninefold (RR = 9.2–10.1) [3].

The prognosis of GBC is extremely poor, most often due to its late diagnosis. Patients with GBC in this study often had advanced stage and grade by the time of diagnosis. The majority of patients presented with either poorly (42.5%) or moderately (38.2%) differentiated disease, and over 85% of patients had lymph node involvement.

The extensive progression of disease can be explained at least in part due to the difficulty in diagnosis [2]. Patients with GBC frequently have nonspecific symptoms such as vague abdominal pain and discomfort [3]. Common complaints include constitutional symptoms, anorexia, and weight loss progressing to painless jaundice [3, 14]. Furthermore, disease progression occurs silently over years [15].

GBC most commonly arises due to the dysplasia-carcinoma sequence but can occasionally occur due to polyps and adenoma-carcinoma progression [1, 14, 16]. Progression from metaplasia to dysplasia may require up to ten years and the development of carcinoma in situ an additional five years [1]. Metaplasia most commonly arises due to inflammation caused by chronic gallstone irritation [14]. Inflammation then leads to increased expression of COX2 and inhibition of tumor suppressor genes such as p53 [14, 17, 18].

The near silent and chronic progression of GBC results in many diagnoses (70%) detected incidentally [2]. Patients with GBC are commonly operated upon for diseases such as gallstones, cholecystitis, or polyps and the cancer is discovered incidentally with a frequency of 0.2% to 3.0% of all cholecystectomies [2, 3]. The recent adoption of laparoscopic surgeries has led to an increase in the frequency of cholecystectomies and therefore an increase in GBC diagnosis [2, 19–22]. This is most apparent in this study in the years between 2000 and 2010, as the number of cholecystectomies and surgical resections doubled.

The tragic consequence of incidental discovery and late diagnosis is a one-year survival of 34%, a cumulative five-year survival of 13%, and a mean overall survival of only 2.7 years. Previous studies have specifically recognized extended disease and the number of positive lymph nodes as important predictors of worsening outcomes [23]. Factors associated with extended disease such as moderately and poorly differentiated tumors are independently associated with increased mortality for GBC.

Surgical resection is the standard of care for GBC patients [24]. In localized disease, simple cholecystectomy may be sufficient, and several studies have demonstrated similar survival with cholecystectomy compared to more radical extended resections [24–27]. In advance disease however, reresection after a simple cholecystectomy or radical resection is associated with significantly improved mortality [25, 28].

The use of radiation as a treatment modality alone has inferior survival rates compared to surgical resection and is typically used in combination with chemotherapy when surgery is not feasible [29]. In the current study, patients undergoing radiation alone survived 9.8 months compared to 3.7 years with surgical resection. The addition of radiation to surgical therapy improved overall survival by a little more than 3 months (4.0 versus 3.7 years with surgical resection alone). Hoehn et al. (2015) conducted a study involving 6,690 GBC patients from the American College of Surgeons National Cancer Data Base and reported that adjuvant chemoradiation significantly improved survival (Hazard Ratio (HR) = 0.77; 95% CI, 0.66–0.90), while adjuvant chemotherapy did not affect survival [30].

Future improvements in therapy are focused on individual processes of carcinogenesis [14]. Current studies are investigating use of small molecule pathway inhibitors and monoclonal antibodies [3, 14, 24]. Several small clinical trials utilizing monoclonal antibodies targeting epidermal growth factor receptor (EGFR), vascular endothelial growth factor receptor (VEGFR), human epidermal growth factor receptor 2 (HER2), and multikinase inhibitors such as sorafenib have been completed or are on-going with demonstrable evidence of treatment effect and improved survival [14].

There are several limitations to this study which need to be considered. The SEER database does not accurately code all clinical factors which may affect patient survival. Secondly, information on chemotherapy received was not provided in detail, limiting this study's ability to evaluate the effect of adjuvant or neoadjuvant therapy. There may also be an element of selection bias, since SEER registries are more likely to sample from urban than from rural areas. Despite these limitations, the SEER database has data obtained a representative sample of the US population and therefore these findings can be generalized to the overall population.

5. Conclusions

GBC is an uncommon malignancy that presents most often among females in their 8th decade of life, with advanced stage of disease and lymph node involvement. The incidence of GBC has doubled in the last decade concurrent with increases in cholecystectomy rates attributable in part to improved histopathological detection, as well as laparoscopic advances and enhanced endoscopic techniques. Surgical resection confers significant survival benefit in GBC patients. The role of radiation therapy remains controversial, and adjuvant radiation therapy in addition to surgical resection has been shown to confer a small survival advantage. Despite treatment, overall and cancer-specific survival remains low. Given its rarity, all GBC patients should be enrolled in clinical trials or registries to optimize treatment and clinical outcomes for these patients.

References

[1] E. C. Lazcano-Ponce, J. F. Miquel, N. Muñoz et al., "Epidemiology and Molecular Pathology of Gallbladder Cancer," *CA: A Cancer Journal for Clinicians*, vol. 51, no. 6, pp. 349–364, 2001.

[2] A. Cavallaro, G. Piccolo, M. Di Vita et al., "Managing the incidentally detected gallbladder cancer: Algorithms and controversies," *International Journal of Surgery*, vol. 12, supplement 2, pp. S108–S119, 2014.

[3] R. Hundal and E. A. Shaffer, "Gallbladder cancer: epidemiology and outcome," *Clinical Epidemiology*, vol. 6, no. 1, pp. 99–109, 2014.

[4] T. Goetze and V. Paolucci, "Does laparoscopy worsen the prognosis for incidental gallbladder cancer?" *Surgical Endoscopy and Other Interventional Techniques*, vol. 20, no. 2, pp. 286–293, 2006.

[5] M. Isambert, C. Leux, S. Métairie, and J. Paineau, "Incidentally-discovered gallbladder cancer: when, why and which reoperation?" *Journal of visceral surgery*, vol. 148, no. 2, pp. e77–84, 2011.

[6] M. Utsumi, H. Aoki, T. Kunitomo et al., "Evaluation of surgical treatment for incidental gallbladder carcinoma diagnosed during or after laparoscopic cholecystectomy: single center results," *BMC Research Notes*, vol. 10, no. 1, article 56, 2017.

[7] B. L. Strom, R. D. Soloway, J. L. Rios-Dalenz et al., "Risk factors for gallbladder cancer. An international collaborative case–control study," *Cancer*, vol. 76, no. 10, pp. 1747–1756, 1995.

[8] G. Randi, S. Franceschi, and C. La Vecchia, "Gallbladder cancer worldwide: geographical distribution and risk factors," *International Journal of Cancer*, vol. 118, no. 7, pp. 1591–1602, 2006.

[9] C. S. M. Lau, K. Mahendraraj, and R. S. Chamberlain, "Hepatocellular carcinoma in the pediatric population: a population based clinical outcomes study involving 257 patients from the surveillance, epidemiology, and end result (SEER) Database (1973--2011)," *HPB Surgery*, vol. 2015, Article ID 670728, 2015.

[10] C. S. M. Lau, A. Ward, and R. S. Chamberlain, "Probiotics improve the efficacy of standard triple therapy in the eradication of Helicobacter pylori: a meta-analysis," *Infection and Drug Resistance*, vol. 9, pp. 275–289, 2016.

[11] D. Fuks, J. M. Regimbeau, Y.-P. Le Treut et al., "Incidental gallbladder cancer by the AFC-GBC-2009 study group," *World Journal of Surgery*, vol. 35, no. 8, pp. 1887–1897, 2011.

[12] I. T. Konstantinidis, V. Deshpande, M. Genevay et al., "Trends in presentation and survival for gallbladder cancer during a period of more than 4 decades: a single-institution experience," *Archives of Surgery*, vol. 144, no. 5, pp. 441–447, 2009.

[13] L. M. Stinton and E. A. Shaffer, "Epidemiology of gallbladder disease: cholelithiasis and cancer," *Gut and Liver*, vol. 6, no. 2, pp. 172–187, 2012.

[14] E. I. Marks and N. S. Yee, "Molecular genetics and targeted therapeutics in biliary tract carcinoma," *World Journal of Gastroenterology*, vol. 22, no. 4, pp. 1335–1347, 2016.

[15] C. Ferreccio, "Salmonella typhi and Gallbladder Cancer," in *Bacteria and Cance*, A. A. Khan, Ed., pp. 117–137, Springer, Dordrecht, The Netherlands, 2011.

[16] V. Trivedi, V. V. Gumaste, S. Liu, and J. Baum, "Gallbladder cancer: adenoma-carcinoma or dysplasia-carcinoma sequence?" *Gastroenterology and Hepatology*, vol. 4, no. 10, pp. 735–737, 2008.

[17] M. Moreno, F. Pimentel, A. F. Gazdar, I. I. Wistuba, and J. F. Miquel, "TP53 abnormalities are frequent and early events in

the sequential pathogenesis of gallbladder carcinoma," *Annals of Hepatology*, vol. 4, no. 3, pp. 192–199, 2005.

[18] T. Asai, E. Loza, G. V.-G. Roig et al., "High frequency of TP53 but not K-ras gene mutations in Bolivian patients with gallbladder cancer," *Asian Pacific Journal of Cancer Prevention*, vol. 15, no. 13, pp. 5449–5454, 2014.

[19] S. B. Choi, H. J. Han, C. Y. Kim et al., "Incidental gallbladder cancer diagnosed following laparoscopic cholecystectomy," *World Journal of Surgery*, vol. 33, no. 12, pp. 2657–2663, 2009.

[20] W.-J. Zhang, G.-F. Xu, and X.-P. Zou, "Incidental gallbladder carcinoma diagnosed during or after laparoscopic cholecystectomy," *World Journal of Surgery*, vol. 33, no. 12, pp. 2651–2656, 2009.

[21] J. Sujata, S. Rana, K. Sabina, M. J. Hassan, and S. J. Zeeba, "Incidental gall bladder carcinoma in laparoscopic cholecystectomy: a report of 6 cases and a review of the literature," *Journal of Clinical and Diagnostic Research*, vol. 7, no. 1, pp. 85–88, 2013.

[22] X. A. de Aretxabala, I. S. Roa, J. P. Mora et al., "Laparoscopic cholecystectomy: its effect on the prognosis of patients with gallbladder cancer," *World Journal of Surgery*, vol. 28, no. 6, pp. 544–547, 2004.

[23] T. B. Tran and N. N. Nissen, "Surgery for gallbladder cancer in the US: a need for greater lymph node clearance," *Journal of Gastrointestinal Oncology*, vol. 6, no. 5, pp. 452–458, 2015.

[24] T. A. Aloia, N. Járufe, M. Javle et al., "Gallbladder Cancer: expert consensus statement," *HPB*, vol. 17, no. 8, pp. 681–690, 2015.

[25] S. P. Shih, R. D. Schulick, J. L. Cameron et al., "Gallbladder Cancer: the role of laparoscopy and radical resection," *Annals of Surgery*, vol. 245, no. 6, pp. 893–901, 2007.

[26] D. M. Hari, J. H. Howard, A. M. Leung, C. G. Chui, M.-S. Sim, and A. J. Bilchik, "A 21-year analysis of stage I gallbladder carcinoma: is cholecystectomy alone adequate?" *HPB*, vol. 15, no. 1, pp. 40–48, 2013.

[27] S. E. Lee, J.-Y. Jang, C.-S. Lim, M. J. Kang, and S.-W. Kim, "Systematic review on the surgical treatment for T1 gallbladder cancer," *World Journal of Gastroenterology*, vol. 17, no. 2, pp. 174–180, 2011.

[28] G. Nigri, G. Berardi, C. Mattana et al., "Routine extra-hepatic bile duct resection in gallbladder cancer patients without bile duct infiltration: a systematic review," *Surgeon*, vol. 14, no. 6, pp. 337–344, 2016.

[29] G. Delaney, M. Barton, and S. Jacob, "Estimation of an optimal radiotherapy utilization rate for gastrointestinal carcinoma: a review of the evidence," *Cancer*, vol. 101, no. 4, pp. 657–670, 2004.

[30] R. S. Hoehn, K. Wima, A. E. Ertel et al., "Adjuvant therapy for gallbladder cancer: an analysis of the national cancer data base," *Journal of Gastrointestinal Surgery*, vol. 19, no. 10, pp. 1794–1801, 2015.

30

Feasibility of Comparing the Results of Pancreatic Resections between Surgeons: A Systematic Review and Meta-Analysis of Pancreatic Resections

Kurinchi Gurusamy,[1] Clare Toon,[2] Bhavisha Virendrakumar,[3] Steve Morris,[4] and Brian Davidson[1]

[1]*Department of Surgery, UCL Medical School, Royal Free Campus, London NW3 2PF, UK*
[2]*Public Health Research Unit, West Sussex County Council, County Hall Campus, West Sussex PO19 1QT, UK*
[3]*Evidence Synthesis, Sightsavers, 35 Perrymount Road, Haywards Heath, West Sussex RH16 3BW, UK*
[4]*Department of Applied Health Research, UCL, London WC1E 7HB, UK*

Correspondence should be addressed to Kurinchi Gurusamy; kurinchi2k@hotmail.com

Academic Editor: Attila Olah

Background. Indicators of operative outcomes could be used to identify underperforming surgeons for support and training. The feasibility of identifying HPB surgeons with poor operative performance ("outliers") based on the results of pancreatic resections is not known. *Methods.* A systematic review of Medline, Embase, and the Cochrane library was performed to identify studies on pancreatic resection including at least 100 patients and published between 2004 and 2014. Proportions that lay outside the upper 95% and 99.8% confidence intervals based on results of the systematic reviews were considered as "outliers." *Results.* In total, 30 studies reporting on 10712 patients were eligible for inclusion in this review. The average short-term mortality after pancreatic resections was 3.1% and proportion of patients with procedure-related complications was 47.0%. None of the classification systems assessed the long-term impact of the complications on patients. The surgeon-specific mortality should be 5 times the average mortality before he or she can be identified as an outlier with 0.1% false positive rate if he or she performs 50 surgeries a year. *Conclusions.* A valid risk prognostic model and a classification system of surgical complications are necessary before meaningful comparisons of the operative performance between pancreatic surgeons can be made.

1. Background

Indicators of operative outcomes could be used to identify underperforming surgeons for support and training. Pancreatic resection is one of the most common major operative procedures performed by Hepato-Pancreato-Biliary (HPB) surgeons. As the procedure is complex with a high associated morbidity and mortality, it may be suitable for comparing the operative performances of HPB surgeons. The major indication for pancreatic resection is pancreatic cancer, the seventh most common cause of cancer-related mortality in the world, resulting in approximately 330 000 deaths worldwide annually [1]. Pancreatic cancer is a biologically aggressive cancer, which is relatively resistant to chemotherapy and radiotherapy and has a high rate of local and systemic recurrence [2–4]. In early pancreatic cancer (with no invasion of adjacent structures such as the superior mesenteric vein, portal vein, or superior mesenteric artery or distal metastases), surgical resection is generally considered the only treatment with the potential for long-term survival and possibility of cure in people likely to withstand major surgery. The overall five-year survival after radical resection ranges from 7% to 25% [4–9], with a median survival of 11 to 15 months [10]. With adjuvant chemotherapy, median survival after radical resection is increased and ranges between 14 and 24 months [11]. However, it should be noted that about half of the patients presenting with pancreatic cancer will have metastatic disease and one-third have locally advanced unresectable disease, leaving about 10% to 20% suitable for resection [12].

Another major indication for pancreatic resection is chronic pancreatitis, a condition associated with long-standing and progressive inflammation of the pancreas resulting in destruction and replacement of pancreatic tissue with fibrous tissue leading to exocrine pancreatic insufficiency and endocrine pancreatic insufficiency (diabetes) [13]. The annual incidence of chronic pancreatitis ranges from 1.5 to 7.9 per population of 100,000 [14–18]. The prevalence of chronic pancreatitis ranges from 17 to 49 per population of 100,000 [15, 16, 18]. The annual mortality rate attributable to chronic pancreatitis is around 1 to 4 per million people [15, 17]. There is no consensus among experts for selecting patients for surgical management but pancreatic pain and other local complications are the major indications for surgical treatment [19]. Other indications for pancreatic resection include ampullary cancers, distal common bile duct cancers, duodenal cancers, intraductal papillary mucinous neoplasm, and neuroendocrine tumours [20–23].

Pancreatic resection is in the form of pancreaticoduodenectomy for cancers of the head of the pancreas, ampullary cancers, distal common bile duct cancers, and duodenal cancers and distal pancreatectomy for cancers of the body and tail of the pancreas [24]. Pancreaticoduodenectomy involves excision of the head of the pancreas and duodenum. The two major types are the classical Whipple operation and the pylorus preserving pancreatoduodenectomy [25]. Surgical excision for chronic pancreatitis can be performed by pancreaticoduodenectomy (standard Whipple's operation or pylorus preserving pancreaticoduodenectomy) or by duodenum preserving pancreatic head resection [19, 26]. Duodenum preserving pancreatic head resection involves resection of the pancreatic head without excision of duodenum. The two major types are Beger's operation and Frey's procedure [26]. The latter involves a drainage procedure anastomosing the duct in the pancreatic remnant to the jejunum by longitudinal pancreatojejunostomy in addition to pancreatic head excision leaving behind a cuff of pancreas on the duodenal wall [26].

In general, pancreaticoduodenectomy is performed by open surgery, although laparoscopic pancreaticoduodenectomy has been reported [27]. Laparoscopic pancreatic resection is more common for distal pancreatectomy [28]. After resection of the body and tail of the pancreas, the cut surface of the pancreatic remnant (pancreatic stump) is closed using staples or sutures [29].

In England, individual surgeon's results of surgery-related complications are being published as part of the drive by NHS England to improve transparency [30, 31] and to allow patients to make informed decisions. This allows patients to identify outliers (a consultant whose clinical outcomes data lies outside the expected range given the national average) [31] and make an informed decision as to whether they would like to be treated by that particular surgeon. The feasibility of identifying HPB surgeons with poor operative performance based on the results of pancreatic resections is not known but it may be the most suited for comparison as the procedures are common and complex and are generally associated with a high morbidity and mortality. The main objectives of this research are to conduct a systematic review of the recent results of pancreatic resections so that it is possible to establish a benchmark for surgeon's performance based on international standards and to assess the feasibility of comparing the results of pancreatic resections between surgeons based on the results of the systematic review.

2. Methods

2.1. Selection of Studies. All studies that reported on pancreatic resections irrespective of whether they were pancreaticoduodenectomies or distal pancreatectomy, the reason for the pancreatic resection (cancer or benign disease), the type of access (open or laparoscopic), the type of anastomosis (pancreaticogastrostomy or pancreatojejunostomy), and the postoperative care provided to the patients were included. Only studies including at least 100 patients, published as full texts or conference abstracts in the previous 10 years from the search date (February 2014), and reporting one or more of the primary outcomes (30-day or in-hospital mortality) or secondary outcomes (12-month mortality, proportion of people with complications, number of complications, the classification system used to report the complications, operating time, and length of hospital stay) were included in the review to ensure that only the recent results on a reasonable number of patients were included in the analysis. Studies were identified by searching Medline, Embase, and the Cochrane library using the Medical Subject Headings (MeSH) search terms "pancreatectomy," "pancreaticoduodenectomy," and "pancreaticojejunostomy." Equivalent free text search terms were used and equivalent search strategies were used in other databases. The search strategies are available in the Appendix. No language restrictions were applied.

Two authors (Clare Toon and Bhavisha Virendrakumar) independently screened titles and abstracts. Full texts were obtained for references that at least one author identified as potentially meeting the inclusion criteria. Further selection was made independently by two authors (Clare Toon and Bhavisha Virendrakumar) by reviewing the full texts. All differences were resolved by discussion and arbitration by another author (Kurinchi Gurusamy).

2.2. Data Collection. Data on patient characteristics including the demographic details, case-mix (risk prognostic models or score to take into account the different anaesthetic and surgical risks in patients), and outcomes were extracted by two authors (Clare Toon and Bhavisha Virendrakumar) independently. Foreign language articles were translated to English before data extraction. When significant overlap of patients between two or more reports was identified based on the authors, centres, and the time period, the report that contained maximum information with regard to the outcomes was included for the analysis. All differences in data extraction were resolved by discussion and arbitration by another author (Kurinchi Gurusamy).

2.3. Meta-Analysis. Meta-analysis was performed using StatsDirect statistical software using a random-effects model. The summary estimates with 95% confidence intervals (CI) have been reported. Heterogeneity was assessed by Higgin's I-square [32] and chi-square test for heterogeneity. Despite exploration of heterogeneity by various subgroup analyses including the reason for pancreatic resection (cancer versus other causes), type of resection (pancreaticoduodenectomy versus distal pancreatic resection), and method of access (laparoscopic versus open access), the data available from the studies were insufficient to allow meaningful subgroup analyses. Publication bias was assessed by funnel plot and Egger's regression test [33].

2.4. Assessment of Feasibility of Comparing the Operative Performance. The short-term mortality and complications which would have been attributable to an individual surgeon for a hypothetical cohort of people undergoing pancreatic resection were calculated based on the summary estimate of the meta-analysis, the lower quartile, and the upper quartile of the proportions observed for these outcomes in the systematic review, thus extrapolating the results of the meta-analysis to an average surgeon. The 95% and 99.8% confidence intervals of these outcomes were calculated using the Wilson score method with continuity correction [34] for samples sizes of 50, 100, and 200 (approximately 1 pancreatic resection a week, 2 pancreatic resections a week, and 4 pancreatic resections a week). Proportions that lay outside the upper 95% and 99.8% confidence limits were considered as outliers with a one-sided false positive rate of 2.5% and 0.1%, respectively. The 95% and 99.8% confidence limits are equivalent to the surgeon having results which are different by two standard deviations and three standard deviations from the average results expected based on the data ("the benchmark"). One-sided false positive rate was calculated since the upper limit of the confidence interval was the main interest of the study; that is, if surgeon-specific mortality and complications were lower than the confidence limits, it was not of any interest since these surgeons are better than other surgeons and there are no concerns on their operative performance.

3. Results

3.1. Search Results. A total of 7193 references were identified by database search. After removing duplicate citations, a total of 6268 unique references were identified. Full text was sought for 41 references [20–23, 35–71]. A total of 6 full texts were excluded (4 studies had less than 100 patients in total [66–69]; one reference was a comment on an excluded article [70]; and one study did not contain any outcomes included in this review [71]). Five references were duplicate reports of other studies or contained a significant proportion of patients included in other reports [61–65]. Data from these studies was not included in the analysis to avoid the same patients being counted multiple times. In total, 30 studies reporting on 10712 patients were eligible for inclusion in this review [20–23, 35–60]. The reference flow is shown in Figure 1.

3.2. Characteristics of Included Studies. The number of patients included in each study, the number and proportion of patients with malignancy, the mean age of patients, the number and proportion of female patients, and different groups within the cohort as reported by the study authors have been tabulated in Table 1. The number of patients included in each study varied from 100 to 2610 patients. Three studies included only patients with chronic pancreatitis [36, 38, 53]. One study included only patients with malignancy [37]. The remaining studies included various proportions of patients with malignancy. The mean age of patients reported in the studies ranged from 42 years to 68 years. Case-mix was assessed using surgical Apgar score (SAS) in one study [39]. None of the remaining studies reported any adjustment for case-mix. The surgical details of patients in terms of the surgeries and the surgical access included in the studies have been tabulated in Table 2. Only three studies included patients undergoing laparoscopic pancreatic resection [20, 22, 41]. It is likely that most of the patients or all the patients in the other studies underwent open pancreatic resection.

3.3. Outcomes

3.3.1. Short-Term Mortality. Short-term mortality (30-day or in-hospital mortality) was reported in 21 studies including 6727 patients [21, 23, 35, 36, 38, 39, 41, 42, 44–48, 50–55, 58]. The 30-day or in-hospital mortality ranged between 0.6% and 10.6% (lower quartile = 1.6%; upper quartile = 4.7%). The mortality proportions in individual studies are shown in Figure 2. The average mortality was 3.1% (95% CI 2.4% to 3.9%; I^2 = 59.6%). There was no evidence of publication bias by Egger's regression test (P = 0.1866).

Depending upon the proportion of short-term mortality used (the meta-analysis summary estimate, lower quartile, or upper quartile), sample size (50, 100, or 200), and the false positive rate (2.5% versus 0.1% for a surgeon to be wrongly identified as an outlier), a surgeon will be called an outlier only when the surgeon-specific mortality is several times the average mortality (Table 3). For example, the surgeon-specific mortality should be more than 5 times the average mortality before he or she can be identified as an outlier with 0.1% false positivity rate (i.e., results lie outside three standard deviations of the average results expected from a surgeon) if he or she performs 50 surgeries a year.

3.3.2. 12-Month Mortality. Twelve-month mortality was reported in 7 studies including 1549 patients [22, 36, 40, 49, 56, 57, 59]. The 12-month mortality ranged between 0.0% and 8.2% (lower quartile = 0.9%; upper quartile = 3.3%). The mortality proportions in individual studies are shown in Figure 3. The average mortality was 2.2% (95% CI 0.7% to 4.5%; I^2 = 83.7%). There was no evidence of publication bias by Egger's regression test (P = 0.1174).

3.3.3. Complications. Complications were reported variably in different studies. Five studies reported complications using the Clavien-Dindo method [72, 73] of classification of complications [20, 37, 39, 48, 60]. One study used the Accordion severity grading system [74] of classification of complications [22]. Two studies used "common terminology criteria for adverse events" system [75] of classification of complications [50, 57]. The remaining studies did not use any specific system of classification of complications.

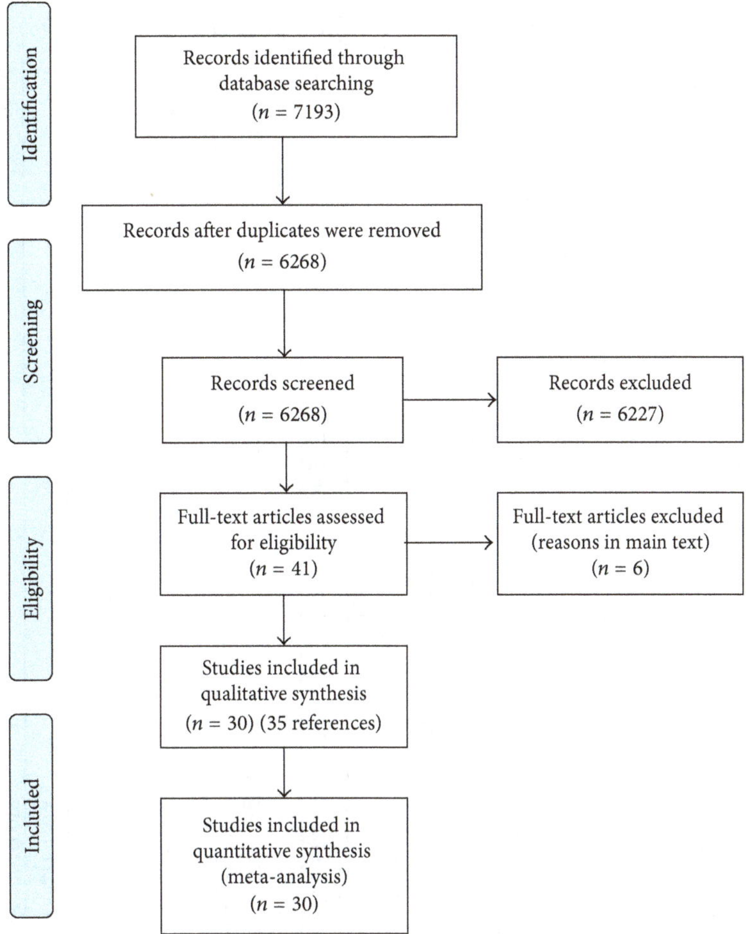

FIGURE 1: Reference flow. Reference flow showing the study selection [77].

The proportion of people with complications was reported in 23 studies including 6712 patients [20, 21, 23, 35–41, 43, 45–50, 52, 54–57, 60]. The proportion of people with complications ranged between 3.3% and 100.0% (lower quartile = 38.3%; upper quartile = 53.4%). The proportions of people with complications in individual studies are shown in Figure 4. The average proportion of people with complications was 47.0% (95% CI 36.0% to 59.0%; I^2 = 98.9%). There was significant publication bias as denoted by Egger's regression test (P = 0.0037) with the funnel plot suggesting that studies with lower complication proportions were more likely to be published.

With regard to comparing the performance of surgeons, a surgeon will be identified as an outlier with 0.1% false positive rate when the proportion of patients who develop complications following surgery by him or her is 1.4 times that of the average even if he or she performs 50 surgeries a year as shown in Table 3.

The number of complications (as opposed to the proportion of people with complications) was reported in 18 studies including 4763 patients [22, 35, 37, 38, 40, 42, 44–49, 52, 54, 55, 57–59]. The number of complications per 100 patients ranged between 40 and 132 (lower quartile = 61 per 100 patients; upper quartile = 95 per 100 patients). The numbers of complications per 100 patients in individual studies are shown in Figure 5. The average number of complications per 100 patients was 80 (95% CI 70 to 90; I^2 = 94.3%). There was no evidence of publication bias by Egger's regression test (P = 0.4189).

3.3.4. Operating Time. The average operating time was reported as mean or median in 22 studies including 5475 patients [20–22, 36, 39–41, 44–49, 52–60]. A meta-analysis was not performed because of insufficient data (i.e., mean and standard deviation were not reported adequately in many studies). The mean or median operating time in the studies ranged between 230 minutes and 492 minutes (median = 337 minutes; lower quartile = 279 minutes; upper quartile = 419 minutes).

3.3.5. Hospital Stay. The average hospital stay was reported as mean or median in 24 studies including 7385 patients [20–23, 35, 36, 38, 40–43, 45–48, 50–52, 54, 55, 57–60]. As for operating time, meta-analysis was not performed for hospital stay because of insufficient data. The mean or median hospital stay in the studies ranged between 6 days and 31 days (median = 15 days; lower quartile = 11 days; upper quartile = 17 days).

TABLE 1: Population characteristics.

Study ID	Number of patients	Cancers (percentage)	Groups* Group 1	Group 2	Group 3	Numbers in each group Group 1	Group 2	Group 3	Average age in years	Females (percentage)
Abu-Hilal et al. 2010 [35]	100	Not reported	Feeding through percutaneous jejunostomy feeding tube	Feeding through percutaneous transgastric jejunal feeding tube	Feeding through nasojejunal feeding tube	25	32	43	67	45 (45%)
Adams et al. 2013 [36]	102	0 (0%)	Total pancreatectomy with islet autotransplant	—	—	102	—	—	42	79 (77.5%)
Addeo et al. 2014 [37]	1325	1325 (100%)	Pancreaticogastrostomy	Pancreaticojejunostomy	—	733	563	—	65	754 (56.9%)
Adham et al. 2013 [20]	242	Not reported	Drain	No drain	—	130	112	—	62	115 (47.5%)
Alexakis et al. 2004 [38]	112	0 (0%)	Opioid use prior to surgery	No opioid use prior to surgery	—	66	46	—	46	35 (31.3%)
Aranha et al. 2006 [21]	396	168 (42.4%)	Pancreaticoduodenectomy	Distal pancreatectomy with splenectomy	—	396	86	—	67	169 (42.7%)
Asbun and Stauffer 2012 [22]	268	130 (48.5%)	Open procedure	Laparoscopic procedure	—	215	53	—	66	144 (53.7%)
Assifi et al. 2012 [39]	597	Not reported	Pancreaticoduodenectomy	Suspension pancreatic duct-jejunum end-to-side continuous suture anastomosis	—	553	65	—	64	284 (47.6%)
Barnett and Collier 2006 [23]	104	85 (81.7%)	Patients undergoing pancreaticoduodenectomy	—	—	104	—	—	63	47 (45.2%)
Bassi et al. 2005 [40]	163	89 (54.6%)	Pancreaticogastrostomy	Pancreaticojejunostomy	—	69	82	—	57	56 (34.4%)
Beane et al. 2011 [41]	230	63 (27.4%)	Endoscopic ultrasound	No endoscopic ultrasound	Distal pancreatectomy	179	51	—	60	143 (62.2%)
Bedi et al. 2011 [42]	248	Not reported	Pancreaticojejunostomy	Pancreaticogastrostomy	—	126	122	—	Not reported	Not reported
Del Chiaro et al. 2012 [43]	367	Not reported	Overweight or obese	Normal weight	—	141	226	—	Not reported	Not reported
Dong et al. 2013 [44]	165	156 (94.5%)	End-to-end/end-to-side invaginated anastomosis	End-to-side mucosal anastomosis	Suspension pancreatic duct-jejunum end-to-side continuous suture anastomosis	52	48	65	51	50 (30.3%)
El Nakeeb et al. 2013 [45]	442	Not reported	Cirrhotic liver	Noncirrhotic liver	—	67	375	—	53	165 (37.3%)
Fang et al. 2007 [46]	377	319 (84.6%)	Pancreaticojejunostomy	Pancreaticogastrostomy	—	188	189	—	68	116 (30.8%)
Fathy et al. 2008 [47]	216	Not reported	Pancreaticoduodenal resection	—	—	216		—	54	85 (39.4%)
Figueras et al. 2013 [48]	130	104 (80%)	Duct-to-duct pancreaticojejunostomy	Double-layer invaginated pancreaticogastrostomy	—	58	65	—	66	42 (32.3%)
Fischer et al. 2010 [49]	209	85 (40.7%)	Acute normovolemic haemodilution	Standard intraoperative management	—	65	65	—	65	61 (29.2%)
Fisher et al. 2011 [50]	100	Not reported	Nasogastric tubes removed in the early postoperative period	Nasogastric tubes removed in the operating room at the conclusion of surgery	—	50	50	—	62	56 (56%)
Haigh et al. 2011 [51]	2610	1828 (70%)	Younger (patients aged under 70 years)	Elder (patients aged over 70 years)	—	1633	799	—	64	1330 (51%)
Kleespies et al. 2009 [52]	182	160 (87.9%)	Cattell-Warren pancreaticojejunostomy	Blumgart anastomosis	—	90	92	—	66	77 (42.3%)
Liu and Zheng 2010 [53]	123	0 (0%)	Pancreaticoduodenectomy	Duodenum preserving pancreatic head resection	—	57	66	—	Not reported	Not reported
Oussoultzoglou et al. 2004 [54]	250	175 (70%)	Pancreaticogastrostomy	Pancreaticojejunostomy	—	167	83	—	59	96 (38.4%)
Peng et al. 2007 [55]	261	194 (74.3%)	Binding pancreaticojejunostomy	Conventional pancreaticojejunostomy	—	106	111	—	52	100 (38.3%)
Qin et al. 2013 [56]	582	Not reported	Pancreaticoduodenectomy		—	582	—	—	Not reported	Not reported
Ross et al. 2013 [57]	200	108 (54%)	No perioperative transfusion	Perioperative transfusion	—	164	36	—	64	113 (56.5%)
Tran et al. 2004 [58]	170	Not reported	Standard Whipple	Pylorus preserving pancreaticoduodenectomy	—	83	87	—	63	62 (36.5%)
Wellner et al. 2012 [59]	267	121 (45.3%)	Pancreaticogastrostomy	Pancreaticojejunostomy	—	59	57	—	66	60 (22.5%)
Williams et al. 2009 [60]	174	172 (71.7%)	Normal weight	Overweight	Obese	103	71	66	65	123 (70.7%)

*Groups according to the way the authors divided the patients.

TABLE 2: Surgery details.

Study ID	Laparoscopic*	Open*	Whipple	Pylorus preserving pancreaticoduodenectomy	Distal pancreatectomy
Abu-Hilal et al. 2010 [35]	Not stated	Not stated	Yes	No	No
Adams et al. 2013 [36]	Not stated	Not stated	Not stated	Not stated	Not stated
Addeo et al. 2014 [37]	Not stated	Not stated	Not stated	Yes	Not stated
Adham et al. 2013 [20]	Yes	Yes	Yes	Yes	Yes
Alexakis et al. 2004 [38]	Not stated	Not stated	Yes	Yes	No
Aranha et al. 2006 [21]	Not stated	Not stated	Yes	Yes	No
Asbun and Stauffer 2012 [22]	Yes	Yes	Yes	Yes	No
Assifi et al. 2012 [39]	Not stated	Not stated	Yes	Yes	No
Barnett and Collier 2006 [23]	Not stated	Not stated	Not stated	Not stated	Not stated
Bassi et al. 2005 [40]	Not stated	Not stated	Not stated	Yes	Not stated
Beane et al. 2011 [41]	Yes	Yes	No	No	Yes
Bedi et al. 2011 [42]	Not stated	Not stated	Yes	No	No
Del Chiaro et al. 2012 [43]	Not stated	Not stated	Not stated	Not stated	Not stated
Dong et al. 2013 [44]	Not stated	Not stated	Not stated	Not stated	Not stated
El Nakeeb et al. 2013 [45]	Not stated	Not stated	Yes	Yes	No
Fang et al. 2007 [46]	Not stated	Not stated	Yes	Yes	Not stated
Fathy et al. 2008 [47]	Not stated	Not stated	Yes	Yes	Not stated
Figueras et al. 2013 [48]	Not stated	Not stated	Yes	Yes	No
Fischer et al. 2010 [49]	Not stated	Not stated	Yes	Yes	Not stated
Fisher et al. 2011 [50]	Not stated	Not stated	Yes	Yes	Yes
Haigh et al. 2011 [51]	Not stated	Not stated	Yes	Yes	Not stated
Kleespies et al. 2009 [52]	Not stated	Not stated	Yes	Yes	Not stated
Liu and Zheng 2010 [53]	Not stated	Not stated	Not stated	Not stated	Not stated
Oussoultzoglou et al. 2004 [54]	Not stated	Not stated	Yes	Yes	Not stated
Peng et al. 2007 [55]	No	Yes	Yes	Yes	Not stated
Qin et al. 2013 [56]	Not stated	Not stated	Not stated	Not stated	Not stated
Ross et al. 2013 [57]	Not stated	Not stated	Not stated	Not stated	Not stated
Tran et al. 2004 [58]	Not stated	Not stated	Yes	Yes	No
Wellner et al. 2012 [59]	Not stated	Not stated	Yes	Yes	Not stated
Williams et al. 2009 [60]	Not stated	Not stated	Yes	Yes	Not stated

*It is likely that the studies that do not report on whether the surgeries were performed by open or laparoscopic method are likely to include open access surgeries.

4. Discussion

In this systematic review and meta-analysis, the recent results of pancreatic resections have been reviewed. Despite significant advances in anaesthetic and surgical techniques in the recent years, pancreatic resection remains a major surgery with significant risk of complications and mortality. The average 30-day or in-hospital mortality after pancreatic resection was approximately 3% (Figure 2) and approximately 47% of patients undergoing pancreatic resection develop one or more complications (Figure 4). However, there was significant variation in the mortality and the complications as evidenced by the I^2 values which demonstrated substantial statistical heterogeneity. The average 12-month mortality was 2.2% (Figure 3) which was less than the average 30-day mortality of 3.1%. This is not clinically possible but was observed in this systematic review because of different studies being included for the different time points. This is further evidence of heterogeneity in mortality between the studies.

One possible reason for this observed heterogeneity in the results is the inclusion of different types of surgeries in different studies. Another possible reason is that the patients included in the different studies had different comorbidities and there was variation in the technical difficulty of surgery ("case-mix"). Use of prognostic models is one of the commonly used methods to adjust for case-mix. A number of prognostic models are available for risk adjustment in pancreatic resections [76], although the accuracy of these models has not been assessed systematically. Only one of the studies included in this review considered a risk prognostic

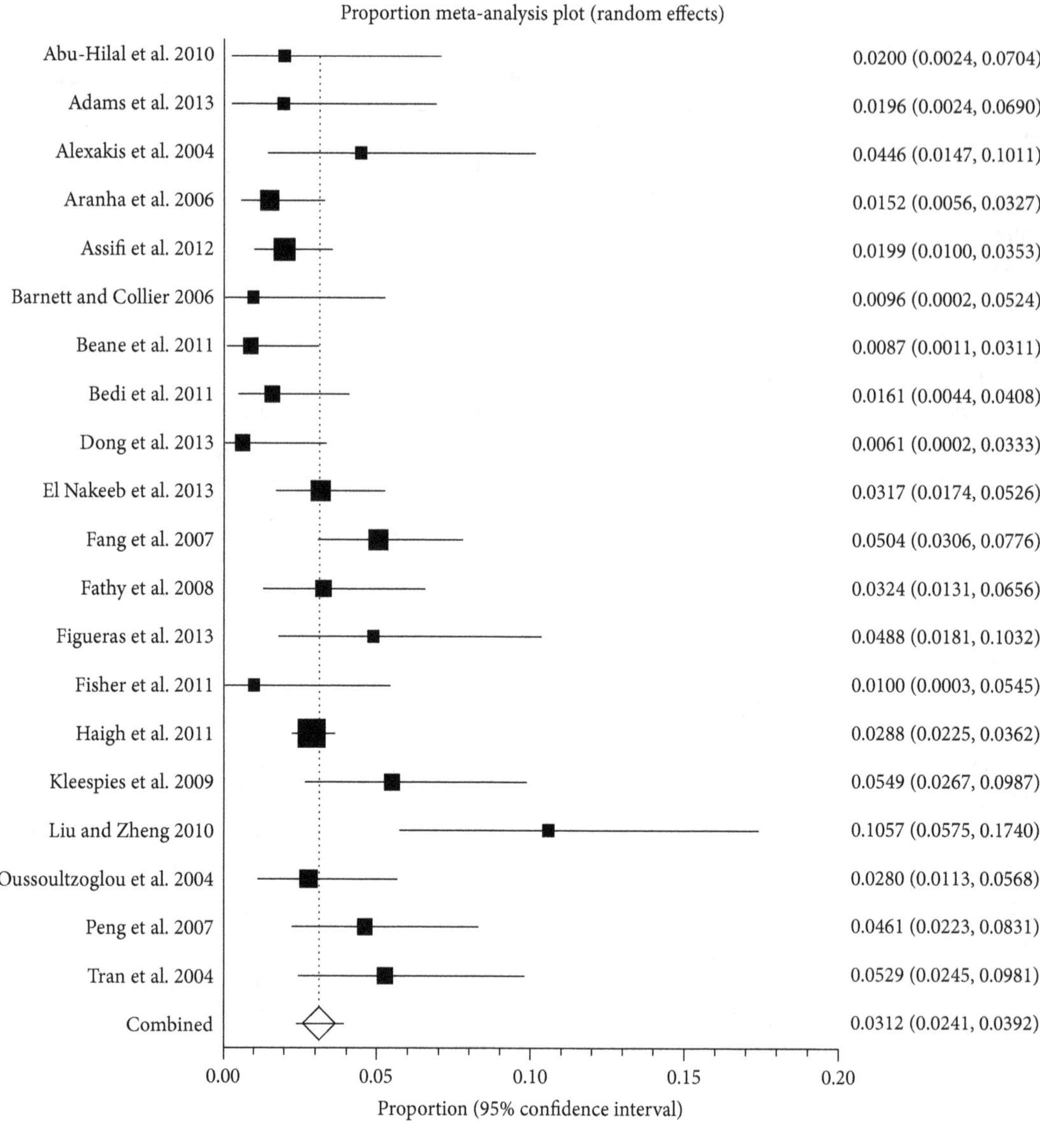

FIGURE 2: 30-day or in-hospital mortality. The figure shows the forest plot of 30-day or in-hospital mortality. The mortality ranged between 0.6% and 10.6%. The average mortality by random-effects model was 3.1%.

model to adjust for case-mix [39]. While the authors used surgical Apgar score as the risk prognostic model, it was not reliable in this study [39].

Prognostic models to adjust for case-mix are essential for comparative audit between specialists to ensure that surgeons are not penalised for accepting to operate on high-risk patients where there is evidence of potential patient benefit. In addition, adequate adjustment for the case-mix is necessary to allow indirect comparison of results obtained in different studies. Thus, a reliable method of adjustment for case-mix (risk prognostic model) is necessary for pancreatic resections.

With regard to complications, in addition to the types of pancreatic resections and case-mix contributing to the heterogeneity in the estimates obtained in the different studies, another reason for heterogeneity is the different methods of classifying complications.

While the mortality rate of 3% is a high perioperative mortality rate, it does not allow comparison of the surgical performance as the surgeon-specific mortality has to be more than 5 times the average mortality before the surgeon is identified as an outlier with 0.1% false positive rate if he or she performs 50 pancreatic resections a year (Table 3). Fifty pancreatic resections per year equates to an average of one resection a week and few surgeons are likely to perform more than this. Thus, using short-term mortality does not appear to be a sensitive way of comparing the performance of HPB or pancreatic surgeons. If, on the other hand, complication rates were used to compare surgeons, an outlier will be identified if the proportion of patients who develop complications following surgery by him or her is only 1.4 times the average complication rates (with 0.1% false positive rate if he or she performs 50 pancreatic resections a year). An evaluation of complication rates following pancreatic resection would therefore

TABLE 3: Identification of outliers.

Outcome and proportion	Sample size	Outlier (2.5% false positive)	Outlier (0.1% false positive)
Mortality: meta-analysis summary (3.1%)	50	>12.2%	>16.7%
	100	>8.6%	>11.2%
	200	>6.5%	>8.1%
Mortality: lower quartile (1.6%)	50	>9.9%	>14.4%
	100	>6.4%	>9.0%
	200	>4.5%	>5.9%
Mortality: upper quartile (4.7%)	50	>14.4%	>19.0%
	100	>10.8%	>13.5%
	200	>8.6%	>10.2%
Complications: meta-analysis summary (47.0%)	50	>60.5%	>64.4%
	100	>56.7%	>59.6%
	200	>53.9%	>56.0%
Complications: lower quartile (38.3%)	50	>52.1%	>56.4%
	100	>48.1%	>51.2%
	200	>45.2%	>47.4%
Complications: upper quartile (53.4%)	50	>66.5%	>70.1%
	100	>62.9%	>65.6%
	200	>60.2%	>62.2%

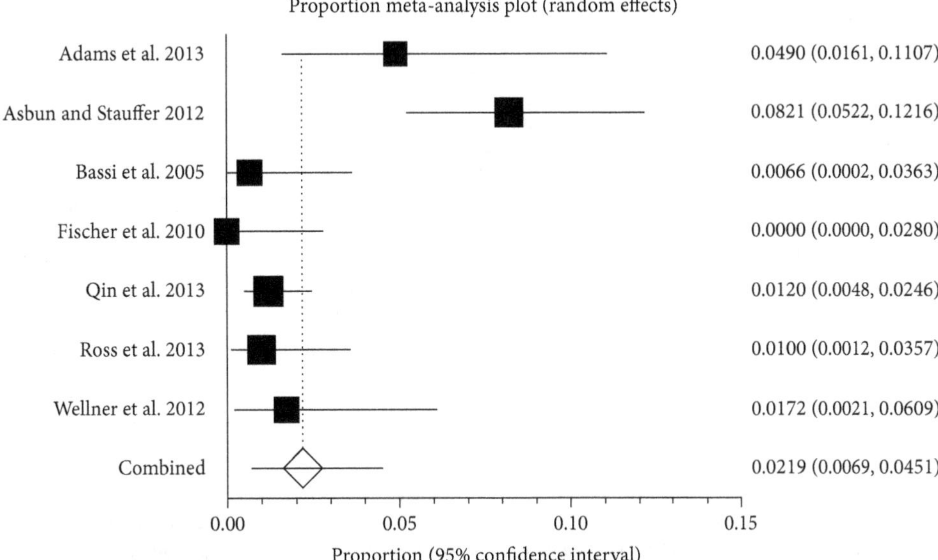

FIGURE 3: 12-month mortality. The figure shows the forest plot of 12-month mortality. The mortality ranged between 0.0% and 8.2%. The average mortality by random-effects model was 2.2%.

allow the comparison of operative performance of surgeons with a reasonable sensitivity. However, the major problem with using complications as the benchmark for assessing surgeons is that they will also depend on the case-mix of the patient cohort. In addition, none of the current classification systems for complications adequately distinguish between complications that result in permanent disability as opposed to those that do not result in permanent disability. While some of these systems include reinterventions and requirement for organ support while classifying complications [72–74], the cost implications of these individual complications to the healthcare funder are not clear. Thus, the existing systems of classification of complications which have been applied to major pancreatic surgery do not appear to be patient outcome oriented or funder oriented and cannot therefore be used as benchmark for assessing surgical performance.

Health-related quality of life (HRQoL) using a validated quality of life scale may be a suitable way of comparing the long-term outcomes of surgeons but is not sensitive enough to capture the severity of the early postoperative complications. This is because the HRQoL is usually impaired immediately after major surgery and hence those developing

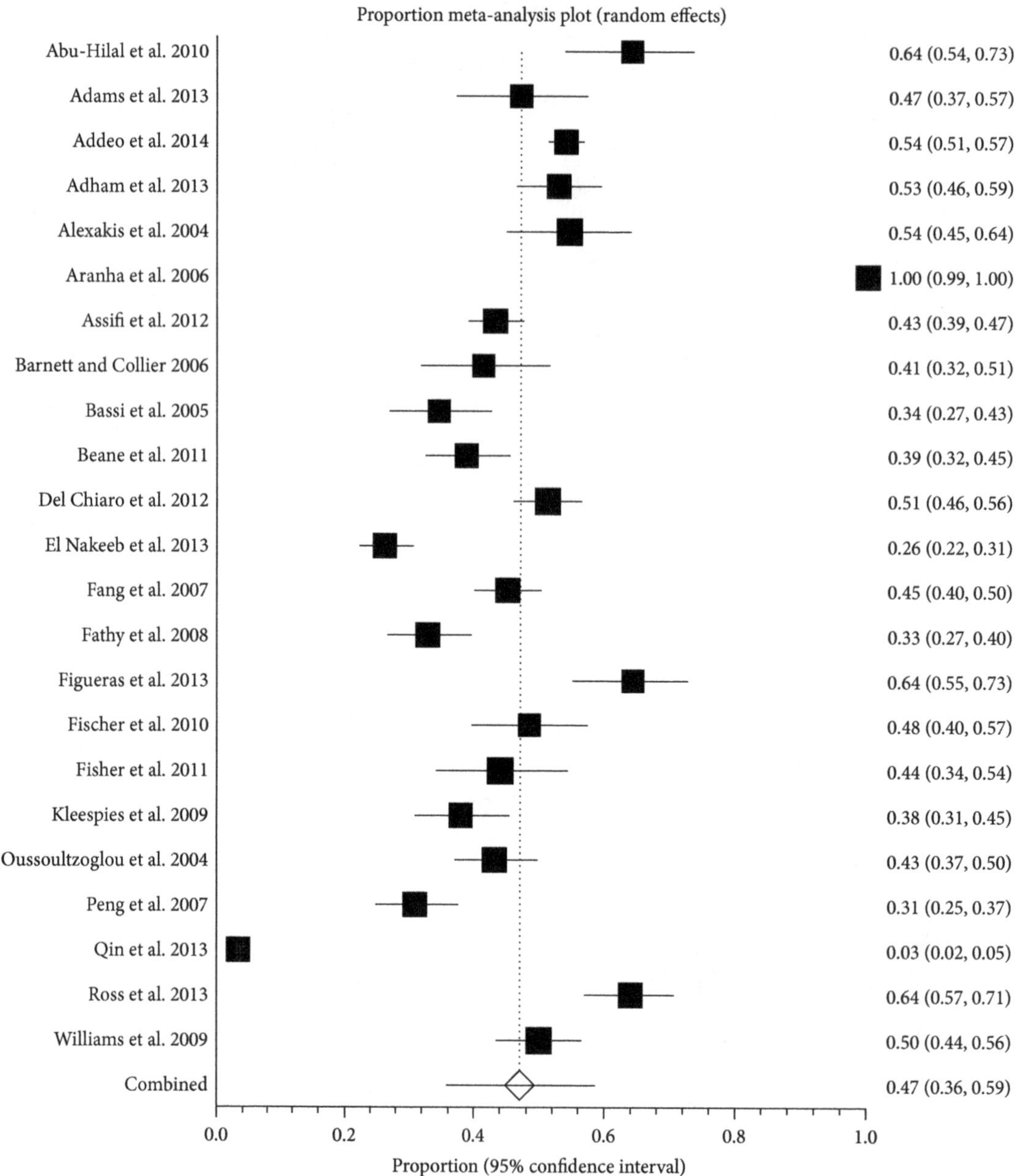

FIGURE 4: Proportion of patients with complications. The figure shows the forest plot of patients with complications. The proportion of people with complications ranged between 3.3% and 100.0%. The average proportion of complications by random-effects model was 47.0%.

major complications shortly after surgery may not have a significant change from the baseline (observed in people without complications) because of the low baseline values. In addition, measurement of long-term HRQoL may necessitate additional follow-up for patients resulting in additional resource utilisation and costs. The likelihood of missing data will increase if long-term follow-up is necessary to assess the outcomes.

Current methods which have been suggested for identifying surgeons with poor operative performance are likely to miss a significant proportion of underperforming pancreatic surgeons. The results of this review are applicable to other surgeries that have similar or lower mortality such as liver resections and colorectal surgeries. Valid risk prognostic model and classification system of surgical complications (which captures long-term disability to patients and the cost implications to funder) are necessary before meaningful comparisons of the operative performance between pancreatic surgeons can be made.

Appendix

A. Search Date: 22 February 2014

A.1. Medline (OvidSP): 3764

(1) exp Pancreatectomy/

(2) (pancreatectomy or pancreatectomies).ti. or (pancreatectomy or pancreatectomies).ab.

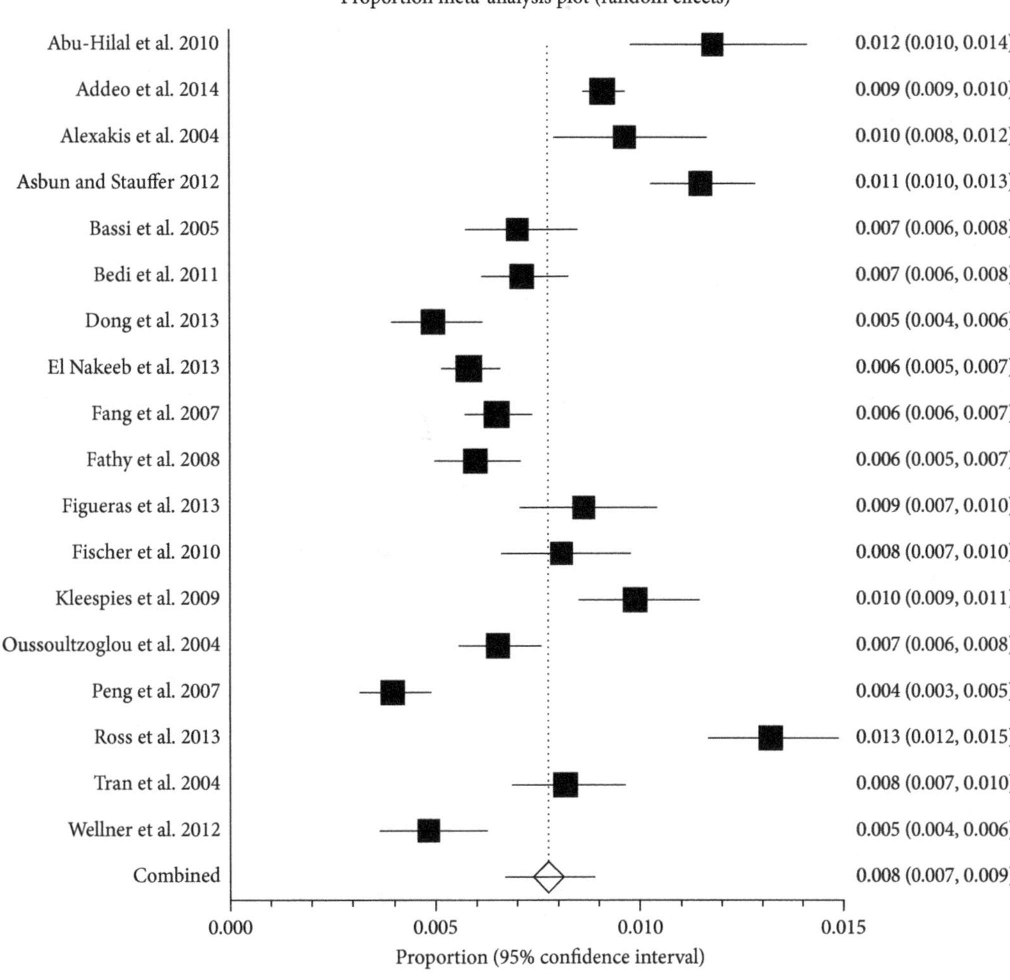

FIGURE 5: Number of complications. The figure shows the forest plot of number of complications. The number of complications per 100 patients ranged between 40 and 132. The average number of complications per 100 patients by random-effects model was 80.

(3) ((pancreas or pancreatic) adj (resection or resections)).ti. or ((pancreas or pancreatic) adj (resection or resections or operation or operations or surgery or surgeries)).ab.

(4) exp Pancreaticoduodenectomy/

(5) (Pancreaticoduodenectomy or pancreaticoduodenectomies or duodenopancreatectomy or duodenopancreatectomies).ti. or (Pancreaticoduodenectomy or pancreaticoduodenectomies or duodenopancreatectomy or duodenopancreatectomies).ab.

(6) ((Whipple adj (procedure or procedures or operation or operations)) or PPPD).ti. or ((Whipple adj (procedure or procedures or operation or operations or surgery or surgeries)) or PPPD).ab.

(7) exp Pancreaticojejunostomy/

(8) (pancreaticojejunostomy or pancreaticojejunostomies or pancreaticogastrostomy or pancreaticogastrostomies).ti. or (pancreaticojejunostomy or pancreaticojejunostomies or pancreaticogastrostomy or pancreaticogastrostomies).ab.

(9) (1) or (2) or (3) or (4) or (5) or (6) or (7) or (8)

(10) randomized controlled trial.pt.

(11) controlled clinical trial.pt.

(12) randomized.ab.

(13) placebo.ab.

(14) drug therapy.fs.

(15) randomly.ab.

(16) trial.ab.

(17) groups.ab.

(18) (10) or (11) or (12) or (13) or (14) or (15) or (16) or (17)

(19) exp animals/not humans.sh.

(20) (18) not (19)

(21) exp cohort studies/

(22) cohort*.tw.

(23) controlled clinical trial.pt.

(24) epidemiologic methods/

(25) limit (4) to yr = 1966–1989
(26) exp case-control studies/
(27) (case$ and control$).tw.
(28) (case$ and series).tw.
(29) (21) or (22) or (23) or (25) or (26) or (27) or (28)
(30) (20) or (29)
(31) (9) and (30)
(32) limit (31) to (humans and last 10 years)

A.2. Embase (OvidSP): 4194

(1) exp pancreas resection/
(2) (pancreatectomy or pancreatectomies).ti. or (pancreatectomy or pancreatectomies).ab.
(3) ((pancreas or pancreatic) adj (resection or resections)).ti. or ((pancreas or pancreatic) adj (resection or resections or operation or operations or surgery or surgeries)).ab.
(4) exp pancreaticoduodenectomy/
(5) (Pancreaticoduodenectomy or pancreaticoduodenectomies or duodenopancreatectomy or duodenopancreatectomies).ti. or (Pancreaticoduodenectomy or pancreaticoduodenectomies or duodenopancreatectomy or duodenopancreatectomies).ab.
(6) ((Whipple adj (procedure or procedures or operation or operations)) or PPPD).ti. or ((Whipple adj (procedure or procedures or operation or operations or surgery or surgeries)) or PPPD).ab.
(7) exp pancreaticojejunostomy/
(8) (pancreaticojejunostomy or pancreaticojejunostomies or pancreaticogastrostomy or pancreaticogastrostomies).ti. or (pancreaticojejunostomy or pancreaticojejunostomies or pancreaticogastrostomy or pancreaticogastrostomies).ab.
(9) (1) or (2) or (3) or (4) or (5) or (6) or (7) or (8)
(10) exp crossover-procedure/or exp double-blind procedure/or exp randomized controlled trial/or single-blind procedure/
(11) (((((random* or factorial* or crossover* or cross over* or cross-over* or placebo* or double*) adj blind*) or single*) adj blind*) or assign* or allocat* or volunteer*).af.
(12) (10) or (11)
(13) exp cohort analysis/
(14) exp longitudinal study/
(15) exp prospective study/
(16) exp follow up/
(17) cohort*.tw.
(18) exp case control study/
(19) (case* and control*).tw.
(20) exp case study/
(21) (case* and series).tw.
(22) (13) or (14) or (15) or (16) or (17) or (18) or (19) or (20) or (21)
(23) (12) or (22)
(24) (9) and (23)
(25) limit (24) to (human and last 10 years)

A.3. Cochrane: 205

(#1) MeSH descriptor: [Pancreatectomy] explode all trees
(#2) (pancreatectomy or pancreatectomies)
(#3) (pancreas or pancreatic) near (resection or resections)
(#4) MeSH descriptor: [Pancreaticoduodenectomy] explode all trees
(#5) (Pancreaticoduodenectomy or pancreaticoduodenectomies or duodenopancreatectomy or duodenopancreatectomies)
(#6) ((Whipple near (procedure or procedures or operation or operations)) or PPPD)
(#7) MeSH descriptor: [Pancreaticojejunostomy] explode all trees
(#8) (pancreaticojejunostomy or pancreaticojejunostomies or pancreaticogastrostomy or pancreaticogastrostomies)
(#9) (#1) or (#2) or (#3) or (#4) or (#5) or (#5) or (#6) or (#7) or (#8) from 2004 to 2014

Authors' Contribution

The project was conceived following a discussion by Kurinchi Gurusamy and Brian Davidson. Data was extracted by Clare Toon and Bhavisha Virendrakumar. Kurinchi Gurusamy wrote the first draft. All authors critically commented on the paper and improved its content. All authors approved the paper.

References

[1] International Agency for Research on Cancer, "GLOBOCAN 2012," 2014, http://globocan.iarc.fr/Default.aspx.

[2] R. A. Abrams, A. M. Lowy, E. M. O'Reilly, R. A. Wolff, V. J. Picozzi, and P. W. T. Pisters, "Combined modality treatment of resectable and borderline resectable pancreas cancer: expert consensus statement," *Annals of Surgical Oncology*, vol. 16, no. 7, pp. 1751–1756, 2009.

[3] P. Ghaneh, E. Costello, and J. P. Neoptolemos, "Biology and management of pancreatic cancer," *Gut*, vol. 56, no. 8, pp. 1134–1152, 2007.

[4] R. K. Orr, "Outcomes in pancreatic cancer surgery," *Surgical Clinics of North America*, vol. 90, no. 2, pp. 219–234, 2010.

[5] J. L. Cameron, H. A. Pitt, C. J. Yeo, K. D. Lillemoe, H. S. Kaufman, and J. Coleman, "One hundred and forty-five consecutive pancreaticoduodenectomies without mortality," *Annals of Surgery*, vol. 217, no. 5, pp. 430–438, 1993.

[6] E. H. Livingston, M. L. Welton, and H. A. Reber, "Surgical treatment of pancreatic cancer: the United States experience," *International Journal of Pancreatology*, vol. 9, pp. 153–157, 1991.

[7] J. E. Niederhuber, M. F. Brennan, and H. R. Menck, "The National Cancer Data Base report on pancreatic cancer," *Cancer*, vol. 76, no. 9, pp. 1671–1677, 1995.

[8] S. S. Nitecki, M. G. Sarr, T. V. Colby, and J. A. Van Heerden, "Long-term survival after resection for ductal adenocarcinoma of the pancreas. Is it really improving?" *Annals of Surgery*, vol. 221, no. 1, pp. 59–66, 1995.

[9] M. Trede and H.-D. Saeger, "Survival after pancreatoduodenectomy: 118 consecutive resections without an operative mortality," *Annals of Surgery*, vol. 211, no. 4, pp. 447–458, 1990.

[10] C. D. Johnson, "Guidelines for the management of patients with pancreatic cancer periampullary and ampullary carcinomas," *Gut*, vol. 54, supplement 5, pp. v1–v16, 2005.

[11] W.-C. Liao, K.-L. Chien, Y.-L. Lin et al., "Adjuvant treatments for resected pancreatic adenocarcinoma: a systematic review and network meta-analysis," *The Lancet Oncology*, vol. 14, no. 11, pp. 1095–1103, 2013.

[12] O. N. Tucker and M. Rela, "Controversies in the management of borderline resectable proximal pancreatic adenocarcinoma with vascular involvement," *HPB Surgery*, vol. 2008, Article ID 839503, 8 pages, 2008.

[13] J. M. Braganza, S. H. Lee, R. F. McCloy, and M. J. McMahon, "Chronic pancreatitis," *The Lancet*, vol. 377, no. 9772, pp. 1184–1197, 2011.

[14] P. Dítě, K. Starý, I. Novotný et al., "Incidence of chronic pancreatitis in the Czech Republic," *European Journal of Gastroenterology & Hepatology*, vol. 13, no. 6, pp. 749–750, 2001.

[15] J. E. Domínguez-Muñoz, A. Lucendo, L. F. Carballo, J. Iglesias-García, and J. M. Tenías, "A Spanish multicenter study to estimate the prevalence and incidence of chronic pancreatitis and its complications," *Revista Española de Enfermedades Digestivas*, vol. 106, no. 4, pp. 239–245, 2014.

[16] M. Joergensen, K. Brusgaard, D. G. Crüger, A.-M. Gerdes, and O. B. S. de Muckadell, "Incidence, prevalence, etiology, and prognosis of first-time chronic pancreatitis in young patients: a nationwide cohort study," *Digestive Diseases and Sciences*, vol. 55, no. 10, pp. 2988–2998, 2010.

[17] B. W. M. Spanier, M. J. Bruno, and M. G. W. Dijkgraaf, "Incidence and mortality of acute and chronic pancreatitis in the Netherlands: a nationwide record-linked cohort study for the years 1995–2005," *World Journal of Gastroenterology*, vol. 19, no. 20, pp. 3018–3026, 2013.

[18] D. Yadav, L. Timmons, J. T. Benson, R. A. Dierkhising, and S. T. Chari, "Incidence, prevalence, and survival of chronic pancreatitis: a population-based study," *The American Journal of Gastroenterology*, vol. 106, no. 12, pp. 2192–2199, 2011.

[19] N. S. Shah and A. K. Siriwardena, "Variance in elective surgery for chronic pancreatitis," *Journal of the Pancreas*, vol. 10, no. 1, pp. 30–36, 2009.

[20] M. Adham, X. Chopin-Laly, V. Lepilliez, R. Gincul, P.-J. Valette, and T. Ponchon, "Pancreatic resection: drain or no drain?" *Surgery*, vol. 154, no. 5, pp. 1069–1077, 2013.

[21] G. V. Aranha, J. M. Aaron, M. Shoup, and J. Pickleman, "Current management of pancreatic fistula after pancreaticoduodenectomy," *Surgery*, vol. 140, no. 4, pp. 561–569, 2006.

[22] H. J. Asbun and J. A. Stauffer, "Laparoscopic vs open pancreaticoduodenectomy: overall outcomes and severity of complications using the accordion severity grading system," *Journal of the American College of Surgeons*, vol. 215, no. 6, pp. 810–819, 2012.

[23] S. A. Barnett and N. A. Collier, "Pancreaticoduodenectomy: does preoperative biliary drainage, method of pancreatic reconstruction or age influence perioperative outcome? A retrospective study of 104 consecutive cases," *ANZ Journal of Surgery*, vol. 76, no. 7, pp. 563–568, 2006.

[24] J. W. Park, J.-Y. Jang, E.-J. Kim et al., "Effects of pancreatectomy on nutritional state, pancreatic function and quality of life," *British Journal of Surgery*, vol. 100, no. 8, pp. 1064–1070, 2013.

[25] P. J. Karanicolas, E. Davies, R. Kunz et al., "The pylorus: take it or leave it? Systematic review and meta-analysis of pylorus-preserving versus standard whipple pancreaticoduodenectomy for pancreatic or periampullary cancer," *Annals of Surgical Oncology*, vol. 14, no. 6, pp. 1825–1834, 2007.

[26] K. Bachmann, A. Kutup, O. Mann, E. Yekebas, and J. R. Izbicki, "Surgical treatment in chronic pancreatitis timing and type of procedure," *Best Practice & Research: Clinical Gastroenterology*, vol. 24, no. 3, pp. 299–310, 2010.

[27] U. Boggi, G. Amorese, F. Vistoli et al., "Laparoscopic pancreaticoduodenectomy: a systematic literature review," *Surgical Endoscopy*, vol. 29, no. 1, pp. 9–23, 2015.

[28] A. Mehrabi, M. Hafezi, J. Arvin et al., "A systematic review and meta-analysis of laparoscopic versus open distal pancreatectomy for benign and malignant lesions of the pancreas: it's time to randomize," *Surgery*, vol. 157, no. 1, pp. 45–55, 2015.

[29] M. K. Diener, C. M. Seiler, I. Rossion et al., "Efficacy of stapler versus hand-sewn closure after distal pancreatectomy (DISPACT): a randomised, controlled multicentre trial," *The Lancet*, vol. 377, no. 9776, pp. 1514–1522, 2011.

[30] NHS England, *Everyone Counts: Planning for Patients 2014/15 to 2018/19*, NHS England, Leeds, UK, 2013, http://www.england.nhs.uk/wp-content/uploads/2013/12/5yr-strat-plann-guid-wa.pdf.

[31] NHS Choices, My NHS. Data for etter Services. Consultant outcome data, 2014, https://www.nhs.uk/Service-Search/performance/Consultants.

[32] J. P. T. Higgins, S. G. Thompson, J. J. Deeks, and D. G. Altman, "Measuring inconsistency in meta-analyses," *British Medical Journal*, vol. 327, no. 7414, pp. 557–560, 2003.

[33] M. Egger, G. D. Smith, M. Schneider, and C. Minder, "Bias in meta-analysis detected by a simple, graphical test," *British Medical Journal*, vol. 315, no. 7109, pp. 629–634, 1997.

[34] R. G. Newcombe, "Two-sided confidence intervals for the single proportion: comparison of seven methods," *Statistics in Medicine*, vol. 17, no. 8, pp. 857–872, 1998.

[35] M. Abu-Hilal, A. K. Hemandas, M. McPhail et al., "A comparative analysis of safety and efficacy of different methods of tube placement for enteral feeding following major pancreatic resection. A non-randomized study," *Journal of the Pancreas*, vol. 11, no. 1, pp. 8–13, 2010.

[36] D. Adams, S. Owczarski, H. Wang, and K. Morgan, "Total pancreatectomy with islet autotransplantation for chronic pancreatitis: the price patients pay for improvements in quality of life," *Pancreatology*, vol. 13, no. 3, p. S17, 2013.

[37] P. Addeo, J. R. Delpero, F. Paye et al., "Pancreatic fistula after a pancreaticoduodenectomy for ductal adenocarcinoma and its association with morbidity: a multicentre study of the French Surgical Association," *HPB*, vol. 16, no. 1, pp. 46–55, 2014.

[38] N. Alexakis, S. Connor, P. Ghaneh et al., "Influence of opioid use on surgical and long-term outcome after resection for chronic pancreatitis," *Surgery*, vol. 136, no. 3, pp. 600–608, 2004.

[39] M. M. Assifi, J. Lindenmeyer, B. E. Leiby et al., "Surgical Apgar score predicts perioperative morbidity in patients undergoing pancreaticoduodenectomy at a high-volume center," *Journal of Gastrointestinal Surgery*, vol. 16, no. 2, pp. 275–281, 2012.

[40] C. Bassi, M. Falconi, E. Molinari et al., "Reconstruction by pancreaticojejunostomy versus pancreaticogastrostomy following pancreatectomy: results of a comparative study," *Annals of Surgery*, vol. 242, no. 6, pp. 767–773, 2005.

[41] J. D. Beane, M. G. House, G. A. Coté et al., "Outcomes after preoperative endoscopic ultrasonography and biopsy in patients undergoing distal pancreatectomy," *Surgery*, vol. 150, no. 4, pp. 844–853, 2011.

[42] M. M. S. Bedi, M. D. Gandhi, A. Venugopal, B. Venugopal, and H. Ramesh, "Pancreaticojejunostomy (PJ) versus pancreaticogastrostomy (PG) in reconstruction after Whipple operation for malignancy," *Pancreatology*, vol. 11, p. 58, 2011.

[43] M. Del Chiaro, E. Rangelova, C. Ansorge, J. Blomberg, and R. Segersvard, "Is the BMI a short and long term prognostic factor for patients undergoing pancreaticoduodenectomy?" *HPB*, vol. 14, p. 90, 2012.

[44] K. Dong, W. Xiong, X.-J. Yu, and C. Gu, "Clinical study on suspension pancreatic-duct-jejunum end-to-side continuous suture anastomosis in pancreaticoduodenectomy," *Chinese Medical Sciences Journal*, vol. 28, no. 1, pp. 34–38, 2013.

[45] A. El Nakeeb, A. M. Sultan, T. Salah et al., "Impact of cirrhosis on surgical outcome after pancreaticoduodenectomy," *World Journal of Gastroenterology*, vol. 19, no. 41, pp. 7129–7137, 2013.

[46] W.-L. Fang, Y.-M. Shyr, C.-H. Su, T.-H. Chen, C.-W. Wu, and W.-Y. Lui, "Comparison between pancreaticojejunostomy and pancreaticogastrostomy after pancreaticoduodenectomy," *Journal of the Formosan Medical Association*, vol. 106, no. 9, pp. 717–727, 2007.

[47] O. M. Fathy, M. Abdel Wahab M, N. Elghwalby et al., "216 Cases of pancreaticoduodenectomy: risk factors for postoperative complications," *Hepato-Gastroenterology*, vol. 55, no. 84, pp. 1093–1098, 2008.

[48] J. Figueras, L. Sabater, P. Planellas et al., "Randomized clinical trial of pancreaticogastrostomy versus pancreaticojejunostomy on the rate and severity of pancreatic fistula after pancreaticoduodenectomy," *British Journal of Surgery*, vol. 100, no. 12, pp. 1597–1605, 2013.

[49] M. Fischer, K. Matsuo, M. Gonen et al., "Relationship between intraoperative fluid administration and perioperative outcome after pancreaticoduodenectomy: results of a prospective randomized trial of acute normovolemic hemodilution compared with standard intraoperative management," *Annals of Surgery*, vol. 252, no. 6, pp. 952–958, 2010.

[50] W. E. Fisher, S. E. Hodges, G. Cruz et al., "Routine nasogastric suction may be unnecessary after a pancreatic resection," *HPB*, vol. 13, no. 11, pp. 792–796, 2011.

[51] P. I. Haigh, K. Y. Bilimoria, and L. A. DiFronzo, "Early postoperative outcomes after pancreaticoduodenectomy in the elderly," *Archives of Surgery*, vol. 146, no. 6, pp. 715–723, 2011.

[52] A. Kleespies, M. Rentsch, H. Seeliger, M. Albertsmeier, K.-W. Jauch, and C. J. Bruns, "Blumgart anastomosis for pancreaticojejunostomy minimizes severe complications after pancreatic head resection," *British Journal of Surgery*, vol. 96, no. 7, pp. 741–750, 2009.

[53] X. Liu and Z. Zheng, "Pancreaticoduodenectomy versus duodenum preserving pancreatic head resection in the treatment of chronic pancreatitis," *Pancreatology*, vol. 10, no. 2-3, p. 303, 2010.

[54] E. Oussoultzoglou, P. Bachellier, J.-M. Bigourdan, J.-C. Weber, H. Nakano, and D. Jaeck, "Pancreaticogastrostomy decreased relaparotomy caused by pancreatic fistula after pancreaticoduodenectomy compared with pancreaticojejunostomy," *Archives of Surgery*, vol. 139, no. 3, pp. 327–335, 2004.

[55] S. Y. Peng, J. W. Wang, W. Y. Lau et al., "Conventional versus binding pancreaticojejunostomy after pancreaticoduodenectomy: a prospective randomized trial," *Annals of Surgery*, vol. 245, no. 5, pp. 692–698, 2007.

[56] R. Y. Qin, M. Wang, F. Zhu et al., "A safe surgical technique for uncinate process resection during pancreaticoduodenectomy using a selective artery or vein first approach and combined blood flow blockage of the mesouncinate: a single-center study," *HPB*, vol. 15, p. 71, 2013.

[57] A. Ross, S. Mohammed, G. Vanburen et al., "An assessment of the necessity of transfusion during pancreatoduodenectomy," *Surgery*, vol. 154, no. 3, pp. 504–511, 2013.

[58] K. T. C. Tran, H. G. Smeenk, C. H. J. van Eijck et al., "Pylorus preserving pancreaticoduodenectomy versus standard whipple procedure: a prospective, randomized, multicenter analysis of 170 patients with pancreatic and periampullary tumors," *Annals of Surgery*, vol. 240, no. 5, pp. 738–745, 2004.

[59] U. F. Wellner, O. Sick, M. Olschewski, U. Adam, U. T. Hopt, and T. Keck, "Randomized controlled single-center trial comparing pancreatogastrostomy versus pancreaticojejunostomy after partial pancreatoduodenectomy," *Journal of Gastrointestinal Surgery*, vol. 16, no. 9, pp. 1686–1695, 2012.

[60] T. K. Williams, E. L. Rosato, E. P. Kennedy et al., "Impact of obesity on perioperative morbidity and mortality after pancreaticoduodenectomy," *Journal of the American College of Surgeons*, vol. 208, no. 2, pp. 210–217, 2009.

[61] G. V. Aranha, J. M. Aaron, and M. Shoup, "Critical analysis of a large series of pancreaticogastrostomy after pancreaticoduodenectomy," *Archives of Surgery*, vol. 141, no. 6, pp. 574–580, 2006.

[62] J. D. Beane, H. A. Pitt, A. Nakeeb et al., "Splenic preserving distal pancreatectomy: does vessel preservation matter?" *Journal of the American College of Surgeons*, vol. 212, no. 4, pp. 651–657, 2011.

[63] M. Del Chiaro, E. Rangelova, C. Ansorge, J. Blomberg, A. Andren-Sandberg, and R. Segersvard, "Results and costs analysis of pancreaticoduodenectomy in elderly patients," *HPB*, vol. 14, pp. 239–240, 2012.

[64] M. del Chiaro, E. Rangelova, C. Ansorge, J. Blomberg, and R. Segersvärd, "Preoperative predictive factors influencing survival after pancreaticoduodenctomi for pancreatic cancer," *Pancreatology*, vol. 12, no. 6, p. 556, 2012.

[65] M. Del Chiaro, E. Rangelova, C. Ansorge, J. Blomberg, and R. Segersvärd, "Impact of bmi on short and long term outcome after oncological pancreaticoduodenectomy," *Pancreatology*, vol. 12, no. 6, pp. 553–554, 2012.

[66] G. Farkas, L. Leidler, and G. Farkas, "Randomised trial of organ- vs. pylorus-preserving pancreatic head resection," *Zeitschrift fur Gastroenterologie*, vol. 43, no. 5, article 418, 2006.

[67] M. B. Farnell, R. K. Pearson, M. G. Sarr et al., "A prospective randomized trial comparing standard pancreatoduodenectomy with pancreatoduodenectomy with extended lymphadenectomy in resectable pancreatic head adenocarcinoma," *Surgery*, vol. 138, no. 4, pp. 618–630, 2005.

[68] M. Sakowska, E. Docherty, D. Linscott, and S. Connor, "A change in practice from epidural to intrathecal morphine analgesia for hepato-pancreato-biliary surgery," *World Journal of Surgery*, vol. 33, no. 9, pp. 1802–1808, 2009.

[69] F.-Z. Tian, L. Shi, L.-J. Tang et al., "Perspective of pre-operational jaundice-reducing indication in carcinoma of head of pancreas," *Chung Hua Wai Ko Tsa Chih*, vol. 44, no. 23, pp. 1614–1616, 2006.

[70] M. B. Farnell, R. K. Pearson, M. G. Sarr, E. P. DiMagno, L. J. Burgart, and T. R. Dahl, "A prospective randomized trial comparing standard pancreatoduodenectomy with pancreatoduodenectomy with extended lymphadenectomy in resectable pancreatic head adenocarcinoma," *Annales de Chirurgie*, vol. 131, no. 2, pp. 171–172, 2006 (French).

[71] U. A. Ali, V. B. Nieuwenhuijs, C. H. van Eijck et al., "Clinical outcome in relation to timing of surgery in chronic pancreatitis: a nomogram to predict pain relief," *Archives of Surgery*, vol. 147, no. 10, pp. 925–932, 2012.

[72] P. A. Clavien, J. Barkun, M. L. de Oliveira et al., "The clavien-dindo classification of surgical complications: five-year experience," *Annals of Surgery*, vol. 250, no. 2, pp. 187–196, 2009.

[73] D. Dindo, N. Demartines, and P.-A. Clavien, "Classification of surgical complications: a new proposal with evaluation in a cohort of 6336 patients and results of a survey," *Annals of Surgery*, vol. 240, no. 2, pp. 205–213, 2004.

[74] S. M. Strasberg, D. C. Linehan, and W. G. Hawkins, "The accordion severity grading system of surgical complications," *Annals of Surgery*, vol. 250, no. 2, pp. 177–186, 2009.

[75] US Department of Health and Human Services, *Common Terminology Criteria for Adverse Events (CTCAE) Version 4.0*, US Department of Health and Human Services, 2009, http://evs.nci.nih.gov/ftp1/CTCAE/CTCAE_4.03_2010-06-14_QuickReference_8.5x11.pdf.

[76] R. S. Lewis Jr. and C. M. Vollmer Jr., "Risk scores and prognostic models in surgery: pancreas resection as a paradigm," *Current Problems in Surgery*, vol. 49, no. 12, pp. 731–795, 2012.

[77] D. Moher, A. Liberati, J. Tetzlaff, D. G. Altman, and The PRISMA Group, "Preferred reporting items for systematic reviews and meta-analyses: the PRISMA statement," *PLoS Medicine*, vol. 6, no. 7, Article ID e1000097, 2009.

Evaluation of Early Cholecystectomy versus Delayed Cholecystectomy in the Treatment of Acute Cholecystitis

Miguel Sánchez-Carrasco,[1] Juan C. Rodríguez-Sanjuán,[2] Fernando Martín-Acebes,[1] Francisco J. Llorca-Díaz,[3] Manuel Gómez-Fleitas,[2] Rocío Zambrano Muñoz,[1] and F. Javier Sánchez-Manuel[1]

[1]*Department of General Surgery, Burgos University Hospital, Avenida Islas Baleares 3, 09006 Burgos, Spain*
[2]*Department of General Surgery, University Hospital "Marqués de Valdecilla", Avenida Valdecilla, s/n, 39008 Santander, Spain*
[3]*Department of Epidemiology, Preventive Medicine and Public Health, School of Medicine, University of Cantabria, Avenida Herrera Oria, s/n, 39011 Santander, Spain*

Correspondence should be addressed to Miguel Sánchez-Carrasco; msanchezc@saludcastillayleon.es

Academic Editor: Shuji Isaji

Objective. To evaluate if early cholecystectomy (EC) is the most appropriate treatment for acute cholecystitis compared to delayed cholecystectomy (DC). *Patients and Methods.* A retrospective cohort study of 1043 patients was carried out, with a group of 531 EC cases and a group of 512 DC patients. The following parameters were recorded: (1) postoperative hospital morbidity, (2) hospital mortality, (3) days of hospital stay, (4) readmissions, (5) admission to the Intensive Care Unit (ICU), (6) type of surgery, (7) operating time, and (8) reoperations. In addition, we estimated the direct cost savings of implementing an EC program. *Results.* The overall morbidity of the EC group (29.9%) was significantly lower than the DC group (38.7%). EC demonstrated significantly better results than DC in days of hospital stay (8.9 versus 15.8 days), readmission percentage (6.8% versus 21.9%), and percentage of ICU admission (2.3% versus 7.8%), which can result in reducing the direct costs. The patients who benefited most from an EC were those with a Charlson index > 3. *Conclusions.* EC is safe in patients with acute cholecystitis and could lead to a reduction in the direct costs of treatment.

1. Introduction

Acute cholecystitis is a pathology of inflammatory origin, usually associated with cholelithiasis, with a high incidence in our environment. The treatment of acute cholecystitis involves an important socioeconomic impact. There are two surgical therapeutic options: early cholecystectomy (EC) during the same admission or delayed cholecystectomy (DC) during a later admission after conservative treatment.

The first studies that assessed EC as a treatment for acute cholecystitis date back to the 1950s [1–3]. In 1970, the first controlled study was published by van der Linden and Sunzel, demonstrating better morbidity and shorter average hospital stay after open EC [4]. The exponential development of laparoscopic surgery occurred during the 1990s. Some of the first publications about laparoscopic EC showed bad results in terms of morbimortality and high percentages of bile duct injuries. Based on these results, laparoscopic EC was deprecated and even considered a contraindication for the treatment of acute cholecystitis, favoring initial conservative treatment followed by a laparoscopic DC. In 1998, Kiviluoto et al. reported similar results in terms of morbimortality between laparoscopic EC and open EC [5]. In that same year, Lo et al. presented the first controlled study that compared laparoscopic EC and laparoscopic DC, with lower morbidity and hospital stay in the laparoscopic EC group [6]. Recently, many studies have reported similar results in favor of laparoscopic EC. It is important to note that the vast majority of these articles only include laparoscopic cases, which could cause a bias in the external validity of these studies, as they exclude many of the less favorable cases involving open EC [7–17].

In spite of many publications that suggest benefits in favor of EC, there is still controversy regarding the timing to perform cholecystectomy. Although literature favors laparoscopic EC, most evidence comes from prospective studies specifically designed to prove this particular aspect [6–11], which probably does not reflect the worldwide clinical practice. In addition, it is well known that laparoscopic EC is not the usual practice in many hospitals [12, 17–23].

Our study aims to compare two treatment protocols for acute cholecystitis, in two similar hospital centers covering two health areas with similar characteristics and with comparable morbimortality results in laparoscopic cholecystectomy for symptomatic cholelithiasis: (A) EC, performed within 48 hours after admission, versus (B) DC, performed 2–4 months after the index episode.

2. Patients and Methods

2.1. Study Population. This is a cohort retrospective study that includes 1043 patients, consecutively treated between January 1, 2005, and December 31, 2010, for acute cholecystitis. The diagnosis was made according to the Tokyo 2013 criteria [24]. The cases of cholecystitis associated with pancreatitis, choledocholithiasis, or cholangitis and those treated with percutaneous cholecystostomy were excluded. In addition, 16 cases from EC group who were treated as DC and 10 cases from DC group who were treated as EC were also excluded due to protocol violation.

The EC group consisted of 531 patients (50.9%), treated at the University Hospital "Marqués de Valdecilla", in Santander. This group was treated with early cholecystectomy, performed within 48 hours after admission to the Surgery Department. 473 patients (89.1%) were operated on within 72 hours of symptoms onset (<72 h) and 54 patients (10.2%) after 72 hours (>72 h). Four patients (0.7%) died before surgery, because of severe cholecystitis and comorbidity.

The DC group consisted of 512 patients (49.1%), treated at the Burgos University Hospital. This group was treated with delayed cholecystectomy, performed 2–4 months after the index episode. A total of 268 patients (52.4%) underwent elective surgery after an average of 105 days, 143 patients (27.9%) required surgery ahead of schedule (urgent surgery), and 101 patients (19.7%) received no intervention.

2.2. Study Variables. There are (1) postoperative hospital morbidity: overall morbidity (medical and surgical complications), surgical morbidity, and the most relevant surgical complications (bleeding, infection, and bile duct injury, according to the Strasberg classification [25]), (the severity of complications was stratified according to the Clavien-Dindo scale [26]), (2) hospital mortality, (3) days of hospital stay, (4) readmissions (note that admission for elective cholecystectomy within the DC group is not regarded as reentry), (5) admissions to the Intensive Care Unit (ICU), (6) type of surgery, (7) operating time, and (8) reoperations.

Additionally, the direct cost savings by implementation of an EC program were estimated.

2.3. Statistical Analysis. Frequency distributions and summary statistics were calculated for all variables; values are expressed as mean or median and range. A Kolmogorov-Smirnov test was used to study the distribution of each variable, and P-P and Q-Q charts were used to confirm it. The majority of variables did follow a normal distribution, and parametric tests were used for comparisons. The independent variable of interest was the variable EC versus DC. The endpoints of this study were the evaluation of morbidity, mortality, days of hospital stay, readmissions, admissions to ICU, type of surgery, operating time, and reoperations. Univariate analysis was performed with logistic or linear regression models or a Mantel-Haenszel chi-square test. A multivariate analysis was performed in order to analyze if the following variables were confounders between the independent and endpoints variables: age, sex, ASA degree [27], Charlson index [28], and severity of the cholecystitis. A significance level of 5% ($p < 0.05$) was accepted in all cases. SPSS software version 19.0 (SPSS, IBM Corp., Armonk, NY) was used for the statistical analysis. Additionally ROC analyses of the risk of death, the risk of complications, and the risk of reoperation are included; the area under the ROC curve shows the ability of any statistical model to predict an event. The closer it gets to 1, the greater its predictive ability will be and thus its reliability.

3. Results

3.1. Comparison of the Groups. The EC and DC groups were compared on the basis of age, sex, medical-surgical risk (ASA), Charlson index, percentage of diabetic patients, and severity of the acute cholecystitis according to the Tokyo 2013 consensus criteria [24]. The EC group had a significantly lower average age, which made the average score for the Charlson index also significantly lower in this group, due to its direct relation with age and comorbidity. Similar results were found for comorbidity (ASA) and severity of acute cholecystitis (Table 1).

3.2. Overall Morbidity. The morbidity in the EC group was lower than in the DC group, with statistically significant differences. Within the EC group, there were no significant differences between the morbidity of patients <72 h and the morbidity of patients >72 h. Of particular note among the DC patients was the low morbidity of patients operated on electively and the high morbidity of patients operated on urgently (Table 2).

Table 3 shows the overall postoperative complications according to the Clavien-Dindo scale, considering mild complications as grades I and II and severe complications as grades III and IV. In the multivariate analysis, we found that EC had a 39% lower risk of complications than DC (OR = 0.61; 95% CI 0.45–0.82; $p < 0.05$) and that the risk of complications increases at a rate of 17% for each point of the Charlson index (OR = 1.17; 95% CI 1.01–1.36; $p < 0.05$) and proportionally with the severity of the cholecystitis: moderate cholecystitis (OR = 2.34; 95% CI 1,70–3,23, $p < 0.05$) and severe cholecystitis (OR = 7.70; 95% CI 4.21–14.07; $p < 0.05$). The area under the ROC curve is 0.73, which indicates that

TABLE 1: Comparison of the groups.

	EC ($n = 531$)	DC ($n = 512$)
Age	66.8	70.0
*Female**, *n* (%)	326 (42.6)	206 (40.2)
*ASA**, *n* (%)		
I	115 (21.6)	120 (23.4)
II	259 (48.8)	242 (47.3)
III	139 (26.2)	129 (25.2)
IV	18 (3.4)	21 (4.1)
Charlson	3.7	4.1
*Diabetics**, *n* (%)	113 (22.1)	87 (17.0)
*Severity of cholecystitis**, *n* (%)		
Mild	229 (43.1)	234 (45.7)
Moderate	262 (49.4)	235 (46.1)
Severe	40 (7.5)	42 (8.2)

*$p > 0.05$.

TABLE 2: Overall and surgical morbidity after surgery; mortality.

	Overall morb.	Surgical morb.	Mortality
EC	**29.9% (158)**	**17.6% (93)**	0.8% (6)
<72 h	29.6% (140)	16.9% (80)	0.4% (2)
>72 h	33.3% (18)	24.1% (13)	0%
No surgery			100% (4)
DC	**38.7% (157)**	**29.9% (123)**	2.7% (14)
Elective	22.4% (60)	18.3% (49)	0.4% (1)
Urgent	69.2% (97)	51.7% (74)	2.8% (4)
No surgery			8.9% (9)

Highlighted in bold font are statistically significant values.

TABLE 3: Overall complications according to the Clavien-Dindo scale.

	I-II	III-IV
EC	**20.4% (108)**	9.3% (49)
<72 h	20.1% (95)	9.3% (44)
>72 h	24.1% (13)	9.3% (5)
DC	**29.7% (122)**	8.3% (34)
Elective	19.0% (51)	3.0% (8)
Urgent	49.7% (71)	18.2% (26)

Highlighted in bold font are statistically significant values.

the predictive ability of the model to foresee complications is not very high.

An analysis of the morbidity in terms of the Charlson index, using univariate logistic regression, was made. We observed that EC patients with Charlson index < 3 had complications in 17.6% (35/199) of cases, while DC patients with Charlson index < 3 had complications in 21.6% (32/148) of cases, (OR = 1.29; $p > 0.05$). On the other hand, EC patients with Charlson index > 3 had a 37.5% (123/328) complications rate and DC patients with Charlson index > 3 had a 47.9% (123/257) complications rate (OR = 1.51; 95% CI 1.32–1.89; $p < 0.05$).

TABLE 4: Surgical complications according to the Clavien-Dindo scale.

	I-II	III-IV
EC	**10.3% (54)**	7.2% (37)
<72 h	9.5% (45)	7.2% (34)
>72 h	16.7% (9)	7.4% (4)
DC	**23.1% (95)**	6.6% (27)
Elective	15.3% (41)	3.0% (8)
Urgent	37.8% (54)	13.3% (19)

Highlighted in bold font are statistically significant values.

TABLE 5: Most relevant surgical complications.

	Infection	Bleeding	Bile injury	Strasberg D-E
EC	**9.7% (51)**	3.0% (16)	2.8% (15)	0.6% (3)
<72 h	9.3% (44)	2.5% (12)	2.7% (13)	0.6% (3)
>72 h	12.9% (7)	7.4% (4)	3.7% (2)	0%
DC	**16.5% (68)**	1.2% (5)	4.6% (19)	1.0% (4)
Elect.	9.3% (25)	0.7% (2)	2.2% (6)	0.8% (2)
Urg.	30.1% (43)	2.1% (3)	9.1% (13)	1.4% (2)

Highlighted in bold font are statistically significant values.

3.3. Surgical Morbidity. When we analyzed only surgical complications after surgery, we observed a lower rate of complications, statistically significant, in the EC group as compared to the DC group. Within the EC group, there were no significant differences between the surgical complications of patients <72 h and the patients >72 h. In the DC group, those operated on electively did not have such low morbidity as would be expected, and of particular note is the high morbidity of the urgent surgery group (Table 2).

Table 4 shows the surgical complications according to the Clavien-Dindo scale, considering mild complications as of grades I and II and severe complications as of grades III and IV.

3.4. Most Relevant Surgical Complications (Table 5)

(1) *Surgical Site Infection.* The proportion of infections was significantly higher in the DC group. We found the risk of postoperative infection to be twice as high in the DC group as the EC group (OR = 1.98; 95% CI 1.78–2.17; $p < 0.05$).

(2) *Bleeding.* There were no significant differences in the frequency of postoperative bleeding.

(3) *Bile Duct Injury.* Both the bile leakage and, more specifically, major injuries of the bile duct (Strasberg D-E) had a greater tendency to occur in the DC group, but the differences were not statistically significant.

TABLE 6: Other results: days of hospital stay, readmissions, ICU stay, type of surgery, operating time, and reoperations.

	Hosp. stay	Readmiss.	ICU	LPS/CONV	Oper. time	Reoperat.
EC	**8.9 (ds 7.6)**	**6.8% (36)**	**2.3% (12)**	**74.8%/21.6%**	90.8 (ds 34.1)	4.6% (24)
<72 h	**8.1 (ds 7.6)**		2.1% (10)	75.1%/20.6%	91.1 (ds 38.6)	4.4% (21)
>72 h	**15.5 (ds 7.8)**		3.7% (2)	72.2%/30.8%	93.5 (ds 25.2)	5.6% (3)
DC	**15.8 (ds 12.2)**	**21.9% (112)**	**7.8% (32)**	**67.9%/9.3%**	89.5 (ds 28.1)	2.4% (10)
Elect.	13.6 (ds 11.9)		0%	91.4%/6.1%	84.2 (ds 18.9)	1.1% (3)
Urg.	19.9 (ds 12.2)		21.7% (31)	23.8%/32.3%	97.0 (ds 22.9)	4.9% (7)
No Surg.	15.8 (ds 12.2)		1% (1)			

Highlighted in bold font are statistically significant values.

3.5. Mortality. In the DC group we found a higher mortality than in the EC group, but the differences were not statistically significant. Of particular note within the DC group was the low mortality of the elective surgery, the high mortality of the patients undergoing urgent surgery, and the very high mortality rate of patients who did not undergo surgery (Table 2).

It is remarkable that, in the DC group, 47 of the 92 patients (51.1%) who did not undergo surgery and did not die in hospital during the treatment died within the next three years.

The multivariate analysis showed that the risk of death was lower in the EC group (OR = 0.71), but without statistical significance ($p > 0.05$). We also found that the risk of death in both groups increased by 13% for each year of age (OR = 1.13; 95% CI 1.05–1.22; $p < 0.05$) and increased by 42% for each point in the Charlson index (OR = 1.42; 95% CI 1.01–1.98; $p < 0.05$). In relation to the severity of the cholecystitis, we found a slight increase in the risk of death in the moderate cholecystitis patients (OR = 1.52), but without statistical significance ($p > 0.05$). For its part, severe cholecystitis was associated with a high mortality (OR = 11.8; 95% CI 2.67–52.27; $p < 0.05$). The area under the ROC curve is 0.94, which confirms that the model has a very high ability to predict the risk of death.

3.6. Days of Hospital Stay. The average hospital stay in the EC group was significantly lower than in the DC group (Table 6).

3.7. Readmissions. For the analysis of hospital readmissions, we established a differentiation between admissions before cholecystectomy and readmissions after surgery. If we analyze all the cases as a whole, the EC group had a 6.8% readmission rate ($n = 36$) (all postsurgical) and the DC group a 21.9% readmissions rate ($n = 112$) ($p < 0.05$) (Table 6). Within the DC group, 18.2% of the patients required at least one readmission before surgery ($n = 93$). The percentage of readmissions after surgery in DC group was 4.6% ($n = 19$), which is not significantly lower than that of the EC group.

3.8. Admission to the Intensive Care Unit. We found that the percentage of EC patients that required admission to the ICU was significantly lower than the DC group. A high proportion of patients who underwent urgent surgery within the DC group required admission to the ICU (Table 6).

3.9. Type of Surgery. There were a greater percentage of conversions from laparoscopic to open surgery in the EC group than in the DC group ($p < 0.05$) (Table 6). On the other hand, there was no significant difference between the percentage of surgeries that were completed by laparoscopy in the EC group (58.6%) and in the DC group (61.6%).

When we matched the type of surgical approach with the severity of the acute cholecystitis, we found that in the EC group, of the 394 patients (74.7%) who underwent laparoscopic surgery, 190 patients had mild cholecystitis (48.2%), 185 patients had moderate cholecystitis (46.9%), and 19 patients had severe cholecystitis (4.8%). For their part, of the 133 patients who underwent laparotomy (25.2%), 37 had mild cholecystitis (27.8%), 76 were admitted with moderate cholecystitis (57.1%), and 20 suffered severe cholecystitis (15.0%). In the DC group, of the 279 patients (67.9%) operated on by laparoscopy, 160 had mild cholecystitis (57.3%), 116 had moderate cholecystitis (41.6%), and 3 were admitted with severe cholecystitis (1.1%). When we looked at the 132 patients who underwent laparotomy (32.1%), we found that 17 were admitted with mild cholecystitis (12.9%), 80 with moderate cholecystitis (60.6%), and 35 with severe cholecystitis (26.5%). In both EC and DC, there was a significantly higher proportion of moderate and severe cases of acute cholecystitis in patients who underwent open surgery than in those with a laparoscopic approach.

The risk of bile duct injury in relation to the surgical approach was calculated. In the EC group, we found 9 cases of bile duct injury in open surgery (6.8%) and 6 cases in the laparoscopic approach (1.52%), ($p < 0.05$). In the DC group, there was a higher tendency towards bile duct injury in open surgery (7.58%) than in laparoscopic surgery (3.22%), but the differences were not statistically significant.

3.10. Operating Time. There were no significant differences in operating time between the EC and DC groups (Table 6). The only factor that influenced the surgical time was the severity of the cholecystitis, with a significant increase in the time for moderate and severe cholecystitis cases ($p < 0.05$).

3.11. Reoperations. There were no significant differences between the percentage of reoperations in the EC group and the DC group (Table 6). In the multivariate analysis, it was noted that the EC group had almost twice the risk of reoperation of the DC group (OR = 1.90), but this ratio was not statistically significant ($p > 0.05$). It also highlighted that severe cholecystitis had a greater risk of reoperation (OR = 2.72), but it was not statistically significant ($p > 0.05$). The model has a low capacity to predict the risk of reoperation, with area under the ROC curve of 0.66.

3.12. Estimated Direct Cost Savings. Faced with the impossibility of assessing, using the data collected in the present study, the exact difference in costs between the treatment options of EC and DC, we instead made an approximation of the same, taking into account the three most important parameters with statistically significant differences between the two study groups: Emergency Department care for readmission, days of stay in ICU, and days of hospital stay.

The EC group had a total of 36 readmissions (0.068 readmissions per patient). The DC group had a total of 112 readmissions (0.219 readmissions per patient). If we subtract both figures we get 0.151, which is the difference in readmissions per patient between EC and DC.

The EC group had a total of 79 days of stay in the ICU (0.149 days of stay in ICU per patient). The DC group had a total of 372 days of stay in ICU (0.727 days of stay in ICU per patient). If we subtract both figures we get 0.578, which is the difference in days of stay in ICU per patient between EC and DC.

The EC group had an average of 8.9 days of hospital stay per patient and the DC group an average of 15.8 days of hospital stay per patient. If we subtract both figures we get 6.9, which is the difference in days of hospital stay per patient between EC and DC.

Therefore, each patient treated with EC would save 0.151 readmissions, 0.578 days of stay in ICU, and 8.9 days of hospitalization.

4. Discussion

In this comprehensive retrospective study, we compared, from a clinical point of view and in relation to the two possible surgical option treatments in the management of acute cholecystitis, the result of the treatment protocols for acute cholecystitis of two nearby hospitals, with very similar profiles in terms of capacity and organizational structure. Both hospitals provide health care to populations with similar demographic characteristics. We have contrasted the reality of the daily practice in the treatment of acute cholecystitis, without a selection of patients according to age, comorbidity, the severity of the acute cholecystitis or the surgical approach. In this way, our study has also included patients who underwent open surgery that had a greater proportion of cases of moderate and severe cholecystitis, factors that most influence, according to our data, the appearance of complications and mortality. This fact means that studies, which only include laparoscopic surgery cases, may have questionable external validity, due to dismissal of cases that have potentially worse evolution.

Of note, in the DC group, patients were operated on after an average of 105 days, an interval which is longer than the ideal 6–8-week period. This was due to the waiting list of a public hospital. We do not think that this influenced the morbidity rate, since fibrosis tends to decrease after several months.

Data from our study in relation to morbidity indicate that DC had a higher rate of complications than EC, due to a higher proportion of minor surgical complications. Many of the previously published studies also showed higher rates of morbidity in patients with DC, but from analyzing the morbidity of some of the most influential studies, such as the meta-analysis of Papi et al. [19] and Gurusamy and Samraj [12], we note that there were no significant differences between both groups. We have observed in our study that the patients who benefit most from EC were those with a Charlson index > 3 (greater age and comorbidity); concordantly, the risk of complications is 50% higher in patients with Charlson index > 3 who underwent DC. This fact has also been highlighted in recent studies [29–32].

We found no significant differences in morbidity among DC patients who underwent surgery during the first 72 hours and those who underwent surgery after 72 hours from the onset of symptoms. This result contrasts with the work published by González-Rodríguez et al. [33], where the morbidity was twice as high in surgery after 72 hours as in surgery within the first 72 hours and with the publication of Banz et al. [15], which notes higher rates of complications as the time increases in the evolution of acute cholecystitis.

The risk of postoperative infection was twice as high in the DC group as in the EC cases, which contrasts with the results of the meta-analysis of Gurusamy and Samraj [12], which notes a higher proportion of infections that required percutaneous drainage in the EC group. With regard to postoperative bleeding, we noted a lesser tendency towards bleeding in DC than in EC, which concurs with the results previously obtained by Norrby et al. [34]. We found that the proportion of bile leakage and major injuries of the bile duct was almost double in DC compared to that in EC, but with no statistically significant differences, which is in line with the results published by Gurusamy et al. in their various meta-analyses [12, 14, 16]. In our experience, the laparoscopic approach seems to be safer than the open surgery in the EC group, but we must consider that the selection of the type of surgery was not randomized in any case, so the results are not conclusive. We must point out that we believe that the ATOM [35] classification is the most appropriate form of assessment of iatrogenic injury to the bile duct, but, given its recent publication and the retrospective nature of the present study, which does not permit us to know certain aspects for the correct characterization of some of the injuries, we have used the Strasberg classification.

In relation to the morbidity analysis, there is a factor that has not been measured, which we believe may be of great interest and, in some way, a crucial factor in supporting the EC as the most optimal treatment for acute cholecystitis. This factor is the assessment, within the DC group, of the medical complications arising during the medical treatment of cholecystitis, as well as the deterioration in health of patients occurring between the index episode and the elective cholecystectomy.

Despite the fact that the mortality rate was more than twice as high in the DC group as in the EC group, the differences were not significant. The majority of the previous studies present similar mortality rates for both groups, with percentages close to 1% [15, 19] or without registered mortality [12, 14, 16].

EC patients had a significantly lower average hospital stay than that of DC patients. All of the articles published to date offer significantly lower results of hospital stay in the EC group, with differences in days of stay ranging from 2 days in the population study of Banz et al. [15] to 10 days in the van der Linden and Sunzel [4] and Papi et al. [19] studies. In addition, many of the works published hospital stay results very close to those of our EC group; among others, Lai et al. showed 7.6 days [7], Papi et al. 10.6 days [19], and Gurusamy et al. 6.7 days [14]. The patients who underwent surgery after 72 hours from the onset of symptoms presented an average stay significantly higher than the patients operated on within the first 72 hours, similar to the DC group, something that was pointed out previously by other studies [6–10, 36–38]; this is explained by the greater average stay prior to the surgery of the patients who underwent surgery after 72 hours of the symptoms onset.

The difference between the percentages of readmissions of the EC and the DC groups is due to the readmissions of the DC group that occur between the first admission for acute cholecystitis and the admission to perform the cholecystectomy (18.2%), which is somewhat lower than the results provided by Lahtinen et al. [39] and Lau et al. [40], with percentages of readmission prior to surgery between 25% and 30%.

We found a greater tendency towards reoperations in the EC group with respect to the DC group, which contrasts with the data published by Banz et al. [15] in their population study, where they highlight a greater proportion of reoperations in DC (27.9%) than in EC (11.9%).

As illustrated in the present study, the worst results of DC as compared to EC are due, in great measure, to the cases operated on earlier than expected and the nonoperated patients, something that is avoided with the EC protocols.

The average hospital stay and the percentage of patients who required a readmission, as well as the percentage of patients who were admitted to the ICU, were all significantly higher in the DC group than in the EC group. All of these factors contribute to ensuring that, with a high probability, the direct costs of EC treatment are lower than those of DC, something also pointed out by other recent studies [17, 41–43].

Main Limitations of the Study. (1) It is retrospective study. (2) Patients are treated in two different hospitals. That could induce variability in the surgical management or perioperative treatment. However, this variability would be minimal, since both hospitals are of the highest standard and both universities. (3) The study just analyzes two different treatment protocols; it is not an "intention to treat analysis" actually.

Conclusion. EC provides better morbidity results, as well as a clear trend toward lower mortality and fewer injuries to the main bile duct. No differences were found in the rate of complications between patients who underwent surgery within the first 72 hours of symptoms and the patients operated on more than 72 hours after the initiation of symptoms. In addition, EC could be of benefit for elderly patients with high comorbidity and lead to a reduction in direct costs due to fewer stays in ICU, fewer readmissions, and fewer days of hospital stay. We would recommend DC only in cases where acute pancreatitis, choledocholithiasis, or cholangitis cannot be ruled out and those with unacceptable anesthetic risk at the time of diagnosis.

Additional Points

This paper is based on the thesis realized by Miguel Sánchez-Carrasco "Evaluation of Early Cholecystectomy versus Delayed Cholecystectomy in the Treatment of Acute Cholecystitis," Department of Surgical Sciences, University of Cantabria, 2014.

Competing Interests

The authors declare that there is no conflict of interests regarding the publication of this paper.

References

[1] J. H. Mulholland, E. H. Ellison, and S. R. Friesen, *Delayed Operative Management of Acute Cholecystitis. Current Surgical Management*, Saunders, Philadelphia, Pa, USA, 1957.

[2] E. H. Ellison, J. H. Miholland, and S. R. Friesen, *Early Operation for Acute Cholecystitis. Current Surgical Management*, Saunders, Philadelphia, Pa, USA, 1957.

[3] B. Pines and J. Rabinowitch, "Perforation of the gallbladder in acute cholecystitis," *Annals of Surgery*, vol. 140, article 170, 1959.

[4] W. van der Linden and H. Sunzel, "Early versus delayed operation for acute cholecystitis. A controlled clinical trial," *The American Journal of Surgery*, vol. 120, no. 1, pp. 7–13, 1970.

[5] T. Kiviluoto, J. Sirén, P. Luukkonen, and E. Kivilaakso, "Randomised trial of laparoscopic versus open cholecystectomy for acute and gangrenous cholecystitis," *The Lancet*, vol. 351, no. 9099, pp. 321–325, 1998.

[6] C.-M. Lo, C.-L. Liu, S.-T. Fan, E. C. S. Lai, and J. Wong, "Prospective randomized study of early versus delayed laparoscopic cholecystectomy for acute cholecystitis," *Annals of Surgery*, vol. 227, no. 4, pp. 461–467, 1998.

[7] P. B. S. Lai, K. H. Kwong, K. L. Leung et al., "Randomized trial of early versus delayed laparoscopic cholecystectomy for acute cholecystitis," *British Journal of Surgery*, vol. 85, no. 6, pp. 764–767, 1998.

[8] C. F. Chandler, J. S. Lane, P. Ferguson, J. E. Thompson, and S. W. Ashley, "Prospective evaluation of early versus delayed laparoscopic cholecystectomy for treatment of acute cholecystitis," *The American Surgeon*, vol. 66, no. 9, pp. 896–900, 2000.

[9] A. S. Serralta, J. L. Bueno, M. R. Planells, and D. R. Rodero, "Prospective evaluation of emergency versus delayed laparoscopic cholecystectomy for early cholecystitis," *Surgical Laparoscopy, Endoscopy and Percutaneous Techniques*, vol. 13, no. 2, pp. 71–75, 2003.

[10] M. Johansson, A. Thune, A. Blomqvist, L. Nelvin, and L. Lundell, "Management of acute cholecystitis in the laparoscopic

era: results of a prospective, randomized clinical trial," *Journal of Gastrointestinal Surgery*, vol. 7, no. 5, pp. 642–645, 2003.

[11] S. B. Kolla, S. Aggarwal, A. Kumar et al., "Early vs delayed laparoscopic cholecystectomy for acute cholecystitis: a prospective randomized trial," *Surgical Endoscopy and Other Interventional Techniques*, vol. 18, no. 9, pp. 1323–1327, 2004.

[12] K. S. Gurusamy and K. Samraj, "Early versus delayed laparoscopic cholecystectomy for acute cholecystitis (review)," *Cochrane Database of Systematic Reviews*, no. 4, Article ID CD005440, 2006.

[13] T. Siddiqui, A. MacDonald, P. S. Chong, and J. T. Jenkins, "Early versus delayed laparoscopic cholecystectomy for acute cholecystitis: a meta-analysis of randomized clinical trials," *The American Journal of Surgery*, vol. 195, no. 1, pp. 40–47, 2008.

[14] K. S. Gurusamy, K. Samraj, C. Gluud, E. Wilson, and B. R. Davidson, "Meta-analysis of randomized controlled trials on the safety and effectiveness of early versus delayed laparoscopic cholecystectomy for acute cholecystitis," *British Journal of Surgery*, vol. 97, no. 2, pp. 141–150, 2010.

[15] V. Banz, T. Gsponer, D. Candinas, and U. Güller, "Population-based analysis of 4113 patients with acute cholecystitis: defining the optimal time-point for laparoscopic cholecystectomy," *Annals of Surgery*, vol. 254, no. 6, pp. 964–970, 2011.

[16] K. S. Gurusamy, C. Davidson, C. Gluud, and B. R. Davidson, "Early versus delayed laparoscopic cholecystectomy for people with acute cholecystitis," *The Cochrane Database of Systematic Reviews*, no. 6, Article ID CD005440, 2013.

[17] C. N. Gutt, J. Encke, J. Köninger et al., "Acute cholecystitis: early versus delayed cholecystectomy, a multicenter randomized trial (ACDc Study, nct00447304)," *Annals of Surgery*, vol. 258, no. 3, pp. 385–393, 2013.

[18] M. Vetrhus, O. Søreide, I. Nesvik, and K. Søndenaa, "Acute cholecystitis: delayed surgery or observation. A randomized clinical trial," *Scandinavian Journal of Gastroenterology*, vol. 38, no. 9, pp. 985–990, 2003.

[19] C. Papi, M. Catarci, L. D'Ambrosio et al., "Timing of cholecystectomy for acute calculous cholecystitis: a meta-analysis," *The American Journal of Gastroenterology*, vol. 99, no. 1, pp. 147–155, 2004.

[20] P. S. P. Senapati, D. Bhattarcharya, G. Harinath, and B. J. Ammori, "A survey of the timing and approach to the surgical management of cholelithiasis in patients with acute biliary pancreatitis and acute cholecystitis in the UK," *Annals of the Royal College of Surgeons of England*, vol. 85, no. 5, pp. 306–312, 2003.

[21] E. H. Livingston and R. V. Rege, "A nationwide study of conversion from laparoscopic to open cholecystectomy," *The American Journal of Surgery*, vol. 188, no. 3, pp. 205–211, 2004.

[22] X. Feliu, E. M. Targarona, A. García et al., "La cirugía laparoscópica en España. Resultados de la encuesta nacional de la Sección de Cirugía Endoscópica de la Asociación Española de Cirujanos," *Cirugía Española*, vol. 74, no. 3, pp. 164–170, 2003.

[23] S. Shikata, Y. Noguchi, and T. Fukui, "Early versus delayed cholecystectomy for acute cholecystitis: a meta-analysis of randomized controlled trials," *Surgery Today*, vol. 35, no. 7, pp. 553–560, 2005.

[24] T. Takada, S. M. Strasberg, J. S. Solomkin et al., "TG13: updated Tokyo Guidelines for the management of acute cholangitis and cholecystitis," *Journal of Hepato-Biliary-Pancreatic Sciences*, vol. 20, no. 1, pp. 1–7, 2013.

[25] S. M. Strasberg, M. Hertl, and N. J. Soper, "An analysis of the problem of biliary injury during laparoscopic cholecystectomy," *Journal of the American College of Surgeons*, vol. 180, no. 1, pp. 101–125, 1995.

[26] D. Dindo, N. Demartines, and P.-A. Clavien, "Classification of surgical complications. A new proposal with evaluation in a cohort of 6336 patients and results of a survey," *Annals of Surgery*, vol. 240, no. 2, pp. 205–213, 2004.

[27] R. D. Dripps, A. Lamont, and J. E. Eckenhoff, "The role of anesthesia in surgical mortality," *The Journal of the American Medical Association*, vol. 178, pp. 261–266, 1961.

[28] M. E. Charlson, P. Pompei, K. L. Ales, and C. R. MacKenzie, "A new method of classifying prognostic comorbidity in longitudinal studies: development and validation," *Journal of Chronic Diseases*, vol. 40, no. 5, pp. 373–383, 1987.

[29] J. C. Rodríguez-Sanjuán, A. Arruabarrena, L. Sánchez-Moreno, F. González-Sánchez, L. A. Herrera, and M. Gómez-Fleitas, "Acute cholecystitis in high surgical risk patients: percutaneous cholecystostomy or emergency cholecystectomy?" *American Journal of Surgery*, vol. 204, no. 1, pp. 54–59, 2012.

[30] Y. Cheng, J. Leng, J. Tan, K. Chen, and J. Dong, "Proper surgical technique approved for early laparoscopic cholecystectomy for non-critically ill elderly patients with acute cholecystitis," *Hepato-Gastroenterology*, vol. 60, no. 124, pp. 688–691, 2013.

[31] A. G. Ferrarese, M. Solej, S. Enrico et al., "Elective and emergency laparoscopic cholecystectomy in the elderly: our experience," *BMC Surgery*, vol. 13, supplement 2, article S21, 2013.

[32] T. Haltmeier, E. Benjamin, K. Inaba, L. Lam, and D. Demetriades, "Early versus delayed same-admission laparoscopic cholecystectomy for acute cholecystitis in elderly patients with comorbidities," *Journal of Trauma and Acute Care Surgery*, vol. 78, no. 4, pp. 801–807, 2015.

[33] F. J. González-Rodríguez, J. P. Paredes-Cotoré, C. Pontón et al., "Early or delayed laparoscopic cholecystectomy in acute cholecystitis? Conclusions of a controlled trial," *Hepato-Gastroenterology*, vol. 56, no. 89, pp. 11–16, 2009.

[34] S. Norrby, P. Herlin, T. Holmin, R. Sjödahl, and C. Tagesson, "Early or delayed cholecystectomy in acute cholecystitis? A clinical trial," *British Journal of Surgery*, vol. 70, no. 3, pp. 163–165, 1983.

[35] A. Fingerhut, C. Dziri, O. J. Garden et al., "ATOM, the all-inclusive, nominal EAES classification of bile duct injuries during cholecystectomy," *Surgical Endoscopy*, vol. 27, no. 12, pp. 4608–4619, 2013.

[36] D. W. Rattner, C. Ferguson, and A. L. Warshaw, "Factors associated with successful laparoscopic cholecystectomy for acute cholecystitis," *Annals of Surgery*, vol. 217, no. 3, pp. 233–236, 1993.

[37] S. Eldar, E. Sabo, E. Nash, J. Abrahamson, and I. Matter, "Laparoscopic cholecystectomy for acute cholecystitis: prospective trial," *World Journal of Surgery*, vol. 21, no. 5, pp. 540–545, 1997.

[38] S. M. Garber, J. Korman, J. M. Cosgrove, and J. R. Cohen, "Early laparoscopic cholecystectomy for acute cholecystitis," *Surgical Endoscopy*, vol. 11, no. 4, pp. 347–350, 1997.

[39] J. Lahtinen, E. M. Alhava, and S. Aukee, "Acute cholecystitis treated by early and delayed surgery. A controlled clinical trial," *Scandinavian Journal of Gastroenterology*, vol. 13, no. 6, pp. 673–678, 1978.

[40] H. Lau, C. Y. Lo, N. G. Patil, and W. K. Yuen, "Early versus delayed-interval laparoscopic cholecystectomy for acute cholecystitis," *Surgical Endoscopy*, vol. 20, no. 1, pp. 82–87, 2006.

[41] D. A. L. Macafee, D. J. Humes, G. Bouliotis, I. J. Beckingham, D. K. Whynes, and D. N. Lobo, "Prospective randomized trial using cost-utility analysis of early versus delayed laparoscopic cholecystectomy for acute gallbladder disease," *British Journal of Surgery*, vol. 96, no. 9, pp. 1031–1040, 2009.

[42] E. Wilson, K. Gurusamy, C. Gluud, and B. R. Davidson, "Cost-utility and value-of-information analysis of early versus delayed laparoscopic cholecystectomy for acute cholecystitis," *British Journal of Surgery*, vol. 97, no. 2, pp. 210–219, 2010.

[43] A. Johner, A. Raymakers, and S. M. Wiseman, "Cost utility of early versus delayed laparoscopic cholecystectomy for acute cholecystitis," *Surgical Endoscopy and Other Interventional Techniques*, vol. 27, no. 1, pp. 256–262, 2013.

Permissions

All chapters in this book were first published in HPB SURGERY, by Hindawi Publishing Corporation; hereby published with permission under the Creative Commons Attribution License or equivalent. Every chapter published in this book has been scrutinized by our experts. Their significance has been extensively debated. The topics covered herein carry significant findings which will fuel the growth of the discipline. They may even be implemented as practical applications or may be referred to as a beginning point for another development.

The contributors of this book come from diverse backgrounds, making this book a truly international effort. This book will bring forth new frontiers with its revolutionizing research information and detailed analysis of the nascent developments around the world.

We would like to thank all the contributing authors for lending their expertise to make the book truly unique. They have played a crucial role in the development of this book. Without their invaluable contributions this book wouldn't have been possible. They have made vital efforts to compile up to date information on the varied aspects of this subject to make this book a valuable addition to the collection of many professionals and students.

This book was conceptualized with the vision of imparting up-to-date information and advanced data in this field. To ensure the same, a matchless editorial board was set up. Every individual on the board went through rigorous rounds of assessment to prove their worth. After which they invested a large part of their time researching and compiling the most relevant data for our readers.

The editorial board has been involved in producing this book since its inception. They have spent rigorous hours researching and exploring the diverse topics which have resulted in the successful publishing of this book. They have passed on their knowledge of decades through this book. To expedite this challenging task, the publisher supported the team at every step. A small team of assistant editors was also appointed to further simplify the editing procedure and attain best results for the readers.

Apart from the editorial board, the designing team has also invested a significant amount of their time in understanding the subject and creating the most relevant covers. They scrutinized every image to scout for the most suitable representation of the subject and create an appropriate cover for the book.

The publishing team has been an ardent support to the editorial, designing and production team. Their endless efforts to recruit the best for this project, has resulted in the accomplishment of this book. They are a veteran in the field of academics and their pool of knowledge is as vast as their experience in printing. Their expertise and guidance has proved useful at every step. Their uncompromising quality standards have made this book an exceptional effort. Their encouragement from time to time has been an inspiration for everyone.

The publisher and the editorial board hope that this book will prove to be a valuable piece of knowledge for researchers, students, practitioners and scholars across the globe.

Contributors

Johanna Laukkarinen, Juhani Sand and Isto Nordback
Department of Gastroenterology and Alimentary Tract Surgery, Tampere University Hospital, Teiskontie 35, FIN-33521 Tampere, Finland

Masanori Matsuda, Hidetake Amemiya, AkiraMaki, Mitsuaki Watanabe, Hiromichi Kawaida, Hiroshi Kono and Hideki Fujii
First Department of Surgery, Yamanashi University School of Medicine, 1110 Shimokato, Chuo City, Yamanashi 409-3898, Japan

Tomoaki Ichikawa, Katsuhiro Sano and Utaroh Motosugi
Department of Radiology, Yamanashi University School of Medicine, 1110 Shimokato, Chuo City, Yamanashi 409-3898, Japan

Fabrizio Romano,Mattia Garancini, Fabio Uggeri, Luca Degrate, Luca Nespoli, Luca Gianotti, Angelo Nespoli and Franco Uggeri
Unit of Hepatobiliary and Pancreatic Surgery, Department of Surgery, San Gerardo Hospital, University of Milan-Bicocca, Via Donizetti 106, 20052 Monza, Italy

R. Ibarra and H. Brunengraber
Departments of Surgery, CaseWestern Reserve University, School of Medicine and University Hospitals, Case Medical Center, 11100 Euclid Avenue, Cleveland, OH44106,USA
Departments of Nutrition, Case Western Reserve University, School of Medicine and University Hospitals, Case Medical Center, 11100 Euclid Avenue, Cleveland, OH44106,USA

J-E. Dazard
Center for Proteomics and Bioinformatics, CaseWestern Reserve University, School of Medicine and University Hospitals, Case Medical Center, Cleveland, OH 44106, USA

Y. Sandlers, R. Kombu and G-F. Zhang
Departments of Nutrition, Case Western Reserve University, School of Medicine and University Hospitals, Case Medical Center, 11100 Euclid Avenue, Cleveland, OH44106,USA

F. Rehman and R. Abbas
Departments of Surgery, Case Western Reserve University, School of Medicine and University Hospitals, Case Medical Center, 11100 Euclid Avenue, Cleveland, OH44106,USA

J. Sanabria
Departments of Surgery, Case Western Reserve University, School of Medicine and University Hospitals, Case Medical Center, 11100 Euclid Avenue, Cleveland, OH44106,USA
Departments of Nutrition, Case Western Reserve University, School of Medicine and University Hospitals, Case Medical Center, 11100 Euclid Avenue, Cleveland, OH44106,USA
Department of Surgery, Cancer Treatment Centers of America, Chicago, IL 60099, USA

Irinel Popescu and Sorin Tiberiu Alexandrescu
Dan Setlacec Center of General Surgery and Liver Transplantation, Fundeni Clinical Institute, Carol Davila University of Medicine and Pharmacy, Fundeni Street No. 258, 022328 Bucharest, Romania

Guillermo P. Sangster, Carlos H. Previgliano, Mathieu Nader, Elisa Chwoschtschinsky and Maureen G. Heldmann
Department of Radiology, LSU Health Shreveport, 1501 Kings Highway, Shreveport, LA 71103, USA

Mesut Sipahi, Ergin Arslan and Hasan Börekci
Department of General Surgery, School of Medicine, Bozok University, 66100 Yozgat, Turkey

Sevinç Fahin
Department of Pathology, School of Medicine, Bozok University, 66100 Yozgat, Turkey

Bayram Metin
Department of Thoracic Surgery, School of Medicine, Bozok University, 66100 Yozgat, Turkey

Nuh Zafer Cantürk
Department of General Surgery, School of Medicine, Kocaeli University, 41000 Kocaeli, Turkey

Ajay K. Khanna, SusantaMeher, Shashi Prakash and Satyendra Kumar Tiwary
Department of General Surgery, Institute of Medical Sciences, Banaras Hindu University, Varanasi, Ultra Pradesh 221005, India

Usha Singh
Department of Pathology, Institute of Medical Sciences, Banaras Hindu University, Varanasi, Ultra Pradesh 221005, India

Arvind Srivastava
Department of Radiodiagnosis, Institute of Medical Sciences, Banaras Hindu University, Varanasi, Ultra Pradesh 221005, India

V. K. Dixit
Department of Gastroenterology, Institute of Medical Sciences, Banaras Hindu University, Varanasi, Ultra Pradesh 221005, India

Lawrence Lau, Christopher Christophi, Mehrdad Nikfarjam, Graham Starkey and Vijayaragavan Muralidharan
Department of Surgery, Austin Health, University of Melbourne, Melbourne, VIC 3084, Australia

Mark Goodwin
Department of Radiology, Austin Health, Melbourne, VIC 3084, Australia

Laurence Weinberg and Loretta Ho
Department of Anaesthesia, Austin Health, University of Melbourne, Melbourne, VIC 3084, Australia

Robert T. Currin and Xing-Xi Peng
Department of Cell and Developmental Biology, University of North Carolina, Chapel Hill, NC 27599, USA

John J. Lemasters
Center for Cell Death, Injury and Regeneration, Departments of Pharmaceutical and Biomedical Sciences and Biochemistry and Molecular Biology, Medical University of South Carolina, Charleston, SC 29425, USA

M. P. Senthil Kuma
The Liver Unit, Queen Elizabeth Hospital Birmingham, Edgbaston, Birmingham B15 2TH, UK
Department of HPB Surgery and Liver Transplantation, Queen Elizabeth Hospital Birmingham, 3rd Floor Nuffield House, Edgbaston, Birmingham B15 2TH, UK

R.Marudanayagam
The Liver Unit, Queen Elizabeth Hospital Birmingham, Edgbaston, Birmingham B15 2TH, UK

Jennifer K. Plichta, Jacqueline A. Brosius, Sam G. Pappas, Gerard J. Abood and Gerard V. Aranha
Department of Surgery, Loyola University Health System, Maywood, IL 60153, USA

Hui Jiang and Cheng Chen
Department of Hepatobiliary Pancreatic Surgery,The Second People's Hospital of Neijiang, Luzhou Medical College, Neijiang, Sichuan 641003, China

Chi Du, Mingwei Cai and Hai He
Department of Cancer,The Second People's Hospital of Neijiang, Luzhou Medical College, Neijiang, Sichuan 641003, China

Jianguo Qiu and HongWu
Department of Hepatobiliary Pancreatic Surgery,West China Hospital, Sichuan University, Chengdu, Sichuan 610041, China

Quirino Lai, Giovanni B. Levi Sandri, Gabriele Spoletini, FabioMelandro, Nicola Guglielmo, Marco Di Laudo, Fabrizio M. Frattaroli, Pasquale B. Berloco and Massimo Rossi
Department of General Surgery and Organ Transplantation, Sapienza University of Rome, Umberto I Policlinic of Rome, Viale del Policlinico 155, 00161 Rome, Italy

Rafael S. Pinheiro
Department of Liver Transplantation, University of São Paulo, 01005 010 São Paulo, SP, Brazil

M. G. Wiggans and D. A. Stell
Hepatopancreatobiliary Surgery, Plymouth Hospitals NHS Trust, Derriford Hospital, Derriford Road, Plymouth, Devon PL6 8DH, UK
Peninsula College of Medicine and Dentistry, University of Exeter and PlymouthUniversity, John Bull Building, Plymouth, Devon PL6 8BU, UK

J. T. Lordan, S. Aroori and M. J. Bowles
Hepatopancreatobiliary Surgery, Plymouth Hospitals NHS Trust, Derriford Hospital, Derriford Road, Plymouth, Devon PL6 8DH, UK

G. Shahtahmassebi
School of Science and Technology, Nottingham Trent University, Nottingham NG1 4BU, UK

Shirin Elizabeth Khorsandi and Nigel Heaton
Institute of Liver Studies, King's College Hospital, Denmark Hill, London SE5 9RS, UK

Sundeep Jain, Mitesh Kaushik and Lokendra Jain
Department of Gastrointestinal Hepatopancreatobiliary Minimal Access and Bariatric Surgery, Fortis Escorts Hospital, Jawahar Lal Nehru Marg, Malviya Nagar, Jaipur, Rajasthan 302017, India

Bharat Sharma
Department of General and Minimal Access Surgery, Soni Manipal Hospital, Sikar Road, Vidhyadhar Nagar, Jaipur, Rajasthan 302013, India

Durairaj Segamalai, Abdul Rehman Abdul Jameel, Naveen Kannan, Amudhan Anbalagan, Benet Duraisamy, Prabhakaran Raju and Kannan Devy Gounder
Institute of Surgical Gastroenterology, Madras Medical College, Chennai 600003, India

Giovanni Dapri and Guy-Bernard Cadiére
Department of Gastrointestinal Surgery, European School of Laparoscopic Surgery, Saint-Pierre University Hospital, 1000 Brussels, Belgium

Livia DiMarco
Department of Anesthesiology, Saint-Pierre University Hospital, 1000 Brussels, Belgium

Vincent Donckier
Liver Unit, Department of Abdominal Surgery, Hôpital Erasme, Université Libre de Bruxelles, 808 Route de Lennik, 1070 Brussels, Belgium

Helge Bruns, Veronika Kortendieck, Hans-Rudolf Raab and Dalibor Antolovic
Department of General and Visceral Surgery, Carl von Ossietzky University of Oldenburg, Oldenburg, Germany

Charalampos Markakis
Department of Surgery, St. Georges' Hospital, Tooting SW17 0QT, UK

Alexandra Tsaroucha, Christina Tsigalou, Konstantinos Romanidis and Constantinos Simopoulos
Department of Surgery and Laboratory of Experimental Surgery, Faculty of Medicine, Democritus University of Thrace, 68100 Alexandroupolis, Greece

Apostolos E. Papalois
Experimental Research Center, ELPEN Pharmaceuticals, Pikermi, 19009 Attica, Greece

Maria Lambropoulou
Laboratory of Histology, Faculty of Medicine, Democritus University of Thrace, 68100 Alexandroupolis, Greece

Eleftherios Spartalis
Second Propaedeutic Department of Surgery, Thoracic Surgery Department, "Laiko" General Hospital, 11527 Athens, Greece

Christel Weiß
Department of Medical Statistics, Medical Faculty Mannheim, University of Heidelberg, Theodor-Kutzer-Ufer 1-3, 68167 Mannheim, Germany

Jochen Schuld
Department of General, Visceral, Vascular and Paediatric Surgery, University Hospital of the Saarland, Kirrberger Straße, 66424 Homburg/Saar, Germany

Malte Weinrich and Bettina M. Rau
Department of General,Thoracic, Vascular and Transplantation Surgery, University Hospital Rostock, Schillingallee 35, 18057 Rostock, Germany
Department of General, Visceral, Vascular and Paediatric Surgery, University Hospital of the Saarland, Kirrberger Straße, 66424 Homburg/Saar, Germany

Ulf Kulik, Joline Kolb, Jürgen Klempnauer and Frank Lehner
General, Visceral and Transplantation Surgery, HannoverMedical School, Germany

Mareike Plohmann-Meyer, Jill Gwiasda, Daniel Meyer and Alexander Kaltenborn
Core Facility Quality Management and Health Technology Assessment in Transplantation, Integrated Research and Treatment Center Transplantation (IFB-Tx), Hannover Medical School, Germany

Harald Schrem
General, Visceral and Transplantation Surgery, HannoverMedical School, Germany
Core Facility Quality Management and Health Technology Assessment in Transplantation, Integrated Research and Treatment Center Transplantation (IFB-Tx), Hannover Medical School, Germany

Kin-Pan Au, See-Ching Chan, Kenneth Siu-Ho Chok, Albert Chi-Yan Chan, Tan-To Cheung, Kelvin Kwok-Chai Ng and Chung-Mau Lo
Department of Surgery,The University of Hong Kong, Hong Kong

Kumar Jayant and Isabella Reccia
Department of Surgery and Cancer, Imperial College London, London, UK

Francesco Virdis
Department of Surgery, Kings College, London, UK

A. M. James Shapiro
Department of Surgery, University of Alberta, Edmonton, Canada

Ayodeji Oluwarotimi Omiyale
Department of General Surgery, Royal Shrewsbury Hospital, Shrewsbury SY3 8XQ, UK

Antonio Siniscalchi, Giulia Tarozzi, Lorenzo Gamberini, Lucia Cipolat and Stefano Faenza
Division of Anesthesiology, Alma Mater Studiorum University of Bologna, Policlinico S. Orsola-Malpighi, Via Massarenti 9, 40138 Bologna, Italy

Giorgio Ercolani and Antonio D. Pinna
Division of Surgery and Transplantation, Policlinico S. Orsola-Malpighi, University of Bologna, Via Massarenti 9, 40138 Bologna, Italy

Natesh Yepuri, Camille Richards, Dilip Kittur, Ajay Jain and Mashaal Dhir
Department of Surgery, SUNY Upstate Medical University, Syracuse, NY 13210, USA

Rana Naous
Department of Pathology, SUNY Upstate Medical University, Syracuse, NY 13210, USA

Christine S. M. Lau and Aleksander Zywot
Department of Surgery, Saint Barnabas Medical Center, Livingston, NJ, USA
School of Medicine, Saint George's University, True Blue, Grenada

Krishnaraj Mahendraraj
Department of Surgery, Saint Barnabas Medical Center, Livingston, NJ, USA

Ronald S. Chamberlain
Department of Surgery, Saint Barnabas Medical Center, Livingston, NJ, USA
School of Medicine, Saint George's University, True Blue, Grenada
Department of Surgery, Banner MD Anderson Cancer Center, Gilbert, AZ, USA
Department of Surgery, New Jersey Medical School, Rutgers University, Newark, NJ, USA

Kurinchi Gurusamy and Brian Davidson
Department of Surgery, UCL Medical School, Royal Free Campus, London NW3 2PF, UK

Clare Toon
Public Health Research Unit,West Sussex County Council, County Hall Campus,West Sussex PO19 1QT, UK

Bhavisha Virendrakumar
Evidence Synthesis, Sightsavers, 35 Perrymount Road, Haywards Heath, West Sussex RH16 3BW, UK

Steve Morris
Department of Applied Health Research, UCL, LondonWC1E 7HB, UK

Miguel Sánchez-Carrasco, Fernando Martín-Acebes, Rocío Zambrano Muñoz and F. Javier Sánchez-Manuel
Department of General Surgery, Burgos University Hospital, Avenida Islas Baleares 3, 09006 Burgos, Spain

Juan C. Rodríguez-Sanjuán and Manuel Gómez-Fleitas
Department of General Surgery, University Hospital "Marqués de Valdecilla", Avenida Valdecilla, s/n, 39008 Santander, Spain

Francisco J. Llorca-Díaz
Department of Epidemiology, Preventive Medicine and Public Health, School of Medicine, University of Cantabria, Avenida HerreraOria, s/n, 39011 Santander, Spain

Index

www.ingramcontent.com/pod-product-compliance
Lightning Source LLC
Chambersburg PA
CBHW061330190326
41458CB00011B/3957
* 9 7 8 1 6 3 2 4 2 8 1 3 4 *